AF333648

WOUND CARE PRACTICE

2ND EDITION

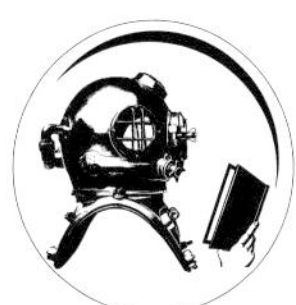

WOUND CARE PRACTICE
2ND EDITION

PAUL J. SHEFFIELD, PhD
Editor

CAROLINE E. FIFE, MD
Co-Editor

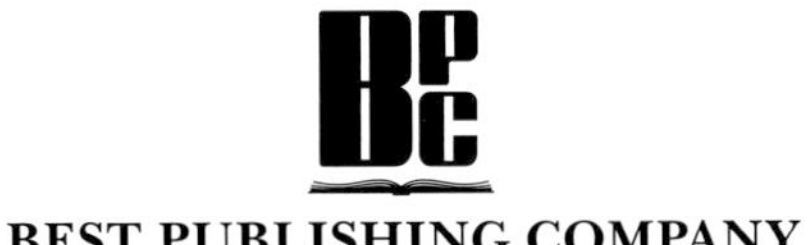

BEST PUBLISHING COMPANY

Cover & Layout Design: William Owen
                        Kelly Phillips

Edited By: James T. Joiner
            Kate Lasky

International Standard Book Number-13:   978-1-930536-38-8
International Standard Book Number-10:   1-930536-38-0
Library of Congress Control Number: 2007925867

For more information contact:
Best Publishing Company
2355 North Steves Boulevard
P.O. Box 30100
Flagstaff, AZ 86003-0100 USA

Tele: 928.527.1055
Fax: 928.526.0370
divebooks@bestpub.com
www.bestpub.com

CONTENTS

SECTION 1. THE PROBLEM WOUND

SECTION 2. PRINCIPLES OF WOUND ASSESSMENT

SECTION 3. PRINCIPLES OF WOUND MANAGEMENT

VOLUME TWO

SECTION 4. PAIN, INFECTION, & ADJUNCTIVE THERAPIES

SECTION 5. COMMUNICATION AND TRUST

SECTION 6. HEALTHCARE DELIVERY

PREFACE

EDITOR

Chronic wounds are a major cause of patient suffering and a profound financial burden to society. The focus of this Second Edition is assessment and management of chronic wounds in a Wound Care Practice. Physicians, podiatrists, nurses, enterostomal therapists, physical therapists, occupational therapists, and other health care professionals will find in this book the principles of modern, moist, interactive wound care, and the application of advanced therapeutic technologies. It represents the combined efforts of 65 authors selected from the basic sciences, clinical sciences, and clinical practice. The reader can examine the principles of managing the wound and treating the underlying cause of pressure sores, vascular insufficiency ulcers, chronic venous insufficiency ulcers, diabetic/neurotrophic foot ulcers, and other chronic wounds.

Section I defines the Problem Wound. It presents the etiology of a problem wound and the basic science of wound healing.

Section II describes the Principles of Wound Assessment. It discusses methods used in patient assessment for wound healing and describes specific assessment methods available to the wound care physician. It also addresses the need for evidence-based wound care.

Section III discusses the Principles of Wound Management. It provides general principles of modern wound care and the rationale for medical and surgical management of a wide variety of problem wounds. The authors were asked to write about what works for them in their various wound care practices. Thus, occasionally there are differences in recommended procedures.

Section IV deals with Pain, Infection and Adjunctive Therapies. It addresses nutrition, glycemic control, pain management, wound infection control, wound dressings, and advanced therapeutic methods, including hyperbaric oxygen therapy. It also describes available support services such as physical therapy, occupational therapy, and orthotics. The biochemistry and biophysical basis of the various classes of wound products are presented in depth.

Section V is about Communication and Trust. It addresses the key elements for comforting the patient, as well as the ethical and legal issues that must be dealt with in a wound care practice.

Section VI pertains to Healthcare Delivery. It offers suggestions for creating and managing a modern, comprehensive wound center and how to deal with issues of infection control and latex allergies. There is advice on documentation necessary for facility accreditation and for professional and technical services reimbursement.

The authors were asked to write each chapter as a stand-alone document for clinicians. Thus, there are redundancies pertaining to basic wound physiology, assessment tools, and principles of wound management. Some of the advanced therapeutic options such as negative pressure wound therapy (NPWT) and hyperbaric oxygen (HBO2) therapy are mentioned by several authors as they describe various treatment methods they have found to be useful. The reader will find that the authors have been generous with color photographs, figures, and tables to give a clear image of the wounds and the various assessment and management options. This will be helful to clinicians and medical students alike who read this book to gain a basic understanding of the wound healing process, both at the cellular level and at the bedside.

At the end of each chapter are review questions regarding key points that the reader will find valuable as a self assessment tool while preparing for specialty certification in wound care.

Following the publication of the classic JC Davis & TK Hunt textbook, *Problem Wounds: Role of Oxygen*, in 1988, the first Clinical Management of Problem Wounds Symposium was held in San Antonio, Texas. Subsequently, ten Symposia followed a natural evolution from research-oriented seminars, to clinical management symposia, to case-based workshops, to specific wound care methodologies. In 2002 it became a basic "hands on" course for clinical practice and certification in wound care. It was renamed, *The Wound Care Course*, and become the nucleus of the first edition of *Wound Care Practice* (2004). Most of the contributors to this book have been faculty members of these wound care symposia and courses that were organized by the Senior Editor. Today, because of the wealth of knowledge and growth in wound care technology this second edition of Wound Care Practice has expanded into two volumes.

The editors are grateful to the contributors to this book, who bring their insights and unique experiences to the text and enhance its value both as a readable volume and as an enduring reference.

Paul J. Sheffield, PhD
San Antonio, Texas
Editor

PREFACE
CO-EDITOR

In the 16th century, Ambroise Pare traveled with the French Army as a barber-surgeon. To counteract the purported poisonous effects of gunpowder, the wounds of injured soldiers were scalded with boiling oil. However, at the Battle of Turin, Pare ran out of boiling oil. In hopes of offering some therapeutic intervention for the doomed soldiers, he mixed a potion of egg yolks, turpentine, and oil of roses, thus creating the first controlled clinical trial in wound healing. To his surprise, not only did the soldiers deprived of boiling oil survive, but their wounds healed faster and with less pain. He coined the now famous phrase, "I dressed the wound, and God healed him."

As with all of medicine, the field of wound healing has been a plodding journey, punctuated by periods of enlightment. An understanding of the germ theory led to sterile, dry dressings and frequent antibiotic scrubs. The original work by Dr. George Winter, published in 1962, demonstrated the value of a moist wound environment. Now recombinant DNA technology and genetic engineering hold out the possibility of growing replacement tissues and blood vessels.

As the complexity of the Wound Management field increases, clinicians come to the field from many diverse specialties. The clinical application of wound care crosses most specialty boundaries, as is apparent from a review of the list of contributing authors. Wound healing issues form a continuum. No disease process recognizes specialty "niches" in its clinical manifestations.

This book is an attempt to cross the specialty boundaries and gain insight from all these perspectives. We are deeply indebted to these clinicians, without whom this book, and this specialty would not be possible. Our understanding of the wound healing process continues to evolve. This book is a snapshot of our current level of understanding, thanks to the work and dedication of many. To paraphrase Sir Isaac Newton—If we have seen farther, it is because we have stood on the shoulders of giants.

Caroline E. Fife, MD
Co-Editor

FOREWORD

During my residency, my program director J. Englebert Dunphy, recognized for his interest in wound healing wrote a well-regarded article for the New England Journal of Medicine entitled, "The Fibroblast, an Ally For the Surgeon." By using the word "for," he told me, he meant to carry forward his belief that this valuable ally would be available to us only if we made conditions right. The rest he felt was immutable. Looking back, it was a rebellious streak in me that led me to challenge him. I felt that healing mechanisms, like any other biologic process, can be rationally influenced, rationally slowed, rationally accelerated. (In those days, our sole ambition was to speed it.) I decided to challenge him. If I had fully appreciated the depth of his pessimism, I probably would have left the subject alone in favor of some other project. However, I took the challenge, and sensing my interest, he asked me to take consultations on wound problems. It took only two or three to realize that I had few answers. Protective dressings, casts, debridement, and lots of vitamin C were about all that I had. This state of "cluelessness" led most physicians of that day to avoid wound problems, and hide them behind dry eschars and dressings. One thing, though, warm, wet dressings were in favor. Ironically, they were effective but then fell almost totally out of use for many years. Now warmth is seeing a rebirth. There was cynicism about what warmth does. Does it even get into the tissue? Does it really enhance perfusion? Yes, local heat elevates subcutaneous temperature and with it perfusion and oxygen. Look it up! (Hint: Rabkin).

My first inklings of a real practical progress in wound care came when Hinman and Maibach found that epithelization (note the preferred spelling) could be hastened by keeping wounds moist. Never mind that it was to be another twenty to thirty years before its power was to be fully appreciated. In the 1960's, first Juha Niinikoski, then I, then the two of us together showed the importance of the perfusion and oxygenation of wounds, also a concept that has not yet reached its maximum contribution.

As we all know, antibiotics quickly reached their maximum contribution to wound care. Nevertheless, antibiotics gave great hope at the time. At that time, controversy about prophylactic use polarized the profession. A great deal of print passed through the presses before our current guidelines for prophylactic antibiotics in surgery were finally accepted.

This forward inertia would have run out of steam, I suspect, if the age of rational care, the clinical trial, had not developed on top of the increasing belief that healing could, in fact, be fostered. Trials on pressure garments for "venous wounds," further examination of moisture, protocols on prevention and care of pressure sores, surgical correction of venous and arterial pathologies have led to a discipline that led, in turn, to optimism and development of special expertise. You will find these developments superimposed on advanced understanding of inflammation and vascular pathology in this book.

One great theoretical advance, growth factors, increased industrial participation and funded research like never before. Their discovery multiplied commercial investment in research and centers of excellence, "wound clinics." In a practical sense administration of growth factors has advanced us relatively little, but it did lead to discovery of the value of "radical excision" of chronic wounds—which began as a result of frustration over the failure of growth factors to work and the new belief that "senescent" tissue could not respond to growth factor stimulation.

So, today, we have gathered together a rationale, a fairly tightly knit concept of how healing works, to promise a better day sometime in the not-too-distant future. Although the development of the concept of growth factors, though leading to relatively little in a human clinical level, convinced us ten years ago that if we only knew how to mix and add, suspend and apply, we would find the happier day just around the corner. The joy, though not realistic, has lasted long enough to allow us to reach some real practical advancement. The greatest benefit of the growth factors has been the conviction that their discovery has given us that healing—tissue repair—is, in fact, a malleable process.

This book is different from many others in the sense that it emphasizes assessment or, if you wish, "wound diagnostics." Many wounds fail to heal from inability to cope with natural wear and tear, drying and contamination, local contamination. In these cases, the most important decision is to enhance perfusion or oxygenation. There is often more than one impediment to healing of chronic wounds. There also needs to be an assessment of resources that the victim's body can offer. Perfusion and malnutrition are the major items. An impairment of the normal inflammatory reaction to injury is also one of the most common. Then, of course, there is the need to assess the degree to which antibacterial therapy will advance the course.

Though it has seemed like terribly painful progress, we've gone a long way since vitamin C. The editors of this book have been long interested in the problem of supplying adequate oxygen, and we should compliment them for their pioneering work on being the first, I think, to measure oxygen in chronic human wounds. Paul Sheffield was the first to note that hyper-oxygenation can enhance angiogenesis in human wounds. I predict for this area an interesting near future.

In this book there is a tacit recognition of the history of our recognition of the special properties of oxygen. Forty years ago when Juha Niinikoski started on oxygen, we knew it as an energy substrate and a nutritional substance for collagen production. More recently we began to see it as a source of antibacterial reactive oxygen species, probably the major "internal antibiotic" against organisms that find vulnerability in wounds. There is little or no specific immunity against staphylococcus for instance. Slowly but surely, we have begun to see hypoxia followed by re-oxygenation as a serious problem especially in non-healing wounds due to venous insufficiency and hyperglycemia.*

---

* High glucose inhibits the enzyme that converts O_2^+ the antibacterial oxidants H_2O_2 and O_2^-.

In the future I think we will find that redox effects that are based on oxygen and lactate constitute a fundamental wound-messaging system. But even at this point, we will have the same problem that has plagued us before. Too little oxygen is obviously bad. Enough oxygen is obviously good, a little more oxygen than normal is almost always helpful, but a lot more is clearly harmful. How do we find the effective range? Can we stay in the effective range? Must we push conditions out of the safe range (hyperbaric) in order to help? We know that inflammation can produce excessive, locally damaging oxidants. Can this flux of oxygen into redox messengers be controlled within the beneficial range? Can we use a combination of antibiotics plus debridement plus moisture retention, plus enhanced perfusion plus supporting oxygen supply to heal wounds that would not otherwise heal? This is the first book that I know to explore the area of oxygen in sufficient detail so that what we know can be exploited in a clinical sense.

Thomas K. Hunt, MD

ACKNOWLEDGEMENTS

Encouragement from Susan and Jim Joiner at Best Publishing Company to produce this book is gratefully acknowledged. In preparing, revising, and editing manuscripts, Suzanne Pack provided excellent technical support.

I am especially thankful for the assistance of Consulting Editor, Caroline E. Fife who is a highly respected wound care specialist at the University of Texas at Houston. She brings a wealth of experience from her wound care practice. As author and consulting editor, she has made major contributions to this book.

Finally, this book is dedicated to Dr. Jefferson C. Davis and—as a surprise—to Dr. Thomas K. Hunt, who introduced the Senior Editor to wound care in the mid 1970s. Dr. Davis was expanding the application of hyperbaric oxygen therapy at the USAF Hyperbaric Center at Brooks Air Force Base, Texas. Dr. T.K. Hunt was the whom of whom when there was no whomer in wound care research. Together, they provided the stimulus for our Center to conduct tissue oxygen studies, which confirmed that respired oxygen was delivered to human wounds and that a course of hyperbaric oxygen therapy elevates basal wound pO_2 as angiogenesis occurs. These pioneers saw the wisdom of adjunctive hyperbaric oxygen therapy to correct severe tissue hypoxia in selected problem wounds, and proposed the creation of wound healing centers. They co-edited Problem Wounds: Role of Oxygen (1988), which was a seminal document, laying the foundation for modern wound care.

DEDICATION

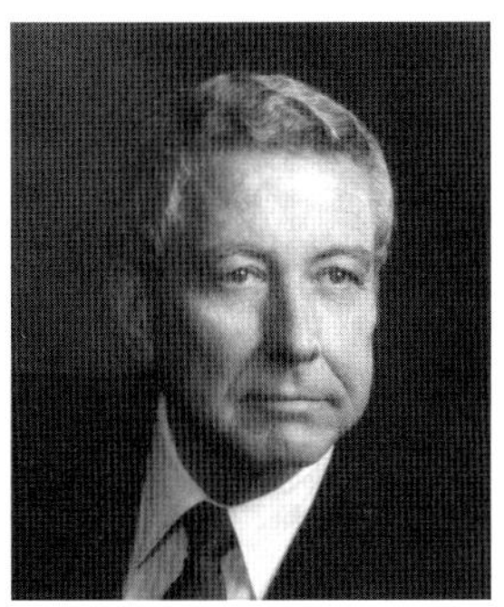

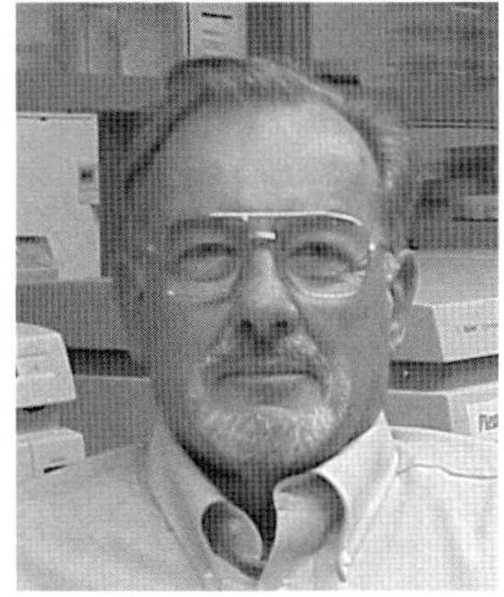

JEFFERSON C. DAVIS, MD

Dr. Jefferson C. Davis was the consummate physician and a pioneer in wound healing and hyperbaric medicine. Through his clinical practice, educational activities, and publications, he inspired several generations of clinicians to provide quality medical service for aviators, divers, and patients with difficult wounds.

Dr. Davis was born December 7, 1932. After receiving his MD at the University of Missouri in 1957, he joined the U.S. Air Force Medical Corps to become a Flight Surgeon. He received his MPH from the University of California and was Board Certified in Aerospace Medicine. In 1974, he founded the USAF Hyperbaric Medicine Center at Brooks Air Force Base in Texas. As the Center's first Director, he created the Davis Hyperbaric Oxygen Protocol for wound healing enhancement. Later, as Medical Director for Medical Seminars' Medicine of Diving Program he taught

THOMAS K. HUNT, MD

Dr. Hunt is Professor Emeritus and Director of the Wound Healing Laboratory, Department of Surgery, University of California at San Francisco.

Dr. Thomas K. Hunt has devoted over 40 years to serving the wound healing community. He has been an inspiration to researchers and clinicians who advance our understanding of the wound healing process and develop methods to improve healing. Much of what is written in this book is the experience of authors who stand on the academic shoulders of Dr. T.K. Hunt.

Dr. Hunt was born August 6, 1930. After receiving his MD from Harvard Medical School in 1956, he served a brief tour in the U.S. Army Medical Corps. He then completed a Surgical Residency at the University of Oregon Medical School and a Research Fellowship at Western Infirmary, University of Glasgow, Scotland. In 1965, he became Director of the Wound Healing Laboratory at University

DAVIS (continued)

civilian physicians from all medical specialties to treat injured divers.

After retiring from the U.S. Air Force in 1979, Dr. Davis and associates founded International ATMO, Inc, the first known contract provider of wound care and hyperbaric medicine services. He established two successful wound care and hyperbaric medicine services in San Antonio Texas hospitals.

Dr. Davis' collaboration with Dr. T.K. Hunt produced the first hyperbaric medicine textbook, *Hyperbaric Oxygen Therapy* (1977); followed in 1988 with *Problem Wounds: Role of Oxygen*, which is a seminal document in wound healing. He authored over 70 papers and book chapters, and produced 5 books.

Dr. Davis was President of the Aerospace Medical Association, the American College of Preventive Medicine, and the Undersea & Hyperbaric Medical Society. Of all his achievements, he was most proud of being "an old country doctor," and his compassion for every patient's well being was legendary. Dr. Davis lost his battle with cancer in his 57th year on July 30, 1989.

HUNT (continued)

of California at San Francisco where his studies of wound healing mechanisms are legendary. These pioneering studies defined the role of oxygen in healing wounds. Several modern therapeutic modalities for wound healing are based on his scientific findings.

Dr. Hunt was a founding member and first President of the American Wound Healing Society, a founding member of three international professional societies, and President of the American Trauma Society, California Division. He has over 430 publications in the scientific literature and has produced 10 books.

PRIMARY CONTRIBUTORS

RONALD P. BANGASSER, MD, FAAP
Medical Director, Wound Care Department, Redlands Community Hospital, Redlands, California Associate Professor, Loama Linda University, Loma Linda, California

350 Terracina Blvd.
Redlands, California 92373
Direct: (909) 335-4123
Office: (909) 335-5615
Fax: (909) 307-5027
Email: rbangass@epiclp.com

FERNANDO BOCCALANDRO, MD, FACC, FASCAD
Odessa Heart Institute

720 N. Golden
Odessa, Texas 79761
Office: (432) 337-3117
Fax: (432) 337-3448
Email: fernbo@pol.net

GORDON W. BOSKER, MED, CPO, CPED,
University of Texas Health Science Center at San Antonio

7703 Floyd Curl Drive
San Antonio, Texas 78284
Office: (210) 567-5346
Fax: (210) 567-5354
Email: bosker@uthscsa.edu

THOMAS M. BOZZUTO, DO, FACEP, FACHM, ABEM/UHM, FCCWS
Medical Director, Phoebe Wound Care & Hyperbaric Center

Phoebe Wound Care & Hyperbaric Center
803 North Jefferson Street, Suite A
Albany, Georgia 31701
Office: (229) 312-7600
Fax: (229) 312-7605
Email: tbozzuto@ppmh.org

CRAIG L. BROUSSARD, PHD, RN, CNS
Clincial Consultants

4228 Atlantic Road
Port Arthur, Texas 77642
Office: (409) 960-7747
Fax: (490) 962-0949
Email: craigB60@swbell.net

PHILOMENA C. BROUSSARD, PT, MPHA, CERT MDT
Director of Rehabilitation Services and Driector of the Wound Care and Hyperbaric Medicine Center

2809 Denny Avenue
Pasagoula, Minnesota 39581
Email: p_Broussard@srshealth.com

CLIFFORD J. BUCKLEY, MD, FACS
Professor of Surgery, Texas A&M University Health Service Center, College of Medicine Director, Division of Vascular Surgery, Scott & White Memorial Hospital

2401 South 31st Street
Temple, Texas 76508
Office: (254) 724-1647
Fax: (254) 724-3173
Email: cbuckley@swmail.sw.org

GLORIA CHIN, MD, MS
Assistant Professor, Division of Plastic and Reconstructive Surgery, Department of Surgery

University of Florida
Gainesville, Florida 32610-0286
Office: (352) 846-0377
Fax: (352) 846-0387
Email: chinga@mail.surgery.ufl.edu

PEGGY NAKAYAMA COE, BSN, RN, CWOCN, CIC
Wound & Ostomy Nurse—Southwestern Medical Center; Wound Ostomy Nurse Consultant—Quantum, Healthcare Lawton, Oklahoma

Southwestern Medical Center
5602 South West Lee Blvd.
Lawton, Oklahoma 73505
Officc: (580) 531-4965
Email: peggy.coe@capellahealth.com

FRANS J. CRONJE, MBCHB (PRET), MSC
President of the South African Wound Healing Association, President of the South African Undersea and Hyperbaric Medical Association, and President-elect of the International Congress of Hyperbaric Medicine. Private practice at the Eugene Marais Hospital Wound Care and Hyperbaric Oxygen Therapy Center. Professor at the University of Pretoria, Faculty of Health Sciences, School of Medicine, Division of Aerospace Medicine, Department of Internal Medicine

AIMEE DENNIS-WAUTERS, MS, RD, CDE
Clinical Dietitian, Diabetes Educator, Diabetes Education Department, Texas Diabetes Institute, San Antonio, Texas

3414 Buckhaven
San Antonio, Texas 78230
Office: (210) 525-1059
Fax: (210) 525-8586
Email: adwauters@hotmail.com

ROBERT F. DIEGELMANN, PHD
Professor of Biochemisty, Anatomy & Emergency Medicine, Virginia Commonwealth University Medical Center

VCU Medical Center—Dept. of Biochemistry; Sanger Hall, Rm 2-007
1101 E. Marshall St.
Richmond, Virginia 23298-0614
Office: (804) 828-9677
Fax: (804) 828-1473
Email: rdieglm@vcu.edu

DUANE A. DIETZ, MD
Wound Treatment Centers of South Texas; Nix Healthcare System; Guadalupe Region Medical Center

414 Navarro, Suite 502
San Antonio, Texas 78205
Office: (210) 223-1145
Fax: (210) 615-7619
Email: hbo2@gvec.net

TIMOTHY A. EMHOFF, MD, FACS
Assistant Professor of Surgery, Tufts University Medical School, Department of Surgery Wound Care and Hyperbaric Medicine Program

WMASS Memorial Medical Center
55 Lake Ave North
Worcester, Massachusetts 01655
Office: (508) 856-1168
Fax: (508) 856-4224
Email: timothy.emhoff@umassmed.edu

JOHN J. FELDMEIER, DO
Toledo Radiation Oncology and The University of Toledo School of Medicine

15044 Kay Circle
Monroe, Michigan 48161
Office: (419) 383-4541
Fax: (419) 383-3040
Email: jfeldmeier@meduohio.edu

HARVEY FERGUSON, JR, RPH, JD, LLM
Gonzales, Hoblit & Ferguson, L.L.P.

One Riverwalk Place
700 N. St Mary's Street, Suite 1800
San Antonio, Texas 78205
Office: (210) 224-9991
Fax: (210) 226-1544
Email: HFerguson@ghf-lawfirm.com

CAROLINE E. FIFE, MD
*Associate Professor, Department of Anesthesiology, University of Texas Health Science
Center, Houston, Director of Clinical Research, Memorial Hermann Center for Wound
Healing & Lymphedema Management*

54 N. Brokenfern Drive
The Woodlands, Texas 77380
Direct: (713) 305-2971
Fax: (281) 364-1121
Email: cfife@intellicure.com

DONALD M. GREER, JR., MD
Plastic Surgeon, Private Practice

335 Upper Cibolo Creek Road
Boerne, Texas 78006
Office: (830) 537-3129
Fax: (830) 537-3134
Email: dmgjgmd@earthlink.net

CLYDE O. HAGOOD, JR., MD, FACS (RETIRED)
*Emeritus Director of Problem Wound and Hyperbaric Medicine Center—Memorial
Hospital, Gulfport, Mississippi*

6103 Grande Cove Court
Granbury , Texas 76049-6360
Office: (817) 326-8288
Fax: (817) 326-8288 [Call first]
Email: copdhago1@alltel.net

THOMAS K. HUNT, MD, FACS, FRCS, DMHC
Professor Emeritus, Department of Surgery, School of Medicine, University of California, San Francisco, California

513 Parnassus Ave, HSW 1619, Box 0522
San Francisco, California 94143-0522
Office: (415) 476-1865
Fax: (415) 476-5190
Email: hanlink@surgery.ucsf.edu

CLYDE IKEDA, MD, FACS

1199 Bush Street, Suite 640
San Francisco, California 94109

KHURRAM H. KHAN, DPM
Chief Resident, Department of Orthopedics, Podiatry Division; University of Texas Health Science Center at San Antonio, Texas

7703 Floyd Curl Drive
San Antonio, Texas 78229

PATRICK N. KIMBRELL, MD
Medical Director, Center for Wound Care, Warm Springs Rehabilitation Hospital Clinical Associate Professor, University of Texas Health Science Center of San Antonio

5101 Medical Drive
San Antonio, Texas 78229
Office: (210) 592-5349
Fax: (210) 592-5462
Email: wound_doc@juno.com

DIANE L. KRASNER, PHD, RN, CWCN, CWS, FAAN
Wound & Skin Care Consultant

212 East Market Street
York, Pennsylvania 17403
Office: (717) 812-1734
Fax: (717) 812-0135
Email: dlkrasner@aol.com

VALERIE LARSON-LOHR, MS, APRN, CWCN, CEN, CHRNC
Director, Centers for Wound Care, Warm Springs Hospitals, Diversified Clinical Services

5101 Medical Drive
San Antonio, Texas 78247
Office: (210) 592-5349
Fax: (210) 592-5462
Email: wound_nurse@juno.com

JACK L. LE FROCK, MD, FACP, FIDSA
Medical Director, 3D Dosing Systems Inc.

647 Waterside Way
Sarasota, Florida 34242
Direct: (941) 809-7559
Office: (941) 349-9863
Fax: (941) 309-6304
Email: doclefrock@aol.com

DAVID L. McCORVEY, MD
Guthrie Clinic

130 Centerway
Pine City Corning
New York 14871

CHARLES P. MOUTON, MD, MS
Professor and Chair, Department of Community and Family Medicine, Howard University College of Medicine

520 West Street, NW Room 2400
Washington, DC 20059
Office: (202) 806-6300
Fax: (202) 806-4898
Email: cmouton@howard.edu

HERBERT B. NEWTON, MD, FAAN
Professor of Neurology, Oncology, and Hyperbaric Medicine, Dardinger Neuro-Oncology Center, Ohio State University Medical Center and James Cancer Hospital

465 Means Hole
1654 Uphem Drive
Columbus, Ohio 43260
Office: (614) 293-8930
Fax: (614) 293-6111
Email: newton.12@osu.edu

JEFFREY A. NIEZGODA, MD, FACEP, FACHM
Medical Director, The Center for Comprehensive Wound Care and Hyperbaric Oxygen Therapy, St. Lukes Medical Center, Milwaukee, Wisconsin

5910 Glen Haven Drive
Greendale, Wisconsin 53129
Office: (414) 385-8724
Fax: (414) 525-0490/0491
Email: niezgoda@execpc.com

LIZA G. OVINGTON, PHD, CWS
Associate Medical Director; Johnson & Johnson Wound Management, Somerville, New Jersey

775 South Dogwood Road
Walnutport, Pennsylvania 18088
Office: (610) 760-1304
Fax: (775) 845-9296
Email: lovingt@ethus.jnj.com

RUDY C. PRUNEDA, PHD (ABMM)
Consultant Services, San Antonio, Texas

9114 Serene Creek
San Antonio, Texas 78230
Office: (210) 525-8070
Email: rpruneda@earthlink.net

CHARLES A. REASNER, MD
University of Texas Health Science Center; Texas Diabetes Institute, San Antonio, Texas

University Center for Community Health; Texas Diabetes Institute
701 S. Zarzamora, Mail Stop 12-5
San Antonio, Texas 78207
Office: (210) 358-7402
Fax: (210) 358-7406
Email: Charles.Reasner@UHS-SA.com

JAYESH B. SHAH, MD, CWS
President, South Texas Wound Associates, PA, Medical Director, Southwest Center for Wound Care and Hyperbaric Medicine, Southwest General Hospital, San Antonio, Texas

7500 Bralie Blvd. #104
San Antonio, Texas 78224
Direct: (210) 408-0117
Office: (210) 921-3493
Fax: (210) 921-3533
Email: drshah@wounddoctors.com

KIMBERLY MOREHOUSE SHEFFIELD, MA-LPC
Licensed Professional Counselor (Texas)

Behavioral Health Department
Family Service Associations of San Antonio, Texas
Email: ksheffield@family-service.org

PAUL J. SHEFFIELD, PHD, CASP, CHT
President and CME Program Director, International ATMO, Inc., San Antonio, Texas

Nix Medical Center
414 Navarro, Suit 502
San Antonio, Texas 78205
Office: (210) 614-3688
Fax: (210) 223-4864
Email: psheffield@hyperbaricmedicine.com

J. BENJAMIN SLADE, JR., MD
Northbay Center for Wound Care

131 Blackwood Court
Vacaville, California 95688-1058
Direct: (707) 332-2005
Office: (707) 451-1491
Fax: (707) 455-8353
Email: jslade1515@aol.com

ADRIANNE P. S. SMITH, MD
Medical Director, Kinetic Concepts, Inc., Assistant Professor, University of Texas Health Science Center of San Antonio, Texas

Medical Department
6203 Farinon Drive
San Antonio, Texas 78249
Office: (210) 255-6640
Email: asmith24@satx.rr.com

MELVIN D. SMITH, MD
Associate Director, Methodist Wound Care and Hyperbaric Oxygen Treatment Center, San Antonio, Texas

Methodist Hospital Wound Care and Hyperbaric Oxygen Service
4499 Medical Drive-SL-2
San Antonio, Texas 78229
Office: (210) 575-4497
Fax: (210) 575-4498
Email: msmith11@satx.rr.com

LENA L. SOTO, RN, BSN, MS, CHRN
Operations Branch Chief, Hyperbaric Medicine Division; USAF School of Aerospace Medicine, 2611 Louis Bauer Dr, Brooks City-Base, Texas 78235-5130

25515 Echo Terrace
San Antonio, Texas 78258-6811
Office: (210) 536-3281
Fax: (210) 536-2944
Email: lena.soto@brooks.af.mil

JOHN S. STEINBERG, DPM
Assistant Professor, Department of Plastic Surgery, Georgetown University School of Medicine, Washington DC

3800 Reservoir Rd, Northwest
1-Main-West
Washington, DC 20007-2113
Office: (202) 444-3059
Fax: (202) 444-5391
Email: steinberg@usa.net

MELLICK T. SYKES, MD, MA, FACS
Peripheral Vascular Associates

7950 Floyd Curl Drive, Suite 109
San Antonio, Texas 78229
Office: (210) 692-9700
Fax: (210) 692-9730
Email: mellicksykes@aol.com

MISTY M. VAUGHN, PT, CWS, FCCWS
Comprehensive Therapy Solutions, Owner; American Medical Technologies, Regional Vice President

615 North Main, #102
Euless, Texas 76039
Office: (817) 681-7875
Fax: (817) 685-7243
Email: mistypt@comcast.net

ROBERT A. WARRINER, III, MD, FACA, FCCP, FCCWS, ABPM/UHM,CWS
Executive Vice President of Medical Affairs, Diversified Clinical Services, Jacksonville, Florida; Emeritus Medical Director and Founder, Southeast Texas Center for Wound Care and Hyperbaric Medicine, Conroe Regional Medical Center, Conroe, Texas

1610 Woodstead Court, Suite 460
The Woodlands, Texas 77380
Office: (281) 298-1400
Fax: (281) 298-1570
Email: rwarriner@diversifiedclinicalservices.com

GREGORY R. WEIR, MD
Vascular Surgeon in private practice at the Eugene Maris and Zuid Afrikaans Hospitals in Pretoria; Fellowship in Vascular Surgery, South African College of Medicine; M. Med (Surgery), University of Pretoria

P.O. Box 26091
Gezina, 0031, South Africa
Office: +27123358651
Fax: +27123358651
Email: gweir@vascular.co.2A

LYNDA T. WELLS, MD, DABPM, FRCA
Associate Professor of Anesthesiology & Pediatrics, University of Virginia Health System

Dept. of Anesthesiology
P.O. Box 800710
Charlottesville, Virginia 22908-0710
Office: (434) 924-2283
Fax: (434) 982-0019
Email: ltw6r@virginia.edu

RANDALL D. WOLCOTT, MD
Southwest Regional Wound Care Center, Lubbock, Texas

2002 Oxford Avenue
Lubbock, Texas 79410
Office: (806) 793-8869
Fax: (806) 793-0043
Email: randy@randallwolcott.com

E. GEORGE WOLF, JR., MD
Wound Care and Hyperbaric Medicine, Private Practice

414 Navarro, Suite 502
San Antonio, Texas 78205
Office: (210) 536-3281
Fax: (210) 536-2944
Email: george.wolf@brooks.af.mil

DISCLAIMER

The views expressed by the authors are their own and do not necessarily reflect the opinion of the editors, International ATMO, Inc, or Best Publishing Company.

While the information in this book is consistent with good medical practice, no responsibility can be assumed by the author or the publisher for any injuries or damage of any nature whatsoever, as a result of product failure, negligence, or from the application of any recommendations or ideas contained in this book.

Medicine is an ever-changing field. Standard safety precautions must be followed, but as new research and clinical experience broaden our knowledge, changes in treatment and drug therapy may become necessary or appropriate. Readers are advised to check the most current product information provided by the manufacturer of each drug, device, or equipment to verify the recommended dose, the method and duration of administration, and contraindications.

TRANCUTANEOUS OXIMETRY

To avoid confusion in terminology, in this book TCOM refers to the equipment (transcutaneous oxygen monitoring) or the procedure (transcutaneous oximetry) used for obtaining tissue oxygen values in the skin. PtcO2, aka $TcpO_2$ (transcutaneous oxygen tension) refers to the tissue pO_2 data obtained by TCOM, and is expressed in mm Hg. Although PtcO2 is the technically correct term it is seldom used by government agencies, insurance carriers, or clinicians, who prefer the term TcpO2. Thus, the authors have used PtcO2 and TcpO2 interchangeably in this book.

NOTES

SECTION 1
THE PROBLEM WOUND

CHAPTER **1**

ETIOLOGY OF THE PROBLEM WOUND

CHAPTER ONE OVERVIEW

ETIOLOGY OF THE PROBLEM WOUND

Adrianne P.S. Smith

Problem wounds are problems because they fail to do as we expect. They fail to heal after adequate surgical and antibiotic management. JC Davis, TK Hunt (1977)

INTRODUCTION

Although exact statistics on the number and total national financial burden of the "problem wound" are difficult to confirm, it has been suggested that patients with nonhealing chronic wounds utilize approximately eighty percent (80%) of national health expenditure. Identifying and eliminating the causes of wound failure should help to ease the financial burden. This task proves difficult since the etiology of wound failure in specific cases usually proves to be multi-factorial. Major impediments to wound healing include: infection/inflammation, recurrent trauma associated with incomplete off-loading, malnutrition, inadequate oxygen and blood supply, underlying debilitating chronic medical diseases, and inadequate medical care because of socio-economic or psychosocial limitations.

As we define a "problem wound" it is easy to see why multiple causes may prevail. The initial insult varies greatly: surgery, burn, severe arterial insufficiency, edema with venous insufficiency, prolonged pressure, and intermittent trauma without protective sensation associated with poor perfusion. While most wounds proceed rapidly through a normal healing sequence, others develop into problem wounds, which fail to progress normally or undergo deterioration. A wound that originally appeared to progress through a normal healing sequence might suddenly arrest to become a "chronic wound." Although various wound types proceed through healing at different rates, a chronic wound is generally defined by failure to progress normally over a 30-day period. It is usually characterized by inadequate granulation tissue, persistent wound exudate, deficient wound contraction and/or absence of neo-epithelialization.

Wound failure may arise in response to disease processes that negatively impact the immune or coagulation processes such as diabetes, hepatitis, or infection. Materials normally generated in the wound base such as slough, eschar, edema fluid, colonizing bacteria, and necrotic tissue, collectively referred to as the "bio-burden," stimulate the release of pro-inflammatory biochemical factors. When generated in excess, these factors negatively impact wound progression. Removing excessive pro-inflammatory materials from the wound base aids in faster wound healing. Other disease states impede wound healing by limiting oxygenation or perfusion to the injured tissue. Cellular and biochemical alterations caused by these disease states must be countered for normal healing to proceed. Developing an understanding of the histological and biochemical changes associated with chronic wound development enables one to more adequately devise strategies to address the problem wound.

Frequently, the nonhealing problem wound arises because of socio-economical encumbrances. Inability to afford recommended nutritious foods, medicines, supplies, or treatment modalities may hamper progression. Repetitive trauma sustained from walking on a diabetic neuropathic foot ulcer or from sitting on a presacral decubitus ulcer underscores the need for appropriate off-loading in wound care treatment. Other patient health choices may negatively impact outcome. Cigarette smoking, alcohol abuse, obesity, sedentary lifestyle, and noncompliance with recommended daily care have all been implicated in poor outcomes. In many cases, clinicians have to identify and correct histological, biochemical and socio-economic impediments to achieve successful wound closure.

ONE GLITCH SAMPLER

Because there are so many factors to evaluate, this author uses a mneumonic, ONE GLITCH SAMPLER, as an assessment tool to identify potential causes of problem wounds (Table 1). Each element of the mneumonic is described below.

TABLE 1. ETIOLOGY OF THE PROBLEM WOUND: ONE GLITCH SAMPLER

Oxygen and Perfusion	**G**lucose Control	**S**ocio-Economical Issues
Nutrition and Hydration	**L**ipid Control	**A**utoimmune Disease
Edema Control	**I**nfection/Inflammation	**M**edications
	Trauma (repetitive)	**P**sycho-Social Issues
	Chronicity	**L**ook-a-Likes (misdiagnosed/undiagnosed)
	Hematological Abnormality	**E**veryday Care
		Rheumatologic Diseases

ONE GLITCH SAMPLER is a simple mnemonic that can be used to identify potential causes of nonhealing or failing wound.

OXYGEN AND PERFUSION

Tissue oxygenation associated with adequate perfusion is vitally important for successful wound healing. Tissue hypoxia exists when the tissues are deprived of oxygen. Hypoxia hampers wound healing and is categorized into four main types.

1. Hypoxemic hypoxia is associated with low partial pressure of oxygen in inspired air as may occur in high altitudes or during inhaled anesthetic treatments.

2. Anemic hypoxia is associated with reduced hemoglobin concentrations secondary to low levels of iron, vitamin B12, and/or copper.
3. Stagnant hypoxia is associated with reduced blood flow as occurs in peripheral arterial occlusive disease (PAOD).
4. Cytotoxic hypoxia is associated with toxic interference in cellular respiration as occurs with poisonous agents (i.e., carbon monoxide or cyanide poisoning). It also is associated during physiological cellular respiration regulation with nitric oxide (NO) after stimulation of inducible nitric oxide synthetase (iNOS).

Hypoxia generates specific proteins, Hypoxia Inducing Factors (HIF), which maintain oxygen homeostasis and regulate hypoxia inducible genes. These genes code for human erythropoietin (EPO), vascular endothelial growth factor (VEGF), inducible nitric oxide synthetase (iNOS), heme oxygenase 1 (OH-l), aldolase A (ALDA), enolase 1 (ENO-1), glucose transporter 1 (GLUT-1), lactate dehydrogenase A (LDHA), and phosphoglycerate kinase 1 (PGK-1). Hypoxia inducing factor-1 (HIF-1) is composed of two subunits; the α-subunit (HE-lα) and the ß-subunit (HIF-1ß), an aryl hydrocarbon receptor nuclear translocator (ARNT). Both subunits are continuously produced; however, in normoxic conditions the α-subunit undergoes proteosomal degradation and is not available. Alternatively, under hypoxic conditions, the ß-subunit becomes stable and then combines with the ß-subunit to promote transcription of the hypoxia inducible genes. Iron chelators, transition metals and antioxidants also stabilize the α-subunit. The ARNT ß-subunit is oxygen independent and appears to be responsible for HIF-1 DNA-binding. Hypoxia inducible genes help to resolve hypoxia through the following mechanisms: 1) formation and development of erythrocytes (EPO and OH-l), 2) development and relaxation of blood vessels (iNOS and VEGF), and 3) adaptation of cellular metabolism to low oxygen conditions (GLUT-1 and most glycolytic enzymes). Through these mechanisms HIF-l improves tissue oxygenation in response to hypoxia by improving the blood oxygen carrying capacity, the tissue blood flow and the local cellular adaptation to a low oxygen state. Although hypoxia signals are required to initiate healing processes, subsequent adequate oxygenation is necessary to support and maintain the proliferative phase of cellular growth.

In injured tissue, oxygen supplies originate from intact vasculature at the margins and base of the wound. Within seconds of an injury, hemostasis is initiated to prevent exsanguinations. Blood vessels contract and retract to control bleeding. Coagulation proceeds over 0–2 hours as platelets exposed to type IV and type V collagen in the injured subendothelial tissue become activated to undergo shape changes, become sticky, aggregate, and secrete contents from their granules (degranulation). Activated platelet membranes and the endothelial cellar membranes both secrete von Willebrand Factor (vWF) that binds to Glb receptors on platelets and allows them to adhere to endothelial cells. Fibrinogen from the plasma is also activated in response to exposed type IV collagen in the epithelial lining. A fibrinous mesh is formed as fibrin attaches to the spiny processes of activated platelets trapping more platelets, leukocytes and erythrocytes. The formation of clot physically plugs the injury defect.

Platelet degranulation releases chemotactic factors and growth factors that attract and activate neutrophils and macrophages. Neutrophils are the first to arrive from sites marginated along the blood vessel wall. They remove necrotic tissue, foreign bodies, bacterium and debris by secreting peroxidase and incorporating material into phagosomes. This process of oxidative killing is oxygen-dependent. The neutrophils secrete growth factors and chemotactic factors that notify the T-cells (when necessary) and attract macrophages to the area of injury. Macrophages ingest bacteria, interact with white blood cells, self-regulate, and help orchestrate the wound healing process. They are predominantly responsible for secreting vascular endothelial growth factor (VEGF), the major factor responsible for vascular network development in the wound site. Vasodilation with resultant edema, warmth, and rubor are the result of factors secreted from the macrophage and other leukocytes present at the wound site.

Although hypoxia and lactic acidosis are chemoattractants for macrophages, lactic acid secreted by macrophages acts in a self-regulatory fashion to attract additional macrophages to the site. This occurs even after VEGF has induced the formation of neovascularization and the wound oxygen content has increased.

Cellular proliferation of leukocytes, fibroblasts and keratinocytes requires adequate oxygen supply. Collagen secretion from fibroblast is rate limited dependent upon the available oxygen content.

In some disease states, microvascular and macrovascular abnormalities preclude the adequate delivery of blood, oxygen, and nutrients to tissue. Noninvasive studies that assess macrovascular perfusion include: pulse palpation, pulse auscultation, perfusion pressures (ankle, toe), ankle-brachial index (ABI), toe-brachial index (TBI), and pulse waveform evaluation. The normal ABI range is between 0.9 and 1.2. At levels less than 0.9 the patient is at risk for increased incidence of myocardial infarction (MI) and cerebral vascular accidents (CVA). Significant peripheral vascular disease is usually associated with ABI values less than 0.8. Critical stenosis is usually seen with ABI values of less than 0.5.

In patients with significant arterial calcification, such as in diabetics, the blood vessels may be non-compressible. Diabetic patients having Monckeberg's sclerosis, calcification of the infrageniculate vessels of the calf, have led to falsely elevated ABI results. Non-compressible vessels lead to falsely elevated ABI results. In diabetic patients the calcification does not extend into the digits. Therefore, a toe-brachial index (TBI) or toe perfusion pressure (TPP) will prove to be a more accurate reflection of distal foot perfusion in diabetic patients. TBI values less than 0.5 are considered abnormal but values less than 0.45 show decreased healing with spontaneous ulcerations developing in patients with TBI < 0.20. In diabetic patients, absolute TPPs of more than 55 mm Hg, are likely to heal, whereas pressures of less than 30 mm Hg are unlikely to heal (see Table 2). For more information about vascular evaluation see the chapter by Buckley and Lee titled, "Non-invasive and Invasive Evaluations for Lower Extremity Arterial Occlusive Disease."

Hyperbaric oxygen therapy (HBO2) has been used to improve wound healing in patients with compromised oxygenation and/or perfusion. Multiple sessions of HBO2 (more than 14 treatments) have increased angiogenesis and new blood vessel growth. Other benefits of HBO2 are listed in Table 4. For more information about HBO2, see the chapter by Fife and Warriner titled, "Hyperbaric Oxygen Applications in Wound Care."

Transcutaneous oxygen ($P_{tc}O_2$ or $TcpO_2$) studies aid in assessing tissue oxygenation. Normal $TcpO_2$ values are 40 mm Hg or above (see Table 3). $TcpO_2$ values of less than 30 mm Hg have been correlated with an increased risk of amputation. Low $TcpO_2$ values may be secondary due to hypoxia of any cause, poor perfusion, vasoconstriction, cigarette smoking, edema, thickened or sclerotic skin, irradiated tissues, probe placement over bony structures, tendons or ligaments, and inappropriate probe temperature. For more information about tissue oxygenation, see the Dietz and Sheffield chapter titled "Non-Invasive Wound Assessment Tools."

TABLE 2. ANKLE–BRACHIAL AND TOE-BRACHIAL INDEX MEASURES

Bedside Non-Invasive Evaluation of Oxygen and Perfusion	
Ankle-Brachial Index (ABI)	**Toe-Brachial Index (TBI)**
> 1.2 Non-compressible (calcified)	> 0.75 Normal
0.9–1.2 Normal range	< 0.5 Abnormal
0.5–0.9 Mixed arterial/venous disease	< 0.25 Critical Occlusive Disease
< 0.5 Critical stenosis	
< 0.2 Ischemic gangrene necrosis likely	**Toe Perfusion Pressure (TPP)**
	> 55 mm Hg Likely to heal
	< 30 mm Hg Unlikely to heal

Diabetics with calcified (non-compressible) blood vessels may have a falsely elevated ankle brachial index (ABI). Medial vascular calcification in diabetes does not extend into the toes; therefore diabetic patients with a falsely elevated ABI are better evaluated with a toe-brachial index (TBI) or a toe perfusion pressure (TPP). Unfortunately, TPP values may vary with skin temperature. A 10°C change in skin temperature may create a 10 mm Hg change in TPP.

TABLE 3. TRANSCUTANEOUS OXYGEN TENSION MEASUREMENTS

Bedside Non-Invasive Evaluation of Oxygen and Perfusion	
Transcutaneous Oxygen Tension ($TcpO_2$)	**Potential Causes of Low $TcpO_2$ Values**
> 40 mm Hg Normal	Poor perfusion
< 30 mm Hg Abnormal	Hypovolemia
	Vasoconstriction
Oxygen Challenge Goals	Cigarette smoking
O_2 (1 ATA) 40–45 mm Hg	Edema
In Chamber	Thick or sclerotic skin (scar, palms, soles)
(2.0–2.5 ATA) 200 mm Hg	Post-irradiated tissues
Flaps/Grafts 50 mm Hg (in-chamber)	Flaps/Grafts (interrupted vasculature)
	Probe placement over bony structures
	Inappropriate probe heat temperature

$TcpO_2$ measurements are predictive of adjunctive improvement using HBO2 therapy when accompanied by an oxygen challenge. The oxygen challenge is done either outside the chamber using a mask (breathing 100% O_2 at 1 ATA) or inside the chamber (breathing 100% O_2 at the recommended treatment pressure of 2.0-2.5 ATA). Before recommending hyperbaric therapy, the oxygen challenge values outside the chamber should increase to 40–45 mm Hg. For inside the chamber at 2.0 ATA, the values should be more than 200 mm Hg. For conditions such as failed skin grafts where there has

TABLE 4. THERAPEUTIC BENEFITS OF HBO

Therapeutic effects of HBO2 are related to the ability of oxygen and/or pressure under hyperbaric conditions to:

1. Reverse hypoxia
2. Alter ischemic effect
3. Influence vascular reactivity
4. Reduce edema
5. Stimulate nitric oxide changes
6. Modify growth factors and cytokine effect by regulating their levels and/or receptors
7. Induce changes in membrane proteins affecting ion exchange and gating mechanisms
8. Promote cellular proliferation
9. Accelerate collagen deposition
10. Stimulate capillary budding and arborization
11. Accelerate microbial oxidative killing
12. Improve selected antibiotic exchange across membranes
13. Interfere with bacterial disease propagation by denaturing toxins
14. Modulate the immune system response
15. Enhance oxygen radical scavengers thereby decreasing ischemia-reperfusion injury

Adapted from PJ Sheffield and APS Smith, Physiological and Pharmacological Basis of Hyperbaric Oxygen Therapy. *In Hyperbaric Surgery-Perioperative Care. Flagstaff, AZ: Best Publishing Company, 2002: 63–110.*

been a disruption of the vascular supply, HBO2 is recommended if in-chamber levels of 50 mm Hg can be achieved. Patients with severe vascular disease that do not achieve these oxygen values may be too compromised to show an appropriate response to hyperbaric therapy. Therefore, a referral for vascular surgical intervention is recommended. For more information on arterial insufficiency, see "Arterial Insufficiency Ulcers" by Biggs, Sykes and Blumoff.

NUTRITION AND HYDRATION

Nutrition is divided into micronutrients (vitamins, mineral and trace elements), and macronutrients (protein, fat, and carbohydrates) that provide required energy. Protein-energy malnutrition is the inadequate intake of macronutrients. This frequently occurs in the elderly populations in specialized living situations, such as: community dwelling (5–12%), hospitalized patients (30-61%) and long-term care facilities (40–85%). Protein-energy malnutrition (PEM) has been linked to involuntary weight loss which is defined as: 1) 5% loss of usual body weight over 30 days, 2) 10% loss over 180 days, or 3) a body mass index below standard or ideal measurements.

TABLE 5. PREALBUMIN RULE OF FIVES

Prealbumin Rule of Fives	
Normal	> 15 mg/dL
Mild Deficiency	< 15mg/dL
Moderate Deficiency	< 10mg/dL
Severe Deficiency	< 5mg/dL

Represents a simplified interpretation of prealbumin levels.

TABLE 6. NUTRITIONAL REQUIREMENTS NORMAL AND WOUND HEALING

Requirements	Healthy Individuals	Patients with Wounds/Stress (loss < 15% LBM)
Calories	1200–200 kcal/d	30 kcal/kg/d
Protein	0.8 g/kg/d lean body mass, 10% of calories average 50 gms	1.5–2.0 g/kg/d lean body mass
Fluids	Average 3 liters/d	1 mL water per calorie
Carbohydrates	60% of calories average 300 gms	50–60% of calories
Fat	30% of calories (10% sat. fat) average 65 gms	25% of calories
Vitamin A	1.0 mg/day for the adult man and 0.8 mg/day for the adult woman. 6 mg of beta-carotene is considered to be the equivalent of 1 mg of vitamin A.	1600–2000 mg per day (1 RE = I micro gm =3.33 IU)
Vitamin B (complex)	100–300 mg	200% RDA
Vitamin C	60 mg	100–1000 mg
Vitamin D	200 International Units (IU) per day (adults)	NA
Vitamin E	10 mg/day for the adult man, 8 mg/day for the adult woman, and 3 mg/day for the infant.	NA
Zinc	15 mg	15–30 mg per day
Iron	10 mg for men and 15 for women	20–30 mg per day elevation
Copper	1.5–3.0 mg	

TABLE 7. LABORATORY STUDIES USED TO ASSESS PROTEIN

Laboratory Study	Usual Values	Levels in Malnutrition	Half life $t_{1/2}$	Influences
Albumin	3.5–5.5 g/dl	< 3.5 g/dl	18–20 days	Hydration status will either dilute or concentrate the measured levels. A late indicator of malnutrition. Levels raise slowly during periods of re-feeding. Reliable changes are seen in 2–3 weeks.
Prealbumin	15–25 mg/dl	<15 g/dl	2 days	Reflects the immune status and the inflammatory state, in addition to the nutritional status. Best used as a monitor of current protein status. Changes with fluid status, but not as greatly as albumin. Usually measured once or twice a week.
Total Lymphocyte Count (TLC)	1500–3000 cells per mm³	< 1500 cells per mm³	NA	Tests immune function and protein status. Also depressed by chemotherapy, autoimmune disease, stress, and infections.
Transferrin (TF)	200–400 mg/dl	< 100 mg/dl	8–10 days	Decreased levels of TF are associated with the acute phase response, chronic inflammation, malnutrition, hemochromatosis, and hereditary transferrin deficiency. Increased levels are associated with iron deficiency, early to mid pregnancy, acute hepatitis, and estrogen use.

TABLE 8. EXPECTED PROTEIN MONITORING PARAMETERS IN NORMAL AND PROTEIN MALNOURISHED STATES

	Normal	Mild	Moderate	Severe
Albumin	3.5–5.0 gm/dl	2.8–3.5	2.1–2.7	< 2.1
Prealbumin	15–25 mg/dl	10–15	5–9	< 5
Transferrin	200–400 mg/dl	151–200	100–150	< 100
Total Lymphocyte Count	1500–3000 cells per mm^3	1200–1500	801–1200	< 800

Wound healing requires both macronutrients and micronutrients. Many patients with nonhealing chronic wounds suffer from involuntary weight loss and protein-energy malnutrition (PEM). Adequate protein, hydration, vitamins (A, B, C, D, E and K) and trace elements (zinc, copper, iron, and manganese) are well recognized for their roles in wound healing, Patients who suffer from wounds utilize more energy and require more calories, protein, vitamins and minerals than people who are healthy. Healthy people require approximately 0.8 g of protein per kilogram per 24 hours. Patients facing wounds and stress may require between 1.5–2.0 g/kg/24hr.

Albumin, prealbumin, total lymphocytes count (TLC), and transferrin are all used to monitor protein levels. Albumin is considered the most helpful for an initial overall screen, providing information reflecting a week of protein intake. Serum albumin level of < 3.5 gm/dL is associated with involuntary weight loss and pressure ulcers. Low serum albumin levels in elderly patients are correlated with the presence and severity of pressure ulcers. Prealbumin, on the other hand, provides information reflecting protein intake over the past several days. Prealbumin, therefore, is best used in the outpatient setting to monitor changes once protein replacement has begun. An easy guide for interpreting prealbumin levels is to follow the Prealbumin Rule of Fives (See Table 5). All parameters that measure protein are altered by the patient's hydration status. Over hydration can dilute the concentrations and lower the value while dehydration tends to hemo-concentrate protein levels and thereby cause false elevations. Some selected nutritional requirements are located in Table 6. Laboratory studies and protein monitoring parameters are found in Tables 7 and 8. For daily nutritional guidelines and requirements, see the Dennis-Wauters chapter titled, "Nutrition and Hydration."

Many supplements are available to provide either single component or combination (protein, vitamin and trace element) component therapy. The packaging is varied to provide a variety of methods for consumption, such as shakes, sodas, puddings, wafers, and powders to be mixed with solid foods. Care should be taken to avoid "over-treating" a patient with vitamins and trace elements when using combination therapy. L-arginine is sometimes used to aid in wound healing by increasing the semi-essential amino acid. In animal studies, L-arginine dietary supplementation shortened the re-epithelization time, increased the amount of hydroxyproline and accelerated the synthesis of reparative collagen. Similar results were found in a human study where L-arginine supplementation improved both wound healing and the immune response.

Consultation with a nutritionist is prudent to assure proper treatment and follow-up in patients at risk for malnutrition.

Many patients and their physicians are beginning to pay closer attention to agents that were previously considered as Alternative Medicine. Aloe vera has undergone more detailed scrutiny in a peer-reviewed fashion. Although the use of oral aloe vera has been touted to reduce glucose levels in diabetic patients, lower lipid levels in hyperlipidemia, and expedite the healing rate of burns, the exact role of this agent is still unclear. Acemannan, a glycoprotein fraction isolated from aloe vera, increases the production of the cytokines IL-6 and TNF-α, and nitric oxide suggesting that aloe vera may exert its effects through macrophage activation.

EDEMA CONTROL

In the face of trauma, edema fluid is released into the wound and periwound tissue as part of the healing process. Processes that support wound healing when acutely activated may become destructive when applied chronically over time. Acutely activated edema fluid activates fibrinogen and initiates peri-capillary cuffing. This prevents further blood loss at the wound site. Chronically applied, the peri-capillary cuffing may starve the tissue by

TABLE 9. CATEGORIZATION OF MATRIX METALLOPROTEINASES (MMPS)

Matrix Metalloproteinase Review
Membrane Bound/Membrane Type (MT-1, -2, -3,-4, -5) achieves membrane attachment with components located at the C-terminal. It activates a variety of secreted products to include other MMPs, growth factors and cytokines.
Membrane Type 1 (MT–1): is activated during migration of human endothelial cells and modulates endothelial motility and matrix remodeling. It clusters in specific areas when activated and modulates endothelial migration, invasion, and formation of capillary tubes during the angiogenic response. MT-1 activates pro-MMP-2 and degrades fibrinogen.
Membrane Type 2 (MT-2)
Membrane Type 3 (MT-3)
Membrane Type 4 (MT-4)
Membrane Type 5 (MT-5)
Soluble Type Matrix Metalloproteinases: secreted into the matrix either as zymogens or activated by membrane-bound (MT-MMP) as they cross during secretion.
Collagenases (MMPs –1, -8, -13, -18): degrade specific fibrillar collagen types in a specific fashion.
Gelatinases (MMPs –2, -9): Gelatinases degrade gelatin, the main residual products of collagen degradation after collagen undergoes lysis by specific collagenases. Additionally, MMP-2 and MMP-9 are the main proteases available to degrade type IV collagen, present only in basement membrane. Basement membranes are sheet-like structures that surround all tissues and organs; therefore, type IV collagen, the major constituent of basement membranes is found in all tissues. Gelatinases may also degrade other collagens (non-specifically) and stromal components. At resting basal states MMP-2 is produced more than MMP-9.
Gelatinase-A: -MMP-2 (72 kD type IV collagenase): gelatin, collagens I, IV, V, VII, and X, fibronectin, laminins, aggrecan, tenascin-C, vitronectin
Gelatinase-B: -MMP-9 (92 kD type IV collagenase)-gelatin, collagens IV, V, and XIV, aggrecan, elastin, tenascin, vitronectin
Stromolysins: degrade non-collagen ECM components; MMPs –3, -10, -11
Stromolysin
Stromolysin
Unclassified MMPs: 7, -12, -19,

Categorization of matrix metalloproteinases (MMPs)

reducing the amount of oxygen and nutrients delivered to the injured tissue. Fibrin plugs formed during coagulation also block local lymphatic channels. Obstructing local lymphatic channels prevents lymphatic drainage from the injury site, thereby, localizing the inflammatory reaction to support healing. A persistent inflammatory process activates factors that bind or inhibit growth factor function and impede further wound healing. Exuded edema fluid is a pro-inflammatory proteinacious mixture that initiates a series of enzymatic processes through the activation of matrix metalloproteinases (MMPs). MMPs (see Tables 9 and 10) are designed to promote remodeling and growth of the tissue matrix. However, MMPs predominant in chronic wound fluid are highly degradative, reduce proper extracellular gel matrix formation, interfere with collagen cross bridging, and/or impede the deposit of vital stromal structures. Additionally, in some patients the loss of protein rich edema fluid serves as an important source of total body protein loss. Obviously, controlling edema fluid should be a major focus to prevent the development of chronic wounds.

Acute vs. Chronic Wound Fluid

Fluid exuded from acute healing wounds differs in content from fluid obtained from chronic non-healing wounds. For research purposes, acute wound fluid is obtained from skin graft donor sites, mastectomy incisions, and fresh punch biopsies. Wound fluid obtained from venous and arterial insufficiency ulcers, decubitus ulcers, and diabetic foot ulcers serves as a source for chronic wound fluid.

Although collagenase and gelatinase activity increases after acute wounding, chronic wound fluid shows a further increase (two to 25-fold) for various matrix metalloproteinases (MMPs). Conversely, Tissue Inhibitors of Metalloproteinases (TIMP) are depressed in chronic wounds. Decrease in TIMP levels may be secondary to binding with activated MMPs, decreased transcription, or enhanced degradation. As a wound heals, the proteolytic activity normalizes. Proinflammatory cytokines interleukin-1 (IL-1), interleukin-6 (IL-6), and tumor necrosis factor-alpha (TNF-α) rapidly revert as a wound progresses through the normal healing responses. Other growth factors such as platelet-derived growth factor (PDGF), epidermal growth factor (EGF), basic fibroblast growth factor (FGF) and transforming growth factor-beta (TGF-ß)

TABLE 10. REGULATION OF MATRIX METALLOPROTEINASES

Inactive Form-zymogen
Specific Tissue Inhibitors of Matrix Metalloproteinases (TIMPs)
Medication Inhibitors of MMPs

Macrolides
1. Tetracycline Derivatives: may block MMP-8 by inhibiting conversion to an active state or inhibiting reactive oxygen species (ROS) that are involved in activation of MMPs. Tetracycline analogues also inhibited keratinocyte migration and growth, an effect not found for the other inhibitors tested.
2. Erythromycin: has an anti-inflammatory effect. Studies show a down regulation in MMP-9 protein and MMP-9 mRNA. Moreover, IL-6 is released in therapeutic levels (approx. 10^6)
3. Clarithromycin: has similar effect to Erythromycin

Non-steroidal Anti-inflammatory Drugs (NSAID)
These agents are thought to inhibit MMP-2 expression by repression of mRNA transcription.

stabilize more slowly. These results suggest that the impaired healing response seen in chronic wounds may be more dependent upon inflammatory mediators in the edema fluid as opposed to an overall deficit in growth factor levels.

In addition to immune system mediation, acute and chronic wounds deposit extracellular matrix molecules differently. Concentrations of extra cellular molecules, such as fibronectin (FN), chondroitin sulfate (CS), and tenascin (TN) persist for only 12–18 months in healing dermal tissue; whereas these stromal components remain elevated even longer in non-healing tissue.

In summary, in comparison to acute wounds, chronic wound fluid contains more collagenase and gelatinase activity. Also, chronic wounds have less TIMP activity, and more proinflammatory mediators associated with an increased number of extra cellular molecules that persist longer in the dermal stomal tissue from which the fluid is released.

Occlusive Compression Therapy Dressings

The use of occlusive dressings for edema control may benefit the patient through several proposed mechanisms. Occlusive dressings reduce loss of exudate related protein, decrease activation of matrix metalloproteinases, reduce formation of peri-capillary fibrinous cuffing, promote fibrinolysis of excessive fibrin deposition, and maintain contact between the wound bed to accumulated wound fluid which is thought to contain growth stimulatory substances.

Treatment for edema usually includes some form of compression therapy. Compression therapy in diabetic patients may be complicated by the presence of macrovascular disease with critical stenosis. Application of compression should always be preceded by an arterial assessment to include palpation of pulses, auscultation of pulses, ABI determination and, if indicated, a TBI determination. It is generally recommended that compression be applied cautiously for patients with ABI < 0.7 and withheld for patients with ABI < 0.5 or a TBI < 3.0.

Additives to Compression Wraps

Zinc paste wraps (Unna's boots) are frequently used to treat edema associated with lower extremity wounds. Zinc therapy may serve a variety of functions: replacement for zinc-deficiency related wound healing impairment, improvement in local immune function, interference with bacterial toxins without interfering with PMN function, and provision of a vital structural component for enzymatic proteins involved in matrix modification and DNA transcription regulation (finger proteins). Although no single universally accepted zinc measurement exists, most researchers agree that many patients suffering from chronic pressure and venous insufficiency ulcers are mild to moderately zinc-deficient, described as a "marginal zinc status." Medical conditions such as sickle cell anemia and age-related malabsorption predispose certain subpopulations towards zinc deficiency. Zinc oxide solubilizes continuously when applied to intact skin and increases blood levels when applied to open wounds. Topically applied zinc oxide may convert some chronic wounds into healing wounds with improved neo-epithelialization. Zinc sulfate, however, does not have the same beneficial effect. Zinc replacement provides cytotoxic protection against bacterial toxins including Staphylococcus alpha-toxin but it does not impair PMN phagocytosis or bacterial killing. The effect of zinc oxide appeared to be related to a local modulation of the immune system as opposed to a direct toxic reaction with the bacterium. Zinc is required for the activity of more than 300 enzymes, including alcohol dehydrogenase, Cu/Zn superoxide dismutase, carbonic anhydrase, and many proteases. Zinc acts as a cofactor in the catalytic area for matrix metalloproteinases and zinc assists in the correct folding of specific domains in transcription factors that regulate DNA transcription such as zinc-dependent DNA-binding motifs, known as zinc fingers and zinc clusters. For more information on edema management see the chapters "Venous Disease" by Kimbrell and Larson-Lohr and "Lymphedema: An Epidemic Hidden in Plainsight" by Fife.

GLUCOSE CONTROL

Although prolonged hyperglycemia impedes wound healing, no correlation exists between a specific glucose level or hemoglobin A1C (HgA1C) value and a specific wound healing outcome. In general, wound-healing outcomes improve as HgA1C values approach normal levels (HgA1C less than 6.0%).

Prolonged exposure to hyperglycemia produces a variety of negative alterations in the vasculature, coagulation pathways, inflammatory response, granulation tissue proliferation, and tissue maturation. Recent or transient corrections in glucose control may improve some complications while other hyperglycemia-derived complications may persist for up to five years after the disease has been corrected with pancreatic transplantation. These pathological alterations arise from several common mechanisms: 1) development of advanced glycosylation end-products (AGE), 2) induction of oxidative stress and pro-inflammatory responses, and 3) protein kinase-C (PKC) activation with subsequent alterations in growth factor expression.

Excessive coagulation leads to necrosis. Deviation from the appropriate inflammatory response impedes host responses to infection. Inhibition in cell phase progression inhibits granulation tissue proliferation. Along with delays in maturation all of these result in wound failure.

Endothelial dysfunction describes several pathological conditions: altered anticoagulant and anti-inflammatory properties of the endothelium, impaired modulation of vascular growth, abnormal regulation of vascular remodeling and impaired endothelium-dependent vasorelaxation caused by a loss of nitric oxide (NO) activity in blood vessel walls. Endothelial dysfunction is a major factor in diabetic-related wound healing delays.

Advanced Glycosylation End-Products (AGE)

Prolonged hyperglycemia generates nonenzymatic glycosylation of proteins and lipids, resulting in adducts, called advanced glycosylation end-products (AGEs). AGEs have been implicated in cellular aging and in the development of diabetic complications associated with endothelial dysfunction. Glycosylated proteins recognize specific receptors for advanced glycosylation end-products (RAGEs), which induce oxidative stress, promote proinflammatory responses, and activate protein kinase-C (PKC). PKC activation ultimately results in altered growth factor expression. While glycosylation predominantly depends upon glucose concentration and time of exposure, localized oxidative stress accelerates glucose deposition. Through interaction with RAGE receptors, stimulating local oxidative stress, the process of AGE formation increases substantially. Early in the process, improved glycemic control and antioxidant usage may facilitate glucose removal; however, some enzymes along blood vessel walls are permanently damaged rendering capillary beds incapable of normal function.

Coagulation Abnormalities

In addition to microvascular endothelial dysfunction, prolonged hyperglycemia promotes a hypercoagulable state associated with macrovascular calcifications and poor wound healing. Microthrombi formation, atherosclerotic deposition, and vascular wall hypertrophy inhibit proper oxygen and nutrient exchange.

In diabetes, elevated levels of coagulation markers and activated factors are present. Elevated markers such as prothrombin activation fragment and thrombin-anti-thrombin complexes, as well as, elevated levels of clotting factors-fibrinogen, factor VII, factor VIII, factor XI, factor XII, kallikrein, and von Willebrand factor (vWF) predispose the diabetic patient to atherosclerotic disease and delayed wound healing. Conversely, the level of the protective anticoagulant protein C (PC) is decreased in diabetic patients.

Platelet hyperactive activity forms another important component of the hypercoagulable state. Platelet aggregates with increased platelet contractile force (PCF) and higher plasma levels of platelet release products, such as,- thromboglobulin, platelet factor 4, and thromboxane B2, stimulate microthrombi formation.

Abnormal clot formation accompanied by an increase in plasminogen activator inhibitor type I (PAI-1) compromises the patient's capability to remove excessive clot deposition. Increased PAI-1 is more prevalent in obese type II diabetic patients than in lean type II diabetic patients. Moreover, obese type II diabetic patients exhibit a more profound lack of fibrinolytic activity than lean diabetic patients and consequently bear more risk for poor outcomes induced by microthrombi complications.

Microvasculature Hypertrophy

A complement regulatory protein, CD59, protects blood vessel walls from inappropriate complement deposition. Reduction of CD59 expression in vasculature membrane permits the deposition of membrane attack complex of complement (MAC). MAC stimulates blood vessel endothelium to release fibroblast growth factor (FGF) and platelet-derived growth factor (PDGF), which in turn stimulates fibroblasts and smooth muscle cell proliferation. Glycosylation inactivates CD59, thereby facilitating MAC deposition, fibroblast and smooth muscle proliferation, and microvasculature dysfunctional hypertrophy. Additionally, glycosylation of matrix components such as collagen VI, laminin, and vitronectin alter interactions between matrix components, transmembrane integrin receptors, and growth factors.

Maximizing Glucose Control

From 1983 to 1993, The National Institute of Diabetes and Digestive and Kidney Diseases (NIDDK) Division of the National Institutes of Health (NIH) compared the effects of either standard therapy or intensive control on the outcome of diabetic complications. The comprehensive review included 1,411 volunteers with type I diabetes at 29 medical centers in the United States and Canada. Researchers concluded that normalizing blood glucose levels retards the onset and progression of diabetic related complications: eye disease (76%), kidney disease (50%), and nerve disease (60%). The largest and longest run study reviewing the complications of type II diabetic patients, the United Kingdom Prospective Diabetes Study (UKPDS), conclusively demonstrated that improved blood glucose control in these patients reduces the risk of developing retinopathy and nephropathy and possibly reduces neuropathy. UKPDS data showed a continuous relationship between the risk of microvascular complications and glycemia, such that for every percentage point decrease in HbA1c (i.e., 9–8%), there was a 35% reduction in the risk of microvascular complications. Uncontrolled diabetes negatively influences all phases of wound healing. Neuropathic and neuroischemic diabetic foot ulcers are the lesions most specifically associated with diabetes; nonetheless, disorders in microvasculature throughout the body lead to delays in healing, post-operative dehiscence, poor flap and graft "take," and amputation. For more information on glucose control, see Reasner's chapter entitled, "Glycemic Control in the Patient with Diabetes."

LIPID CONTROL

Dyslipidemia, in particular, hypertriglyceridemia is associated with accelerated vascular plaque formation and a prothrombotic state. Elevated triglyceride (TG) levels, small low-density lipoprotein (LDL) particles, and depressed levels of high-density lipoprotein cholesterol (HDL-C) characterize the "atherogenic lipoprotein phenotype" or "triad" of atherogenic dyslipidemia. A metabolic syndrome has been described that includes the coexistence of the lipid triad, elevated blood pressure, insulin resistance (plus glucose intolerance), and a prothrombotic state. Atheromatous plaques emanate from oxidative stress, a process that generates reactive oxygen species (ROS) from respiring cells that exceed local antioxidant defenses. ROS bind DNA, proteins, carbohydrates, and lipids preventing these basic molecules from functioning normally; thereby, producing endothelial dysfunction. Patients suffering from atheromatous plaque formation and endothelial dyslipidemia are at risk for developing non-healing wounds.

Additionally, hyperlipidemia, arising from either dietary or from diabetic origins, has the potential to change macrophage phenotype and function. Influenced by hypertriglyceridemia, monocytic differentiation leads to a non-progressive inflammatory macrophage phenotype rather than a reparative, proliferative phenotype. Decreased production of several notable factors, such as interleukin-1 beta (IL-1ß), tumor necrosis factor-alpha (TNFα), platelet-derived growth factor (PDGF), and transforming growth factor beta 1 (TGF-ß1) may represent another cellular mechanism responsible for delayed wound healing.

Diabetes and Dyslipidemia

Diabetes is frequently associated with dyslipidemia in the form of elevated cholesterol and elevated triglycerides. The elevated lipid levels may arise from a combination of overproduction and poor clearance. This abnormality leads to an accelerated development of atherosclerotic disease. Levels greater than 240 mg/dl have been associated with increase strokes and heart attacks. Therefore, previous recommendations supported maintaining cholesterol levels below 200 mg/dl. Special emphasis is placed on lowering LDL-C, which reduces coronary risk by 30%. The latest guideline released from the Third Report of the Expert Panel on Detection, Evaluation, and Treatment of High Blood Cholesterol in Adults (Adult Treatment Panel III) emphasizes risk modifications that promotes earlier detection and intervention:

1. Sets optimal level for total cholesterol at less than 200 mg/dL
2. Places more emphasis on the role of low-density lipoproteins (LDL)
3. Raises the normal cholesterol high-density lipoprotein (HDL) level from > 35 mg/dL to > 40 mg/dL for men, and > 50 mg/dL for women; to emphasize the protective role of HDL
4. Lowers the hypertriglyceride classification cutoff points to give more attention to moderate elevations; LDL < 100 mg/dL is optimal, > 130 mg/dL is high
5. Total cholesterol/HDL ratio < 4.0

Omega-6 vs. Omega-3 Fatty Acids

Omega-6 fatty acids, such as arachidonic acid, serve as precursors for prostaglandin E2 (PGE-2) and leukotriene B4 (LTB4), bioactive compounds with inflammatory and vasodilatory effects. These compounds are chemotatic and stimulatory for normal fibroblast function in wound healing and extracellular connective tissue matrix formation. In overproduction, prostaglandins and leukotrienes produce chronic inflammation and impair wound healing. Elevated levels of PGE-2 may inhibit wound healing by blocking fibroblast proliferation and chemotaxis. On the other hand, omega-3 fatty acids suppress omega-6 fatty acid production, reduce prostaglandin E2 (PGE-2) generation and alter the T cell proliferative response. Omega-3 fatty acids stimulate cell migration during wound healing. Diets high in omega-3 fatty acids are associated with lower postoperative infection rates, restoration of normal postoperative tissue function, and prevention of systemic inflammatory response syndrome (SIRS). SIRS is a systemic inflammatory response to a wide variety of severe clinical insults, manifested by two or more of the following conditions:

- Temperature > 38°C or < 36°C (>100°F or <96.8 °F)
- Heart rate > 90 beats/min
- Respiratory rate > 20 breaths/min or PaCO2 < 32 mm Hg
- WBC count > 12,000/mm3, < 4000/mm3, or > 10% immature (band) forms

These correlations highlight the relationship between fat and the inflammatory process. The type of fat consumed is relevant to the level of inflammation generated.

INFECTION AND INFLAMMATION

Infection and inflammation robs tissue of vital oxygen and nutrients. The lack of oxygen and nutrients coupled with chronic activation of cytokines, matrix metalloproteinases, and other inflammatory mediators reduce the ability of wounds to heal effectively. All chronic wounds are colonized with bacteria. Initially normal flora covers the wound after migrating from adjacent tissue. Subsequently, organisms that are common in the environment as well as adjacent skin will be cultured for *S. aureus* and *Beta-hemolytic Strep. Group B Strep* and *S. aureus* are common isolates in diabetic foot wounds. After several weeks to months, facultative anaerobic and gram-negative organisms, *Proteus, E. Coli, Klebsiella,* appear to predominate. Wound deterioration and the presence of devitalized tissue increases the likelihood of harboring these organisms. Deeper wounds favor infection with anaerobes. Most chronic wounds commonly are infected with more than four to five organisms in a polymicrobial fashion in addition to the anaerobic organisms. Environmental exposure that occurs with soaking one's foot in a bath or shower usually is associated with the development of aerobic gram-negative rods such as *Pseudomonas, Acinetobacter and Stenotrophomonas (Xanthomonas)*.

Bacteria may inhibit or promote wound healing depending upon the mediators they provoke. Host-bacteria interaction influences how bacteria affect wound healing with the host response to the bacterium being the most important determinant towards wound healing. The presence of necrotic tissue in the wound bed, eschar, debris, fibrinous slough, bacterial toxins, as well as, proteins secreted from bacterium or displayed upon the surface of organisms collectively is referred to as the wound bioburden. Foreign bodies such as suture material, dirt or grass, splinters, or insect parts are also commonly associated with the development of an inflammatory reaction. The bioburden promotes the release of inflammatory mediators. Constant bombardment with a variety of immune factors may down regulate some cells at the margin of the wound into a dormant phenotype (senescent cell). Contamination occurs when non-replicating organisms are present on the wound. All chronic wounds are contaminated with indigenous microflora or environmental related microflora. Host immune response is not engaged with contamination. Colonization occurs when replicating microorganisms adhere to the wound but do not injure the host. Colonization usually involves normal skin flora. Although the host immune system becomes engaged and surveillance is initiated no invasion of the organisms occurs. *Staphylococcus epidermidis, Corynebacterium, Brevibacterium, Proprionibacterium,* and *Pityrosporum* are frequently seen as colonizing organisms. Replicating invasive microorganisms that injure the host is the hallmark of infection. *Staphylococcus aureus, Beta hemolytic Streptococcus (S. pyogenes, S. agalactiae), E. coli, Proteus, Klebsiella, anaerobes, Pseudomonas, Acinetobacter,*

TABLE 11. COMMON VIRULENCE FACTORS

- Endotoxins: gram negatives
- Toxins: *Streptococcus pyogenes, Staphylococcus aureus*
- Proteases: *Staphylococcus aureus, Pseudomonas aeruginosa*
- Hyaluronidase: *Streptococcus pyogenes*
- Synergy
- Biofilm

and *Stenotrophomonas (Xanthomonas)* are frequently isolated from infected wounds. Infection is measured at 1.0 x 10^5 - 10^6 CFU organisms on biopsy, although injection with virulent organisms or compromised hosts may render tissue invasion at a fewer number of organisms. The organisms have the ability to work together to create an advantage over the host (synergism), or in the development of a biofilm through factors such as high virulence (invasiveness) or secreted toxins. Common Virulence Factors are listed at Table 11.

Wound Bioburden

The bioburden is the combination of organic and inorganic materials in the wound bed that stimulate an inflammatory response. Necrotic tissue, debris, slough, senescent cells, proteinacious secretions, eschar, and foreign bodies will activate a host immune response. The bioburden usually adds to the physical barrier in the wound base. In addition to promoting the presence of senescent cells (fibroblast and keratinocytes) the bioburden creates a metabolic stress load. Copious amounts of proteinacious drainage can rob an individual of vital nutrient stores. These factors collectively lead to a delay in wound healing.

Synergy

Synergy occurs when microorganisms work together to create an advantage over the host organism. The process may be initiated when one organism influences the host organism to alter the target tissue's cellular or immune response such that the second organism may exert or invade the tissue at lower numbers as occurs with HIV and cryptococcal infections. Alternatively the first organism may upgrade or down grade various receptors, or promote membrane structural changes such that the second organism may gain access to a cell such as occurs with adenoviral throat infections and bacterial suprainfections.

Biofilms

Biofilms exist on wounds with similar characteristics to those found in other fluid-organic medium interfaces. A biofilm is a community of organisms located in a slime matrix at a fluid surface interface that work together to support survival of the community. Examples of important "organic surfaces" that harbor biofilms are wound beds, implants and prostheses, the bronchial-alveolar tubes, structures within the oral cavity and bones. Disease processes such as non-healing wounds, infected implants, cystic fibrosis, dental plaque, and osteomyelitis represent biologic biofilms. Organisms secrete the polysaccharide coat that encases the organisms and protects them from host defenses. Biofilms therefore are a mixture of glycosaminoglycans, proteins, and fibrinous debris. The bacterium, yeast, fungus and viruses that are encased in the biofilm secrete toxins into the wound bed. These toxins promote a prolonged proinflammatory state, supporting tissue destruction and may create chronic non-healing wounds. Incorporation of the organisms within the biofilm protects them from concentrations of biocides that would otherwise kill or inhibit those organisms. Some antibiotics may require a 1000–5000 fold increased concentration to eradicate a biofilm. Factors that contribute to biofilm resistance include: poor gel penetration, nutrient-limited physiology, antimicrobial neutralization, adaptation, and cells that survive a stressor. Antibiotic effectiveness is increased in the presence of even a weak, intermittent electrical field. The combination of electricity plus antibiotic is more effective against biofilm cells than either is alone. Using mechanical, sharp, chemical, or biological debridement may be helpful in disrupting the biofilm, thereby decreasing its effectiveness in impeding wound healing. For more information on biofilms see Wolcott's chapter "Bio-film Based Wound Care," and for infection control, see "Skin Structure and Muscle Infections" and "Post-Operational Surgical Site Infections (SSIs) and Non-Necrotizing Skin and Soft Tissue Infections" by LeFrock.

TRAUMA (REPETITIVE)

Repetitive trauma, in the form of intermittent pressures and continuous pressure has been associated with the development of diabetic foot ulcers (neuropathic and neuroischemic), arterial insufficiency ulcers, decubitus ulcers, and venous ulcers. Pressure related injury develops with three types of force: direct pressure, shear, and friction. Direct pressure insult occurs when tissue is compressed between a bony prominence and an immobile surface such as occurs with lying directly on the trochanteric prominence. Unrelieved pressure for more than two hours can cause pressure ulcers in sites with poor mobility. Diabetic foot ulcers develop from predisposing peripheral neuropathy associated with continuous pressure inside a tight shoe or under a prominent metatarsal head that bears the majority of the body weight with each step. Therefore, ulceration from direct pressure may occur with continuous or intermittent forces.

Direct pressures of 65 n/m^2 or greater are considered sufficient to generate ulcerations in the diabetic foot. The higher weight (force) placed upon the tissue will shorten the time for the tissue to become exposed. Patients sitting upright in a chair should be shifted every 15 minutes to relieve pressure upon the buttocks and presacral regions. Moisture from sweat or incontinence, malnutrition, and reduced subcutaneous tissue diminish the

TABLE 12. MANAGING TISSUE LOAD

Proper Steps to Take
• Keep head of bed at or below 30 degrees
• Reposition patients (2h bed, 15 min chair)
• Rotate patient onto buttock at 15 degrees off trochanter
• Use lift devices to assist with patient movement
• Use pressure reducing surfaces
• Site specific support surfaces on extremities
• Keep skin dry and well lubricated
• Increase mobility and activity (if possible)

Problems to Avoid
• Do Not use "donut" type devices
• Do Not rub bony prominences
• Do Not drag patient skin across linens
• Do Not position patients on greater trochanter
• Do Not reapply pressure until completely healed

level of tolerance to pressure loads. Skin that has thinned because of steroids or age, likewise, is at risk to breakdown with minimal pressure exposure. Shear pressure occurs when the skin is adherent to a surface and the underlying supportive vascular structures are pulled or molded to limit adequate local blood supply. An example of this type of injury is the decubitus ulcer that occurs on the back of an individual with the head of the bed elevated more than 30 degrees. The skin sticks to moist sheets while the weight of the body distorts the underlying tissue in a downward motion. Friction can cause blisters, skin tears, and erosion when the skin is drawn across a surface which occurs when a patient is repositioned without lifting.

Offloading Pressure

Pressure ulcers generally will not heal until adequate offloading has been achieved. Appropriate management to tissue loads is associated with some recommended dos and don'ts as shown at Table 12.

Neuropathy and Loss of Protective Sensation (LOPS)

Loss of protective sensation secondary to neuropathy predisposes diabetic patients to developing diabetic foot ulcerations. Patients with recurrent foot ulcerations tend to have higher vibration perception threshold values as compared to patients without recurrent ulcers. High vibration perception threshold (> 50 mV) is the only risk factor correlating independently with ulcer development, irrespective of age, sex, hemoglobin Alc, presence of retinopathy and nephropathy, plasma creatinine, and total nitric oxide vascular content. Loss of protective sensation allows patients to load their feet with high plantar pressures. Diabetic neuropathic ulcers occur on the plantar surface and diabetic neuroischemic ulcers more often occur on foot margins.

Multiple devices are available to aid with reducing pressure. These devices may focus on reducing the pressure of a surface (i.e., bed inlays, mattresses, seat cushions). Other devices are used as adjunctive with appliances (i.e., insoles, prosthesis linings). Other devices replace clothing articles to alter the distribution of forces when the patient is in motion (i.e., total contact casts, CAM walkers, Darco® shoes). For more information on pressure relief devices, see chapter entitled "Orthotics and Prosthetics in Wound Care" by Bosker and La Fontaine

CHRONICITY

The term "wound chronicity" implies that the wound failed to proceed through a normal healing sequence in a timely fashion. Alternatively, the term is used to implicate the underlying medical, biological, or biochemical factors that functionally delayed wound progression. Protease imbalance, bacterial burden, insufficient angiogenesis, and cellular aging have been listed as causes for the development of a chronic state. Still others use the term to indicate a permanent or irreversible process that has impaired health, mental capacity or physical capabilities. This predisposes the patient to non-healing such as a spinal cord injury patients at risk for decubitus ulcers or diabetic patients with limited range of ankle motion and anteriorly displaced plantar fat pads at risk for neuropathic plantar ulcers.

The onset of chronicity is difficult to diagnose. Projected healing rates differ depending upon type of original insult and associated co-morbidities. Wounds in diabetic patients heal more slowly than non-diabetic patients. Patients with systemic lupus erythematosus (SLE) do not heal as quickly as patients who do not have a rheumatoid condition. Likewise, patients with sickle cell anemia leg ulcers heal slowly but at rates that may differ from those with patients with SLE or diabetes. Reliable estimates of healing times are not readily available but wound healing trajectories for the major wound types have been proposed from several centers. Trajectories are created by pooling data from several wound healing studies of a given wound type. Evaluating those patients that healed separately from those that did not heal allows researchers to develop a healing and a nonhealing time line or trajectory. Without a comparable healing trajectory, providers who anticipate a slower healing rate in certain subpopulations of wounds may lull a provider into overlooking the chronicity of the wound.

Medical providers who practice in wound healing must be careful to closely trend progression. Several groups are working on mathematical modeling in order to provide a better way to detect the onset of delayed healing so that alternative interventions may be attempted sooner. Information in the neuropathic diabetic foot model suggests that the size, duration, and grade can be used to aid in the prediction of likelihood to heal in 20 weeks.

Protease Imbalance

A group of serine, neutral endopeptidases called matrix metalloproteinases (MMPs) modify the extracellular matrix and modulate the chemical messages important in cell-to-cell communication. The MMP gene family contains a zinc2+ binding domain in their active sites and calcium ions to interconnect folds and maintain structure. Enzymes are divided into subfamilies of secretory enzymes (collagenases, gelatinases, stromelysins, unclassified) and membrane-bound type enzymes (MT-MMPs) based upon structural characteristics and the substrates they preferentially bind.

During normal skin repair, keratinocytes, fibroblasts, macrophages and endothelial cells secrete MMPs and express MT-MMPs on their surfaces. In chronic wounds, excessive protease activity from elevated levels of collagenase and gelatinase interfere with proper granulation tissue formation. MMPs support wound healing, morphogenesis, tissue resorption and remodeling, nerve growth and hair follicle development.

MMPs direct wound healing processes by controlling platelet aggregation, macrophage and neutrophil function, cell migration and proliferation, angiogenesis and collagen secretion. MMPs exert their effect by modulating enzyme cascades and by either activating or inactivating matrix proteins, cytokines, growth factors and adhesion molecules. MMPs change cell adherence to gel, which influences cell migration. MMPs promote cellular proliferation apoptosis or morphogenesis and can dictate the number and type of cellular concentration in tissue. MMPs modulate biological active molecules, such as growth factors (GF) and growth factor receptors (GFR).

Pathologic MMP expression has been implicated in a variety of disease processes such as chronic wound ulceration, rheumatoid arthritis, osteoarthritis, cancer invasion, cancer metastasis, periodontal diseases, fibrotic diseases, atherosclerosis, epidermolysis bullosa and aortic aneurysm. Multiple factors dictate the type and amount of MMP expression. These factors include available cytokines, growth factors, hormones, oncogenes, and changes in cell-cell interactions, cell-matrix interactions as well as feedback from inflammatory mediators. Tumor necrosis factor (TNF), interleukin-2, (IL-2) interleukin-6 (IL-6) and interleukin-8 (IL-8) have been shown to have specific MMP links.

MMP proteolytic activity is controlled by three mechanisms: 1) regulation of the transcription process, 2) enzymes are transcribed as zymogens, and 3) interaction with specific tissue inhibitory matrix proteins (TIMPs). MMPs are synthesized as preproenzymes and subsequently bind to the cell surface or secreted into the extracellular space. Interaction of a cysteine amino acid residue with the zinc2+ moiety at the catalytic site maintains the enzyme in a latent state. Zinc2+ has four binding sites and the cysteine-zinc bond produces a fold that conceals the catalytic site. Disruption of the bond exposes the catalytic site and expresses the "active" state. This process is called the "Cysteine Switch." TIMP -1, -2, -3, and -4 inhibit MMP activity by inserting their terminal amino acid residue into the fourth zinc2+ site.

Additionally, some macrolide antibiotics (erythromycin, azithromycin, tetracycline) and non-steroidal anti-inflammatory drugs (NSAID) inhibit MMPs. Macrolide antibiotics retard tissue breakdown independent of their antibiotic effect. More than thirteen new macrolide-based MMP inhibitors are under investigation. Moreover, some non-steroidal anti-inflammatory drugs (NSAIDs) inhibit MMP activity with transcription repression as the proposed mechanism.

Bacterial Balance

The bacterial burden in the wound refers to the biofilm, planktonic organisms and toxins in the wound. Growth factors are degraded in the presence of significant quantities of bacterium in the wound. Protease activity arising from bacterial proteases and matrix metalloproteinases secreted in response to bacterial antigen or toxins inactivate local growth factors.

The presence of fibroblasts enhances the degradation suggesting they may be the source of the MMP production. All chronic wounds have a bacterial load, usually consisting of normal flora, Although not an invasive infection, colonization may impede wound healing by creating a proinflammatory environment with secreted proteases decreasing available growth factor effect.

Bacterial virulence, pathogenicity, bacterial load, and toxins in association with host defense determine the extent of inhibition created by colonizing organisms. The term, critical colonization, describes the situation where there are no systemic signs of colonization but wound healing fails to progress along the anticipated trajectory. In the presence of replicating organisms, the wound may exhibit excessive drainage, pain, odor, bright red fleshy friable granulation tissue, epithelial islands or epithelial bridging. For adequate wound healing to progress, bacterial balance must be established by decreasing organisms to a level easily managed by host defenses.

Insufficient Angiogenesis

New blood vessel growth is a vital factor in the development of healthy granulation tissue. At least 20 angiogenic factors have been identified. Some promote blood vessel growth as their primary function, such as VEGF; while others, appear to promote neovascularization as an additional process, such as follistatin. In addition to VEGF, angiogenic factors commonly encountered in the healing wound include-fibroblastic growth factor acidic and basic (FGF-a, FGF-b), interleukin-8 (IL-8), platelet-derived growth factor beta/beta (PDGF-ßß), transforming growth factor-alpha (TGF-α), transforming growth factor-beta (TGF-ß), and tumor necrosis factor-alpha (TNF-α). When angiogenic factors are produced in excess of inhibitors wound healing occurs. In proinflammatory states some angiogenic factors are produced in excess, which might account for the production of granulomatous tissue in infected wounds. However, when angiogenic factor production decreases in response to decreased production or inhibition, granulation tissue does not develop.

There are at least 30 angiogenic inhibitors. Angiogenic inhibitor-interferon (IF-α, ß, and γ), fibronectin fragment, matrix metalloproteinase inhibitors (TIMPs), plasminogen activator inhibitor, retinoids, and thrombospondin-1 (TSN-1) balance wound angiogenesis. Interestingly, TGF-ß exerts opposing effects both as an angiogenic stimulator and as an angiogenic inhibitor.

Cellular Aging

Cellular aging is a term used to describe the phenotypical changes that occur in cells that are slow to function and secondary to oxidation of cellular components. Typically, these changes are seen in older cells that have encountered oxidative stress over time. The term has also been used to refer to cells that are obtained from older individuals. These cells now function less aggressively because of the genetic changes that occur in older individuals which is secondary to lifetime exposures to reactive oxygen species. More recently the term has been used to refer to senescent cells that function as though they were older cells or were obtained from an older individual. These macrophages, fibroblasts, and keratinocytes found at the margin of wound beds respond sluggishly to stimulation with appropriate chemotatic agents or growth factors.

Investigators are researching this senescent response or cellular aging response to determine how it effects wound healing outcomes. Whether the oxidative stress occurs cumulative over decades as in elderly patients or gradually over weeks as with a chronic wound, cellular oxidation confers changes that preclude RNA and protein synthesis. The inability to aggressively respond to stressors with appropriately synthesized protein (enzymes) confers the phenotype of a non-functional or poorly functioning cell.

Characteristically, elderly skin becomes thin, wrinkles, develops increased fragility and becomes more susceptible to ulceration. Decreased dermal turnover, slowed toxin clearance, and inadequate skin immune dysfunction are also noted. Inflammatory cells migrate more slowly into wound beds and a generalized decline in cellular function is observed in aged skin of the elderly. On the other hand, cells residing in the base and margin of wound beds fail to properly migrate, secrete, and divide when given the usual level and type of stimuli. It is unclear if the failure is related to an inability to acquire the message at the level of the cell receptor, a malfunction in the transmission of the information within the cell, or a direct blockage at the level of RNA and protein synthesis. Alternatively, the abnormality may arise from chemical inhibitors present at the receptors or within the cell.

Reversing the phenotypical changes of cellular aging in the wound base may be difficult until a better understanding of the inciting problem has been fully elucidated. Current recommendations include removing the cells through a debridement process, adding local antioxidants to convert any reversible component of the oxidant stress, inhibiting MMPs that may be the source of chemical impedance to wound healing, over-flooding the receptors with exogenous growth/chemotatic factors to override an inhibitory blockade. Additional recommendations include performing gene therapy by infecting senescent cells with viron coupled DNA or RNA, or by introducing phenotypically healthy, "young-profile" cells into the wound.

Phenotypically young cell profiles are found in exogenous grafts (Apligraf® and Stem cell therapy). Omnipotent stem cells develop into whole organisms, whereas, pluripotent cells develop into specialized tissue. Both types of stem cells are being studied as potential adjunctive agents to wound healing. For more information on the effects of aging, see "Wound Healing in the Geriatric Patient" by Mouton, et al. For more information about biochemical differences in healing and chronic wounds, see "Biochemistry of Wound Healing in Wound Care Practice" by Chin, et al.

HEMATOLOGICAL ABNORMALITIES

The two hematological abnormalities most commonly associated with poor wound healing are anemia and hypercoagulability.

Anemia

Anemia is frequently associated with diabetic patients. It is more prevalent and develops early in the course of chronic renal insufficiency associated with diabetic nephropathy. Use of erythropoietin is helpful in effecting a better outcome in diabetic complications. Fatouros (68) performed studies in rats with colonic surgery and demonstrated faster anastomotic healing with enhancement of the fibroblast and a faster rate of maturation.

Hypercoagulability

The ability of the blood to clot, or coagulate depends upon the presence of a favorable prothrombotic state derived from any combination of Virchow's triad: 1) blood vessel wall abnormalities, 2) abnormalities within the circulating blood, or 3) stasis of blood flow. Various medical conditions increase the likelihood of a prothrombotic state with resultant myocardial infarction, stroke, pulmonary embolism, deep venous thrombosis (DVT), and peripheral arterial obstructive disease (PAOD). Aging is associated with increased thromboembolic events, particularly after the age of 55 years. Women have a lower rate than do men but their advantage dissipates as their age approaches 60 years to approximate the male rate.

Trauma, atherosclerosis and vasculitis create focal abnormalities within the blood vessel wall to promote platelet adherence, aggregation,

TABLE 13. DEFICIENT FACTORS ASSOCIATED WITH HYPERCOAGULABLE STATES

Antithrombin III Deficiency	binds and inhibits thrombin; accelerated effectiveness with exogenous heparin and endogenous heparin sulfate
Protein C Deficiency	binds and inhibits activated clotting factors Va and VIIIa; type I—low amount; type II—poor quality/function
Protein S Deficiency	combines with Protein C to inhibit Va and VIIIa

TABLE 14. ANTIBODIES ASSOCIATED WITH HYPERCOAGULABLE STATES

Antiphospholipid Antibody Syndrome (Hughes Syndrome)	associated with arterial and venous clots; multiple types of antibodies; primary (idiopathic) and secondary (i.e., SLE)
Lupus Anticoagulant Antibodies **Anticardiolipin Antibodies** **Other Specific Molecule Antibodies**	

activation, and fibrin deposition with promulgation of a clot. Prothrombotic abnormalities within the circulating blood relates to excessive clotting factor activation or defective factor deactivation once the processes has begun. Fibrinogen levels increase with age, pregnancy and with some disease states like diabetes. Interestingly, Acang's (67) investigation into the hypercoagulable state in diabetic patients showed a relationship between the higher levels of fibrinogen when compared to normal persons, associated with shorter PT and APTT. The fibrinogen appears to be more aggressively deposited with a lower rate of fibrinolytic activity. The hypercoagulable state of diabetes may correlate with the poor wound healing seen in diabetes (see Tables 13 and 14). Antibodies may stimulate factors that activate or deactivate clotting sequences. Rheumatologic diseases, with associated vasculitis and antibodies that activate clotting factors, provide them with a focus on the blood vessel wall for deposit. Abnormalities in clotting factor V (factor V Leiden) may render it resistant to activated protein C neutralization.

Hyperhomocysteinemia increases the atherogenic properties of LDL and stimulates smooth muscle proliferation while also accelerating blood coagulation. Increased homocysteine levels are found in advanced age, heavy smoking, renal insufficiency, psoriasis, acute lymphoblastic leukemia, breast cancer, and deficiency of B vitamins, B6, B12, and folic acid. Drugs that interact with vitamin B6, vitamin B12, and folic acid (i.e., methotrexate, carbamazepine, phenytoin) or that interfere with the absorption of homocysteine (i.e., colestipol, niacin) or with its metabolism (i.e., isoniazid) may lead to elevated homocysteine levels. Stasis of blood flow may occur in either the arterial or venous system. Both types of stasis are related to poor wound healing.

SOCIOECONOMIC ISSUES

Social and economical circumstances exert a significant influence upon the overall health of an individual. Lower socioeconomic status is associated with limited financial resources for securing proper food, shelter, clothing, medications, medical supplies, transportation to medical visits and medical insurance. The number of uninsured and underinsured individuals in the United States during 2001–2002 peaked at 75 million individuals, over one fourth of the nation.

Uninsured individuals are less likely to have a regular source of care outside the emergency room, often go without screenings and preventive care, and often delay or forego needed medical care. They often are subject to avoidable hospital stays, frequently present for care when they are sicker, and die earlier than those who have insurance. Social behaviors such as smoking, drinking alcohol and using illegal drugs negatively impact wound healing. The risk for developing pressure ulcerations is positively correlated with unemployment, low level of education, drug or alcohol abuse, and poverty. Delays in wound healing may arise when an individual's work capacity is taken into consideration. At either end of the extreme, some patients will return to work too soon while others will use their medical condition for "secondary gain" as a means to avoid work.

Alcohol

Alcoholism delays wound healing and increases the risk of opportunistic infections. Heavy alcohol consumption functionally alters all three types of blood cells: erythrocytes, leukocytes, and platelets. It interferes with folate storage and release from liver cells, which leads to impaired red blood cell development. In addition, megablastic hypochromic anemia may ensue. Alcohol consumption alters cytokine release and predisposes the individual to infection by negatively influencing leukocyte migration, aggregation and adherence. Acute ethanol ingestion decreases mesenteric lymph node immunoglobulin M (IgM) synthesis in response to trauma. IgM confers immune protection through resistance to bacterial infection. Consistent suppression of IgM synthesis as seen in chronic alcoholism may contribute to the increased incidence and severity of acute infection seen in chronic alcoholism. Thrombocytopenia is a commonly associated hematologic finding which does not allow the remaining platelets to aggregate normally. Coupled with deficiencies in clotting factors and fibrinogen, the bleeding risk is greatly accentuated in heavy drinkers, especially those with ascites. Thus, alcohol interferes with both the cellular and humoral protective components of host defense.

Delays in wound healing develop as a consequence of this breakdown in cellular and humoral protective response. Acute ethanol ingestion inhibits the cytokine function responsible for the proliferation of fibroblast cells that are a source of collagen in a healing wound. Although basal collagen secretion is not affected, TGF-β induced bursts of collagen secretion are also suppressed. Ethanol inhibits osteoblast function and supports systemic bone loss thereby increasing the risk of fracture. The etiology of alcohol-associated bone disease is multifactorial. Nutritional deficiencies, liver damage, hypogonadism, and transitory hypoparathyroidism with resultant hypocalcemia and hypercalciuria have been implicated. Recidivism rates for diabetic foot ulcerations are higher in patients who have poor glycemic control, more neuropathy and increased alcohol intake. Smoking and alcohol abuse are known predictive factors for anastomotic leakage after colonic and rectal resection.

Alcohol intervention often is not possible in the office setting on the first visit. However, the amount and type of alcohol ingestion should be documented with a discussion of alcohol cessation at the time of the first visit. Additional intervention should follow. Liver disease associated with acute ingestion interferes with proper drugs and nutrient metabolism. The metabolism of drugs normally occupying the microsomal system (P450), such as phenytoin, barbiturates and anticoagulants will be impaired during alcohol intoxication, and their dosage will require modification accordingly. Caution must be taken in prescribing new medications for pain, as some medications such as a non-steroidal anti-inflammatory agent may increase the risk of gastrointestinal bleeding. Alcohol ingestion may also increase the inebriation that occurs with narcotics. Dehydration should be treated with oral or intravenous replacement as dictated by the patient's condition. B-vitamin replacement with folic acid (1 mg per day) and thiamine (100 mg per day x 3 days) may be considered. Thiamine replacement should also be given when glucose replacement is required.

Alcohol withdrawal syndrome occurs in 40% of patients who significantly alter or stop consuming alcohol. Symptoms typically include any combination of generalized hyperactivity, anxiety, tremor, sweating, nausea, retching, tachycardia, hypertension and mild pyrexia- peaking between 10–30 hours and subsiding by the end of the second day. Mental status changes with confusion occurring in the first 12–48 hours. Auditory and visual hallucinations, which are much less common, typically last for 5–6 days. Delirium tremens (DTs), seen in less than 5% of individuals withdrawing from alcohol, usually begins within 48–72 hours after the alcohol consumption change and are characterized by coarse tremor, agitation, fever, tachycardia, profound confusion, delusions and hallucinations. Convulsions do not typically accompany this condition except at the onset. Hyperpyrexia, ketoacidosis and profound circulatory collapse may develop if alcohol withdrawal is not recognized and appropriately addressed.

Tobacco

Smoking is most prevalent in the young (age 18–24 years) men, minorities, and persons of low educational background and socioeconomic status. Tobacco usage correlates with an increased infection risk in general and orthopedic surgical cases and increased amount of postoperative wound rupture when compared with never-smokers. Cigarette smoking-dependent poor wound healing is popularly attributed to the vasoconstrictive effects of nicotine on the vascular endothelium with resultant transient local poor oxygenation. A clearer understanding of smoking related impediment to wound healing emerges as our understanding of pro-oxidant stressors develops. In addition to local hypoxia there appears to be a correlation with more long-term endothelial vasomotor alterations, endothelial dysfunction, accelerated atherosclerosis effects, platelet activation, and inhibition of collagen synthesis with alterations of the cytokine and matrix metalloproteinase levels. Tobacco smoke and aqueous extracts from tobacco have been demonstrated to contain reactive species that generate glycation products that rapidly react with proteins to form advanced glycation end-products (AGEs), Glycation products whether from cigarettes, diabetes, or dietary sources are called "glycotoxins." Smoking tobacco-derived glycotoxins are mutagenic and have been associated with elevated levels of blood AGE apolipoprotein-B and serum AGE levels in smokers. As such, these glycotoxins accelerate the rate of atherosclerotic deposition. Microcirculation vasoconstriction occurs within 5–20 minutes of smoking a single cigarette with approximately a 30–38% reduction in microvascular flow after smoking two cigarettes, as measured through laser Doppler flow of reimplanted digits. The effects were more pronounced with shorter durations from time of surgery in prior smokers as opposed to non-smokers. The delay in recovery from smoking related vasoconstriction likewise is more pronounced in older smokers. Additionally, the vasodilatory response of forearm skin microvasculature showed impairment in the older but not the younger subjects who had smoked cigarettes for many years. The blunted vasodilatory response was noted in both endothelium-dependent and endothelium-independent responses when laser Doppler flow was measured in response to iontophoretically applied acetylcholine (endothelium-dependent vasodilator), sodium nitroprusside, and post-occlusive forearm reactive hyperemia (endothelium-independent vasodilation). Platelet-derived nitric oxide (NO) release is significantly impaired in long-term smokers, resulting in the augmentation of platelet aggregability.

Cigarette smoking predisposes to wound development, delayed wound closure, increased wound dehiscence, and wound infections. Subcutaneous collagen synthesis is impeded in smokers indicating an impaired wound healing process. No difference in wound rupture between continuous and abstinent smokers suggests that tissue hypoxia induced by smoking is not necessarily the only cause for reduced collagen production and wound dehiscence in smokers. Guerrero-Romero (76) showed a strong correlation between microalbuminuria, diabetes duration, cigarette smoking, and aging with the development of diabetic foot ulcers. Sorenson (93, 94, 95) found that both light and heavy cigarette smoking predicted post-mastectomy wound infection, skin flap necrosis, and epidermolysis as an independent risk factor when adjustments were made for confounding factors such as diabetes, obesity, alcohol, NSAIDs, duration of surgery, and surgical experience.

Many patients are placed on a protocol to stop smoking for some variable number of pre-operative and post-operative days. These durations typically range between six to 28 days total depending upon the type and extent of surgery being performed. Patient compliance with a perioperative smoking cessation request is also variable depending upon the age, sex, matrimonial status, number of medical conditions, presence of social support systems, and long-term smoking history. Improved post-operative complications in 120 patients who underwent either hip or knee arthroplasty showed a positive correlation with a cessation in smoking, an established exercise program exceeding four hours per week, and having a higher education level. A four-week pre-operative abstinence from smoking reduced post-operative infection risk to that of never-smokers; however, abstinence did not affect the incidence of wound rupture. Patients report a desire to stop smoking in 70% of cases, one-third attempt to stop, but only 5% are successful (cold turkey) without medical intervention. Sorensen completed a study at the University of Copenhagen that demonstrated that male patients and patients with good social network were more likely to successfully stop smoking. Physician advice, given repetitively and clearly, was a major factor in successful outcome. Patient factors such as high personal motivation, confidence, and lower levels of nicotine addiction also improve the likelihood of smoking cessation. Smoking cessation recommendations should include: 1) written materials with a strong "pro-health" message directed specifically at the concerns of the individual being treated, 2) direct advice to quit with a planned date, 3) smoking cessation programs, 4) nicotine replacement therapy, and 5) follow up and follow through by the physician.

Intervention with an antidepressant of the aminoketone class, Welbutrin SR® (buproprion HC1 100 mg/150 mg qd or bid) has been shown to have a higher likelihood of success. Vitamin C, ascorbic acid, the main water-soluble antioxidant in human plasma, protects against lipid peroxidative damage by scavenging superoxide and other reactive oxygen species. Smoking decreases both plasma and tissue vitamin C levels. Vitamin C improves endothelium-dependent vasodilation in the forearm skin and coronary arteries of smokers.

Illicit Drug Abuse

The effect of illicit drug abuse and addiction on wound healing has not been widely studied. It presents an arduous task due to the vast number of agents abused, increasing numbers of new "designer" drugs becoming available, the multiple means of intake, the predilection for drug abusers to use emergency services to access medical care and the poor follow-up. The initial wounding pattern, co-morbidities, amount of active metabolites and their effect upon the immune system all influence wound healing differently. Vascular perfusion complications related to drug abuse may affect venous, arterial and lymphatic districts.

Following intra-arterial injections, arterial and venous pseudo-aneurysm, vasculitis, aneurysms, aortic dissections, abscesses complicated by erosions of vessels, arteriovenous fistulas, compartment syndrome, superficial and deep venous thrombosis, septic thrombophlebitis, and puffy hand syndrome have all been described. The prevalence of soft tissue infections (abscesses, cellulitis, and infected ulcers) among injection drug users ranges between 21% and 32%. In a retrospective review of soft tissue infections among intravenous drug abusers collected in a Seattle, Washington emergency department over a three-month period from November 1999 through April 2000, Takahashi (98) found 242 patients who were predominantly male (63.6%), Caucasian (69.4%), without health insurance (52.0%), and most had abscesses (72.3%). Patients with only cellulitis were more likely to be hospitalized compared to those with abscesses who underwent emergency department incision and drainage prior to discharge. Forty percent of the patients were hospitalized with deltoid abscesses due to the likeliness of receiving an operative procedure. Follow-up to closure was not reported.

Individuals that use intravenous heroin and/or cocaine are more susceptible to human immunodeficiency acquisition than non-intravenous users. The susceptibility rates correlate with higher levels than those predicted by intravenous exposure alone. The immunodeficiency associated with this behavior is thought to confer the defect in host defense.

In reviewing the effect of addiction on wound healing, major themes that emerge include malnutrition, higher risk of infection, higher number of drug induced medical co-morbidities, higher number of associated mental co-morbidities, lower economical status, and lack of medical insurance and social support. In illicit drug addiction calorie and protein malnutrition are common with a higher correlation with the female sex, intensity of drug addiction, anorexia and poor food and drink consumption, and disturbance of the social and familial links. In cases where drug usage persists it becomes important to note that acute organic pathology leads to a significant worsening of the nutritional status of drug addicts. Heroin and non-heroin addiction appear to have similar impact on social and nutritional status, but heroin addicts are seven times more likely to develop hepatitis B or C infection; whereas, non-heroin addicts were more prone to develop depressed cellular immunity. Intravenous cocaine inhibits neutrophil phagocytosis and phagolysosomal acidification in vitro. Cocaine acts directly on lymphoid cells and indirectly modulates the immune response by affecting the level of neuroendocrine hormones. However, published in vivo studies reviewing the different means of intake and formulation report contradictory results, showing stimulatory, suppressive or no effect. Among adults in year 2001, mental health co-morbidity with substance abuse to include alcohol and illicit drugs was 20.3% whereas substance abuse in patients without serious mental health issues was only 6.3%. These conditions of medical and mental health co-morbidities, immune deficiencies, malnutrition, poor social support systems, and lack of financial means combine to impede the ability to optimize outcome in the wound care center. For more information about wound prevention, see Wolf's chapter, "Prevention: The Sixth Phase of Wound Healing."

AUTOIMMUNE DISORDER

Autoimmune diseases develop when the protective component of the immune system mounts an attack upon normal structures. Women (75%), predominantly of childbearing ages, are most frequently affected with a predilection for certain diseases to occur more commonly in certain minority populations. More than 80 autoimmune disorders have been described. Some common autoimmune disorders that have been associated with poor wound healing include: rheumatoid arthritis, autoimmune hemolytic anemia, pernicious anemia, Crohn's disease, autoimmune thrombocytopenia, ulcerative colitis, type I or immune mediated diabetes mellitus, autoimmune hepatitis, anti-phospholipid syndrome, Grave's disease, Behcet's disease, Wegener's granulomatosis, Reiter's disease, psoriasis, autoimmune diseases of the adrenal gland, Hashimoto's thyroiditis, rheumatoid arthritis (RA), systemic lupus erythematosus (SLE), scleroderma, polymyositis, dermatomyositis, Sjogren's syndrome, and ankylosing spondylitis. Because of the presence of poorly healing wounds in association with these syndromes, patients with the more common disorders, such as diabetes, rheumatoid arthritis, SLE, and scleroderma, tend to be referred to the wound center. The more rare conditions such as Wegener's granulomatosis may be referred from specialists in dermatology and rheumatology for assistance with local wound care.

Antibodies are generated against normal body structures or abnormal materials secreted or deposited upon normal structures. The antibodies may mark cells, tissues, or organs for destruction by neutrophil and macrophages. Autoimmune disorders, such as rheumatoid arthritis (RA) cartilaginous tissue of the joints are frequently affected while the pancreas may be targeted as in Latent Autoimmune Diabetes in Adults (LADA). Neutrophil and macrophages may be hypersecretory, releasing cytotoxic chemicals or compounds that destroy the tissue. Alternatively, humoral components released from host T-cell or B-cell lymphocytes may be the source of the "self destruction." Depending upon the disease process, the autoantibodies may be continuously, intermediately, or transiently produced to create the damage. In syndromes with waxing and waning symptomatology the antibodies may be intermittently produced giving periods of exacerbation as occurs with rheumatoid arthritis. Also they may be produced at the initiation of the insult and resolve after permanent damage has occurred as with type I diabetes.

Aging, chronic stress, hormones, and pregnancy can exacerbate an autoimmune condition. Although RA seems to improve with pregnancy, SLE tends to worsen, and both flare-up in the postpartum period. Sunlight has been found to exacerbate SLE. Treatment of the underlying disease process usually helps in wound resolution. Steroids commonly are employed during flare-ups.

MEDICATIONS

Many medication used to treat patients may produce secondary undesirable side effects such as vasoconstriction, hypoperfusion, inhibition of white blood cell function, poor collagen production or deposit, or depletion of vital nutrients that may ultimately cause delays in wound healing rates (Table 15). Glucocorticosteroids, antineoplastic agents, chemotherapeutic agents used to prevent transplant rejection, and anti-coagulants are the most common agents encountered in most wound care centers. For more information about pain management, see Well's chapter entitled "Acute and Chronic Pain Management."

Glucocorticoids

Glucocorticoids (corticosteroids) cause a delay in wound healing by altering the metabolism of L-arginine, a semi-essential amino acid that plays a vital role in developing an inflammatory response and in collagen synthesis and deposition. Glucocorticoids have been linked to dehiscence of surgical incisions, increased risk of wound infection, and delayed healing of open wounds. Proposed mechanisms for these effects include interference with inflammation, fibroblast proliferation, collagen synthesis and degradation, deposition of connective tissue ground substances, angiogenesis, wound contraction, and re-epithelialization. L-arginine is the only substrate for nitric oxide synthesis and when metabolized through the urea cycle it produces ornithine, the precursor to polyamine and proline.

Nitric oxide synthetase (iNOS) regulates collagen formation, cell proliferation and wound contraction.

Treatment with a common glucocorticoid, methylprednisolone, significantly decreases TGF-ß and IGF-I levels in the wound fluid and hydroxyproline content in the tissue. In an animal model, retinoic acid partially reversed the reduction in TGF-beta and IGF-I and significantly increased hydroxyproline content toward normal levels with enhanced collagen deposition. Vitamin A treatment restores the inflammatory response in patients and promotes epithelialization and the synthesis of collagen and ground substances; however, vitamin A does not reverse the detrimental effects of glucocorticoids on wound contraction and infection. In clinical practice, vitamin A is dosed in 20,000 IU per day given as an oral, topical, or periwound injection. Although generally accepted in clinical practice some controversy still exists. vitamin A given in large doses to patients who continue to smoke has been associated with higher risk of heart disease and arteriosclerosis (results from the Beta Carotene and Retinol Efficacy Trial [CARET]). Vitamin E, another anti-oxidant, inhibits collagen synthesis and should be avoided.

Antineoplastic Agents

Cancer chemotherapy is associated with severe side effects including the destruction of normal cells, tissues, and organs. Stimulating granulation tissue development in the presence of agents designed to attack all fast growing tissue can be difficult. Using medications to counter the inhibition conferred by some of these agents may interfere with the drug's antineoplastic activity. Understanding the mechanism of action for wound healing inhibition may offer strategies for intervention. For example, levamisole is an effective antihelminthic drug with immunomodulatory and anticancer augmenting activities when used in combination with fluorouracil (5-FU) as adjuvant treatment following resection of Dukes' stage C colon carcinomas. Although the combination is very effective in treating colon cancer, combined therapy with levamisole and 5-FU compromises healing at the anastomotic site in the intestine when taken in the immediate postoperative period. Independently, each of the drugs decreases fibroblast proliferation and collagen production in a dose dependent fashion. In combination, the two drugs work synergistically to further decrease fibroblast and collagen formation. Inhibition of dephosphorylation of regulatory phosphoproteins may be related to the therapeutic efficacy of the combination. Through this mechanism, the potential to affect multiple immunoparameters expands. Alone, 5-FU binds thymidilate synthetase and inhibits DNA synthesis (S-phase specific). Through this mechanism, mRNA transcription is reduced. Levamisole, on the other hand, increases mRNA and provides protection against the generalized inhibition in protein synthesis associated with global mRNA transcription inhibition. Leucovorin another antineoplastic modulator used in conjunction with 5-FU enhances the binding of 5-FU to the thymidilate synthetase enzyme with prolongation in the activity of 5-FU. The use of other chemotherapeutic agents in the immediate postoperative period has been associated with rupture at the anastomotic site. Bleomycin does not affect collagen synthesis in colon fibroblasts but inhibits synthesis in skin fibroblasts.

Alternatively, collagen synthesis in colon fibroblasts is inhibited by cisplatin while synthesis in skin fibroblasts is minimally affected.

Transplant Rejection Prevention Agents

Cyclosporine A is a powerful immunosuppressive agent that is widely used for the prevention of allograft rejection and for the treatment of autoimmune diseases. Cyclosporine A may delay wound healing by down regulating and modulating cytokines that regulate connective tissue and immune system interactions. Cyclosporine A is a cyclic peptide blocks the synthesis of interleukin-2 and other cytokines produced by CD4+ lymphocytes. In the healing dental socket of an animal model, it was demonstrated that Cyclosporine A exerted an immunosuppressive response by inhibiting the activity of matrix metalloproteinases 2 and 9 in the early phase of granulation tissue. These observations suggest that Cyclosporine A may exert some of its inhibitory effects in wound healing by interfering with these enzymes. Side effects of Cyclosporine A treatment include chronic nephrotoxicity, hepatotoxicity and neurotoxicity, lymphoproliferative neoplasms, hypertension, thromboembolic complications and gingival overgrowth.

PSYCHOSOCIAL ISSUES

Psychosocial issues influence how a patient perceives, understands and complies with instructions given. Depression of chronic illness affects many wound healing patients and prevents them from protecting their ability to heal. Some patients intentionally wound themselves in an effort to maintain a social relationship with their providers.

Friis (119) assessed 102 subjects in Orange County, California for depression including 56 diabetic patients and 56 without diabetes. Diabetes was associated with a higher level of both depression and unemployment. The subject's employment status more significantly predicted depressive symptomatology. Level of education, type of diabetes, blood sugar level, and required medications were not significant predictors of depression. Therefore, unemployment among diabetic persons might warrant special counseling programs.

Type II diabetic patients are also known to have poor cognitive function in relation to verbal memory. Cognitive studies in Type II diabetics support a correlation between the duration of diabetes and cognitive performance on measures of verbal memory. Macrovascular disease, hypertension and depression, might contribute to observed cognitive decrements in Type II diabetics. Irrespective of socio-demographic, health status, and treatment differences, Rost et. al. (123) found a 1.6-fold likelihood of not remembering all of the medication recommendations immediately after a follow-up primary care visit.

Stress can significantly delay wound healing. The biochemical mechanisms have not been fully elucidated but there is an interaction between stress and some of the pro-inflammatory cytokines. Stress decreases the production of interleukin-1 beta (IL-1ß) in response to lipopolysaccharide (LPS) stimulation. In a suction-induced blister model, both interleukin-1 alpha

TABLE 15. SELECTED AGENTS THAT IMPAIR WOUND HEALING

Agents	Mechanism of Action
Immunosuppressants	
Steroids (glucocorticoids): (Prednisone, hydrocortisone, methylprednisolone)	Inhibits phospholipase A2, inhibits synthesis of inflammatory mediators: Inhibits transcription of IL-1 and IL-6 encoding m-RNA in macrophages Blocks antigen recognition, decrease IL-1 and IL-6 driven effects Redistributes lymphocytes
Dapsone	Produces methemoglobinemia by oxidizing iron in hemoglobin from ferrous to ferric form. This renders hemoglobin unable to carry oxygen to tissues. Bacteriostatic action of dapsone is probably similar to that of the sulphonamides as both are inhibited by para-aminobenzoic acid (PABA).
Cyclosporine A-	Inhibits interleukin-2 (IL-2), and induces transforming growth factor-beta (TGF-beta).
Tacrolimus (FK-506)	Inhibits mRNA transcription of interleukin-2 (IL-2)
Azathioprine	Inhibits mRNA transcription of interleukin-2 (IL-2)
Methotrexate (MTX)	Inhibits purine biosynthesis, creates folic acid deficiency within the target cells. Leucovorin can be used as a "rescue" medication
Antineoplastic Agent	
Cyclophosphamide	Inhibits both purine and pyrimidine biosynthesis
5-Fluorouracil (5-FU)	Inhibits DNA synthesis (S-phase specific), binds Thymidilate Synthetase; Leucovorin enhances the binding and prolongs 5 FU action
Ergamisol® (levamisole)	Antineoplastic adjunct, biological response modifier, immunostimulatory properties
Doxorubicin	Inhibits fibroblast proliferation and collagen production by inactivating prolyl hydroxylase
Mitomycin C	Generates DNA fragmentation which inhibits DNA and protein synthesis causing cell membrane disruption
Interferon –gamma (If-γ)	Inhibits fibroblast motility, proliferation and collagen synthesis
Anticoagulants	
Tissue Plasminogen Activator (TPA)	Converts plasminogen to plasmin to degrade fibrin and fibronectin
Heparin	Inhibit the synthesis of fibrin and fibronectin
Radiation Therapeutic Intervention	
Beta radiation	Promotes vascular occlusion, causes ischemia, and inhibits fibroblast proliferation and collagen remodeling

(IL-lα) and interleukin-8 (IL-8) levels were produced at lower rates in women who scored higher on the Perceived Stress Score tests. Salivary cortisol levels were used as an objective measure to confirm the subject's subjective sense of being in a stressful situation. In relation to stress experienced by individuals recovering from addiction vs non-addicted individuals, the mean for the Stress Symptoms Scale and the means for all symptoms subscales were also significantly higher for the recovering drug addicts, with the highest values for cognitive and muscular symptoms. Whether the stress is secondary to co-morbid medical conditions or other social demands, the perception of elevated stressful situations may impede wound healing.

Self-injurious behaviors such as "skin picking" has been reviewed in relation to teenage behaviors with mean onset at age 15 and mean duration of illness for 21 years. The most common co-morbid Axis I diagnosis was obsessive-compulsive disorder, 52%, alcohol abuse or dependency, 39%, body dysmorphic disorder, 32%, and major mood disorder, 48%. The most common associated Axis II disorders were obsessive-compulsive personality disorder, 48%, and borderline personality disorder, 26%. In a population of mentally challenged patients there is no correlation with depression and self-injurious behavior. There is a higher correlation with male patients suffering from severe, profound mental retardation. As with teenagers, adults who injure themselves usually use the behavior as a means of expression. Research into self-inflicted dermatoses is not largely reported in the psychiatric literature. Studies are available in the dermatologic literature under the topics of dermatitis artefacta, neurotic excoriations, and trichotillomania. Larger wounds are generally discussed in the realm of Munchausen's Syndrome.

Depression is commonly associated with chronic medical conditions. Severe depression is associated with anorexia and weight loss. Depressed patients exhibit significantly lower albumin and transferrin levels than healthy individuals. Melancholia correlates strongly with a decrease in the plasma proteins. Therefore, depression may affect the wound healing on a variety of different levels.

LOOK-A-LIKE DISORDERS

Neuropathy diabetic foot ulcers result from repetitive trauma occurring after the patient suffers a loss of protective sensation (LOPS). Arterial vascular insufficiency ulcers develop secondary to poor tissue oxygenation and perfusion. Neuroischemic ulcers develop predominantly on the lateral and dorsal aspects of the foot; whereas, neuropathic ulcers are found most commonly on the plantar surface. Several conditions may be misdiagnosed as diabetic foot ulcers when located on the foot of a diabetic patient. More frequently, misdiagnosis occurs when the lesion is on the calf. Unfortunately, the misnomer "leg ulcer" without respect to the true underlying etiology is used or the generic "venous ulcer" is applied because the lesion is located on the lower extremity. This common occurrence may explain some of the chronic lower extremity wounds that persist secondary to misdirection in therapy. Pursuing the true diagnosis usually leads to a more appropriate therapeutic intervention. Sometimes biopsy may be required to diagnose the unusual infection, vasculitic disorder, or cancer that may be

TABLE 16. DIFFERENTIAL DIAGNOSIS FOR LOWER EXTREMITY ULCERATION

Etiology of Wound	Differential	Method of Investigation
Infectious Conditions	Mycobacterial Fungal Bacterial Treponemal/spirochetic	Wound biopsy with special stains and cultures. VDRL, PPD, CBC, SED CRP, CXR, Wound X-ray
Malignancy	Basal cell carcinoma, Squamous cell carcinoma, Kaposi's Sarcoma Lymphoma Mycosis fungoides	Wound biopsy for pathologic evaluation
Macrovascular Arterial Insufficiency	Arteriosclerosis Post-traumatic Thrombosis	Non-invasive vascular studies (NIVS) Bi-directional Color Doppler $TcpO_2$ Arteriography Magnetic resonance arteriogram (MRA)
Vasculitis/Vasculopathy (Microvascular Arterial Insufficiency)	Diabetic microangiopathy Hypertensive microangiopathy Thromboangiitis obliterans Raynaud's Disorder	$TcpO_2$ Laser Doppler Possible Biopsy
Venous Insufficiency (Deep and Superficial)	Deep vein thrombosis (DVT) Extrinsic compression (tumors) Deep valve insufficiency Perforator valve insufficiency Superficial venous insufficiency (varicosity)	Pneumoplethysmography (maximum venous outflow) Venous photoplethysmography Bi-directional color Doppler
Lymphatic Obstruction/ Lymphedema	Veno-lymphatic disease (secondary to congestive heart failure, hepatic failure, renal failure, other overload states) Primary lymphatic insufficiency Lymphangiosarcoma	Clinical diagnosis, Hx/PE CXR, LFT, Chemistries Lymphangiography
Hematological Abnormalities	Anemia (sickle cell disease) Polycythemia Dysproteinemia	CBC, Fe Studies (Fe, TIBC, Folate, B12) Sickle cell prep
Collagen Vascular Disorders	Systemic Lupus Erythematosus Scleroderma Polyarteritis nodosum Wegener's granulomatosis	FANA RA prep Serum complement Rheumatologic Work-up
Excessive Pressure	Diabetic neuropathy Alcoholic neuropathy Decubitus Post-operative deformity Bone spurs	Monofilament (10 gm) Vibratory sensation (>25mV) X-rays

masquerading as a routine "leg ulcer." Table 16 lists some of the disorders to consider when lower extremity wounds are not responding as anticipated.

Pyoderma Gangrenosum

A painful, rapidly enlarging ulcer with undermined bluish and purplish-red margins with extensive necrosis around the edges of the lesions characterizes pyoderma gangrenosum. It is usually but not always, found in association with an inflammatory disease. Associations with rheumatoid arthritis, ulcerative colitis, Crohn's disease, chronic inflammatory bowel disease, diabetes mellitus, chronic active hepatitis and systemic lupus erythematosus are common. They are not caused by bacterial disease but may show some limited response to antibiotics if suprainfections are present. Biopsy typically reveals a massive neutrophilic infiltration, in the absence of vasculitis and granuloma formation. Untreated ulcers may enlarge, slowly heal, or remain unchanged. Systemic steroids or immunosuppressive agents are used to treat these patients.

Malignant Transformation

The most common skin tumor, basal cell carcinoma, arises from cells at the base of the epidermis. Basal cell carcinoma usually starts as a slow-growing, small, shiny (or pearly) bump that develops into an open sore. The sore takes longer than three weeks to heal. Squamous cell carcinoma, the second most common skin cancer arises from cells in the medial portion of the epidermis. Both cancers usually develop in areas of ultraviolet sun damaged face, arms, and hands. However, primary cancers may be found on the lower extremities of women who sunbathe. Skin cancers may also develop as a malignant degeneration of chronic wounds. Malignant transformation of squamous cells in the face of osteomyelitis is the most common recognized mechanism. Malignant transformation has also been found in wounds from burns, traumatic insults, radiation exposure and diabetic origins. Squamous cell carcinoma, and more rarely, basal cell carcinoma, malignant melanoma, sarcoma and fibrous histiocytoma have been reported. In cases of malignant transformation, conservative treatment consists of amputation of the affected limb. Alternative considerations include Mohs micrographic surgery (MMS) as a limb saving procedure for squamous cell carcinoma arising from osteomyelitis, with less extensive disease.

Calciphylaxis

A highly morbid syndrome of vascular calcification and skin necrosis that occurs most commonly in the lower extremities of patients with chronic renal failure, hypercalcemia, hyperphosphatemia, an elevated calcium-phosphate product, secondary hyperparathyroidism, or uremia. Most patients with calciphylaxis are patients with end-stage renal disease on dialysis. Sepsis from infected, necrotic skin lesions is the leading cause of death. Mortality is high (60–80%). Surgical intervention, total or subtotal parathyroidectomy, is thought to be helpful in some cases. Aggressive debridement, judicious antibiotic use, and in some cases, hyperbaric oxygen may be beneficial. For more information on misdiagnosed wounds, see Shah's chapter entitled "Approach to Commonly Misdiagnosed Wounds and Unusual Leg Ulcers."

EVERYDAY CARE

The selection of dressing, cleansing, debriding, and off-loading device used as part of the everyday care may either enhance or hinder a successful outcome in wound healing. Education of the patient, family visiting nurse support team as well as the clinician and his staff is vital. Many clinicians have developed regional patterns of wound care practice. In some regions, the use of hydrogen peroxide, turpentine, Betadine, Dakin's solution, and acetic acid 0.25% are commonplace practices. These agents tend to destroy granulation tissue. Although they may have a role in controlling infection, when the tissue begins to show granulation these agents may prove toxic enough to destroy healthy granulation tissue.

Many diabetic patients are still treated with whirlpool sessions leading to maceration of the wound and periwound tissue. Heating lamps are also sometimes employed. These tend to desiccate the tissue and impede granulation tissue development. There are products available to protect the wound while maintaining a warm "body temperature" environment. Unfortunately, many patients devise their own therapies using vinegar to simulate acetic acid, diluted bleach to simulate Dakin's solution, and a whole host of other culturally derived home remedies that may prove detrimental to progressive healthy tissue growth. Pribitkin (133) suggests that up to 70% of patients do not reveal their use of herbal products to their surgical providers. Identifying and correcting problems with everyday care will improve the likelihood of a successful outcome.

RHEUMATOLOGICAL ABNORMALITIES

Rheumatological disorders may affect wound healing through changes in autoimmune function as reviewed above; as well as, through deformity of joints, pain, poor GI absorption, and stress. As an example, a patient with diabetes may develop limited range of motion at the ankle joint, hammertoe deformities, and tendon contractions. The anterior fat pad is displaced anteriorly, and the metatarsal joints are left with minimal protection on the plantar surface. Ulcerations typically occur at these deformities.

Diseases commonly seen in wound healing centers that have a rheumatologic component include: diabetes mellitus, rheumatoid arthritis, system lupus erythematosus (SLE), scleroderma, and Behcet's disease.

CONCLUSION–OPTIMIZING WOUND HEALING

Optimal wound healing is achieved by maintaining a moist clean wound bed, minimizing the effect of co-morbid diseases, providing adequate oxygenation, affording proper off-loading, reducing the bio-burden, and ensuring adequate nutrition for the wound to heal. Creation of a moist wound environment facilitates granulation tissue development through increased gel-matrix secretion, new blood vessel growth, collagen secretion, fibroblast proliferation, and epidermal migration. Maintaining a "clean" wound environment free of pro-inflammatory factors helps to achieve and maintain the proliferative phase of wound healing by maximizing the presence of the fibroblast, preventing the formation of fibrin slough, and avoiding reentry into the inflammation stage of wound healing.

Overall goals for wound healing should be directed at:

- Reducing the biological burden of necrotic tissue and debris,
- Reducing callous formation,
- Controlling edema and periwound maceration,
- Eradicating infections,
- Maintaining "body" temperature at the wound site,
- Eliminating dead space with packing material,
- Wicking deep fluid filled cavities to prevent abscess pocket formation,
- Controlling odor,
- Promoting granulation tissue in a moist wound environment,
- Promoting re-epithelialization, and
- Restoring function.

Treatments selected to meet these goals should be uncomplicated methods of cleansing, dressings, debriding medication, antibiotic medication, or devices that the patient or his/her caretaker can easily apply. Table 17 is a convenient guide to consider for optimizing wound healing.

TABLE 17. WOUND CENTER GUIDE FOR OPTIMIZING WOUND HEALING

1. Assess and treat systemic illness (History, Focused Exam, Vital Signs)
2. Assess for diabetes, maintain HbAIC < 6.5
3. Identify and improve anemia
4. Minimize lipid and cholesterol levels
5. Evaluate nutritional status and correct deficiencies (Hydration, Protein, Vitamins)
6. Identify and treat infection (oral/PIC line)
7. Utilize laboratory and radiological assessment for proper diagnosis. (Wound biopsy or aspiration, X-ray studies, sedimentation rate, C-reactive protein, Duplex scan, Doppler, $TcpO_2$, arteriogram, etc.)
8. Upgrade Tetanus (rabies prophylaxis)
9. Develop and maintain a moist, warm, debris-free wound base
10. Assess the wound for hypoxia/ischemia ($TcpO_2$, NIVS, Doppler, A-gram, MRA)
11. Correct major ischemic compromise when possible (surgical or transcutaneous vascular intervention)
12. Provide appropriate edema reduction
13. Provide method for adequate off-loading
14. Address smoking, alcohol, illicit drug use
15. Identify and address depression
16. Educate patient and/or care taker about appropriate daily wound care
17. Facilitate appropriate off-site wound care
18. Ensure patient has primary care physician and refer to specialist care as indicated

REFERENCES

Introduction

1. Zeman F, Ney D. *Applications of Clinical Nutrition* pp 27. New Jersey: Prentice-Hall, 1988.

2. Bergstrom N, Bennett MA, Carlson CE, et al. Treatment of Pressure Ulcers. Clinical Practice Guideline, No. 15. Rockville, MD: US Department of Health Care and Policy and Research. AHCPR Publication No. 95-0652. December 1994.

3. Zacur H; Kirsner RS. Debridement: Rationale and Therapeutic Options. Wounds- A Compendium of Clinical Research and Practice. Vol 14. No. 7, 2002. (Supplement E). *http://woundsresearch.com/wnds/hpsupp03.cfm*

4. Falanga V, Wound Bed Preparation and the Role of Enzymes: A Case for Multiple Actions of Therapeutic Agents, *Wounds* 14(2):47-57, 2002. © 2002 Health Management Publications, Inc.

Oxygen and Perfusion

5. Brown GC, Cooper CE. Nanomolar concentrations of nitric oxide reversibly inhibit synaptosomal respiration by competing with oxygen at cytochrome oxidase. *FEBS Lett* 1994; 356: 295-298.

6. Brown GC, Foxwell N, Moncada S. Transcellular regulation of cell respiration by nitric oxide generated by activated macrophages. *FEBS Lett* 1998; 439:321-324.

7. Cohen HJ, Ashima M, Sushama V. "Co-Transactivation of the 3' Erythropoietin Hypoxia Inducible Enhancer by the HIF-1 Protein." *Blood Cells, Molecules, and Diseases* 31 May 1997: 169-176.

8. Kimura H, Weisz A, Ogura T, et al. "Identification of Hypoxia-Inducible Factor-1 (HIF-1) Ancillary Sequence and Its Function in Vascular Endothelial Growth Factor Gene Induction by Hypoxia and Nitric Oxide." *The Journal of Biological Chemistry* 2000 Oct 30.

9. Mukhopadhyay CK, Mazumder B, Fox PL. "Role of Hypoxia-inducible Factor-1 in Transcriptional Activation of Ceruloplasmin by Iron Deficiency" *Journal of Biol. Chem* 2000; 275(28): 21048-21054.

10. Kimure H, Weisz A, et al. Hypoxia Response Element of the Human Vascular Endothelial Growth Factor Gene Mediates Transcriptional Regulation by Nitric Oxide: Control of Hypoxia-Inducible Factor-1 Activity by the Nitric Oxide. *Blood* 2000; 95(1):189-97.

11. Chilov D, Camenisch G, Kvietikova I, et al., Induction and nuclear translocation of hypoxia-inducible-factor-l (HIF-1: heterodimerization with ARNT is not necessary for nuclear accumulation of HIF-1 alpha. *J Cell Sci* 1999 Apr; 112 (Pt 8):1203-12.

12. Marx RE, Ehler W, Tayapongsak P, et al. Relationship of Oxygen Dose to Angiogenesis Induction in Irradiated Tissue. *Am J Surgery* 1990; 160, 519-24.

13. Ballard JL, Eke CC, Bunt TJ, et al. A prospective evaluation of transcutaneous oxygen measurements in the management of diabetic foot problems. *J Vasc Surg* 1995; 22:485-92.

14. Sheffield PJ, Smith APS. Physiological and pharmacological basis of hyperbaric oxygen therapy. In *Hyperbaric Surgery-Perioperative Care* DJ Bakker, FS Cramer (eds). Flagstaff, AZ: Best Publishing, 2002; 63-110.

Nutrition and Hydration
Protein

15. Brugler, L, DiPrinzio MJ, Bernstein L. The five-year evolution of a malnutrition treatment program in a community hospital. *JT Comm J Qual Improv* 1999;r:191-206.

16. Flanigan KH: Nutritional aspects of wound healing, *Adv Wound Care* 1997; 10(2):48.

17. Morley JE, Silver AJ. Nutritional issues in nursing home care. *Ann Int Med* 1995; 123:850-859.

18. Collins N. The difference between Albumin and Prealbumin, *Adv Skin & Wound Care* 2001; 14 (5): 235-236.

19. Demling RH, DeSanti L. Protein-energy malnutrition, and the nonhealing cutaneous wound. medscape from the web MD, *www,medscape.com*

20. Sullivan DH, Sun S, Walls RC. Protein-energy under-nutrition among elderly hospitalized patients. *JAMA* 1999; 281:2013-9.

21. Thomas DR, Causes of protein-energy malnutrition. *Z Gerontol Geriat* 32 (1999); 7,S38-S44.

Alternative Medicines

22. Chithra P, Sajithlal GB, Chandrakasan G. Influence of Aloe Vera on collagen characteristics in healing dermal wounds in rats. *Mol Cell Biochem* 1998 Apr; 181 (1-2):71-6.

23. Vogler BK, Ernst E. Aloe Vera: a systematic review of its clinical effectiveness. *Br J Gen Pract* 1999 Oct; 49(447):823-8.

24. Somboonwong J, Thanamittramanee S, Jariyapongskul A, et al. Therapeutic effects of Aloe Vera on cutaneous microcirculation and wound healing in second degree burn model in rats. *J Med Assoc Thai* 2000 Apr; 83 (4):417-25.

25. Zhang L, Tizard IR. Activation of a mouse macrophage cell line by acemannan: the major carbohydrate fraction from Aloe Vera gel. *Immunopharmacology* 1996; Nov;35(2):119-28.

Edema Control

26. Agren MS. Studies on zinc in wound healing. *Acta Derm Venereol Suppl (Stockh)* 1990; 154:1-36.

27. Agren MS, Steenfos HH, Tarnow P, et al. Zinc oxide augments endogenous expression of insulin-like growth factor-1 (IGF-1) and activates matrix metalloproteinases (MMPs) in wounds. Paper presented at EWMA Stockholm 2000. EWMA J. 2001; 1 (1):16-7.

28. Andrews M, Gallagher-Allred C, The role of zinc in wound healing. *Adv Wound Care* 1999 Apr; 12(3):137-8.

29. Katz MH, Alvarez AF, Kirsner RS, et al. Human wound fluid from acute wounds stimulates fibroblast and endothelial cell growth. *J Am Acad Dermatol* 1991; Dec; 25(6 Pt 1):1054-8.

30. Lauer G, Sollberg S, Cole M, et al. Expression and proteolysis of vascular endothelial growth factor is increased in chronic wounds. *J Invest Dermatol* 2000 Jul; 115(1):12-8.

31. Lobmann R, Ambrosch A, Schultz G, et al. Expression of matrix-metalloproteinases and their inhibitors in the wounds of diabetic and non-diabetic patients. *Diabetologia* 2002; Jul; 45 (7) :1011-6.

32. Loots MA, Lamme EN, Zeegelaar J, et al. Differences in cellular infiltrate and extracellular matrix of chronic diabetic and venous ulcers versus acute wounds. *J Invest Dermatol* 1998 Nov;111(5):850.

33. Moore K. The scientific basis of wound healing. *Advances in Tissue Banking* 2001; 5: 379-397

34. Nezu R, Takagi Y, Ito T, et al. The importance of total parenteral nutrition-associated tissue zinc distribution in wound healing. *Surg Today* 1999; 29(1):34-41.

35. Rojas AI, Phillips TJ. Patients with chronic leg ulcers show diminished levels of vitamins A and E, carotenes, and zinc. *Dermatol Surg* 1999; Aug;25(8):601-4.

36. Saarialho-Kere UK. Patterns of matrix metalloproteinase and TIMP expression in chronic ulcers. *Arch Dermatol Res* 1998 Jul; 290 Suppl:S47-54.

37. Sunzel B, Holm S, Reuterving CO, et al. The effect of zinc on bacterial phagocytosis, killing and cytoprotection in human polymorphonuclear leucocytes. *APMIS* 1995 Sep;103(9):635-44.

38. Trengove NJ, Stacey MC, MacAuley S, et al. Analysis of the acute and chronic wound environments: the role of proteases and their inhibitors. *Wound Repair Regen* 1999 Nov-Dec; 7(6):442-52.

39. Wood RJ. Assessment of marginal zinc status in humans, *Journal of Nutrition* 2000; 130:1350S-1354S.

40. Wysocki AB, Staiano-Coico L, Grinnell F. Wound fluid from chronic leg ulcers contains elevated levels of metalloproteinases MMP-2 and MMP-9. *J Invest Dermatol* 1993 Jul; 101 (1):64-8.

41. Yager DR, Zhang LY, Liang HX, et al. Wound fluids from human pressure ulcers contain elevated matrix metalloproteinase levels and activity compared to surgical wound fluids. *J Invest Dermatol* 1996 Nov; 107(5):743-8.

Clucose Control

42. Aronson D, Rayfield EJ. How hyperglycemia promotes atherosclerosis: molecular mechanisms. *Cardiovasc Diabetol* 2002; 1 (1):1.

43. Aso Y, Matsumoto S, Fujiwara Y, et al. Impaired fibrinolytic compensation for hypercoagulability in obese patients with type 2 diabetes: association with increased plasminogen activator inhibitor-1. *Metabolism* 2002 Apr; 51 (4):471-6.

44. Carr ME. Diabetes mellitus: a hypercoagulable state. *J Diabetes Complications* 2001 Jan-Feb; 15(1):44-54.

45. Cerami C, Founds H, Nicholl I, et al. Tobacco smoke is a source of toxic reactive glycation products. *Proc Natl Acad Sci USA* 1997; December, 9; 94(25): 13915 - 13920.

46. Jude EB, Tentolouris N, Appleton I, et al. Role of neuropathy and plasma nitric oxide in recurrent neuropathic and neuroischemic diabetic foot ulcers. *Wound Repair Regen* 2001 Sep-Oct; 9 (5) :353-9.

47. Koschinsky T, He CJ, Mitsuhashi T, et al. Orally absorbed reactive glycation products (glycotoxins): An environmental risk factor in diabetic nephropathy. *Proc Natl Acad Sci USA* 1997 June 10; 94(12): 6474 - 6479.

48. The Diabetes Control and Complications Trial Research Group. The effect of intensive treatment of diabetes on the development and progression of long-term complications in insulin-dependent diabetes mellitus. *N Engl J Med* 1993 Sep 30; 329(14):977-86.

49. Vlassara H, Fuh H, Makita Z, et al. Exogenous advanced glycosylation end products induce complex vascular dysfunction in normal animals: a model for diabetic and aging complications. *Proc Natl Acad Sci* USA 1992 Dec 15; 89(24):12043-47.

Lipid Control

50. Albina JE, Gladden P, Walsh WR. Detrimental effects of an omega-3 fatty acid-enriched diet on wound healing. *J Parenter Enteral Nutr* 1993; 17:519-21.

51. Chu X, Newman J, Park B, et al. In vitro alteration of macrophage phenotype and function by serum lipids. *Cell & Tissue Research:* ISSN: 0302-766X (printed version);ISSN: 1432-0878 (electronic version) Abstract Volume 296 Issue 2 (1999) pp 331-337.

52. National Institutes of Health, Interpretation and adaptation of the third ATP (Adult Treatment Panel) report Detection, Evaluation, and Treatment of High Blood Cholesterol in Adults (Adult Treatment Panel III) prepared by the National Cholesterol Education Program, National Heart, Lung, and Blood Institute. (National Institutes of Health NIH Publication No. 01-3670 May 2001).

53. Hua Cai, Harrison DG. Endothelial dysfunction in cardiovascular diseases: the role of oxidant stress. *Circulation Research* 2000; 87:840. Mini-review.

54. Weitz JI, Byrne J, Clagett GP, et al. Diagnosis and treatment of chronic arterial insufficiency of the lower extremities: a critical review, *Circulation* 1996; 94:3026-3049.

Infection and Inflammation

55. Crout RJ, Lee HM, Schroeder K, et al. The "cyclic" regimen of low-dose doxycycline for adult periodontitis: a preliminary study. *J Periodontol* 1996; 67:506-14.

56. Hashimoto N, Kawabe T, Hara T, et al. Effect of erythromycin on matrix metalloproteinase-9 and cell migration. *J Lab Clin Med* 2001 Mar; 137(3):176-83.

57. Van Winkelhoff AJ, Ramos TE, Slots J. Systemic antibiotic therapy in periodontitis. *Periodontol* 2000. 1996; 10:45-78.

58. Williams RC, Paquette DW. Periodontal disease diagnosis and treatment: an exciting future. J *Dent Educ* 1998; 62:871-81.

Trauma (Repetitive)

59. Chong PH, Kezele B. Periodontal disease and atherosclerotic cardiovascular disease: confounding effects or epiphenomenon? *Pharmacotherapy* 2000, 20(7):805-18.

60. Frykberg RG, Lavery LA, Pham H, et al. Role of neuropathy and high foot pressures in diabetic foot ulceration. *Diabetes Care* 1998 Oct; 21(10):1714-9.

Chronicity

61. Castronuovo JJ Jr. Effects of chronic wound fluid on the structure and biological activity of becaplermin (rhPDGF-BB) and becaplermin gel. *Am J Surg* 1998 Aug;176(2A Suppl):61S-67S.

62. Raffetto JD, Mendez MV, Marien BJ, et al. Changes in cellular motility and cytoskeletal actin in fibroblasts from patients with chronic venous insufficiency and in neonatal fibroblasts in the presence of chronic wound fluid. *J Vasc Surg* 2001 Jun; 33(6):1233-41.

63. Page RC. Milestones in periodontal research and the remaining critical issues. *J Periodont Res* 1999; 34:331-9.

64. Takizawa H, Desaki M, Ohtoshi T, et al. Erythromycin suppresses interleukin 6 expression by human bronchial epithelial cells: a potential mechanism of its anti-inflammatory action. *Biochem Biophys Res Commun* 1995 May 25; 210(3):781-6.

65. Trengove NJ, Analysis of the acute and chronic wound environments: the role of proteases and their inhibitors. *Wound Repair Regen* 1999 Nov-Dec; 7(6):442-52.

66. Wysocki AB, Grinnell F, Fibronectin profiles in normal and chronic wound fluid. *Lab Invest* 1990 Dec; 63(6):825-31.

67. Acang N, Jalil FD. Hypercoagulation in diabetes mellitus. *Southeast Asian J Trop Med Public Health* 1993; 24 Suppl 1:263-6.

Hematologic Abnormalities

68. Fatouros MS, Vekinis G, Bourantas KL, et al. Influence of growth factors erythropoietin and granulocyte macrophage colony stimulating factor on mechanical strength and healing of colonic anastomoses in rats. *Eur J Surg* 1999 Oct; 165 (10):986-92.

69. Hughes A, McVerry BA, Wilkinson L, et al. Diabetes, a hypercoagulable state? Hemostatic variables in newly diagnosed type 2 diabetic patients. *Acta Haematol* 1983; 69 (4):254-9.

70. Jones RL, Jovanovic L, Forman S, et al. Time course of reversibility of accelerated fibrinogen disappearance in diabetes mellitus: association with intravascular volume shifts. *Blood* 1984 Jan; 63(1):22-30.

71. Kazmi WH, Kausz AT, Khan S, et al. Anemia: an early complication of chronic renal insufficiency. *Am J Kidney Dis* 2001 Oct; 38(4):803-12.

72. Matsuda T, Morishita T, Jokaji E, et al. Mechanism on disorders of coagulation and fibrinolysis in diabetes. *Diabetes* 1996 Jul; 45 Suppl 3:S109-10.

Socio–Economical Issues

73. Abalkhail BA. Social status, health status and therapy response in heroin addicts. *East Mediterr Health J* 2001 May; 7(3):465-72.

74. Cerami C, Founds H, Nicholl I, et al. Tobacco smoke is a source of toxic reactive glycation products. *Proc Natl Acad Sci USA* 1997 Dec 9; 94(25):13915-20.

75. Chakkalakal DA, Novak JR, Fritz ED, et al. Chronic ethanol consumption results in deficient bone repair in rats. *Alcohol Alcoholism* 2002 Jan-Feb; 37(1):13-20.

76. Guerrero-Romero F, Rodriguez-Moran M. Relationship of microalbuminuria with the diabetic foot ulcers in type II diabetes. *J Diabetes Complications* 1998 Jul-Aug; 12(4):193-6.

77. Jorgensen LN, Kallehave F, Christensen E, et al. Less collagen production in smokers. *Surgery* 1998 Apr; 123(4):450-5.

78. Laitinen K, Valimaki M. Alcohol and bone. *Calcif Tissue Int* 1991; 49 Suppl:S70-3.

79. Makela JT, Kiviniemi H, Juvonen T, et al. Factors influencing wound dehiscence after midline laparotomy. *Am J Surg* 1995 Oct; 170 (4):387-90.

80. Manassa ER, Hertl CH, Olbrisch RR. Wound healing problems in smokers and nonsmokers after 132 abdominoplasties. *Plast Reconstr Surg* 2003 May; 111 (6) 2082-7; discussion 2088-9.

81. Mantey I, Foster AV, Spencer S, et al. Why do foot ulcers recur in diabetic patients? *Diabet Med* 1999 Mar; 16(3):245-9.

82. Moller AM, Pedersen T, Villebro N, et al. Impact of lifestyle on perioperative smoking cessation and post-operative complication rate. *Prev Med* 2003 Jun; 36(6):704-9.

83. Monfrecola G, Riccio G, Savarese C, et al. The acute effect of smoking on cutaneous microcirculation blood flow in habitual smokers and nonsmokers. *Dermatology* 1998; 197(2):115-8.

84. Mukunda BN, Callahan JM, Hobbs MS, et al. Cocaine inhibits human neutrophil phagocytosis and phagolysosomal acidification in vitro. *Immunopharmacol Immunotoxicol* 2000 May; 22(2):373-86.

85. Nyquist F, Berglund M, Nilsson BE, et al. Nature and healing of tibial shaft fractures in alcohol abusers. *Alcohol Alcoholism* 1997 Jan-Feb; 32 (1):91-5.

86. Pellaton C, Kubli S, Feihl F, et al. Blunted vasodilatory responses in the cutaneous microcirculation of cigarette smokers. *Am Heart J* 2002 Aug; 144(2):269-74.

87. US Department of Health and Human Services. Prevalence of Substance Use Among Racial & Ethnic Subgroups in the U.S., SAMHA, Substance Abuse and Mental Health Services, US Department of Health and Human Services, National Household Survey on Drug Abuse. Accessed 11 July, 2003. On line at *http://www.samhsa.gov/oas/nhsda/2klnhsda/voll/highlights.htm*

88. Raso AM, Visentin I, Zan S, et al. [Vascular pathology of surgical interest in drug addicts] [Article in Italian] *Minerva Cardioangiol* 2000 Oct; 48(10) :287-96.

89. Santolaria-Fernandez FJ, Gomez-Sirvent JL, Gonzalez-Reimers CE, et al. Nutritional assessment of drug addicts. *Drug Alcohol Depend* 1995 Apr; 38 (1):ll-8.

90. Schryvers OI, Stranc MF, Nance PW. Surgical treatment of pressure ulcers: 20-year experience. *Arch Phys Med Rehabil* 2000 Dec; 81 (12):1556-62.

91. Shin VY, Liu ES, Koo MW, et al. Cigarette smoke extracts delay wound healing in the stomach: involvement of polyamine synthesis. *Experimental Biology and Medicine* 227:114-124 (2002).

92. Smith AJ, Shepherd JP, Hodgson RJ. Brief interventions for patients with alcohol-related trauma. *Br J Oral Maxillofac Surg* 1998 Dec; 36(6):408-15.

93. Sorensen LT, Jorgensen T, Kirkeby LT, et al. Smoking and alcohol abuse are major risk factors for anastomotic leakage in colorectal surgery. *Br J Surg* 1999 Jul; 86(7) 927-31.

94. Sorensen LT, Horby J, Friis E, et al. Smoking as a risk factor for wound healing and infection in breast cancer surgery. *Eur J Surg Oncol* 2002 Dec; 28(8):815-20.

95. Sorensen LT, Karlsmark T, Gottrup F. Abstinence from smoking reduces incisional wound infection: a randomized controlled trial. *Ann Surg* 2003 Jul; 238(1):1-5.

96. Stephens P, al-Khateeb T, Davies KJ, et al. An investigation of the interaction between alcohol and fibroblasts in wound healing. Int. *Journal of Oral & Maxillofacial Surgery* 1996; 25(2):161-164.

97. Tabata T, Meyer AA. Immunoglobulin M synthesis after burn injury: the effects of chronic ethanol on post-injury synthesis. *J Burn Care Rehabil* 1995 Jul-Aug; 16 (4):400-6.

98. Takahashi TA, Merrill JO, Boyko EJ, et al. Type and location of injection drug use-related soft tissue infections predict hospitalization. *J Urban Health* 2003 Mar; 80(1):127-36.

99. van Adrichem LN, Hovius SE, van Strik R, et al. Acute effects of cigarette smoking on microcirculation of the thumb. *Br J Plast Surg* 1992 Jan; 45(1):9-11.

100. van Adrichem LN, Hovius SE, van Strik R, et al. The acute effect of cigarette smoking on the microcirculation of a replanted digit. *J Hand Surg* [Am]. 1992 Mar; 17(2):230-4.

101. Watzl B, Watson RR. Immunomodulation by cocaine-a neuroendocrine mediated response. *Life Sci* 1990; 46(19):1319-29.

102. Zhang J, Ying X, Lu Q, et al. A single high dose of vitamin C counteracts the acute negative effect on microcirculation induced by smoking a cigarette. *Microvasc Res* 1999 Nov; 58 (3):305-11.

Autoimmune Diseases

103. Davidson A. Keiser, HD. Diagnosing and treating the predominantly female problems of systemic autoimmune diseases. *Medscape General Medicine* 1(2), 1999. © 1999 Medscape Posted 02/20/1997.

104. Pozzilli P, Di Mario U. Autoimmune diabetes not requiring insulin at diagnosis (latent autoimmune diabetes of the adult): definition, characterization, and potential prevention. *Diabetes Care* 2001 Aug; 24(8):1460-7.

105. Matejkova-Behanova M. Latent autoimmune diabetes in adults (LADA) and autoimmune thyroiditis (Mini review). *Endocr Regul* 2001 Sep; 35 (3):167-72.

106. National Institutes of Health. Understanding autoimmune diseases. May 1998 NIH Publication No. 98-4273. Online access: *http://www.niaid.nih.gov/publications/autoimmune/autoimmune.htm*

Medication the Impede Wound Healing

107. Anstead GM. Steroids, retinoids, and wound healing. *Adv Wound Care* 1998 Oct; 11(6):277-85.

108. News Release: Beta Carotene and Vitamin A Halted in Lung Cancer Prevention Trial. News Release Date: Thurs., Jan. 18, 1996. For Release: 12:00 p.m. ESTContact: NCI (301) 496-6641 or Fred Hutchinson Cancer Center (206) 667-2896.

109. de Waard JW, de Man BM, Wobbes T, et al. Inhibition of fibroblast collagen synthesis and proliferation by levamisole and 5-fluorouracil. *Eur J Cancer* 1998 Jan; 34(1):162-7.

110. Goodman GE, Thornquist MD, Balmes J, et al. The Beta-Carotene and Retinol Efficacy Trial: incidence of lung cancer and cardiovascular disease mortality during 6-year follow-up after stopping beta-carotene and retinol supplements. *J Natl Cancer Inst* 2004 Dec 1; 96(23):1743-50.

111. Hendricks T, Martens MF, Huyben CM, et al. Inhibition of basal and TGF beta-induced fibroblast collagen synthesis by antineoplastic agents. Implications for wound healing. *Br J Cancer* 1993 Mar; 67(3):545-50.

112. Hunt TK, Ehrlich HP, Garcia JA, et al. Effect of vitamin A on reversing the inhibitory effect of cortisone on healing of open wounds in animals and man. *Ann Surg* 1969 Oct; 170(4):633-41.

113. Sasaki T. The effects of basic fibroblast growth factor and doxorubicin on cultured human skin fibroblasts: relevance to wound healing. *J Dermatol* 1992 Nov; 19(11):664-6.

114. Silva HC, Coletta RD, Jorge J, et al. The effect of cyclosporin A on the activity of matrix metalloproteinases during the healing of rat molar extraction wounds. *Arch Oral Biol* 2001 Sep; 46(9):875-9.

115. Ulland AE, Shearer JD, Coulter C, et al. Altered wound arginine metabolism by corticosterone and retinoic acid. *J Surg Res* 1997 Jun; 70(1):84-8.

116. Wicke C, Halliday B, Allen D, et al. Effects of steroids and retinoids on wound healing. *Arch Surg* 2000 Nov; 135 (11):1265-70.

117. Yamamoto T, Nishioka K. Animal model of sclerotic skin. V: Increased expression of alpha-smooth muscle actin in fibroblastic cells in bleomycin-induced scleroderma. *Clin Immunol* 2002 Jan; 102(1):77-83.

Psycho–Social Issues

118. Cosway R, Strachan MY, Dougall A, et al. Cognitive function and information processing in Type 2 diabetes. *Diabet Med* 2001 Oct; 18(10).803-10.

119. Friis R, Nanjundappa G. Diabetes, depression and employment status. *Soc Sci Med* 1986; 23(5):471-5.

120. Glaser R, Kiecolt-Glaser JK, Marucha PT, et al Stress-related changes in proinflammatory cytokine production in wounds. *Archives of General Psychiatry* 1999; 56: 450-456.

121. Lamon BC, Alonzo A. Stress among males recovering from substance abuse. *Addict Behav* 1997 Mar-Apr; 22 (2): 195-205.

122. Maes M, Vandewoude M, Scharpe S, et al. Anthropometric and biochemical assessment of the nutritional state in depression: evidence for lower visceral protein plasma levels in depression. *J Affect Disord* 1991 Sep; 23(1):25-33.

123. Rost K, Roter D, Quill T, et al. Capacity to remember prescription drug changes: deficits associated with diabetes. Collaborative Study Group of the Task Force on the Medical Interview. *Diabetes Res Clin Pract* 1990 Oct; 10(2):183-7.

124. Tsiouris JA, Mann R, Patti PJ, et al. Challenging behaviours should not be considered as depressive equivalents in individuals with intellectual disability. *J Intellect Disabil Res* 2003 Jan; 47(Pt 1):14-21.

125. Wilhelm S, Keuthen NJ, Deckersbach T, et al, Self-injurious skin picking: clinical characteristics and co-morbidity. *J Clin Psychiatry* 1999 Jul; 60 (7):454-9.

126. Rennie D, Fontanarosa PB. Theme issue on access to health care. *JAMA* 2006; 295:2182-2183.

127. Holahan J, Cook A. Changes in economic conditions and health insurance coverage, 2000-2004 [Epub ahead of print]. *Health Aff* (Millwood). 2005;W5:498-508.

Look-a-Likes
(Undiagnosed and Misdiagnosed Medical Conditions)

128. Milas M, Bush RL, Lin P, et al. Calciphylaxis and nonhealing wounds: the role of the vascular surgeon in a multidisciplinary treatment. *J Vasc Surg* 2003 Mar; 37(3):501-7.

129. Basile C, Montanaro A, Masi M, et al, Hyperbaric oxygen therapy for calcific uremic arteriolopathy: a case series. *J Nephrol* 2002 Nov-Dec; 15(6):676-80.

130. Kirsner RS, Spencer J, Falanga V, et al, Squamous cell carcinoma arising in osteomyelitis and chronic wounds. Treatment with Mohs micrographic surgery vs amputation. *Dermatol Surg* 1996 Dec; 22(12):1015-8.

131. Trent JT, Kirsner RS. Wounds and malignancy. *Adv Skin Wound Care* 2003 Jan-Feb; 16(1):31-4.

132. Wines N, Wines M, Byman W. Understanding Pyoderma Gangrenosum: A Review. June 27, 2001 *Medscape General Medicine* 3(2), 2001. © 2001 Medscape Portals, Inc.

Everyday Care Issues

133. Pribitkin ED, Boger G. Herbal therapy: what every facial plastic surgeon must know. *Arch Facial Plast Surg* 2001 Apr-Jun; 3(2):127-32.

Rheumatologic Diseases

134. Yocum D. Sharpe J. Maini RN. et al. Structural Damage in Rheumatoid Arthritis, Feb 20, 2001: *Medscape.com*. Copyright at Arizona Board of Regents for the University of Arizona College of Medicine.

135. Öien RF; Håkansson A.; Hansen BU. Leg ulcers in patients with rheumatoid arthritis a prospective study of aetiology, wound healing and pain reduction after pinch grafting. *Rheumatology* 2001; 40: 816-820 © 2001 British Society for Rheumatology.

REVIEW QUESTIONS

1.) One Glitch Sampler is
   a. A mnemonic assessment tool
   b. An antibiotic
   c. A nutritional supplement
   d. An administrative oversight

2.) A chronic wound is characterized by all of the following EXCEPT:
   a. Inadequate granulation tissue
   b. Persistent wound exudates
   c. Deficient wound contraction
   d. Absence of neo-epithelialization
   e. Fails to progress

3.) Which of the following statements about serum prealbumin levels is FALSE?
   a. It is most helpful for an initial overall screen of nutritional status.
   b. It reflects protein intake over the past several days.
   c. It is altered by the patients; hydration status.
   d. It is best used in the outpatient setting to monitor changes once protein replacement has begun.

4.) Optimal wound healing is achieved by all the following EXCEPT:
   a. Keeping the wound dry
   b. Minimizing the effect of co-morbid diseases
   c. Providing adequate oxygenation
   d. Reducing the bio-burden
   e. Ensuring adequate nutrition for the wound to heal

5.) Treatments selected to heal the wound should be uncomplicated methods of cleansing, dressings, debriding medication, anitbiotic medication, or devices that the patient or his/her caretaker can easily apply.
   a. True
   b. False

Answers: 1a, 2e, 3a, 4a, 5a

BIOCHEMISTRY OF WOUND HEALING IN WOUND CARE PRACTICE

CHAPTER TWO OVERVIEW

Biochemistry of Wound Healing in Wound Care Practice

Gloria A. Chin, Gregory S. Schultz, Robert F. Diegelmann, Nasser Chegini

INTRODUCTION

Normal healing of acute skin wounds proceeds through four distinct, but overlapping phases that can be described as hemostasis, inflammation, proliferation and remodeling (Figure 1). Multiple types of specialized cells participate in these phases including platelets, neutrophils, macrophages, fibroblasts, epithelial and vascular endothelial cells. The actions of these cells are regulated by a relatively small number of key proteins, perhaps less than 50 that include cytokines, chemokines, growth factors, receptors, proteases, and their inhibitors. Thus, as healing progresses through the sequential stages, the patterns of regulatory proteins and the actions of the wound cells change. Eventually, the damaged skin tissue is repaired with scar tissue that approximates the original architecture and functions of normal skin. Therefore, the key to influencing wound healing at the bedside is to understand and utilize the basic cellular and molecular principles that regulate healing.

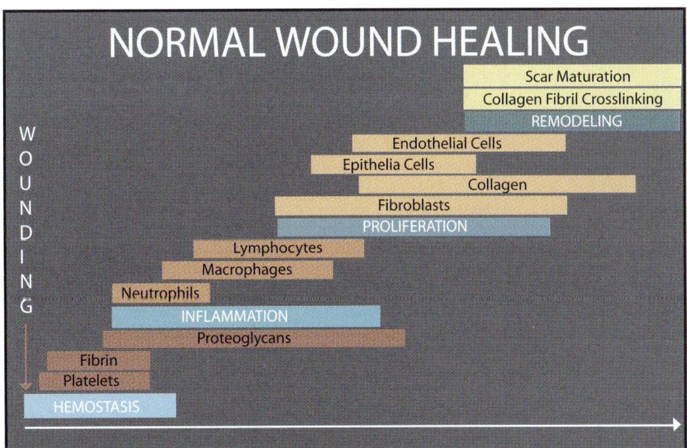

Figure 1. Phases of normal wound healing. Cellular and molecular events of normal wound healing progress through four major, integrated, phases of hemostasis, inflammation, proliferation and remodeling (Reprinted with permission).

PHASES OF ACUTE WOUND HEALING
Hemostasis
Blood clotting

The process of hemostasis begins immediately following a skin injury that extends into the dermis. The clotting cascade is rapidly triggered when inactive proteases in plasma (factors VII and X of the extrinsic pathway and factors XI and XII of the intrinsic pathway) contact extracellular matrix (ECM) components (i.e., type I collagen) that are exposed when tissues are damaged. The proteases become activated, and in a series of proteolytic activation steps, activate prothrombin to thrombin, which proteolytically activates fibrinogen to fibrin. The fibrin molecules self assemble into a large polymer network that entraps red blood cells and platelets, forming a plug in the wound that blocks flow from blood vessels. Capillary endothelial cells and vascular smooth muscle cells in damaged vessels contract, which further reduces blood flow through vasoconstriction.

TABLE 1. MAJOR GROWTH FACTOR FAMILIES

Growth Factor Family	Cell Source	Actions
Transforming Growth Factor B TGF-b1, TGF-b2, TGF-b3	Platelets Fibroblasts Macrophages	Fibroblast Chemotaxis and Activation ECM Deposition • Collagen Synthesis • TIMP Synthesis • MMP Synthesis Reduces Scarring • Collagen • Fibronectin
Platelet Derived Growth Factor PDGF-AA, PDGF-BB, VEGF	Platelets Macrophages Keratinocytes Fibroblasts	Activation of Immune Cells and Fibroblasts ECM Deposition • Collagen Synthesis • TIMP Synthesis • MMP Synthesis Angiogenesis
Fibroblast Growth Factor Acidic FGF, Basic FGF, KGF	Macrophages Endothelial Cells Fibroblasts	Angiogenesis Endothelial Cell Activation Keratinocyte Proliferation and Migration ECM Deposition
Insulin-like Growth Factor IGF-I, IGF-II, Insulin	Liver Skeletal Muscle Fibroblasts Macrophages Neutrophils	Keratinocyte Proliferation Fibroblast Proliferation Endothelial Cell Activation Angiogenesis • Collagen Synthesis ECM Deposition Cell Metabolism
Epidermal Growth Factor EGF, HB-EGF, TGF-a, Amphiregulin, Betacellulin	Keratinocytes Macrophages	Keratinocyte Proliferation and Migration ECM Deposition
Connective Tissue Growth Factor CTGF	Fibroblasts Endothelial Cells Epithelial Cells	Mediates Action of TGF-bs on Collagen Synthesis

Platelet degranulation

As platelets become entrapped in the fibrin network of the blood clot, they are stimulated to release the contents of their granules. Contained in the alpha granules are high concentrations of numerous growth factors, including platelet derived growth factor (PDGF), transforming growth factor beta (TGF-b), transforming growth factor alpha (TGF-a), basic fibroblast growth factor (bFGF), and vascular endothelial growth factor (VEGF) (1–7) (Table 1). PDGF and TGF-b are chemotactic for neutrophils and monocytes and recruit them from the vasculature to initiate the inflammatory response. VEGF, bFGF, and TGF-a stimulate endothelial cells to initiate angiogenesis. PDGF is also chemotactic for fibroblasts, which migrate toward the wound from uninjured tissue around the wound and begin synthesizing new collagen. Thus, platelets provide an immediate supply of growth factors that are released in the wound site and initiate key cellular responses in the phases of wound healing.

Provisional wound matrix

The fibrin clot that forms at the site of an injury is necessary to stop bleeding. However, it plays other important roles in wound healing by serving as the provisional wound matrix. As fibroblasts migrate from the collagen-rich matrix of normal dermis surrounding the wound into the fibrin-rich provisional wound matrix in response to the chemotactic growth factors released by platelets, their integrin receptors detect the change in ECM environment (Figure 2). The integrin receptors then generate new intracellular signals that cause the fibroblasts to stop migrating, in combination with growth factors in the provisional wound matrix, stimulate the fibroblasts to begin proliferating and synthesizing new collagen and other ECM components. Initially, activated wound fibroblasts predominately synthesize type III collagen, which is slowly replaced over weeks and months by type I collagen molecules that are found in normal skin and mature scar. Thus, the fibrin-rich provisional wound matrix is much more than an inert scaffold in which scar tissue is deposited. It acts as a reservoir to help trap growth factors and it actively signals fibroblasts, epidermal cells and vascular endothelial cells via their integrin receptors to transform into activated wound cells that will repair the injury.

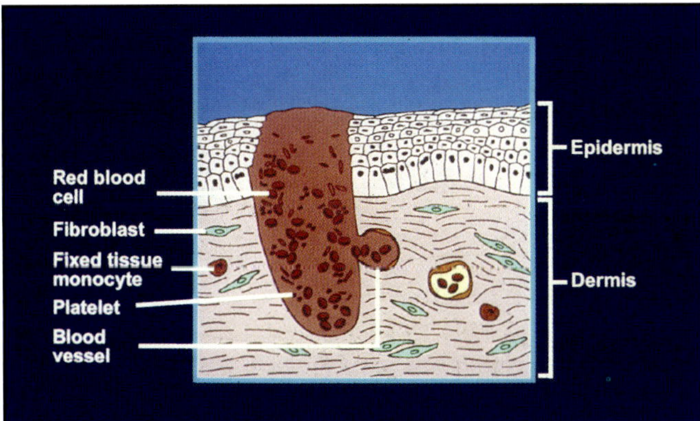

Figure 2. Hemostasis Phase. At the time of injury, the fibrin clot forms the provisional wound matrix and platelets release multiple growth factors that initiate the repair process (Reprinted with permission).

Inflammation
Chemokines

Inflammation begins within 24 hours after injury and can last for up to two weeks in normal wounds. All the major types of white cells in blood (mast cells, neutrophils, macrophages, T and B lymphocytes) may become involved in wound inflammation. Chemokines, cytokines and growth factors can all regulate important aspects of wound inflammation (1–7). Chemokines, named from a contraction of chemoattractive cytokine, are the newest type of these regulatory molecules. In general, chemokines have two primary functions: 1) they regulate the trafficking of leukocyte populations during normal health and development, and 2) they direct the recruitment and activation of neutrophils, lymphocytes, macrophages, eosinophils, and basophils during inflammation. The structural and functional similarities among chemokine molecules were not initially appreciated, and this led to an idiosyncratic nomenclature consisting of many acronyms that were based on their biological functions, their source for isolation, or their biochemical properties. For example, monocyte chemoattractant protein 1 (MCP-1) and macrophage inflammatory protein 1 (MIP-1) were named on biological functions, whereas platelet factor 4 (PF-4) was named for its source of isolation. *Interferon-Inducible Protein* of 10 kDa (IP-10) and *Regulated Upon Activation Normal T-cell Expressed* and *Secreted* (RANTES) were named for their biochemical properties. As the biochemical structures of different chemokines were established, it was recognized that the approximately 40 chemokines could be grouped into four major classes based on the pattern of cysteine residues located near the N-terminus. In fact, there has been a recent trend to re-establish a more organized nomenclature system based on these four major classes, as shown in Table 2.

TABLE 2. CHEMOKINE FAMILIES INVOLVED IN WOUND HEALING

Chemokines	Cell Affected
a-CHEMOKINES (CXC) with glutamic acid-leucine-arginine near the N-terminal Interleukin-8 (IL-8)	Neutrophils
a-CHEMOKINES (CXC) without glutamic acid-leucine-arginine near the N-termal Interferon-inducible protein of 10kd (IP-10) Monokine induced by interferon-g (MIG) Stromal-cell-derived factor 1 (SDF-1)	Activated T lymphocytes
b-CHEMOKINES (CC) Monocyte chemoattractant proteins (MCPs): MCP-1,-2,-3,-4,-5 Regulated upon activation normal T-cell expressed and secrete (RANTES) Macrophage inflammatory protein (MIP-1a) Eotaxin	Eosinophils Basophils Monocytes Activated T lymphocytes
g-CHEMOKINES (C) Lymphotactin	Resting T lymphocytes
d-CHEMOKINES (CXXXC) Fractalkine	Natural killer cells

Cytokines

Cytokines are small polypeptides that were initially identified due to their powerful action on chemotaxis, proliferation and differentiation of inflammatory cells. It is now recognized, however, that cytokines also have important actions on non-inflammatory wound cells such as fibroblasts, epithelial cells and vascular endothelial cells. For example, IL-1a and TNFa stimulate production of proteases by fibroblasts, and TNFa induces apoptosis of epithelial cells. Nevertheless, cytokines are major signaling molecules in the immune system.

To understand the actions of cytokines in inflammation and wound healing, it is helpful to review the basic immunobiology of inflammation. As shown in Figure 3, there are two basic types of inflammatory cell responses: the humoral-mediated response (antibody), and the cell-mediated response. The cellular response involves two major subtypes of cells: the helper T-cells (TH) and cytotoxic T-cells (TC). The cytokines that regulate the humoral and cell mediated responses are grouped into two classes, designated as TH1 and TH2 cytokines. TH1 cytokines, such as IL-2, INF-gamma, and TNF-a are generally expressed after a viral infection, and they a promote TC response. When a virus infects a cell, the viral proteins are digested by enzymes in the cell and are presented with the major histocompatibility complex (MHC) proteins on the cell's surface. The viral peptide/MHC complex is recognized by TH and TC cells, the TH cells secrete TH1 cytokines, which stimulate macrophages and neutrophils to kill the infected cells, thus limiting viral replication and spreading of the infection.

The TH2 cytokines, including IL-4, IL-5, and IL-10, are synthesized by TH2 cells, and are generally expressed after a bacterial infection. The TH2 cytokines promote the synthesis of antibodies by activating B-cells. The antibodies bind to the bacteria and target them for destruction by phagocytic cells, thus limiting the bacterial infection.

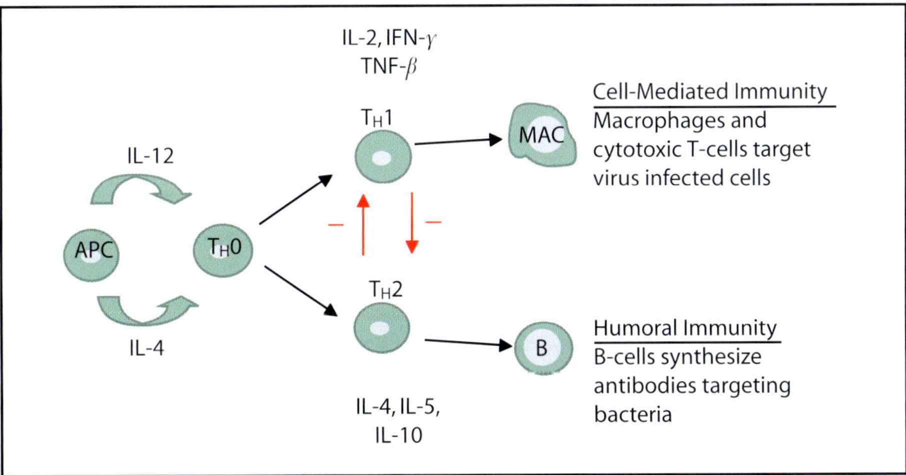

Figure 3. TH1 and TH2 Cytokine Regulation of Cellular and Humoral Immune Responses. TH1 cytokines stimulate cellular inflammation to limit viral infections, while TH2 cytokines stimulate humoral inflammation (antibody) to control bacterial infections. In addition, TH1 and TH2 cytokines are cross-regulatory, i.e., TH1 cytokines down regulate TH2 cytokines, and TH2 cytokines down regulate TH1 cytokines (Reprinted with permission).

Another important property of TH1 and TH2 cytokines is that they are cross-regulatory: TH1 cytokines tend to suppress antibody production, and TH2 cytokines tend to suppress the cellular response. For example, IL-10 is a TH2 cytokines that is produced at high levels during a bacterial infection, and it reduces synthesis of TH1 cytokines by TH1 cells, thereby reducing cell-mediated inflammation. IL-12, which is produced by TH1 cells, promotes differentiation of immature T-cells (TH0) into TH1 cells when they are presented a viral antigen by an antigen presenting cell (APC). Increased numbers of TH1 cells increases synthesis of TH1 cytokines at the expense of TH2 cytokines. Table 3 lists cytokines that have important actions in wound healing and some of their biochemical properties.

TABLE 3. CYTOKINES INVOLVED IN WOUND HEALING

Cytokine	Cell Source	Biological Activity
Pro-Inflammatory Cytokines		
TNF-a	Macrophages	PMN margination and cytotoxicity, ± collagen synthesis; provides metabolic substrate
IL-1	Macrophages Keratinocytes	Fibroblast and keratinocyte chemotaxis, collagen synthesis
IL-2	T lymphocytes	Increases fibroblast infiltration and metabolism
IL-6	Macrophages PMNs Fibroblasts	Fibroblast proliferation, hepatic acute-phase protein synthesis
IL-8	Macrophages Fibroblasts	Macrophage and PMN chemotaxis, keratinocyte maturation
IFN-g	T lymphocytes Macrophages	Macrophage and PMN activation; retards collagen synthesis and cross-linking; stimulates collagenase activity
Anti-Inflammatory Cytokines		
IL-4	T lymphocytes Basophils Mast cells	Inhibition of TNF, IL-1, IL-6 production; fibroblast proliferation, collagen synthesis
IL-10	T lymphocytes Macrophages Keratinocytes	Inhibition of TNF, IL-1, IL-6 production; inhibits macrophage and PMN activation

Neutrophils

Neutrophils are the first inflammatory cells to respond to the soluble mediators released by platelets and the coagulation cascade. They serve as the first line of defense against infection by phagocytosing and killing bacteria, and by removing foreign materials and devitalized tissue. During the process of extravasation of inflammatory cells into a wound, important interactions occur between adhesion molecules (selectins, cell adhesion molecules (CAMs) and cadherins) and receptors (integrins) that are associated with the plasma membranes of circulating leukocytes and vascular endothelial cells (8, 9). Initially, leukocytes weakly adhere to the endothelial cell walls via their selectin molecules which causes them to decelerate and begin to roll on the surface of endothelial cells. While rolling, leukocytes can become activated by chemoattractants (chemokines, cytokines, growth factors or bacterial products). After activation, leukocytes firmly adhere to endothelial cells as a result of the binding between their integrin receptors and ligands such as VCAM and ICAM that are expressed on activated endothelial cells. Chemotactic signals present outside the venule then induce leukocytes to squeeze between endothelial cells of the venule and migrate into the wounded tissue using their integrin receptors to recognize and bind to extracellular matrix components. The inflammatory cells release elastase and collagenase to help them migrate through the endothelial cell basement membrane and to migrate into the ECM at the site of the wound. Neutrophils also produce and release inflammatory mediators such as TNF-a and IL-1 that further recruit and activate fibroblasts and epithelial cells. After the neutrophils migrate into the wound site, they generate oxygen free radicals, which kill phagocytized bacteria, and they release high levels of matrix metalloproteinases (MMPs) proteases. These proteases include neutrophil elastase and neutrophil collagenase (MMP-8) which remove components of the extracellular matrix that were damaged by the injury. The persistent presence of bacteria in a wound may contribute to chronicity through continued recruitment of neutrophils and their release of proteases, cytokines and reactive oxygen species. Usually neutrophils are depleted in the wound after 2–3 days by the process of apoptosis, and they are replaced by tissue monocytes.

Macrophages

Activated macrophages play pivotal roles in the regulation of healing, and the healing process does not proceed normally without macrophages (10). Macrophages begin as circulating monocytes that are attracted to the wound site beginning about 24 hours after injury (Figure 4). They extravasate by the mechanism described for neutrophils, and are stimulated to differentiate into activated tissue macrophages in response to chemokines, cytokines, growth factors and soluble fragments of extracellular matrix components produced by proteolytic degradation of collagen and fibronectin. Similar to neutrophils, tissue macrophages have a dual role in the healing process. They patrol the wound area ingesting and killing bacteria, and removing devitalized tissue through the actions of secreted MMPs and elastase. Macrophages differ from neutrophils in their ability to more closely regulate the proteolytic destruction of wound tissue by secreting inhibitors for the proteases. As important as their phagocytic role, macrophages also mediate the transition from the inflammatory phase to the proliferative phase of healing. They release a wide variety of growth factors and cytokines including PDGF, TGF-b, TGF-a, FGF, IGF-1, TNFa, IL-1, and IL-6. Some of these soluble mediators recruit and activate fibroblasts, which will then synthesize, deposit, and organize the new tissue matrix, while others promote angiogenesis (11–14). The absence of neutrophils and a decrease in the number of macrophages in the wound is an indication that the inflammatory phase is nearing an end, and that the proliferative phase is beginning.

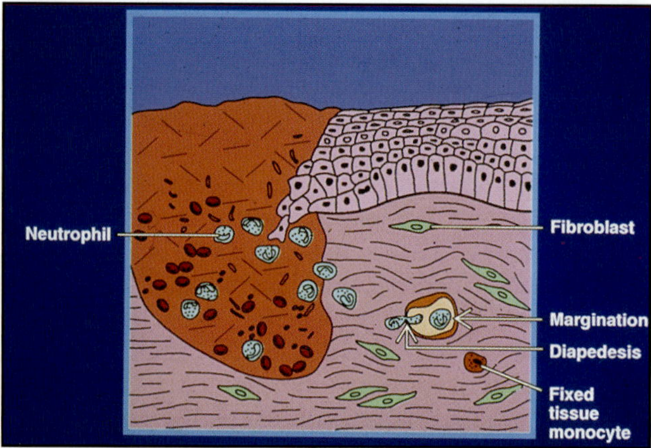

Figure 4. Inflammation Phase. Within a day following injury, the inflammatory phase is initiated by neutrophils that attach to endothelial cells in the vessel walls surrounding the wound (margination), change shape and move through the cell junctions (diapedesis), and migrate to the wound site (chemotaxis) (Reprinted with permission).

Proliferation

The final outcome of the proliferative phase is the replacement of the fibrin-rich provisional wound matrix with scar tissue that consists of new collagen fibers, proteoglycans, and elastin fibers that partially restore the structure and function of the tissue (Figure 5). This is accomplished by the migration, proliferation and differentiation of epithelial cells, dermal fibroblasts and vascular endothelial cells into the wound from uninjured tissue (15, 16).

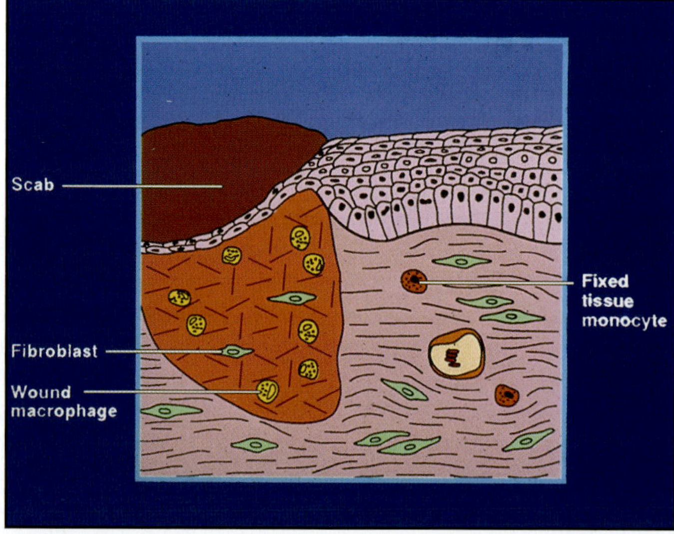

Figure 5. Proliferation Phase. Fixed tissue monocytes activate, move into the site of injury, transform into activated wound macrophages that kill bacteria, release proteases that remove denatured ECM, and secrete growth factors that stimulate fibroblast, epidermal cells and endothelial cells to proliferate and produce scar tissue (Reprinted with permission).

Fibroblast migration

Fibroblasts in normal dermis are typically quiescent and sparsely distributed, whereas in the provisional wound matrix and in granulation tissue, they are numerous and are quite active synthetically. Fibroblasts migrate into the wound in response to several soluble cytokines and growth factors that are released initially from platelets when they degranulate, and later by macrophages in the wound. These include PDGF, TGF-b and bFGF. The direction of fibroblast movement is determined by the concentration gradient of chemotactic factors, and by the alignment of the fibrils in the ECM and provisional matrix. Fibroblasts tend to migrate along these fibrils as opposed to across them. Fibroblasts begin moving by first binding to matrix components such as collagen, fibronectin, vitronectin and fibrin via their cell surface integrin receptors. Integrin receptors bind to specific amino acid sequences (such as arginine-glycine-aspartic acid or R-G-D) or carbohydrates that are part of the matrix proteins. While one end of the fibroblast remains bound to the matrix component, the cell extends a cytoplasmic projection to find another binding site. When the next site is found, the attachment to the original site is broken, apparently by local protease activity, and the cell uses its cytoskeleton network of actin fibers to pull itself forward. The MMPs are essential for migration of cells through the ECM. The most important of these MMPs are: collagenase (MMP-1), which cut intact collagen at a single site; gelatinases (MMP-2 and MMP-9) which degrade gelatin substrates; and stromelysin (MMP-3) which degrades multiple protein substrates in the ECM.

Synthesis of scar matrix

After the fibroblasts have migrated into the fibrin-rich provisional wound matrix, they proliferate and begin synthesizing new collagen, proteoglycans and other components that comprise granulation tissue. PDGF and TGF-b are two of the most important growth factors that regulate fibroblast activity. PDGF, which originates predominantly from platelets and macrophages, stimulates several fibroblast functions including migration, proliferation, and collagen expression. TGF-b, also secreted by platelets and macrophages, appears to be the dominant regulatory signal for extracellular matrix deposition. TGF-b increases the overall production of matrix proteins by stimulating transcription of collagen, proteoglycan and fibronectin genes. At the same time, TGF-b down-regulates the synthesis of MMPs, which break down the ECM components, and also stimulates synthesis of tissue inhibitors of metalloproteinases (TIMPs), which further prevent breakdown of the new matrix. Recent data indicate that a new growth factor, named connective tissue growth factor (CTGF), mediates many of the effects of TGF-b on the synthesis of extra-cellular matrix.

Different types ECM components must be synthesized to repair the damaged matrix, and the molecular composition of the initial scar ECM is not identical to normal dermis. Type III collagen is initially synthesized at high levels and is slowly replaced by type I collagen molecules as the scar matrix matures. Other types of specialized collagen molecules are synthesized to replace damaged structures such as the basement membrane of the epidermis. Unlike the straight rod-like shape of types I and III collagen that assemble to form fibers in dermis, type IV collagen molecules are bent, which causes them to assemble into a planar, chicken wire-like web like structure that is the major component of the basement membranes. Type VII collagen molecules form tail-to-tail dimmers that anchor epidermal cells to the basement membrane. Other ECM components that must be replaced include laminin, tenascin, elastin and multiple types of proteoglycans and glycosaminoglycans.

Synthesis of functional collagen molecules and their organization into fibrils involves multiple steps. After transcription and splicing of collagen mRNA, it associates with ribosomes on the endoplasmic reticulum where the new collagen chains are synthesized. During this process, hydroxylation of proline and lysine residues occurs. Hydroxylation of proline is important because it plays a major role in stabilizing the triple helical conformation of collagen molecules. Three collagen chains associate and begin to form the characteristic triple helical structure of the fibrillar collagen molecule, and the nascent chains undergo further modification by the process of glycosylation. Fully hydroxylated collagen has a higher melting temperature. When levels of hydroxyproline are low, which occurs in vitamin C-deficient conditions (scurvy), the collagen triple helix has an altered structure and denatures (unwinds) at lower temperatures. To ensure optimal wound healing, wound care specialists should be sure patients are receiving good nutritional support with a diet with ample protein and vitamin C.

Finally, procollagen molecules are secreted into the extracellular space where they undergo further processing by proteolytic cleavage of the short, non-helical segments at the N- and C-termini. The collagen molecules then spontaneously associate in a head-to-tail and side-by-side arrangement forming collagen fibrils, which associate into larger bundles that form collagen fibers. In the extra-cellular spaces an important enzyme, lysyl oxidase, acts on the collagen molecules to form stable, covalent, cross-links. As the collagen matures and becomes older, more and more of these intramolecular and intermolecular cross-links are placed in the molecules. This important cross-linking step gives collagen its strength and stability, and the older the collagen the more cross-link formation has occurred.

Dermal collagen on a per weight basis approaches the tensile strength of steel. In normal tissue, it is a strong molecule and highly organized into a basket-weave pattern. In contrast, collagen fibers that form in scar tissue are much smaller and have a more random orientation. Scar tissue is always weaker and will break apart before the surrounding normal tissue. During the early phases of scar formation, the collagen molecules tend to be arranged in bundles that are orientated parallel to the edges of the wound rather than the more complex basket weave pattern of collagen bundles that is characteristic of normal dermis. As the initial scar tissue remodels over many months, the architecture and composition of the scar matrix begins to resemble non-wounded skin, but never fully regenerates non-wounded ECM.

Angiogenesis

Ischemia is a major impediment to healing of injured tissue. The process of angiogenesis is stimulated by local factors of the microenvironment including low oxygen tension, low pH, and high lactate levels. Also, certain soluble mediators are potent angiogenic signals for endothelial cells. Many of these are produced by epidermal cells, fibroblasts, vascular endothelial cells and macrophages, and include bFGF, TGF-b, and VEGF. It is now recognized that oxygen levels in tissues directly regulate angiogenesis by interacting with oxygen sensing proteins that regulate transcription of angiogenic and anti-angiogenic genes. For example, synthesis of VEGF by capillary endothelial cells is directly increased by hypoxia through the activation of the recently identified transcription factor, hypoxia-inducible factor (HIF), which binds oxygen. When oxygen levels surrounding capillary endothelial cells drop, levels of HIF increase inside the cells. HIF-1 binds to specific DNA sequences and stimulates transcription of specific genes such as VEGF that promote angiogenesis (13). When oxygen levels in wound tissue increase, oxygen binds to HIF, leading to the destruction of HIF molecules in cells and decreased synthesis of angiogenic factors. Regulation of angiogenesis involves both stimulatory factors like VEGF and anti-angiogenic factors like angiostatin, endostatin, thrombospondin, and pigment epithelium-derived factor (PEDF).

The cells that form the new capillaries have been assumed to arise from the pre-existing capillary endothelial cells, and it is clear from animal experiments that angiogenic factors cause endothelial cells of the capillaries adjacent to an ischemic site to begin to migrate into the matrix and proliferate, forming buds or sprouts. However, new data suggest that some of the cells that form new capillaries actually come from bone marrow stem cells, called hemangioblasts, that circulate in the blood stream. When an injury or ischemia occurs and angiogenic factors are released, the hemangioblasts migrate into the ECM and differentiate into capillary endothelial cells (14). Once again the migration of these cells into the matrix requires the local secretion of proteolytic enzymes, especially MMPs. As the tip of the sprouts extend from endothelial cells and encounter another sprout, they develop a cleft that subsequently becomes the lumen of the evolving vessel and complete a new vascular loop. This process continues until the capillary system is sufficiently repaired and the tissue oxygenation and metabolic needs are met. It is these new capillary tuffs that give granulation tissue its characteristic bumpy or granular appearance.

Granulation tissue and contraction

Dermal wounds that remain open typically fill in by a combination of granulation tissue formation and contraction. Granulation tissue is a transitional replacement for normal dermis, which eventually matures into a scar during the remodeling phase of healing. It differs from unwounded dermis by having an extremely dense network of blood vessels and capillaries, a high density of fibroblasts and macrophages, and randomly organized collagen fibers. It also has an elevated metabolic rate compared to normal dermis, which reflects the activity required for cellular migration and division and protein synthesis. Contraction is the movement of tissue toward the center of the wound. It is produced by highly differentiated cells called myofibroblasts that arise from the dermal fibroblasts. Growth factors, including TGF-b, CTGF, or PDGF stimulate the transformation of fibroblasts into myofibroblasts by inducing fibroblasts to synthesize large amounts of the contractile protein called alpha smooth muscle actin. The myofibroblasts then attach to the ECM by their integrin receptors, and contract the matrix as they generate intracellular forces with the alpha smooth muscle actin.

Epithelialization

Epithelialization is the process where epithelial cells around the margin of the wound or in residual skin appendages, such as hair follicles, sweat glands, and sebaceous glands, proliferate and migrate onto the wound surface and differentiate into a multilayered epidermis (15). The normal, intact, mature epidermis consists of 5 layers of differentiated epithelial cells ranging from the cuboidal basal keratinocytes nearest the dermis up to the flattened, hexagonal, terminally differentiated cells filled with keratin in the uppermost layer. Only the basal epithelial cells are capable of proliferation. These basal cells are normally attached to their neighboring cells by intercellular structures called desmosomes and to the basement membrane by hemi-desmosomes. When growth factors such as EGF, TGF-a, and keratinocyte growth factor (KGF) are released during the healing process, they bind to receptors on epithelial cells and stimulate migration and proliferation. The binding of the growth factors triggers the desmosomes and hemi-desmosomes to dissolve so the cells can detach in preparation for migration. New types of integrin receptors are then expressed by the basal cells, and the normally cuboidal basal epithelial cells flatten in shape and begin to migrate as a monolayer over the newly deposited granulation tissue, following along collagen fibers. Proliferation of the basal epithelial cells near the wound margin supply new cells to the advancing monolayer apron of cells (cells that are actively migrating are incapable of proliferation). Epithelial cells in the leading edge of the monolayer produce and secrete proteolytic enzymes (MMPs) which enable the cells to penetrate scab, surface necrosis, or eschar. Migration continues until the epithelial cells contact other advancing cells to form a confluent sheet. Once this contact has been made, the entire epithelial monolayer enters a proliferative mode and the stratified layers of the epidermis are re-established and begin to mature to restore barrier function. TGF-b is one growth factor that can speed up the maturation (differentiation and keratinization) of the epidermal layers. The intercellular desmosomes and the hemi-desmosome attachments to the newly formed basement membrane are also re-established. Epithelialization is the clinical hallmark of healing but it is not the final event—remodeling of the granulation tissue is yet to occur.

Remodeling

Remodeling is the final phase of the healing process in which the granulation tissue matures into scar and tissue tensile strength is increased (Figure 6). The maturation of granulation tissue also involves a reduction in the number of capillaries via aggregation into larger vessels and a decrease in the amount of glycosaminoglycans and the water associated with the GAGs and proteoglycans. Cell density and metabolic activity in the granulation tissue decrease during maturation. Changes also occur in the type, amount, and organization of collagen, which enhance tensile strength. Initially, type III collagen was synthesized at high levels, but it becomes replaced by type I collagen, the dominant fibrillar collagen in skin. The tensile strength of a newly epithelialized wound is only about 25% of normal tissue. Healed or repaired tissue is never as strong as normal tissues that have never been wounded. Tissue tensile strength is enhanced primarily by the reorganization of collagen fibers

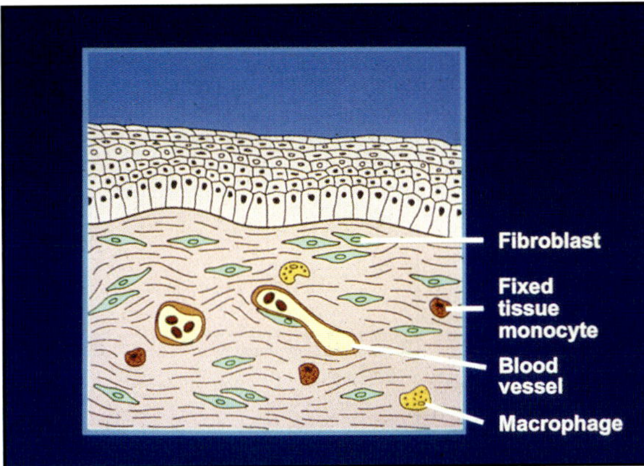

Figure 6. Remodeling Phase. The initial, disorganized scar tissue is slowly replaced by a matrix that more closely resembles the organized ECM of normal skin (Reprinted with permission).

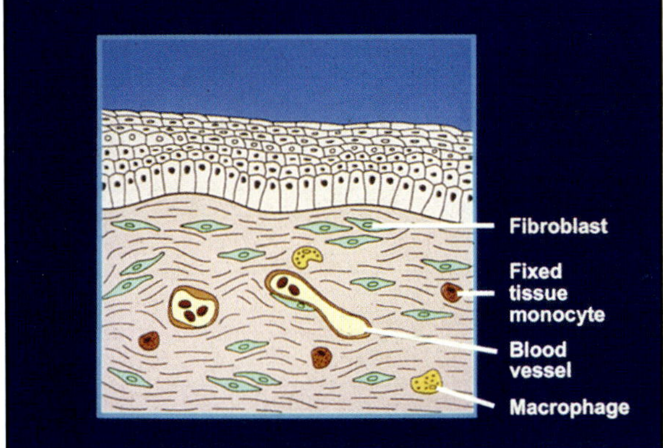

Figure 7. Mature Scar. The final mature scar contains ECM that resembles normal dermis, but only reaches 80% of normal skin tensile strength and is devoid of specialized structures such as hair follicles (Reprinted with permission).

that were deposited randomly during granulation and increased covalent cross-linking of collagen molecules by the enzyme, lysyl oxidase, which is secreted into the ECM by fibroblasts. Over several months or more, changes in collagen organization in the repaired tissue will slowly increase the tensile strength to a maximum of about 80% of normal tissue (Figure 7).

Remodeling of the extracellular matrix proteins occurs through the actions of several different classes of proteolytic enzymes produced by cells in the wound bed at different times during the healing process. Two of the most important families are the MMPs and serine proteases (Table 4). Specific MMP proteases that are necessary for wound healing are the collagenases (which degrade intact fibrillar collagen molecules), the gelatinases (which degrade damaged fibrillar collagen molecules) and the stromelysins (which very effectively degrade proteoglycans). An important serine protease is neutrophil elastase which can degrade almost all types of protein molecules. Under normal conditions, the destructive actions of the proteolytic enzymes are tightly regulated by specific enzyme inhibitors, which are also produced by cells in the wound bed. The specific inhibitors of the MMPs are the tissue inhibitors of metalloproteinases (TIMPs) and specific inhibitors of serine protease are a 1-protease inhibitor (a 1-PI) and a 2 macroglobulin.

TABLE 4. MATRIX METALLOPROTEINASES AND TISSUE INHIBITORS OF METALLOPROTEINASES

Protein	Pseudonym	Substrates
MMP-1	Interstitial Collagenase Fibroblast Collagenase	Type I, II, III, VII, and X Collagens
MMP-2	72 kDa Gelatinase Gelatinase A Type IV Collagenase	Type IV, V, VII, and X Collagens
MMP-3	Stomelysin-1	Type III, IV, IX, and X Collagens Type I, III, IV, and V Gelatins Fibronectin, Laminin and Pro-Collagenase
MMP-7	Matrilysin Uterine Metalloproteinase	Type I, III, IV, and V Gelatins Casein, Fibronectin and Pro-Collagenase
MMP-8	Neutrophil Collagense	Type I, II, and III Collagens
MMP-9	Type I, II, III Collagens	Type IV and V Collagens Type I and V Gelatins
MMP-10	Stromelysin-2	Type III, IV, V, IX, and X Collagens Type I, III, and IV Gelatins Fibronectin, Laminin and Pro-Collagenase
MMP-11	Stromelysin-3	Not Determined
MMP-12	Macrophage Metalloelastase	Soluble and Insoluble Elastin
MT-MMP-1	Membrane Type MMP-1	PRO-MMP-2
MT-MMP-2	Membrane Type MMP-2	Not Determined
TIMP-1	Tissue Inhibitor of Metalloproteinases-1	Collagenases
TIMP-2	Tissue Inhibitor of Metalloproteinases-2	Tissue Inhibitor of Metalloproteinases-2
TIMP-3	Tissue Inhibitor of Metalloproteinases-3	Collagenases

SUMMARY OF ACUTE WOUND HEALING
Four Phases of Wound Healing:
- Hemostasis—establishes the fibrin provisional wound matrix and platelets provide initial release of cytokines and growth factors in the wound
- Inflammation—mediated by neutrophils and macrophages remove bacteria and denatured matrix components that retard healing, and are the second source of growth factors and cytokines.

Prolonged, elevated inflammation retards healing due to excessive levels of proteases and reactive oxygen that destroy essential factors.

- Proliferation—fibroblasts, supported by new capillaries, proliferate and synthesize disorganized ECM and myofibroblasts contract scar. Basal epithelial cells proliferate and migrate over the granulation tissue to close the wound surface.
- Remodeling—fibroblast and capillary density decreases, and initial scar tissue is removed and replaced by ECM that is more similar to normal skin. ECM remodeling is the result of the balanced, regulated activity of proteases.

Cellular functions during the different phases of wound healing are regulated by key chemokines, cytokines, and growth factors. Cell actions are also influenced by interaction with components of the ECM through their integrin receptors and adhesion molecules. MMPs produced by epidermal cells, fibroblasts and vascular endothelial cells assist in migration of the cells, while proteolytic enzymes produced by neutrophils and macrophages remove denatured ECM components and assist in remodeling of initial scar tissue.

BIOCHEMICAL DIFFERENCES IN THE MOLECULAR ENVIRONMENTS OF HEALING AND CHRONIC WOUNDS

Chronic wounds all begin as acute wounds, but they fail to progress through the sequential phases of healing. The key question is why? Data from numerous animal and human studies now suggest that wounds fail to heal because molecular and cellular abnormalities develop in the wound due to prolonged inflammation. The result is a cascade of elevated levels of cytokines and proteases that result in decreased levels of growth factors and poorly responding wound cells.

The first major concept to emerge from analysis of wound fluids is that the molecular environments of chronic wounds have reduced mitogenic activity compared to the environments of acute wounds (16–20). Fluids collected from acute mastectomy wounds when added to cultures of normal human skin fibroblasts, keratinocytes or vascular endothelial cells, consistently stimulated DNA synthesis of the cultured cells. In contrast, addition of fluids collected from chronic leg ulcers typically did not stimulate DNA synthesis of the cells in culture. Also, when acute and chronic wound fluids were combined the mitotic activity of acute wound fluids was inhibited. Similar results were reported by several groups of investigators who also found that acute wound fluids promoted DNA synthesis while chronic wound fluids did not stimulate cell proliferation.

The second major concept to emerge from wound fluid analysis is the elevated levels of pro-inflammatory cytokines observed in chronic wounds as compared to the molecular environment of acute wounds (19, 20). The ratios of two key inflammatory cytokines, TNF a and IL-1 a, and their natural inhibitors, P55 and IL-1 receptor antagonist, in mastectomy fluids were significantly higher in mastectomy wound fluids than in chronic wound fluids. Trengove and colleagues (20) also reported high levels of the inflammatory cytokines IL-1, IL-6, and TNF a in fluids collected from venous ulcers of patients admitted to the hospital. More importantly, levels of the cytokines significantly decreased in fluids collected two weeks after the chronic ulcers had begun to heal. Harris and colleagues (19) also found cytokine levels were generally higher in wound fluids from non-healing ulcers than healing ulcers (20). These data suggest that chronic wounds typically have elevated levels of pro-inflammatory cytokines, and that the molecular environment changes to a less pro-inflammatory cytokine environment as chronic wounds begin to heal.

The third important concept that emerged from wound fluid analysis was the elevated levels of protease activity in chronic wounds compared to acute wounds (21–36). For example, the average level of protease activity in mastectomy fluids determined using the general MMP substrate, Azocoll, was low (0.75 μg collagenase equivalents/ml) with a range of 0.1–1.3 μg collagenase equivalents/ml. This suggests that protease activity is tightly controlled during the early phase of wound healing. In contrast, the average level of protease activity in chronic wound fluids (87 μg collagenase equivalents/ml) was approximately 116-fold higher (p < 0.05) than in mastectomy fluids. Also, the range of protease activity in chronic wound fluids is rather large (from 1–584 μg collagenase equivalents/ml). More importantly, the levels of protease activity decrease in chronic venous ulcers two weeks after the ulcers begin to heal. The Tissue Repair Laboratory in Richmond found ten-fold higher levels of MMP-2 protein, 25-fold higher levels of MMP-9 protein, and ten-fold higher collagenase activity in fluids from pressure ulcers compared to surgical wound fluids using gelatin zymography and cleavage of a radioactive collagen substrate. Other studies using immunohistochemical localization observed elevated levels of MMPs in granulation tissue of pressure ulcers along with elevated levels of neutrophil elastase and cathepsin-G. TIMP-1 levels were found to be decreased while MMP-2 and MMP-9 levels were increased in fluids from chronic venous ulcers compared to mastectomy wound fluids. Recently, Ladwig and colleagues (27) reported that the ratio of active MMP-9/TIMP-1 was closely correlated with healing outcome of pressure ulcers treated by a variety of protocols (27).

It is interesting to note that the major collagenase found in non-healing chronic pressure ulcers was MMP-8, the neutrophil-derived collagenase. Thus, the persistent influx of neutrophils releasing MMP-8 and elastase appears to be a major underlying mechanism resulting in tissue and growth factor destruction and thus impaired healing. This suggests that chronic inflammation must decrease if pressure ulcers are to heal.

Other classes of proteases also appear to be elevated in chronic wound fluids. It has been reported that fluids from skin graft donor sites or breast surgery patients contained intact a 1-antitrypsin, a potent inhibitor of serine proteases, very low levels of neutrophil elastase activity, and intact fibronectin. In contrast, fluids from the chronic venous ulcers contained degraded Alpha 1-antitrypsin, and ten-fold to 40-fold higher levels of neutrophil elastase activity, and degraded fibronectin. Chronic leg ulcers were also found to contain elevated MMP-2 and MMP-9, and that fibronectin degradation in chronic wounds was dependent on the relative levels of elastase, a1-proteinase inhibitor, and a2-macroglobulin.

Besides being implicated in degrading essential extracellular matrix components like fibronectin, proteases in chronic wound fluids also have been reported to degrade exogenous growth factors in vitro such as EGF, TGF-b, or

PDGF. In contrast, exogenous growth factors were stable in acute surgical wound fluids in vitro. Supporting this general concept of increased degradation of endogenous growth factors by proteases in chronic wounds, the average immunoreactive levels of some growth factors such as EGF, TGF-b, PDGF were found to be lower in chronic wound fluids than in acute wound fluids while PDGF-AB, TGF-b and IGF-1 were not lower.

Some chronic wounds may also be deficient in the TGF-b receptor, presumably due to degradation of the receptor by proteases.

In general, these results suggest that many chronic wounds contain elevated MMP and neutrophil elastase activities. The physiological implications of these data are that elevated protease activities in some chronic wounds may directly contribute to the failure of wounds to heal by degrading proteins which are necessary for wound healing such as extracellular matrix proteins, growth factors, their receptors and protease inhibitors.

BIOLOGICAL DIFFERENCES IN THE RESPONSE OF CHRONIC WOUND CELLS TO GROWTH FACTORS

The biochemical analyses of healing and chronic wound fluids and biopsies have suggested that there are important molecular differences in the wound environments. However, these data only indicate half of the picture.

The other essential component is the capacity of the wound cells to respond to cytokines and growth factors. Interesting new data are emerging which suggest that fibroblasts in skin ulcers which have failed to heal for many years may not be capable of responding to growth factors and divide as fibroblasts in healing wounds. Agren and colleagues (35) reported that fibroblasts from chronic venous leg ulcers grew to lower density than fibroblasts from acute wounds from uninjured dermis (35). Also, fibroblasts

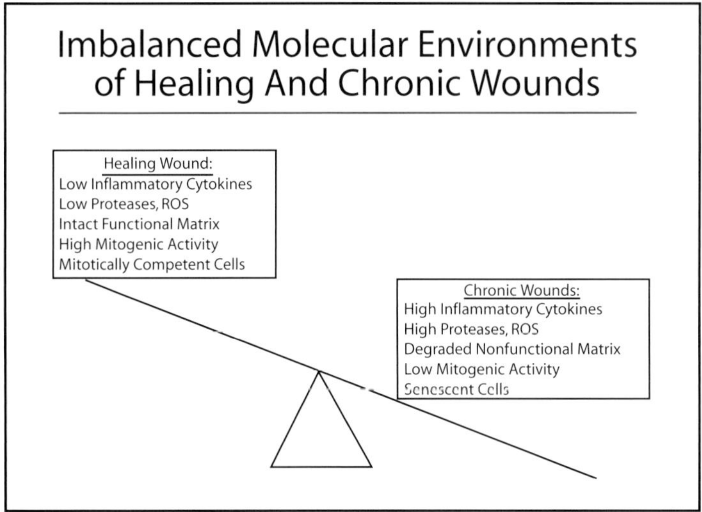

Figure 8. Comparison of the Molecular and Cellular Environments of Healing and Chronic Wounds. Elevated levels of cytokines and proteases in chronic wounds reduce mitogenic activities and response of wound cells, impairing healing (Reprinted with permission).

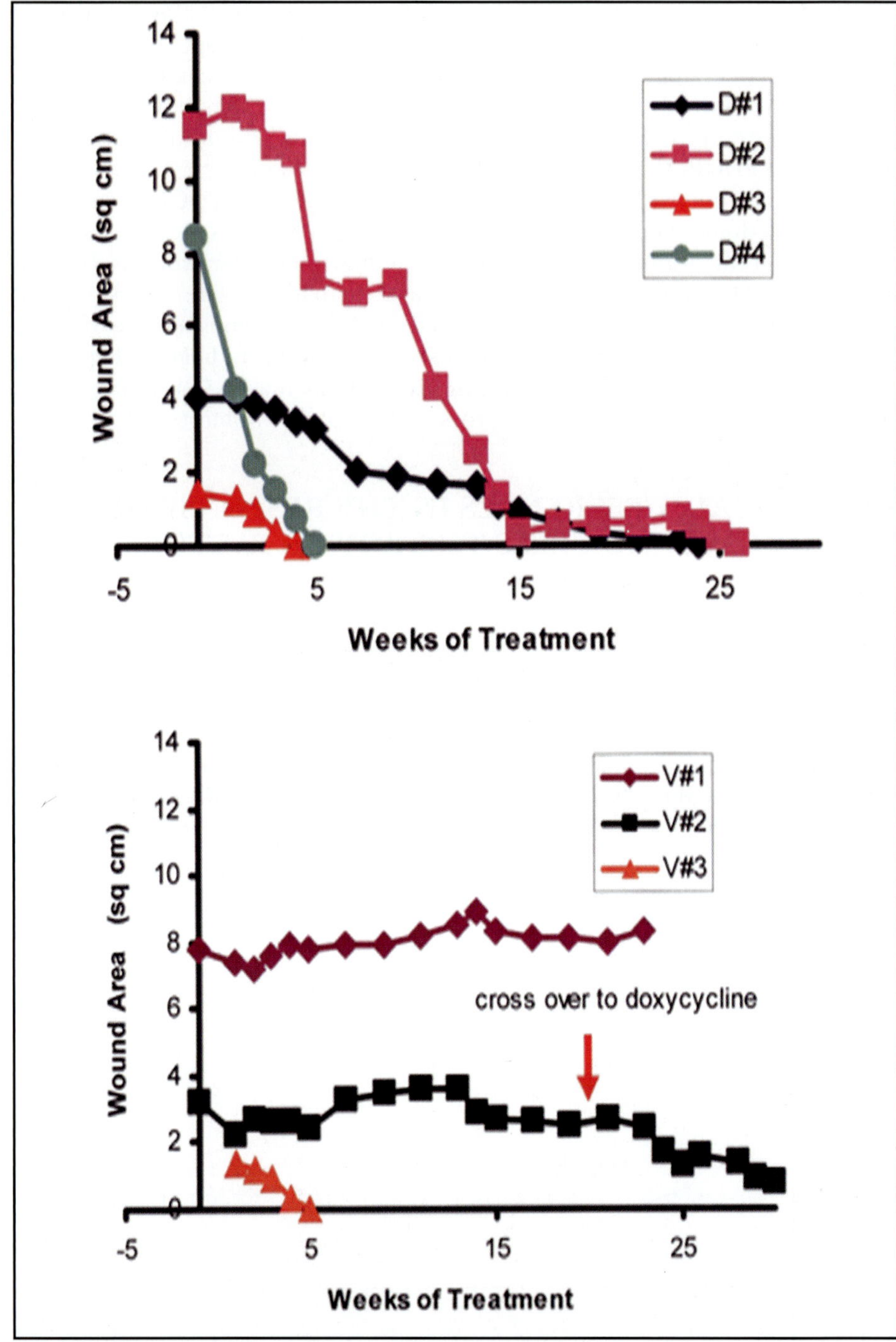

Figure 9. Topical Doxycycline Treatment of Diabetic Foot Ulcers. A randomized controlled trial of 1% doxycycline treatment of diabetic patients with chronic foot ulcers found that all four ulcers treated daily with doxycycline in a carboxy methyl cellulose vehicle healed in less than the 20 week treatment period. In contrast, only one of the three ulcers treated with vehicle healed in 20 weeks (50). One patient treated with vehicle elected to receive doxycycline treatment after the 20 week study, and the ulcer began healing during the 12 week cross-over treatment period. Importantly, no adverse events occurred that were attributable to doxycycline treatment.

from venous leg ulcers that had been present greater than three years grew more slowly and responded more poorly to PDGF than fibroblasts from venous ulcers that had been present for less than three years. These results suggest that fibroblasts in ulcers of long duration may approach senescence and have a decreased response to exogenous growth factors.

Based on these biochemical analyses of the molecular environments of acute and chronic human wounds, it is possible to propose a general model of differences between healing and chronic wounds. As shown in Figure 8, the molecular environment of healing wounds promotes mitosis of cells, has low levels of inflammatory cytokines, low levels of proteases and high levels of growth factors and cells capable of rapid division. In contrast, the molecular environments of chronic wounds generally have the opposite characteristics, i.e., the molecular environment does not promote mitosis of cells, has elevated levels of inflammatory cytokines, has high levels of proteases and low levels of growth factors and cells that are approaching senescence. If these general concepts are correct, then it may be possible to develop new treatment strategies which would re-establish in chronic wounds the balance of cytokines, growth factors, proteases, their natural inhibitors and competent cells found in healing wounds.

CLINICAL STRATEGIES TARGETING MOLECULAR ABNORMALITIES OF CHRONIC WOUNDS

The concept that chronic wounds fail to heal because of molecular and cellular abnormalities in the wound environment implies that therapies that correct these imbalances should promote healing. Several new treatment strategies for chronic wounds are being developed that are based on these concepts.

One of the first approaches to correcting the molecular imbalance in chronic wounds targeted the elevated levels of inflammatory cytokines. The simplest approach to correcting this condition is to prepare the wound bed using debridement and moisture control (37, 38). This concept has been more thoroughly described in a recent supplement that unites wound bed preparation under a TIME acronym that stands for Tissue, Infection, Moisture, and Epidermal treatments. The importance of proper wound debridement was clearly demonstrated in the clinical study performed by David Steed's group in Pittsburgh who showed that healing of chronic diabetic foot ulcers that were treated at ten different centers was closely correlated with the frequency of debridement (38). The benefit was seen both in patients that received standard care and in patients who were treated with topical PDGF. Thus, wound debridement is a vital adjunct in the care of patients with chronic diabetic foot ulcers. It is likely that frequent sharp debridement of diabetic ulcers helps to reduce the level of inflammation in the chronic wound by converting it into a pseudo-acute wound molecular environment.

Another approach to correcting the abnormal molecular environment of chronic wounds is to add recombinant growth factors to the wound (39–47). Several clinical studies have reported improved healing of various types of chronic wounds with recombinant human growth factors and cytokines, including PDGF, KGF-2, TGF- b, bFGF, and GM-CSF. It is important to recognize that growth factors can only function well in chronic wounds when the environment is similar to that found in acute wounds. In other words, growth factors cannot resurrect dead, inflamed, protease laden tissue. Thus, the principles of wound bed preparation must be used in conjunction with topical growth factor treatments.

Since chronic wounds typically contain elevated levels of proteases, especially MMPs, another targeted approach to correcting the abnormal molecular environment of chronic wounds is to add topical protease inhibitors. Relatively few clinical studies have investigated this approach. One study currently underway is investigating topical treatment of diabetic foot ulcers with doxycycline. Doxycycline is a member of the tetracycline family of antibiotics, and is a moderately effective inhibitor of metalloproteinases, including MMPs and the TNFa converting enzyme (TACE). As shown in Figure 9, a randomized control trial of 1% topical doxycycline treatment of diabetic patients with chronic foot ulcers found that all four ulcers treated daily with doxycycline in a carboxymethyl cellulose vehicle healed in less than the 20 week treatment period. In contrast, only one of three ulcers treated with vehicle healed in 20 weeks. One patient treated with vehicle elected to receive doxycycline treatment after the 20 week study, and the ulcer began healing during the 12 week cross-over treatment period. Importantly, no adverse events occurred that were attributable to doxycycline treatment.

A new wound dressing has been introduced that contains denatured collagen (gelatin) and oxidized regenerated cellulose (Promogran). The gelatin in the dressing acts as a "decoy substrate" for proteases, especially MMPs, and resulted in reduced levels of protease activities in fluids from chronic human wounds measured in vitro. Results of a 12-week clinical study of chronic diabetic plantar surface ulcers found that 31% of 51 patients treated with Promogran added to conventional dressings had complete wound closure compared with 28% of 39 patients treated with conventional dressings (p = 0.12). Analysis of healing rates in subcategories of patients suggested that the effect of Promogran was more dramatic in healing in ulcers of less that 6 months duration. Other "smart dressings" are under development that are capable of sequestering the damaging proteases that are found in many chronic ulcers (48, 49).

Acticoat® Absorbent dressing consists of a silver coated calcium alginate fiber designed to remove excess ulcer fluid and at the same time release ionic silver to provide a broad-spectrum antibacterial activity. It is recommended for use in moderate to highly exudative ulcers and does not adhere to newly forming granulation tissue. Some dressing materials are available that deliver various forms of iodophore. However caution must be taken when using these materials because they may cause damage to the wound granulation tissue if used too frequently. One must consider the potential benefits with possible harm these dressing may cause. After all compounds that are strong enough to kill bacteria can also damage host tissue when they are presented to the ulcer site in a concentrated form and for extended periods of time.

In contrast to dressings that release antimicrobial agents, another new approach in advanced dressings that is currently under development utilizes a technology (NIMBUS) that permanently binds an antimicrobial

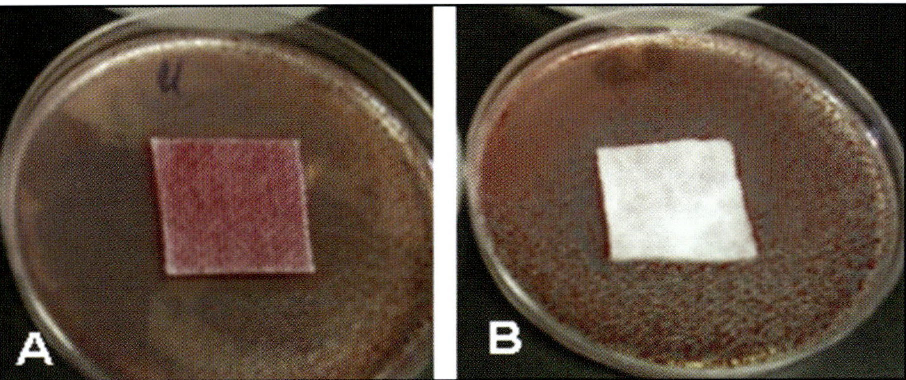

Figure 10. Samples of cellulosic (rayon) dressing material treated with NIMBUS antimicrobial (panel B) were inoculated with 2 ml of PBS containing 10,000 cfu of E. coli then incubated for 15 hours at 37°C on nutrient supplemented agar. The red color indicates areas of bacterial growth on the control non-treated dressing (panel A), but not on the NIMBUS-treated, dressing. Also, there is no zone of inhibition surrounding the NIMBUS-treated dressing demonstrating the antimicrobial is bound to the dressing and does not diffuse into the surrounding agar.

polymer containing quaternary nitrogen groups to the dressing material. The bound antimicrobial polyquat prevents bacteria from penetrating the surface of the wound, enhances absorption of wound exudate, and inhibits growth of bacteria in the dressing, which prevents shedding of large numbers of bacteria back onto the wound surface from a fouled dressing. Another theoretical advantage of this approach is that the bound antimicrobial agent does not diffuse into the wound, thus avoiding the possibility of damaging wound cells and slowing healing. As shown in Figure 10, panel B, bacteria inoculated into a NIMBUS-treated cellulosic dressing fail to grow (white), and there is no zone of inhibition of bacterial growth surrounding the dressing, showing no diffusion of the antimicrobial polymer out of the dressing into the agar. Bonding the quaternary nitrogen polymer to the cellulose (gauze or rayon) creates a high density of positive charges on the surface of the fibers, which produces a sustained release system for negatively charged small molecules that are added to the NIMBUS dressing as counter ions. For example, in vitro tests showed that replacing chloride counter ions in NIMBUS-treated gauze dressing with ampicillin or doxycycline anions produced sustained release of the antibiotics at high microbicidal levels over seven days (48).

CONCLUSION

Normal healing of skin wounds progresses through four phases that are regulated by the integrated actions of chemokines, cytokines, growth factors, and proteases. The failure of some acute wounds to complete these phases of healing leads to molecular imbalances of these key regulator molecules, and the wound becomes chronic. The molecular environment of chronic wounds characteristically contains elevated levels of inflammatory cytokines and proteases, low levels of mitogenic activity, and cells that are often senescent and respond poorly to growth factors. As chronic wounds begin to heal, this molecular pattern shifts to one that resembles a healing wound. As more information is learned about the molecular and cellular profiles of healing and chronic wounds, new therapies will be developed that selectively correct the abnormal aspects of chronic wounds and promote healing of these costly clinical problems. These new therapies work well only when the principles of wound bed preparation are applied to the wound bed.

REFERENCES

1. Bennett NT, Schultz GS. Growth factors and wound healing: Part II. Role in normal and chronic wound healing. *The American Journal of Surgery* 166(July), 74-81. 1993.

2. Bennett NT, Schultz GS. Growth factors and wound healing: Biochemical properties of growth factors and their receptors. *The American Journal of Surgery* 165(June), 728-737. 1993.

3. Lawrence WT. Physiology of the acute wound. Clin.Plast.Surg., 25: 321-340, 1998.

4. Schultz GS. Molecular Regulation of Wound Healing. In R.A.Bryant (ed.), *Acute and Chronic Wounds: Nursing Management, 2nd ed*, pp. 413-429. Philadelphia, PA: Mosby, 2000.

5. Luster AD. Chemokines—chemotactic cytokines that mediate inflammation. N.Engl.J.Med., 338: 436-445, 1998.

6. Gillitzer R, Goebeler M. Chemokines in cutaneous wound healing. *J Leukoc Biol* 69: 513-521, 2001.

7. Dinarello CA, Moldawer LL. Chemokines and Their Receptors. *Proinflammatory and Anti-inflammatory Cytokines in Rheumatoid Arthritis, 1st ed*, pp. 99-110. Thousand Oaks, CA: Amgen Inc., 2000.

8. Frenette PS, Wagner DD. Adhesion molecules, blood vessels and blood cells. *New England J Med* 335, 43-45. 1996.

9. Frenette PS, Wagner DD. Molecular medicine, adhesion molecules. *New England J Med* 334, 1526-1529. 1996.

10. Diegelmann RF, Cohen IK, Kaplan AM. The role of macrophages in wound repair: a review. *Plast Reconstr Surg* 68: 107-113, 1981.

11. Duncan MR, Frazier KS, Abramson S, et al. Connective tissue growth factor mediates transforming growth factor beta-induced collagen synthesis: down-regulation by cAMP. *FASEB J* 13: 1774-1786, 1999.

12. Bhushan M, Young HS, Brenchley PE, et al. Recent advances in cutaneous angiogenesis. *Br J Dermatol* 147: 418-425, 2002.

13. Semenza GL. HIF-1 and tumor progression: pathophysiology and therapeutics. *Trends Mol Med* 8: S62-S67, 2002.

14. Grant MB, May WS, Caballero S, et al. Adult hematopoietic stem cells provide functional hemangioblast activity during retinal neovascularization. *Nat. Med.*, 8: 607-612, 2002.

15. O' Toole EA. Extracellular matrix and keratinocyte migration. *Clin Exp Dermatol* 26: 525-530, 2001.

16. Mast BA, Schultz GS. Interactions of cytokines, growth factors, and proteases in acute and chronic wounds. *Wound Repair and Regeneration* 4, 411-420. 1996.

17. Bucalo B, Eaglstein WH, Falanga V. Inhibition of cell proliferation by chronic wound fluid. *Wound Repair and Regeneration* 1: 181-186, 1993.

18. Katz MH, Alvarez AF, Kirsner RS. Human wound fluid from acute wounds stimulates fibroblast and endothelial cell growth. *J Am Acad Dermatol* 25: 1054-1058, 1991.

19. Harris IR, Yee KC, Walters CE, et al. Cytokine and protease levels in healing and non-healing chronic venous leg ulcers. *Experimental Dermatology* 4, 342-349. 1995.

20. Trengove NJ, Bielefeldt-Ohmann H, Stacey MC. Mitogenic activity and cytokine levels in non-healing and healing chronic leg ulcers. *Wound Repair and Regeneration* 8: 13-25, 2000.

21. Yager DR, Nwomeh BC. The proteolytic environment of chronic wounds. *Wound Repair and Regeneration* 7: 433-441, 1999.

22. Nwomeh BC, Yager DR, Cohen IK. Physiology of the chronic wound. *Clin Plast Surg* 25: 341-356, 1998.

23. Trengove NJ, Stacey MC, Macauley S, et al. Analysis of the acute and chronic wound environments: the role of proteases and their inhibitors. *Wound Repair and Regeneration* 7: 442-452, 1999.

24. Yager DR, Zhang LY, Liang HX, et al. Wound fluids from human pressure ulcers contain elevated matrix metalloproteinase levels and activity compared to surgical wound fluids. *J Invest Dermatol* 107: 743-748, 1996.

25. Rogers AA, Burnett S, Moore JC, et al. Involvement of proeolytic enzymes-plasminogen activators and matrix metalloproteinases-in the pathophysiology of pressure ulcers. *Wound Repair and Regeneration* 3, 273-283. 1995.

26. Bullen EC, Longaker MT, Updike DL, et al. Tissue inhibitor of metalloproteinases-1 is decreased and activated gelatinases are increased in chronic wounds. *The Journal of Investigative Dermatology* 104, 236-240. 1995.

27. Ladwig GP, Robson MC, Liu R, et al. Ratios of activated matrix metalloproteinase-9 to tissue inhibitor of matrix metalloproteinase-1 in wound fluids are inversely correlated with healing of pressure ulcers. *Wound Repair and Regeneration* 10: 26-37, 2002.

28. Rao CN, Ladin DA, Liu Y Y, et al. Alpha 1-antitrypsin is degraded and non-functional in chronic wounds but intact and functional in acute wounds: the inhibitor protects fibronectin from degradation by chronic wound fluid enzymes. *J Invest Dermatol* 105: 572-578, 1995.

29. Wysocki AB, Staiano-Coico L, Grinnell F. Wound fluid from chronic leg ulcers contains elevated levels of metalloproteinases MMP-2 and MMP-9. *J Invest Dermatol* 101: 64-68, 1993.

30. Grinnel F, Zhu M. Fibronectin Degradation in Chronic Wounds Depends on the Relative Levels of Elastase, a1-Proteinase Inhibitor, and a2-Macroglbulin. *J Invest Dermatol* 106: 335-341, 1996.

31. Tarnuzzer RW, Schultz GS. Biochemical analysis of acute and chronic wound environments. *Wound Repair and Regeneration* 4, 321-325. 1996.

32. Yager DR, Chen SM, Ward SI, et al. Ability of chronic wound fluids to degrade peptide growth factors is associated with increased levels of elastase activity and diminished levels of proteinase inhibitors. *Wound Repair and Regeneration* 5, 23-32. 1997.

33. Baker EA, Leaper DJ. Proteinases, their inhibitors, and cytokine profiles in acute wound fluid. *Wound Repair and Regeneration* 8: 392-398, 2000.

34. Cowin AJ, Hatzirodos N, Holding CA, et al. Effect of healing on the expression of transforming growth factor beta(s) and their receptors in chronic venous leg ulcers. *J Invest Dermatol* 117: 1282-1289, 2001.

35. Agren MS, Eaglstein WH, Ferguson MW, et al. Causes and effects of the chronic inflammation in venous leg ulcers. *Acta Derm Venereol Suppl* (Stockh), 210: 3-17, 2000.

36. Trengove NJ, Langton SR, Stacey MC. Biochemical Analysis of Wound Fluid From Nonhealing and Healing Chronic Leg Ulcers. *Wound Repair and Regeneration* 4, 234-239. 1996.

37. Schultz GS, Sibbald RG, Falanga V, et al. Wound bed preparation: a systematic approach to wound management. *Wound Repair and Regeneration* 11 Suppl 1: S1-S28, 2003.

38. Steed DL, Donohoe D, Webster MW, et al. Effect of extensive debridement and treatment on the healing of diabetic foot ulcers. Diabetic Ulcer Study Group. *J Am Coll Surg* 183: 61-64, 1996.

39. Steed DL, and the Diabetic Ulcer Study Group. Clinical evaluation of recombinant human platelet-derived growth factor for the treatment of lower extremity diabetic ulcers. *Journal of Vascular Surgery* 21, 71-81. 1995.

40. Smiell JM, Wieman TJ, Steed DL, et al. Efficacy and safety of becaplermin (recombinant human platelet-derived growth factor-BB) in patients with nonhealing, lower extremity diabetic ulcers: a combined analysis of four randomized studies. *Wound Repair and Regeneration* 7: 335-346, 1999.

41. Rees RS, Robson MC, Smiell JM, et al. Becaplermin gel in the treatment of pressure ulcers: a phase II randomized, double-blind, placebo-controlled study. *Wound Repair and Regeneration* 7: 141-147, 1999.

42. Robson MC, Phillips TJ, Falanga V, et al. Randomized trial of topically applied repifermin (recombinant human keratinocyte growth factor-2) to accelerate wound healing in venous ulcers. *Wound Repair and Regeneration* 9: 347-352, 2001.

43. Robson MC, Phillip LG, Cooper DM, et al. Safety and effect of transforming growth factor-B2 for treatment of venous stasis ulcers. *Wound Repair and Regeneration* 3(2), 157-167. 1995.

44. Robson MC, Hill DP, Smith PD, et al. Sequential cytokine therapy for pressure ulcers: clinical and mechanistic response. *Ann Surg* 231: 600-611, 2000.

45. Robson MC, Phillips LG, Lawrence WT, et al. The safety and effect of topically applied recombinant basic fibroblast growth factor on the healing of chronic pressure sores. *Annals of Surgery* 216(4), 401-408. 1992.

46. Cullen B, Smith R, McCulloch E, et al. Mechanism of action of PROMOGRAN, a protease modulating matrix, for the treatment of diabetic foot ulcers. *Wound Repair and Regeneration* 10:16-25, 2002.

47. Veves A, Sheehan P, Pham HT. A randomized, controlled trial of Promogran (a collagen/oxidized regenerated cellulose dressing) vs standard treatment in the management of diabetic foot ulcers. *ArchSurg* 137:822-827, 2002.

48. Edwards, J.V., Montante, S.J, Cohen, I.K., et al. Modified cotton gauze dressings that reduce elastase activity in solution. *Wound Repair & Regeneration* 9:50-58, 2001.

49. Liesenfeld B, Toreki B, Batich C, et al. An advanced wound dressing with superabsorbent, microbicidal and hemostatic properties. *Wound Repair & Regeneration* 13:A37 abstract 134, 2006.

50. Chin, G.A. Thigpin, T.G. Perrin, K.J., et al. Treatment of Chronic Ulcers in Diabetic Patients with a Topical Metalloproteinase Inhibitor, Doxycycline. *Wounds* 15:315-323, 2003

REVIEW QUESTIONS

1.) The initial inflammatory cell to arrive at the scene of acute tissue injury that provides the first line of defense against infection is the

________________________________.

    a. Platelet
    b. Neutrophil
    c. Macrophage
    d. Mast Cell
    e. Fibroblast

2.) The most important Vitamin required for proper collagen synthesis during tissue repair is Vitamin _________.

    a. A
    b. B
    c. C
    d. D
    e. E

3.) Data from numerous studies suggest that chronic wounds fail to heal because molecular and cellular abnormalities develop in the wound due to prolonged ________________________.

    a. hemostasis
    b. platelet degranulation
    c. contraction
    d. angiogenesis
    e. inflammation

4.) Chronic wound care strategies employing the application of topical growth factors to the ulcer bed have met with limited success because of excessive levels of _____________________.

    a. proteases
    b. platelets
    c. PDGF
    d. extracellular Matrix
    e. albumin

5.) In order for any new therapeutic strategy, growth factor application, hyperbaric oxygen or high tech dressing to succeed in the healing of chronic ulcers, optimal ___________________________must be accomplished first.

    a. elevation
    b. wound bed preparation
    c. pressure application
    d. temperature control
    e. neutrophil diapedesis

Answers: 1b, 2c, 3e, 4a, 5b

Section 2
Principles of Wound Assessment

CHAPTER 3

WOUND ASSESSMENT

CHAPTER THREE OVERVIEW

NOTES

WOUND ASSESSMENT

Robert A. Warriner III

INTRODUCTION

The Wound Healing Society published in 1994 (8) the first attempt to organize a common language for defining a wound, wound healing, and the factors and processes felt to be important in wound healing. Key concepts introduced in that initial statement of definitions and guidelines included the differentiation between acute (healing) and chronic (failing) wounds and the importance of orderliness and timeliness in tissue repair following injury. An attempt was made to define minimum standards for wound assessment that have been included and elaborated on in the paragraphs to follow. These guidelines and the advances in our understanding of wound assessment serve as the basis for this chapter.

INTEGRATING THE FINAL COMMON PATHWAYS FOR WOUND HEALING FAILURE INTO WOUND ASSESSMENT

The cause of wound healing failure is usually multifactorial (Figure 1). Successful treatment involves completing a thorough evaluation of the wound and the wound patient. The evaluation addresses those factors that we know or suspect to be contributors to wound healing failure. Typically those contributing factors have been defined as local (Figure 2) or systemic (Figure 3) factors affecting wound healing. While this differentiation may provide a complete listing of factors that impair healing, it does little to provide a framework around which to evaluate the wound and the wound patient. It is both more flexible and more satisfying to consider wound healing failure from a pathophysiologic perspective and to develop an evaluation plan that identifies clinically significant final common pathways to wound healing failure. The concept of "final common pathways" as shown in Figure 1 focuses attention on critical factors leading to and sustaining impaired wound healing, such as infection, malperfusion and hypoxia, cellular failure, and unrelieved pressure or repetitive trauma. The value of this approach will be apparent as the wound and wound patient assessment process is presented.

The Goals of Wound and Wound Patient Assessment:
- Identify and define the wound etiology
- Identify and define the specific pathophysiology of wound healing failure
- Identify and define associated co-morbidities impacting wound healing or selecting treatment options
- Define the wound as to category and classification

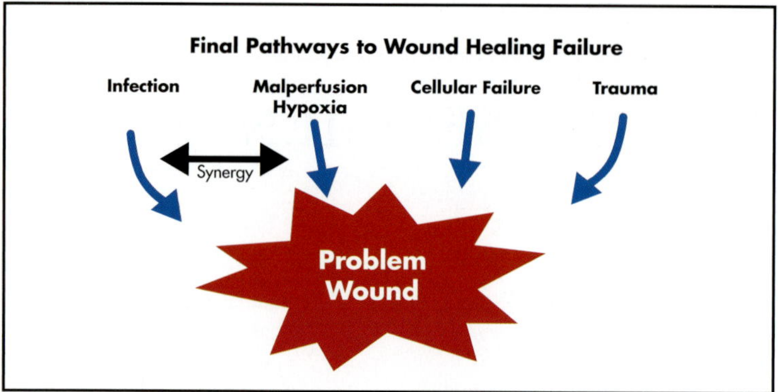

Figure 1. Final common pathways to wound healing failure (Used with permission, Warriner, 2003).

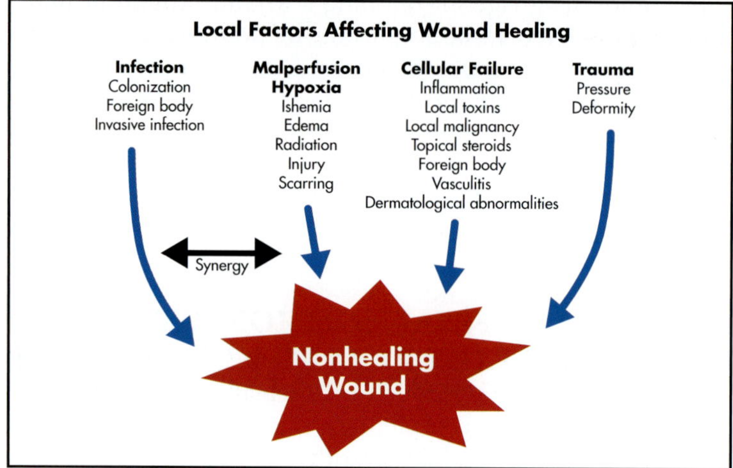

Figure 2. Local factors affecting wound healing associated with each of the final common pathways (Used with permission, Warriner, 2003).

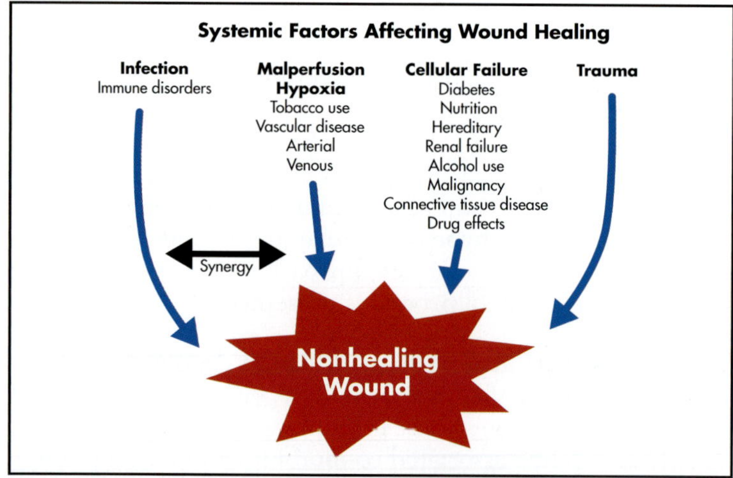

Figure 3. Systemic factors affecting wound healing associated with final common pathways (Used with permission, Warriner, 2003).

"Assessment of any wound should begin with the extent of the wound. A wound can be further described by various attributes, which include the following: duration, blood flow, oxygen tension, infection, edema, inflammation, repetitive trauma and/or insult, innervation, wound metabolism, nutrition, prior wound manipulation, and systemic factors. These attributes are clues to the cause, pathophysiology, and status of the wound" (8).

The goals of assessing the patient presenting with a problem wound (Table 1) are to identify the specific wound etiology, the specific pathophysiology of wound healing failure, and those co-morbidities or associated medical conditions affecting the host's response to the wound and possible treatment interventions. Finally, the wound is staged or classified according to appropriate national guidelines allowing comparison of wound incidence and outcomes statistics across treatment settings.

The first component of wound assessment is to identify which of the final common pathways leading to wound healing failure are present in the wound under evaluation. Infection, malperfusion and hypoxia, cellular failure, and unrelieved pressure or repetitive trauma may be obvious from a simple inspection of the wound. But frequently, critical information is missed unless the evaluator completes a thorough physical assessment of the wound, a complete wound-focused history and review of systems of the wound patient, and a history-directed physical examination. The second component of the wound assessment is to identify co-morbid conditions or contributing underlying medical conditions and other host factors that limit an effective response to the wound or may impact the choice of options for wound treatment. The third component of the wound evaluation is to categorize the

TABLE 1. THREE COMPONENTS OF THE INITIAL PROBLEM WOUND EVALUATION

Identify Final Common Pathways to Non Healing	Identify Co-Morbidities	Identify Wound Diagnosis
• Infection • Malperfusion and/or hypoxia • Cellular failure • Unrelieved pressure, repetitive trauma	• Diabetes mellitus • End stage renal disease, dialysis • Cardiac disease, congestive heart failure • Chronic arterial insufficiency (secondary) • Edema (secondary) • Smoking • Pulmonary disease • Vasculitis (secondary), Reynaud's, other collagen vascular disease • Wound contamination continence • Mobility impairment, cerebral vascular accident, spinal cord injury, other musculoskeletal deformity • Steroid therapy, other chemotherapy • Distant malignancy • Malnutrition • Psychosocial issues	• Diabetic ulcer • Arterial insufficiency ulcer • Venous leg ulcer • Pressure ulcer • Surgical wound dehiscence, failing flap or graft • Progressive soft tissue infection, osteomyelitis • Laceration, acute traumatic injury, crush injury • Burn • Abrasion, skin tear • Contact dermatitis • Dermatological condition, rash • Vasculitis ulcer • Radiation wound • Stoma wound • Other

Used with permission, Warriner, 2003.

wound on the basis of presumed etiology. While it is not always possible and sometimes misleading in the case of unusual presentations of lower extremity ulcerations, it is helpful to identify a preliminary wound category. This enables an appropriate wound classification system to be applied and a treatment plan to be structured that takes into account published standards for care of various wound types.

WOUND ASSESSMENT

- History of wounding event
- Location of the wound (useful in differential diagnosis)
- Edge of the wound and surrounding skin
- Undermining of the wound edges
- Exudate quantity and quality
- Appearance of the wound bed
- Measurement of wound size and depth
- Suffering (patient pain assessment)
- Wound grading and classification
- Re-evaluation on a periodic basis
- Assessment of infection

The structured evaluation process, demonstrated in Table 2 and Figure 4, is necessary to accomplish full and accurate characterization of the wound and wound patient. Each of those component steps is discussed in more detail in the information that follows.

This consistent pattern of evaluation should be followed even when there are strikingly obvious features present. Keast, et al. (6) has validated an algorithmic assessment tool for the wound itself, "MEASURE," which has been incorporated into this process. Structured assessment prevents subtle but significant factors from being overlooked. Remember that in a referral-based wound care practice, the obvious has usually (but not always) already been addressed. A number of tools are also required to complete the wound assessment including a documentation sheet, a ruler and flexible tape measure, calipers for extremely accurate measurement, metal or cotton-tipped probes, gloves, a magnifying glass, good lighting, and a camera for photo documentation. Surgical instruments may also be necessary for limited debridement in order to adequately evaluate the wound.

History of Wounding

The initial step in wound assessment is obtaining the history of the initial wounding event. A chronological history of the occurrence and progression of the wound including previous diagnostic testing and treatment interventions should be obtained and documented. Did the wound occur suddenly (trauma, insect bite) or develop gradually over time (neuropathic foot ulcer, venous leg ulcer)? Is this the first wound at this location or a recurrent wound or pattern of wounding? Is the wound painful, and if so, what is the character and nature of the pain? Are there precipitating or ameliorating factors? Has the patient had chills, fever, or night sweats? Is there any history of unusual environmental or occupational exposures? Does the patient have known diabetes

TABLE 2. COMPONENTS OF WOUND ASSESSMENT

History	• Initial wounding event • Previous wound healing problems • Recurrent wounding • Prior diagnostic testing • Prior treatment
Location	May be important in differential diagnosis
Exudate	• Quantity • Quality
Edge and Surrounding Skin	• Condition • Static vs. dynamic undermining • Extension color • Pigmentation • Inflammation, induration • Dermatologic abnormalities • Satellite lesions • Suppleness • Edema
Undermining	• Presence • Absence
Appearance of Wound Bed	• Eschar • Foreign bodies • Inflammation, infection • Tunneling, sinuses, abscesses • Odor • Necrosis • Granulation tissue • Exposed structures • Fibrin
Measure: Size and Depth	• Length, width • Depth • Circumference, area, volume • Extent
Suffering	Pain level using validated pain scale
Classify the Wound	Use validated wound classification system
Re-Evaluate	All parameters monitored regularly. (1–4 week interval)

Used with permission, Warriner, adapted from Keast et al. Wound Rep Reg 2004; 12:S1–S17. MEASURE algorithm... Measure, Exudate, Appearance, Suffering, Undermining, Reevaluate, Edge.

mellitus, collagen vascular disease, peripheral arterial occlusive disease, or chronic venous insufficiency (evaluated in more detail during the patient assessment section)? What diagnostic studies have already been completed including radiographic or nuclear medicine studies, cultures, biopsies, or vascular studies? What treatments have been applied including debridements, local wound cleansing and wound dressings, offloading and protection, compression wraps or devices to control edema, vascular (arterial or venous) surgical or radiographic interventions, hyperbaric oxygen treatment, electrical stimulation, topical growth factors, bioengineered tissue grafts, or tertiary interventions. Has reconstructive surgery been attempted? What were the results of these interventions and were there any complications?

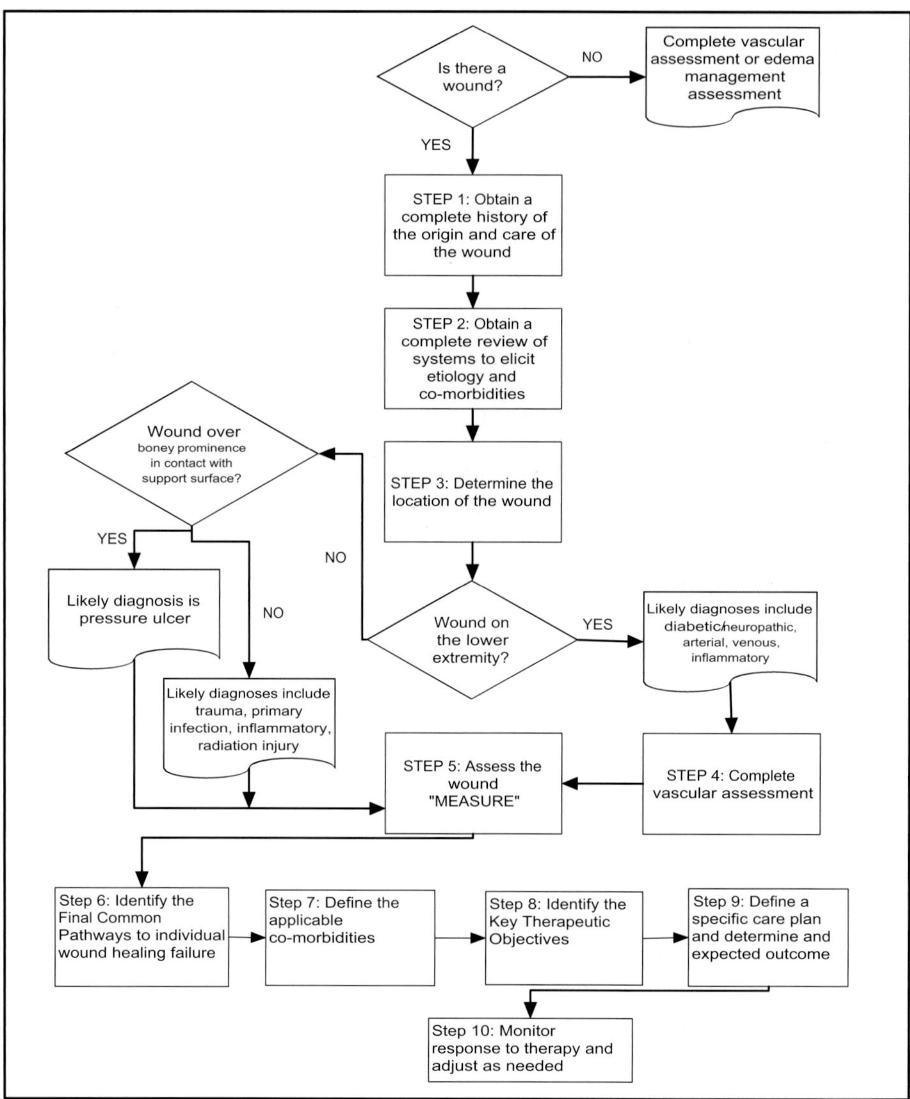

Figure 4. Initial evaluation of the problem wound patient. (Used with permission. Copyright 2006 Diversified Clinical Services) (18).

Location of the Wound

The wound location is often important in identifying possible wound etiologies and may play a critical role in differential diagnosis of lower extremity ulcers as discussed below. Wounds over boney prominences are often directly related to unrelieved pressure while malleolar ulcers are often due to hypertension, peripheral arterial occlusive disease, or vasculitis.

Condition of the Wound Edge and Surrounding Skin

Avoid the temptation to look immediately at the wound itself. The surrounding skin should first be examined and palpated beginning at the periphery and working towards the wound itself (Figure 5). The skin should be examined for color (erythema, rubor, cyanosis, other discoloration) and the presence or absence of normal pigmentation. Signs of inflammation and induration should be identified and the effects of position noted. Dermatologic abnormalities including rashes, purpura, and livedo reticularis should be noted. The presence of satellite lesions or distant necrosis should be described. Palpation of the surrounding skin should reveal the presence of induration, subcutaneous nodules, fibrosis, fluctuance, tenderness, or edema. Skin temperature should be evaluated using an infrared temperature probe to help in identifying local inflammation or cellulites. Local perfusion to the skin surrounding the wound can also be assessed by transcutaneous dermal PO_2 measurement, cutaneous laser Doppler skin blood flow measurement, and skin perfusion pressure measurement. Since wound healing is initiated and

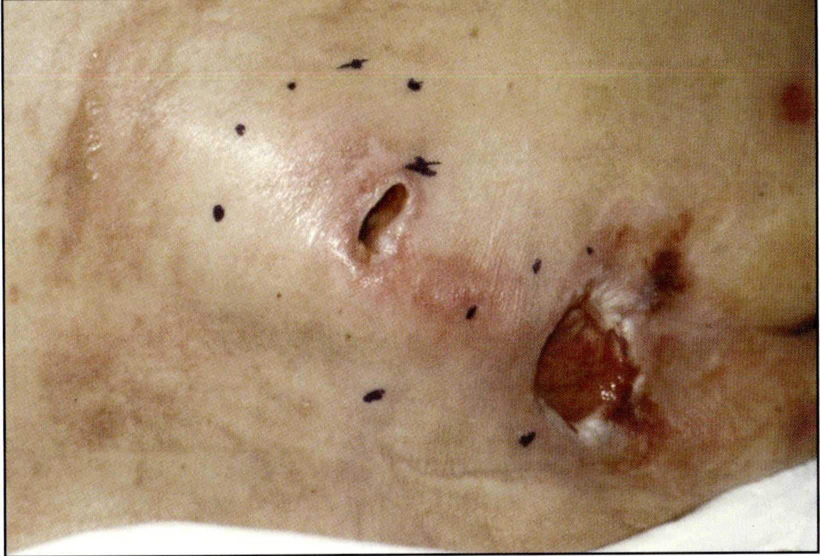

Figure 5. Observe the condition of the surrounding skin for erythema, induration, maceration, and presence of satellite lesions (Photo courtesy of Craig Broussard, Ph.D.).

sustained at the edges of the wound, evaluation of the wound edges provides valuable insight into the condition and response of the wound. Examine the wound margins to identify the presence of undermining under the wound edges, which is characteristic of ulcers subjected to shear stress or in certain vasculitis disorders such as pyoderma gangrenosum. Is there evidence of extension of the wound at the edges? Is the edge static and stable, or dynamic and healing, or failing?

Exudate Quantity and Quality

Exudate volume and character help define wound moisture balance and may point to inflammatory or infectious processes present in the wound bed. Evaluate the exudate on both the removed dressing and the wound bed itself (Figures 6 and 7). Observe for odor, color, and consistency. Remember that quality and quantity of exudate may be misleading. While increased exudate volume may be associated with infection, the amount of drainage may also be increased by hydrating dressings and efforts to mechanically control local edema. Also, topical agents may alter appearance and consistency of exudate.

Exudate is typically described on the basis of increased or decreased quantity and increased or decreased purulence.

Appearance of the Wound Bed

The wound bed is typically described in qualitative terms. Evaluation of the wound bed should be performed after surface cleansing (usually with saline low pressure irrigation and occasionally requiring limited local sharp

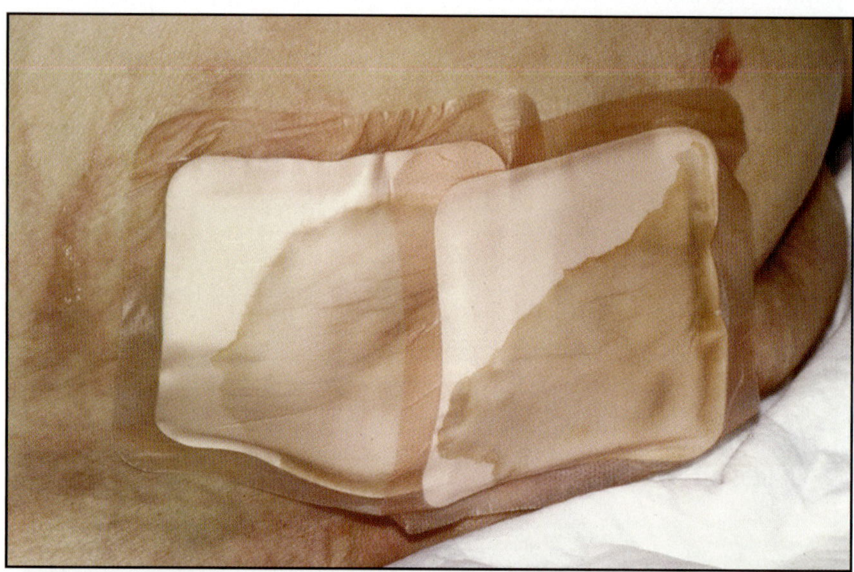

Figure 6. Observe and record exudate strike through the wound dressing before removal (Photo courtesy of Craig Broussard, Ph.D.).

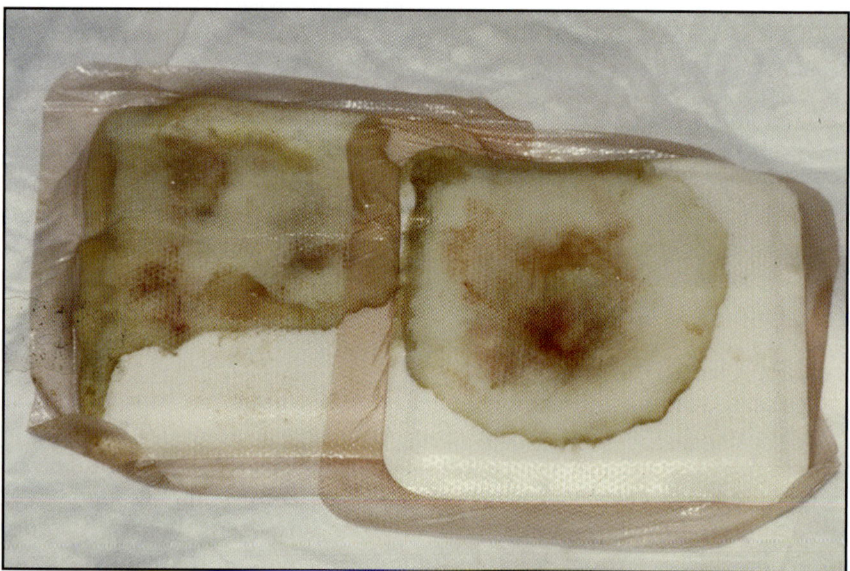

Figure 7. Observe and record exudate volume on the wound contact surface of the dressing (Photo courtesy of Craig Broussard, Ph.D.).

debridement). Removal of old dressing material and loosely adherent exudate allows for more accurate assessment of the wound bed. Evaluation of the wound bed may also involve palpation with a gloved finger or non-surgical exploration using a cotton swab or metal probe. Occasionally, formal surgical exploration or initial debridement is required before the wound bed can be adequately described. Wound odor assessment is helping in assessing bacterial bioburden.While foul odor may represent the presence of tissue necrosis or anaerobic infection, all wounds will have an odor, particularly those that have been occluded under a moisture retentive dressing. The type of wound dressing material can significantly impact the presence and character of any odor from the wound bed. Once cleaned, the wound bed is then assessed for the presence of densely adherent exudate, fibrin, and obvious necrosis that may be present as slough or eschar. The presence of eschar implies some degree of local ischemia. The wound bed is then evaluated for the presence of any exposed deep structures (fascia, tendon, joint capsule, bone, neurovascular structures) and their condition. Any tunneling or sinus tracts should be identified at this time as well as the presence and type of foreign material that may be present in the wound (Figure 8). Finally, the amount and quality of granulation tissue should be described. Typically these characteristics are described as present or absent. Potentially useful attempts to quantify each of these characteristics as predictors of wound healing progress or healing outcomes have not been validated. Assessing the condition of the wound bed may also involve taking a biopsy of tissue (14) for culture in the assessment of infection and for histopathology for the identification of occult malignancy or local or systemic vasculitis. Radiographic studies including plain x-rays and specialized studies such as nuclear scans, CT or MRI may be necessary to define the presence and extent of deep tissue involvement or infection.

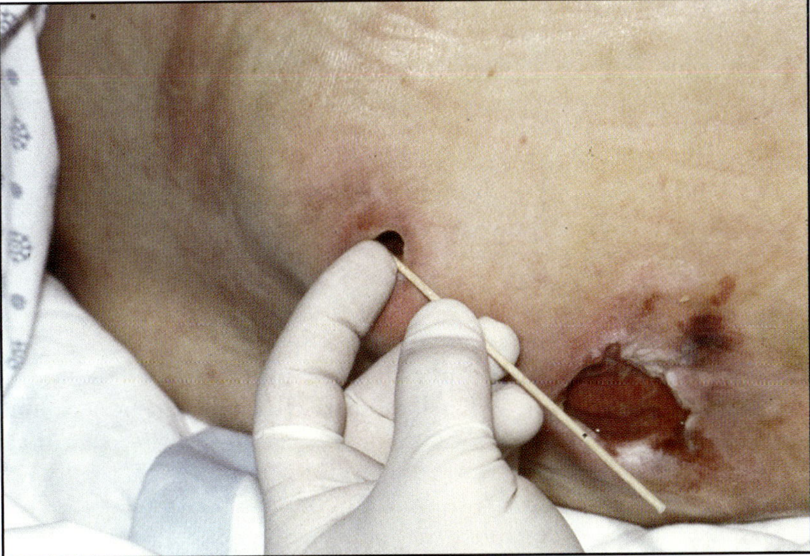

Figure 8. Identify and measure tunneling or undermining using a probe or cotton tipped applicator (Photo courtesy of Craig Broussard, Ph.D.).

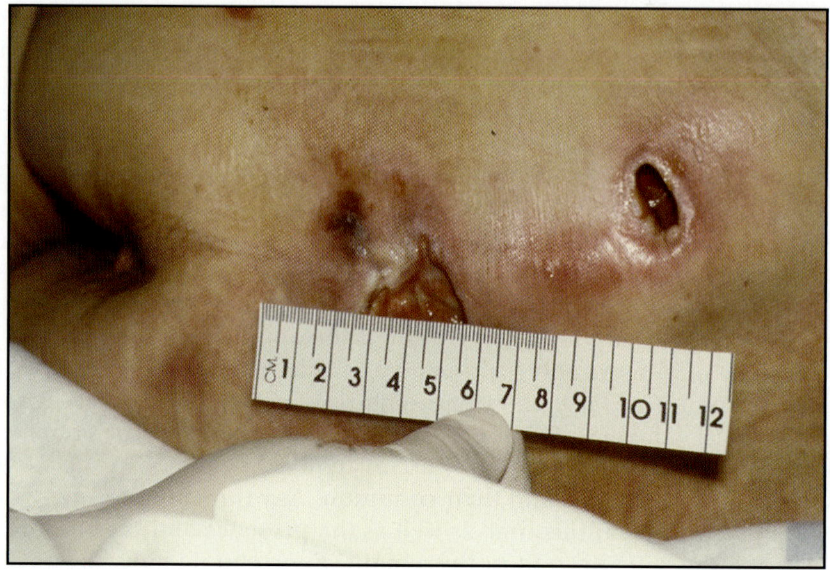

Figure 9. Measure wound length (perpendicular axis of the body) and width (horizontal axis of the body) using a ruler and record in centimeters (Photo courtesy of Craig Broussard, Ph.D.).

Measurement of Size and Depth of the Wound

Next examine the wound to determine its size. Typically wounds are sized according to greatest length, greatest width along the perpendicular to the length, and the greatest depth (Figure 9). Calculations based on these simple linear measures are frequently made to estimate wound surface area or volume. However, there are inherent inaccuracies in such calculations (10). Wound size can be more accurately defined by planimetry that measure wound perimeter length or circumference and make much more accurate wound surface area calculations. While visual overlay of wound tracings is readily available (Figure 10) and may provide qualitative descriptions of wound healing progression or regression, computer assisted planimetry is still required to obtain accurate circumference measurements or surface area calculations (6). These calculations are much more accurate than those obtained from simple length and width measurement. A number of commercially available software programs provide wound data and wound image storage as well as planimetry.

Suffering (Patient Pain Assessment)

Pain should be specifically addressed and can be quantified by a variety of specific pain definition scales. Pain should be characterized by location and quality (sharp, dull, aching, throbbing, burning), and severity. Duration and reproducibility should be ascertained as well as timing of the pain and the associated environmental factors that may precipitate or exacerbate the pain should also be defined. Remember that neuropathic patients may experience deep pain, and pain in this circumstance should be considered a serious symptom warranting further assessment.

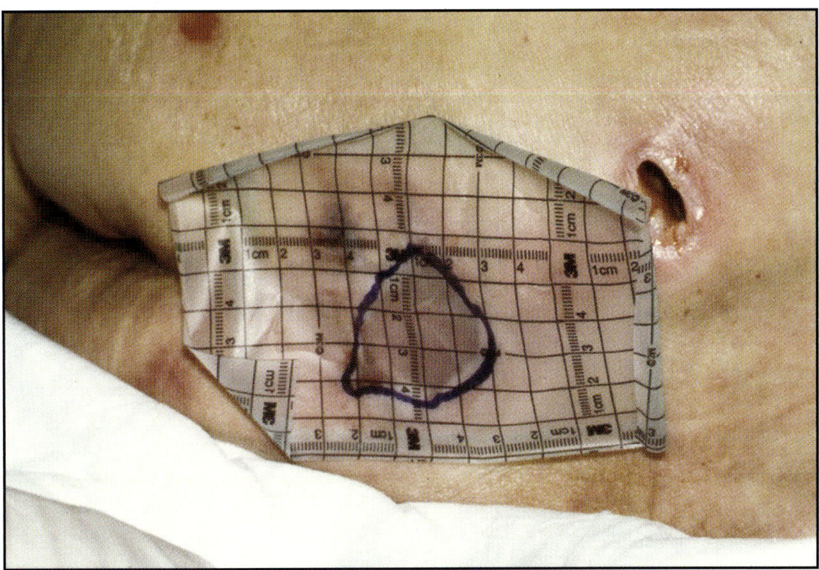

Figure 10. Perimeter or circumferential tracings can be made with a soft fine tipped marking pen and a plastic grid. Surface area can be calculated in various ways using this technique (Photo courtesy of Craig Broussard, Ph.D.).

Classification or Staging of the Wound

This final step allows us to define a wound in comparative and sometimes predictive terms improving comparisons of wound intervention outcomes. A variety of wound classification systems have been developed. Wound staging and classification systems are also used to establish parameters for reimbursement for advanced wound care interventions including pressure relief surfaces and adjunctive hyperbaric oxygen treatment. Some examples of clinically useful classification systems are described below.

Partial and full thickness

The simplest staging system for wounds is to define the level of tissue involvement based upon depth (Table 3) (15).

TABLE 3. PARTIAL AND FULL THICKNESS WOUND CLASSIFICATION

Stage	Depth	Example
Superficial	Involving but not through the epidermis	Blister
Partial Thickness	Through the epidermis into but not through the dermis	Wagner 1 diabetic foot ulcer, Stage 2 pressure ulcer, split thickness skin graft donor site
Full Thickness	Through the epidermis and dermis into the subcutaneous tissue, fascia, etc.	Wagner 2 or greater diabetic foot ulcer, Stage 3 or greater pressure ulcer, surgical wound dehiscence

TABLE 4. WAGNER CLASSIFICATION OF DIABETIC FOOT ULCERS

Grade	Description
0	Intact skin (although there may be evidence of old healed ulcerations or deformity)
1	Superficial ulcer without penetration to deeper layers
2	Deeper ulcer which reaches tendon, bone, or joint capsule
3	Deeper ulcer with abscess, osteomyelitis, or tendonitis extending to tendon or bone
4	Gangrene of some portion of the toe, toes, and/or forefoot which may be wet or dry
5	Gangrene involves the whole foot or enough of the foot that no local procedures are possible

Diabetic foot wound classification systems

Although many classification systems exist for diabetic foot ulcerations, the classic and most widely referenced classification system for diabetic foot wounds was developed and reported by Wagner in 1981 in an attempt to define therapeutic algorithms based on wound characteristics (Table 4) (17).

The Wagner classification system does not provide for specific differentiation of the contribution of infection and vascular compromise to diabetic foot ulcer outcomes. The University of Texas Health Science Center San Antonio classification system (1) (Table 5) provides for four grades of depth (from intact skin to exposed bone or joint) and four stages (clean, infected, ischemic, or infected and ischemic) that can be applied to each grade.

TABLE 5. THE UNIVERSITY OF TEXAS SAN ANTONIO CLASSIFICATION OF DIABETIC FOOT ULCERS

	Grade 0	Grade I	Grade II	Grade III
Stage A	Pre- or post-ulcerative lesion completely epithelialized	Superficial wound, not involving tendon, capsule, or bone	Wound penetrating to tendon or capsule	Wound penetrating to bone or joint
Stage B	Infection	Infection	Infection	Infection
Stage C	Ischemia	Ischemia	Ischemia	Ischemia
Stage D	Infection and ischemia	Infection and ischemia	Infection and ischemia	Infection and ischemia

Venous insufficiency staging and classification

A detailed discussion of the classification of lower extremity venous disease is beyond the scope of this chapter. The CEAP (Clinical, Etiology, Anatomic, Pathophysiological) classification system endorsed by the American Venous Forum (7) (Table 6) provides not only for a grading of the amount of edema, peri-ulcer skin changes, and ulcer characteristics. It also addresses etiology of the underlying venous disease, anatomic location, and pathophysiology. It concludes with a disability score giving it some characteristics of a total patient wound grading system.

TABLE 6. VENOUS DYSFUNCTION—CLINICAL SCORE (PARTIAL)

Clinical Description	Score
Pain	0=none; 1=moderate, not requiring analgesics; 2=severe, requiring analgesics
Edema	0=none; 1=mild/moderate; 2=severe
Venous claudication	0=none; 1=mild/moderate; 2=severe
Pigmentation	0=none; 1=localized; 2=extensive
Lipodermatosclerosis	0=none; 1=localized; 2=extensive
Ulcer size (largest)	0=none; 1= <2 cm diameter; 2= >2 cm diameter
Ulcer duration	0=none; 1= <3 months; 2= >3 months
Ulcer recurrence	0=none; 1= once; 2= more than once

Pressure ulcer classification systems

The most widely used classification system for describing pressure ulcers was first reported in 1989 by the National Pressure Ulcer Advisory Panel (11) (Table 7) and has been generally adopted as the standard for reporting pressure ulcer depth and extent.

With the exception of the Wagner diabetic foot ulcer classification scheme that was originally intended to be bidirectional, (13) these classification systems are intended to describe the initial or presenting stage of the wound. They are not intended to be bi-directional or to be used to describe improvement of the wound during healing or treatment.

The findings obtained during wound assessment should be documented for comparison to subsequent monitoring and re-evaluation during treatment. Wound photographs including a reference number for identification of the patient and a ruler or scale for size comparison provides the best and probably most useful documentation tool. Wound measurements and other characteristics as well as wound treatment interventions and dressing can be recorded on a form such as the one shown in Figure 11.

TABLE 7. NATIONAL PRESSURE ULCER ADVISORY PANEL (NPUAP) PRESSURE ULCER CLASSIFICATION

Stage	Ulcer Description
Stage 1	Non-blanchable erythema of intact skin; the heralding lesion of skin ulceration
Stage 2	Partial thickness skin loss involving epidermis and/or dermis. The ulcer is superficial and presents clinically as an abrasion, blister, or shallow crater.
Stage 3	Full thickness skin loss involving damage or necrosis of subcutaneous tissue which may extend down to, but not through, underlying fascia. The ulcer presents clinically as a deep crater with or without undermining of adjacent tissue.
Stage 4	Full thickness skin loss with extensive destruction, tissue necrosis, or damage to muscle, bone, or supporting structures (i.e. tendon, joint capsule, etc.)

WOUND EVALUATION AND CARE RECORD

Patient Identification

CENTER FOR WOUND CARE AND HYPERBARIC MEDICINE

TYPE OF VISIT: [ ] NEW   [ ] FOLLOWUP   [ ] HBO   [ ] OTHER: [ ] INPATIENT   [ ] OUTPATIENT

VITAL SIGNS: T/P/R: BP: GLUCOSE: mg/dl (meter #) _______   [ ] See NDDR

WOUND EVALUATION

Wd. Location						
Wd. Number						
Length		mm		mm		mm
Width		mm		mm		mm
Depth		mm		mm		mm
Undermining		mm		mm		mm
Exudates	[ ] None [ ] Serous [ ] Purulent [ ] Bloody	[ ] Color [ ] Serosanguineous [ ] Odor Present [ ] Other:	[ ] None [ ] Serous [ ] Purulent [ ] Bloody	[ ] Color [ ] Serosanguineous [ ] Odor Present [ ] Other:	[ ] None [ ] Serous [ ] Purulent [ ] Bloody	[ ] Color [ ] Serosanguineous [ ] Odor Present [ ] Other:
Necrosis?	[ ] Yes	[ ] No	[ ] Yes	[ ] No	[ ] Yes	[ ] No
Gangrene?	[ ] Yes	[ ] No	[ ] Yes	[ ] No	[ ] Yes	[ ] No
Eschar?	[ ] Yes	[ ] No	[ ] Yes	[ ] No	[ ] Yes	[ ] No
Fibrin?	[ ] Yes	[ ] No	[ ] Yes	[ ] No	[ ] Yes	[ ] No
Exposed:						
1) Bone?	[ ] Yes	[ ] No	[ ] Yes	[ ] No	[ ] Yes	[ ] No
2) Tendon?	[ ] Yes	[ ] No	[ ] Yes	[ ] No	[ ] Yes	[ ] No
3) Muscle?	[ ] Yes	[ ] No	[ ] Yes	[ ] No	[ ] Yes	[ ] No
4) Fat?	[ ] Yes	[ ] No	[ ] Yes	[ ] No	[ ] Yes	[ ] No
Granulation Tissue?	[ ] Yes	[ ] No	[ ] Yes	[ ] No	[ ] Yes	[ ] No
1) Quantity:	[ ] Base Covered	[ ] Epithelium	[ ] Base Covered	[ ] Epithelium	[ ] Base Covered	[ ] Epithelium
2) Color:	[ ] Gray [ ] Pink	[ ] Brt Red	[ ] Gray [ ] Pink	[ ] Brt Red	[ ] Gray [ ] Pink	[ ] Brt Red
3) Texture:	[ ] Spongy	[ ] Firm	[ ] Spongy	[ ] Firm	[ ] Spongy	[ ] Firm
Debrided?	[ ] Yes [ ] No Anesthesia [ ] Y [ ] N		[ ] Yes [ ] No Anesthesia [ ] Y [ ] N		[ ] Yes [ ] No Anesthesia [ ] Y [ ] N	

PERIWOUND EVALUATION

Skin Color / Attributes	[ ] Normal [ ] Pallor [ ] Cyanosis [ ] Erythema [ ] Induration	[ ] Dry/Scaly [ ] Rash [ ] Edema [ ] Other:	[ ] Normal [ ] Pallor [ ] Cyanosis [ ] Erythema [ ] Induration	[ ] Dry/Scaly [ ] Rash [ ] Edema [ ] Other:	[ ] Normal [ ] Pallor [ ] Cyanosis [ ] Erythema [ ] Induration	[ ] Dry/Scaly [ ] Rash [ ] Edema [ ] Other:

Figure 11. Wound Evaluation and Care Record (Used with permission, Southeast Texas Center for Wound Care and Hyperbaric Medicine).

Assessment of Infection

Assessing the possible presence of infection can be problematic in many chronic wounds. Wound microbiology has been well described elsewhere (2). Wound infection may be obvious with signs of rubor, callor, dolor, and tumor present although these classical signs may be masked by the presence of systemic disease, topical medications, or wound dressings. More often wound infection presents more subtly or may even be unapparent. Look for any change in the appearance or quality of wound bed granulation tissue, the character or frequency of pain, the development of a foul odor or discharge, or a failure of the wound to demonstrate consistent healing progress (4). Frank purulence may be seen without infection as in pyoderma gangrenosum or may be absent with significantly proteolytic infections such as in necrotizing fasciitis.

The definitive diagnosis of infection in chronic wounds is by a properly taken culture of tissue. Swab cultures may be used but must be properly taken and will not distinguish actual tissue infection from colonization. Cultures of pus rarely yield useful results. Quantitative tissue culture in many institutions is impractical, but a biopsy taken from viable tissue in the wound bed and immediately cultured will usually yield equivalently useful clinical information to the quantitative tissue culture. Remember to also obtain an adjacent biopsy sample in difficult cases to be submitted for histopathology and special stains to identify the presence of leukocyte infiltration, to identify bacterial and fungal forms in the tissue, and to culture for "unusual" organisms including anaerobic, acid-fast, and fungal organisms. Early recognition of rapidly progressive necrotizing soft tissue infections is essential to the effective application of surgical debridement, systemic antibiotic therapy, and, in some cases, adjunctive hyperbaric oxygen treatment (9) (Table 8).

TABLE 8. DIFFERENTIAL DIAGNOSIS OF COMMON NECROTIZING SOFT TISSUE BACTERIAL INFECTIONS

	Crepitant Anaerobic Cellulitis	Progressive Bacterial Synergistic Gangrene	Necrotizing Fasciitis	Nonclostridial Myonecrosis
Incubation	> 3 days	2 weeks	1–4 days	Variable, 3–14 days
Onset	Gradual	Gradual	Acute	Acute
Toxemia	None or slight	Minimal	Moderate to marked	Marked
Pain	Absent	Moderate	Moderate to severe	Severe
Exudate	None or slight	None or slight	Profuse serosanguinous	Dishwater pus
Odor to Exudates	+/– Foul	+/– Foul	Foul	+/– Foul
Gas	Abundant	May be present	Usually not present	Not pronounced
Muscle	No change	No change	Viable	Marked change
Skin	Little change	Shaggy ulcer, gangrenous margins	Pale red cellulitis	Minimal change
Mortality	5–10%	10–25%	30%	75%

Adapted from Mader (9).

Diagnosing the presence of osteomyelitis can be particularly challenging and is often delayed, adversely impacting wound healing outcome, and increasing morbidity. The less the density of tissue between the wound bed and underlying bone, the greater the likelihood that osteomyelitis will eventually develop. Also, the longer the duration of the wound, the more likely osteomyelitis will develop. In patients presenting with plantar diabetic foot ulcers, the presence of exposed bone should be considered as diagnostic of osteomyelitis (12). Long bone osteomyelitis once identified can be classified

TABLE 9A. CIERNY–MADER CLASSIFICATION OF OSTEOMYELITIS —ANATOMICAL DESCRIPTION

Anatomic Stage	Description
Stage I	Medullary osteomyelitis
Stage II	Superficial osteomyelitis
Stage III	Localized osteomyelitis
Stage IV	Diffuse osteomyelitis

Anatomic staging is accomplished by physical inspection of the wound and radiographic studies (3).

TABLE 9B. CIERNY–MADER CLASSIFICATION OF OSTEOMYELITIS —PHYSIOLOGIC (HOST) DESCRIPTION

Physiologic (Host) Type	Description
A Host	Good immune system and delivery
B Host	Compromised locally (Bl) or systemically (Bs)
C Host	Treatment worse than the disease

The host is classified on the basis of the presence or absence of factors affecting immune surveillance and response, metabolism, local vascularity, etc. (3).

Systemic Factors (Bs)	Local Factors (Bl)
Malnutrition	Chronic lymphedema
Renal or hepatic failure	Venous stasis
Diabetes mellitus	Major vascular compromise
Immune deficiency	Local hypoxia
Malignancy	Vasculitis
Extremes of age	Extensive local scarring
Immunosuppression	Radiation fibrosis
Smoking	Peripheral neuropathy

according to a system developed by Cierny and Mader in 1984 (3). The Cierny-Mader Classification System (Table 9A and B) is additionally useful in selecting affected patients for adjunctive hyperbaric oxygen treatment. Like the classification systems for venous leg ulcer disease, it involves more than assessment and description of the wound alone addressing patient systemic factors as well. The Cierny-Mader classification system for osteomyelitis has also been used to describe infection and/or osteomyelitis associated with prosthetic joint infections, infection of nonunion tibial fractures, and osteomyelitis of the mandible. At the completion of the wound assessment those local factors affecting wound healing should be identified.

Re-Evaluation of the Wound

The wound should be reevaluated at periodic intervals as determined by the severity of the wound at presentation, the complexity of treatment provided, and the response to treatment. Typically, wound re-evaluation is performed on a once weekly basis initially with the interval for physician reassessment extending as the wound stabilizes and improves. At re-evaluation an abbreviated process that mimics what was done at the time of initial assessment should be completed and documented.

WOUND PATIENT ASSESSMENT

- General health status
- Presence of associated systemic disease
- Define factors affecting selection of treatment options
- Focused physical examination
- Laboratory studies
- Defining wound severity and impact on the patient
- At the completion of patient assessment all of the systemic factors affecting wound healing should be identified and co-morbidities defined

A wound cannot be adequately discussed in isolation from its effect on the patient and from the response of the patient to the wound. Ultimately understanding the overall health status of the wound patient is essential to adequately address the etiologies of wound healing failure in a particular circumstance and to understand the likely impact of treatment interventions. Assessment of the wound patient addresses co-morbidities that may affect wound healing or the response to and effectiveness of treatment.

General Health Status

The first step in assessing the wound patient involves evaluation of mental status and overall health. What is the overall health of the patient? Has the patient been febrile or been suffering recently from some other intercurrent illness. How well can the patient see? What is the patient's ability to understand the nature of his/her problem and to participate in his/her own care? What was the patient's pre-wound functional and ambulatory capacity? It is helpful to use an objective scale to define pre-wounding capability. The Volpicellim, Chambers, and Wagner ambulatory status grading system (16) (Table 10), while developed to describe function in amputees, is equally useful in assessing wound patients, particularly those with lower extremity wounds.

Other appropriate information to gather at this time includes any history of medications, smoking, alcohol, or illicit drug use. Also, any unusual exposures to animals or to potential toxins, whether inhaled, ingested, or contact, should also be noted. Medication and contact allergy history, particularly any history of latex allergy, should also be obtained at this time. The environment in which the wound patient functions must also be assessed. A social history should be obtained to assess living arrangements, hygiene in the home environment, educational level of the patient and family members or others who might be caregivers (i.e., providing assistance with dressing changes or

TABLE 10. GRADING OF AMBULATORY STATUS

Grade	Ambulatory Status
Grade VI	Unlimited community ambulator: Walks at least 5 blocks; uses a wheelchair for longer distances; may use a cane or crutches; and is able to negotiate independently on stairs without rails, on curbs, on rough terrain, and on public transportation.
Grade V	Limited community ambulator: Walks 1–5 blocks; uses a wheelchair for longer distances; may use a cane or crutches; and is able to negotiate independently on stairs without rails, on curbs, on rough terrain, and on public transportation.
Grade IV	Unlimited household ambulator: Walks at least 30.5 meters (100 feet) in the house; uses a wheelchair for longer distances; may use a cane, crutches or a walker; and is able to negotiate independently on stairs with rails, on carpets, and in and out of chairs.
Grade III	Limited household ambulator: Walks less than 30.5 meters (100 feet) in the house; uses a wheelchair for longer distances outside the house; may use a cane, crutches or a walker; and is able to negotiate independently on stairs with rails, on carpets, and in and out of chairs.
Grade II	Supervised household ambulator: Needs supervision during limited walking in the house.
Grade I	Wheelchair ambulator: Uses a wheelchair at all times and is able to transfer and to propel the wheelchair.
Grade 0	Bedridden: Confined to bed or unable to transfer or to propel a wheelchair.

other care requirements), cultural background, and willingness or ability of the patient to participate in his/her care plan. An occupational history should also be obtained, particularly if the patient must continue to work during the treatment period.

History of Presenting Complaint

The history of wounding and prior diagnostic testing and treatment intervention has already been obtained during the evaluation of the wound and is described above.

Past Medical History and Review of Systems

The purpose of this portion of the patient assessment is to identify clinically significant co-morbidities that may impact wound healing, or selection of and response to potential treatment options. Identification of these co-morbidities from the patient assessment also directs the selection of secondary diagnostic testing and directs the extent of the physical examination that is required. Specifically those items that need to be addressed include:

Diabetes Mellitus: Diabetes plays a major role in wound healing failure as well as being a risk factor for wounding and a contributor to other organ system dysfunction. If present, a detailed history of the onset and progression of diabetes should be obtained including any complications such as recurrent hypo or hyperglycemia, neuropathy, nephropathy, retinopathy, and vasculopathy. The current regimen for glycemic control should be defined and its effectiveness assessed. Concomitant lipid disorders should also be identified.

End Stage Renal Disease, Dialysis: The second most significant contributor to wound healing failure is probably renal disease, particularly chronic renal failure requiring dialysis. Not only does renal dysfunction impact wound healing and response to treatment interventions, but the requirement for regular dialysis whether peritoneal or hemodialysis will impact the patient's ability to comply with regularly recurring wound care interventions such as hyperbaric oxygen treatment. Other issues include the location of vascular access.

Cardiac Disease, Congestive Heart Failure: Cardiac disease may point to the presence of peripheral arterial occlusive disease, may give an indication of general functional status, and may represent a risk factor for hyperbaric oxygen treatment.

Chronic Arterial Insufficiency (Secondary): Peripheral arterial occlusive disease plays a major role in lower extremity wound healing failure either as a primary or secondary contributor. Any history of claudication, ischemic rest pain, prior vascular assessment, or prior surgical intervention should lead to a more detailed assessment. Remember that patients with severe cardiac disease may lack the exercise capacity to experience claudication in spite of having hemodynamically significant disease. Remember also to look for risk factors including hypertension and hyperlipidemia. Also, remember to carefully assess the adequacy of circulation in the contra lateral limb.

Edema (Secondary): Local edema is a frequent contributor to wound healing impairment and may be due to cardiac, venous, lymphatic, or metabolic disorders.

Smoking: The impact of tobacco use on wound healing is well established. Any history of smoking should prompt a more detailed assessment of potential end organ dysfunction including chronic skin changes, pulmonary, and vascular disease.

Pulmonary Disease: Pulmonary disease rarely constitutes a major risk factor for wound healing failure unless accompanied by severe resting hypoxemia but may represent a significant risk factor for certain treatment interventions.

Vasculitis (Primary or Secondary), Raynaud's, Other Collagen Vascular Disease: Look for any history of temperature sensitivity (cryoglobulinemias), hematological disorders (sickle cell anemia, polycythemia vera), microthrombotic disorders (antiphospholipid syndromes, cryoglobulinemia), liver disease including hepatitis, unusual drug exposures, and autoimmune disorders (rheumatoid arthritis, systemic lupus erythematosis, scleroderma).

Wound Contamination Including Incontinence: Is there any risk for recurrent wound contamination on the basis of personal hygiene, home environment, or the presence of urinary or fecal incontinence?

Mobility Impairment, Cerebral Vascular Accident, Spinal Cord Injury, Other Musculoskeletal Deformity: These disorders of mobility impairment may make offloading and protection difficult. What pressure relief surfaces or devices or mobility assistive devices are available, what are their conditions, and are they consistently used?

Steroid Therapy, Other Chemotherapy: A complete drug and exposure history should be obtained.

Distant Malignancy: Any history of malignancy and the history of any radiation, surgical, or chemotherapeutic treatments provided. Also, any history of Crohn's disease or ulcerative colitis should be identified as well as any treatment provided.

Malnutrition: Has there been any difficulty with chewing, eating, swallowing, vomiting, or diarrhea for more than one week? Any unplanned weight loss (greater than ten pounds in the last four months), obesity, any previous diagnosis of malnutrition or malabsorption, any special diet, or use of nutritional supplements, vitamins, or weight loss medications? Finally, what is the level of alcohol and caffeine consumption?

Physical Examination

A focused physical examination is performed, directed largely by the findings obtained during the identification of co-morbidities above. Specific attention is paid to the assessment of the skin, vascular disease, and neuromuscular and neurosensory status. A general overview of the patient should include assessment of gait or mobility, general appearance, skin turgor, state of hydration and nutrition, and vital signs including height and weight. It is important to look for physical signs of underlying systemic diseases or co-morbidities described above. It is particularly important to evaluate the condition of the skin in general, not just adjacent to the wound in question, and identify other skin abnormalities, assess muscle mass and muscle tone, joint mobility, and joint deformity.

Arterial System: In the case of lower extremity wounds, a thorough assessment of the vascular system is essential, particularly if risk factors have been identified in the patient history and systems review. Skin changes consistent with peripheral arterial occlusive disease including decreased temperature, dryness, loss of distal hair growth, and dependent rubor, cyanosis, or pallor on elevation should be assessed. At a minimum, peripheral pulses should be palpated. A handheld Doppler is useful to identify pulses when they cannot be palpated, and an ankle/brachial index can be obtained on each lower extremity. All patients with a lower extremity wound should undergo a screening ABI (ankle:brachial index) or TBI (toe:brachial index in diabetics). Any abnormalities detected should prompt further assessment by formal arterial Doppler studies including pressures and pulse volume recording of the major vessels and the digits. Transcutaneous measurement of dermal oxygen tension and/or skin perfusion pressure measurement can also be performed at this stage of the evaluation to look for occult hypoxia or to quantify the degree of ischemia present distal to a pulse deficit. If warranted, referral for magnetic resonance angiography or peripheral arteriography should be done.

Venous and Lymphatic System: In the presence of lower extremity edema, the skin should be inspected for abnormal pigmentation or lipodermato-sclerosis. The degree of pitting should be defined and foot, ankle and calf circumferences measured. Venous varicosities should also be identified. In a setting consistent with chronic venous insufficiency and venous stasis a more detailed venous system examination should be completed and venous Doppler or venous duplex scanning obtained.

Neurosensory/Neuromuscular Status: If risk factors for peripheral neuropathy or mobility deficit have previously been identified, a thorough neurological examination should be completed. All patients with plantar foot ulcers and those with a history of diabetes or other peripheral neuropathy should have screening for loss of protective sensation using the Semmes-Weinstein 5.07 monofilament and deep tendon reflex testing. Two point discrimination and vibratory (128 Hz tuning fork) sensory testing should also be done along with joint mobility assessment if the sensory screening examination is abnormal. It

TABLE 11. SUGGESTED LABORATORY TESTS IN WOUND EVALUATION

Hemoglobinopathy	• Sickle cell screen • Hemoglobin electrophesis
Coagulopathy	• PT, PTT • Antithrombin III • Protein C, protein S • Factor V Leiden • IgG, IgM • Lupus anticoagulants
Local, Systemic Infections	• CBC, ESR • VDRL • Hepatitis screen • HIV • PPD
Immunologic Disorders	• CBC, ESR • Rheumatoid factor • Antinuclear antibodies • Protein electrophoresis • Immune complexes • Complement • A-ANCA, p-ANCA
Nutrition	• Serum albumin • Pre albumin • Transferrin • Absolute lymphocyte count
Wound Biopsy	• Culture • Histopathology

is also useful to observe gait in ambulatory patients looking for foot drop and instability. The feet should be examined for loss of intrinsic musculature. The condition of the skin and nails and any deformity should be noted.

Laboratory Studies

Selection of laboratory studies for further evaluation is based upon the medical history, the review of systems, and the findings obtained on physical examination (5). These tests typically address the presence and control of diabetes, renal failure, nutritional status, collagen vascular disease/vasculitis, and the complications of therapy. Laboratory testing may include but is not limited to those shown on Table 11.

Wound Severity

A complete assessment of the wound and the wound patient must also address wound severity. Is the wound limb or life threatening? Is inpatient care required, or can care be safely and appropriately completed on an outpatient basis? What is the impact of the wound on functional and ambulatory capacity and the likelihood that recovery to pre-wounding functional levels be achieved? What alterations in self image are present, and to what extent will they play in the patient's acceptance of and response to an optimal treatment plan? Are realistic outcome goals acceptable to the patient and achievable

TABLE 12. DIFFERENTIAL DIAGNOSIS OF COMMON LOWER EXTREMITY ULCERS

History of intermittent claudication History of rest pain, improves with dependency History previous vascular surgery Abnormal pulse examination Temperature differential Cyanosis, rubor Smoking Diabetes Hypertension Hyperlipidemia Aging	Chronic edema Lipodermatosclerosis Previous DVT and/or varicosities Previous venous surgery Decreased mobility Obesity Traumatic injury Family history Previous venous ulcer Pain when extremity is dependent for prolonged periods. Decreased pain and swelling with elevation	Deformity Callous Previous history of ulceration Loss of protective sensation Peripheral vascular disease Duration of diabetes Poor glycaemic control Impaired functional abilities
Arterial Ulcer	**Venous Ulcer**	**Neuropathic Ulcer**
Confirmation by: • Arterial Doppler • Arterial duplex scan • Transcutaneous PO_2 MRA • Arteriogram	Confirmation by: • Venous Doppler • Venous duplex scan • Phethysmography	Confirmation by: • Compatible history • Abnormal sensory exam
Location: Generally at the ankle or below, Over bony prominence or area exposed to pressure; Interdigital spaces **Appearance:** *Color:* wound base pale, may see dry necrotic tissue (eschar) *Size:* tend to be small round ulcers with smooth wound edges "punched out" *Drainage:* minimal, unless infected *Edema:* generally not present unless co-morbid CHF *Skin temperature:* decrease, cool and may have dependent rubor and pallor on elevation *Surrounding skin:* shiny, taut, thin, dry, scaly, no hair on lower extremity, thick brittle toe nails **Perfusion:** Pulses diminished, may only be audible with Doppler or absent, ABI 0.7 or lower, Capillary refill > 3 seconds **Caveat:** Large vessel arterial occlusive disease may coexist with venous insufficiency and stasis, neuropathic, and other causes of lower extremity ulceration.	**Location:** Gaiter area (lower calf area and above the ankle), Most frequent is medial aspect of lower leg superior to malleolus **Appearance:** *Color:* wound base fibrinous or granular *Size:* shallow in depth, small to large in surface area, irregular margins *Drainage:* moderate to heavy *Edema:* frequently present and often associated with dermatitis *Skin temperature:* normal *Surrounding skin:* brown staining called hemosiderosis **Perfusion:** Typically palpable pulses, ABI > 0.8 (if lower may be of mixed etiology), Capillary refill normal < 3 seconds **Caveat:** Arterial disease may coexist and should always be assessed.	**Location:** Plantar or lateral aspect of the foot, Metatarsal heads, Site of repetitive pressure and/or friction **Appearance:** *Color:* wound base granular *Size:* variable, usually small, well defined wound margins but may be large. *Drainage:* minimal, unless infected *Edema:* generally not present *Skin temperature:* warm *Surrounding skin:* periwound has thick callous, skin is dry often with fissures. May see structural changes and bony deformities **Perfusion:** ±Palpable pulses, ABI may not be reliable in diabetic patients, Capillary refill normal < 3 seconds **Caveat:** Remember that diabetes mellitus has numerous specific effects on wound healing making it a unique category of neuropathic ulcer.

Evidence of erythema or Induration Purulent exudates Exuberant granulation tissue	History of systemic inflammatory disease Disproportionate pain Blanching dermal infarcts	Chronic edema	History of trauma	Unusual ulcer appearance History of coexisting malignancy
Infectious Ulcer	**Vasclitis Ulcer**	**Lymphedema**	**Traumatic Ulcer**	**Malignent Ulcer**
Confirmation by: • Culture of tissue • Gram stain of tissue • Histopathology	Confirmation by: • Venous Doppler • Venous duplex scan • Phethysmography	Confirmation by: • Lymphangiogram • MRI/CT scan	Confirmation by: • History of injury • History of bite, sting	Confirmation by: • Biopsy for histopathology
Caveat: Remember that unusual causes of infection may be present, obtain careful history of exposures, travel, etc. • Bacterial • Fungal • Mycobacterial • Treponemal • Viral • Parasitic	**Caveat:** Remember that secondary, local vasculitis may be present in any other wound presentation, particularly ulcers associated with chronic venous insufficiency and stasis. **Caveat:** Remember to look for associated systemic diseases such as Crohn's, ulcerative colitis, collagen vascular disease, malignancy.	**Caveat:** Lymphedema may be a secondary finding in chronic ulcers of other primary etiology, may also be post inflammatory present in about 30% of patients with venous insufficiency and stasis. **Caveat:** Arterial disease may coexist and should always be assessed.	**Caveat:** Remember that unusual patterns of physical activity may produce pressure/traumatic ulcerations in unusual locations. **Caveat:** Remember that neuropathy may coexist as enabler of traumatic injury. **Caveat:** Remember that most vasculitic ulcers are precipitated by minor trauma.	**Caveat:** Diagnosis often missed because it is not considered and ulcer not biopsied.

given the socio-environmental status of the patient? Are there specific contraindications to the optimal treatment plan, and must other less effective alternatives be utilized? Finally, is the proposed treatment worse than the disease?

A few brief survey questions and an initial inspection of the wound may allow a preliminary etiologic classification of the wound that can more quickly direct the types of secondary diagnostic studies that will be required. Table 12 demonstrates how identifying characteristics of lower extremity wounds can lead to more specific primary and secondary assessments that will ultimately fully characterize the wound and the wound patient. However, the etiology and diagnostic category of some lower extremity wounds is not quite so easily determined and may required a more detailed review of the differential diagnostic options.

CONCLUDING THE ASSESSMENT AND DEVELOPING A TREATMENT PLAN
  • Setting key therapeutic goals
  • Monitoring the response to treatment

Setting Key Therapeutic Goals
While not all of the steps of evaluation are required for every wound and every wound patient, the process outlined in this chapter does define the essential steps in assessing any problem wound. The nature of the wound should be identified as early in the assessment process as possible enabling a more focused evaluation. All applicable final common pathway components of wound healing failure should be identified, and co-morbidities impacting patient response to the wound or potential treatment interventions should be defined. This information enables the wound care practitioner to develop an effective treatment plan that takes into account key therapeutic goals (18) including the following:

• Resolution of infection	• Enhancement of nutrition
• Enhancement of perfusion	• Exudate control
• Resolution of edema	• Odor control
• Relief of pressure	• Pain control
• Ambulatory off-loading	• Preservation of function
• Mechanical stabilization	• Patient/caregiver education
• Enhancement of tissue growth	• Patient compliance

Not all key therapeutic goals are applicable to all patients, but proper goals will not be established without a complete evaluation of the problem wound patient.

Monitoring the Response To Treatment
Although already introduced in the section on wound assessment, an additional important consideration is ongoing monitoring and evaluating the response of the wound to treatment interventions. Evaluation of healing

requires the analysis of qualitative and quantitative wound assessments. It is made more difficult because of the dynamic nature of the wound healing process. Regular, periodic wound assessment should be performed using an appropriately abbreviated version of the pattern described above. Monitoring can be provided by any trained healthcare provider. However, periodic re-evaluation requires the particular skills and judgment of the physician. The frequency of such assessments is determined by the nature and seriousness of the wound, the condition of the patient, and the early responses to treatment interventions.

CONCLUSION

A simple declarative that the "wound is healed" is probably an insufficient description. As defined by the Wound Healing Society, an ideally healed wound exhibits restoration of skin providing a return to normal anatomic structure, function, and appearance with an intact barrier function. An acceptably healed wound exhibits epithelialization capable of sustaining functional integrity during normal activity. A minimally healed wound exhibits epithelial covering which is restored without a sustained functional result and with a high probability of rewounding (8). Adopting this terminology will greatly aid our ability to comparatively assess outcomes and the interventions that produce them.

REFERENCES

1. Armstrong DG, Lavery LA, Harkless LB. Treatment-based classification system for assessment and care of diabetic feet. *Ostomy/Wound Management* 1996; 86(7):311-316.

2. Bowler PG, Duerden BI, Armstrong DG. Wound microbiology and associated approaches to wound management. *Clin Microbiol Rev.* 2001; 14(2): 244-269.

3. Cierny G, Mader JT. Adult chronic osteomyelitis. *Orthopedics* 1984; 10:557-564.

4. Gardner SE, Frantz RA, Doebbeling BN. The validity of the clinical signs and symptoms used to identify localized chronic wound infection. *Wound Rep Reg.* 2001; 9:178-186.

5. Hess CT, Trent JT. Incorporating laboratory values in chronic wound management. *Adv Skin Wound Care* 2004; 17(7):378-386.

6. Keast DH, et al. MEASURE: a proposed assessment framework for developing best practice recommendations for wound assessment. *Wound Rep Reg* 2004; 12:S1-S17.

7. Kistner RL, Eklof B. Classification and diagnostic evaluation of chronic venous disease. In: Gloviczki P, Yao JST (eds). *Handbook of Venous Disorders, Guidelines of the American Venous Forum, 2nd ed.* New York: Oxford University Press; 2001: 94-103.

8. Lazarus GS, Cooper DM, Knighton DR, et al. Definitions and guidelines for assessment of wounds and evaluation of healing. *Arch Dermatol* 1994; 130:489-493.

9. Mader JT. Mixed anaerobic and aerobic soft tissue infections. In Davis JC, Hunt TK (eds) *Problem Wounds the Role of Oxygen* New York; Elsevier; 1988: 173-186.

10. Maklebust J, Margolis D. The goodness of measurement. *Advances in Wound Care* 1996; 9(3):6.

11. National Pressure Ulcer Advisory Panel. Pressure ulcers: Incidence, economics, risk assessment. Consensus Development Conference Statement, West Dundee, IL, S-N Publications Inc., 1989.

12. Newman LG, Waller J, Palestro CJ, et al. Unsuspected osteomyelitis in diabetic foot ulcers. *JAMA* 1991; 266:1246-1251.

13. Smith RG. Validation of Wagner's classification: A literature review. *Ostomy/Wound Management* 2003; 49(1):54-62.

14. Trent JT, et al. Skin and wound biopsy: when, why, and how. *Adv Skin Wound Care* 2003; 16(7):372-375.

15. van Rijswijl L. Wound assessment and documentation. In: Krasner LD, Rodeheaver GT, Sibbald RG (eds). *Chronic Wound Care: A Clinical Source Book for Healthcare Professionals, 3rd ed.* Wayne PA: HMP Communications: 2001;101-115.

16. Volpicelli LJ, Chambers RB, Wagner FW. Ambulation levels of bilateral lower-extremity amputees. Analysis of one hundred and three cases. *J Bone Joint Surg* 1983; 65A:599-605.

17. Wagner FW. The dysvascular foot: A system for diagnosis and treatment. *Foot & Ankle* 1981; 2(2):64-122.

18. Warriner RA (ed). *Clinical Practice Guidelines 2006 Edition.* Diversified Clinical Services, Jacksonville, FL.

REVIEW QUESTIONS

1) The cause of wound healing failure is usually:
   a. Multifactorial
   b. A single local contributing factor
   c. A single systemic contributing factor
   d. Due to infection

2) Goals of wound and wound patient assessment include all of the following EXCEPT:
   a. Identify and define the wound etiology
   b. Identify and define the specific pathophysiology of wound healing failure
   c. Identify and define associated co-morbidities impacting wound healing
   d. Define the wound as to category and classification
   e. Identify the medical specialist responsible for creating the wound

3) In the wound assessment process which of the following statements is TRUE?
   a. Taking a history of the wounding event has little value.
   b. The location of the wound is useful in differential diagnosis.
   c. The center of the wound should be examined before the edge of the wound and surrounding skin.
   d. Exudate quantity and quality is never misleading as an assessment tool.
   e. Measuring wound size and depth only applies to large wounds.

4) In the wound assessment process which of the following statements is TRUE?
   a. Neuropathic patients cannot experience pain.
   b. A single classification system is used for all wounds.
   c. The wound patient should be reevaluated on a periodic basis
   d. Usually wound infection is very apparent and easily recognized.

5) For classifying or staging wounds, which of the following statements is FALSE?
   a. The simplest staging system for wounds is to define the level of tissue involvement based on depth.
   b. The Wagner scale is a classification system for diabetic foot wounds.
   c. The CEAP (clinical, etiology, anatomic, pathophysiological) classification system is for classifying lower extremity venous disease.
   d. The Cierny-Mader classification system for osteomyelitis has also been adopted as the standard for reporting pressure ulcer depth and extent.

Answers: 1a, 2e, 3b, 4c, 5d

NOTES

CHAPTER 4

NON-INVASIVE AND INVASIVE EVALUATIONS FOR LOWER EXTREMITY ARTERIAL OCCLUSIVE DISEASE

CHAPTER FOUR OVERVIEW

NOTES

Non-Invasive and Invasive Evaluations for Lower Extremity Arterial Occlusive Disease

Clifford J. Buckley, Shirley D. Lee

INTRODUCTION

Until the advent and availability of arteriography, the diagnosis of arterial insufficiency in the lower extremities was based solely on a careful history and physical examination. Arteriography showed stenoses and occlusions within blood vessels and sometimes identified the degree to which collateral blood vessels developed for purposes of providing arterial flow beyond these obstructions. While arteriography provided the anatomic localization of specific arterial lesions, it offered little physiologic information regarding the effect of the lesions on limb blood flow. Clinicians noted that arterial obstruction produced inconsistent symptoms in patients who had similar arterial lesions. The need for acquiring a means of measuring the physiologic effects of arterial stenoses or occlusions and their associated collateral circulation on limb blood flow became obvious. Non-invasive lower extremity arterial testing was developed to meet this need.

The purpose of a non-invasive arterial vascular evaluation is to define the presence or absence of peripheral arterial disease. It also provides an assessment of the severity of the disease process and localizes it to either the aortoiliac, femoral popliteal or tibioperoneal segments of the lower extremity arterial tree. Single level disease can usually be localized into one of these categories. Multi-level disease is more difficult to localize into a dominant component. It is better characterized by the overall severity of impairment of arterial perfusion which it produces.

Non-invasive arterial testing should not be considered a substitute for a thorough history and physical examination. However, simple notation of presence or absence of pulses and grading pulse quality are generally considered to be inadequate for a modern vascular evaluation. Objective physiologic information regarding the adequacy of lower extremity arterial perfusion is standard of care when evaluating and managing patients with problems related to impaired arterial perfusion.

Lower extremity arterial testing offers the advantages of being non-invasive, quite reproducible, and provides physiologic and some anatomic information for disease localization. This chapter will discuss the main diagnostic procedures both, non-invasive and invasive, used to evaluate patients for lower extremity arterial insufficiency. It will identify the limitations of each method and give an estimation of costs associated with these procedures (1). It is important to know that certain non-invasive vascular studies must be performed in the vascular laboratory or by a certified technologist.

STANDARD NON-INVASIVE ARTERIAL STUDIES
Segmental Systolic Pressure Measurements

The earliest efforts for evaluating the arterial system were measuring limb blood pressures using a sphygmomanometer and stethoscope. Unfortunately, this was not useful for the lower extremity below the knee or the upper extremity below the elbow. Windsor (13) used a plethysmograph to measure systolic pressures in the extremities and described the relationship between arm and lower extremity systolic blood pressure. He noted that lower extremity systolic pressure was higher than arm systolic pressure in normal persons and developed a blood pressure index comparing leg to arm pressure. The ratio which resulted from dividing leg systolic pressure by arm systolic pressure has been called the ankle-brachial index or ABI and is always a value of 1 or more in normal persons. Strandness, Sumner and others (14) refined these extremity systolic blood pressure measurements using the Doppler ultrasonic velocity detector as the device for detecting arterial flow instead of the stethoscope or plethysmograph. A continuous wave Doppler consists of a probe with two separate crystals—one transmitting and one receiving continuous high frequency sound waves (2–10 MHz). When the transmitted ultrasound wave intersects a moving column of blood, the frequency shift caused by this event is recorded by the receiving crystal. This frequency shift is converted to an audible signal (1).

Segmental Doppler acquired systolic pressure measurements are usually made at multiple levels in an extremity. A complete lower extremity evaluation normally includes high thigh, low thigh, calf, ankle and sometimes digital pressure measurements. When only one thigh measurement is done, it is best done with the 18 cm thigh cuff. Calf and ankle measurements are made with the standard 12 cm wide adult arm cuff. If two thigh measurements are made, high thigh and low thigh, the 12 cm wide cuff is used for pressure measurements at these two levels. When smaller cuffs are used in the thigh it creates a 20–30 mm Hg artifact falsely elevating the thigh pressures and this needs to be taken into account when interpreting test results. The two thigh cuff technique has been helpful in separating aortoiliac from femoral-popliteal

TABLE 1. INTERPRETATION OF ANKLE BRACHIAL INDICES

ABI	Interpretation
0.95 and above	Normal arteries
0.5 to 0.9	Intermittent claudication
0.4 and below	Severe lower extremity ischemia

disease in some patients. A gradient of 20 mm Hg or more between measuring locations indicates the presence of a lesion which is impairing blood flow (1).

Ankle-brachial indices of 0.95 or more are considered normal. An index less than 0.9 and greater than 0.5 is usually typical for patients with intermittent claudication. Ankle-brachial indices of less than 0.4 indicate severe lower extremity ischemia and are frequently obtained in patients with rest pain, non-healing soft tissue lesions or threatened viability (2, 3, 12).

The simplest rapid assessment technique for evaluating adequacy of lower extremity arterial perfusion is to measure ankle systolic blood pressure and compare it to brachial pressure. The best Doppler signal obtained from either the dorsalis pedis, posterior tibial or peroneal artery at the ankle or foot is used as the reference vessel (Figure 1).

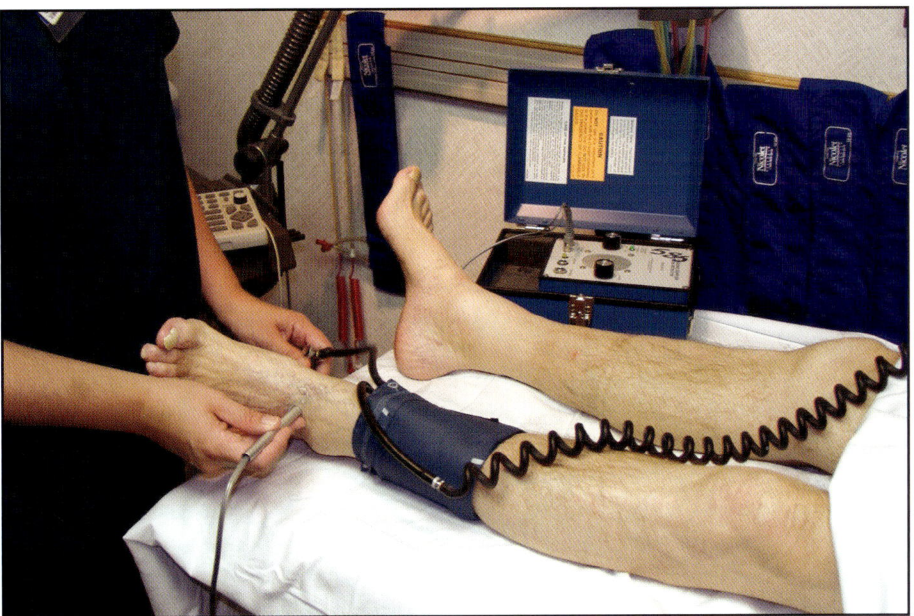

Figure 1. Ankle Systolic Blood Pressure Measurement Technique.

Abnormal arterial stiffness, as seen in patients with femoral-popliteal or tibioperoneal arterial wall calcification, will artificially elevate segmental systolic pressure measurements and will render ABI measurements inaccurate. This is seen in patients with diabetes mellitus and also in individuals who have consumed high mineral content water for most of their adult life. When heavy vascular calcification is present, toe pressure measurements can be useful but, in the normal person there is a 20–30 mm Hg gradient between ankle systolic pressure and toe pressure—the toe pressure being lower. This gradient must be taken into account when toe pressures are used. Approximately 20–25% of segmental systolic pressure studies obtained at rest may be inaccurate because of vessel wall calcification or the presence of lesions which only produce their hemodynamic effects during exercise. The cost for this type of study ranges from approximately $25.00 for a simple ABI measurement to $125.00–$300.00 for full multi-level lower extremity pressure testing. The cost of a good quality hand held Doppler for office use should be less than $500.00.

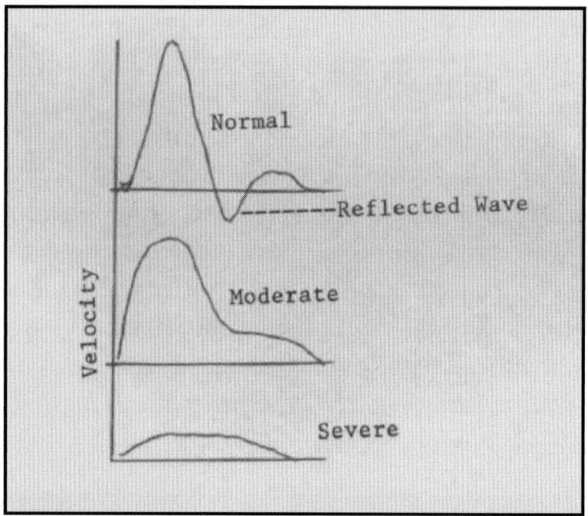

Figure 2. Doppler Wave Form Showing Changes in Normal and Diseased Arteries.

Doppler Wave Form Evaluation

Most Doppler ultrasonic velocity detectors provide an analog signal that is proportional to the velocity of the blood in the vessel being evaluated with the Doppler probe. This analog signal can be displayed on a chart recorder or other type of display screen and is qualitatively analyzed with respect to the shape of the wave form. The Doppler wave form from a normal vessel is quite similar to an intra-arterial pressure wave form. It has a triphasic appearance with rapid systolic upstroke in the anacrotic limb of the tracing and rapid down slope during diastole noted in the catacrotic limb. There is reversed flow in the normal vessel in early diastole. This reversed flow is often referred to as the "reflected wave" part of the Doppler wave form. Loss of the reflected wave or reversed flow is the first Doppler wave form change noted when there is a stenosis proximal to the site where the vessel is being evaluated (Figure 2). As the degree of arterial occlusive disease increases in severity, the Doppler wave form becomes more blunted or rounded and broadens. Flat wave forms indicate severe occlusive disease and near absence of Doppler detected blood flow. Arterial lesions distal to the site where the wave form is being recorded can also influence the wave form appearance because of their affect on resistance in the vascular outflow bed (6).

Doppler wave form evaluations are usually obtained at the common femoral, superficial femoral, popliteal, posterior tibial, anterior tibial and peroneal levels in a lower extremity. The advantages of this test are that it may be more sensitive to milder forms of occlusive disease and can be more vessel specific than simple segmental systolic pressure measurements. The limitations of this test are numerous. It is extremely operator dependent in that the Doppler probe must be held at an approximate 60° angle of incidence with the blood vessel being evaluated. If too much pressure is applied to the probe, the vessel beneath it can be compressed simulating a stenosis or occlusion. Patients who are obese or who have scarred extremities from previous surgical intervention on their blood vessels, produce wave form studies which are difficult to interpret. Finally, in patients with advanced diffuse arterial occlusive disease, the wave forms become so distorted that they loose their usefulness for disease localization. The cost of a standard resting multi-level wave form study is approximately $200.00.

Segmental Plethysmography

Plethysmography has been used for more than 50 years to evaluate segmental limb blood flow. It is based on a principal that during systole, the blood entering an extremity produces an increase in the total volume of the extremity. During diastole the limb volume returns to base line. These changes in limb volume with each cardiac cycle can be measured at specific locations. The earliest form of plethysmography was the oscillometer which was a type of blood pressure cuff placed on an extremity and partially inflated to the point where changes in volume beneath it were detected on a gauge. Silastic mercury strain gauge, water displacement, impedance and capacitance plethysmographs have all been used to evaluate arterial perfusion. Most, however, need frequent meticulous calibration, are cumbersome to use and may require a constant temperature environment for accurate interpretation. In the early 1970s, Raines and associates (2) developed a segmental air plethysmograph or pulse-volume recorder (PVR) for use in evaluating the peripheral arterial system. The PVR uses air filled cuffs of various sizes which are inflated to 65 mm Hg for the larger portions of the limb and 35–40 mm Hg for digits. The reason for inflating the cuffs to 65 mm Hg is to compress the underlying venous channels so that the change in volume detected by the air filled cuff represents only the effect of arterial inflow during systole. An extremely sensitive transducer detects the pressure change in the cuff produced by the corresponding segmental limb systolic volume increase.

Pulse-volume recordings are usually obtained at high thigh, low thigh, calf, ankle, transmetatarsal and digital levels in each extremity (Figure 3). Hard copy pulse wave forms are generated by the PVR and are qualitatively compared at various levels in the extremity as well as comparing one limb to another (Figure 4). Patients with normal arteries show PVR's which are similar to intra-arterial pressure tracings in that they have a rapid anacrotic rise during systole, a dicrotic notch during early diastole and a rapid down slope in the catacrotic limb of the wave form during diastole. Pulse-volume recordings are usually reported as category I-V. Category I is normal and Category V is essentially flat and indicates severe impairment of segmental limb blood flow (2, 3, 12). Loss of the dicrotic notch is similar to loss of the reflected wave in Doppler wave form studies and is usually indicative of a mild occlusive process (Figure 5).

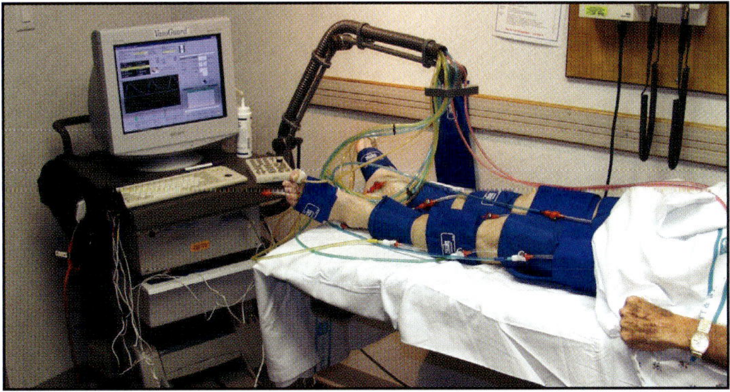

Figure 3. Complete Segmental Pulse Volume Recording Lower Extremity Evaluation Procedure.

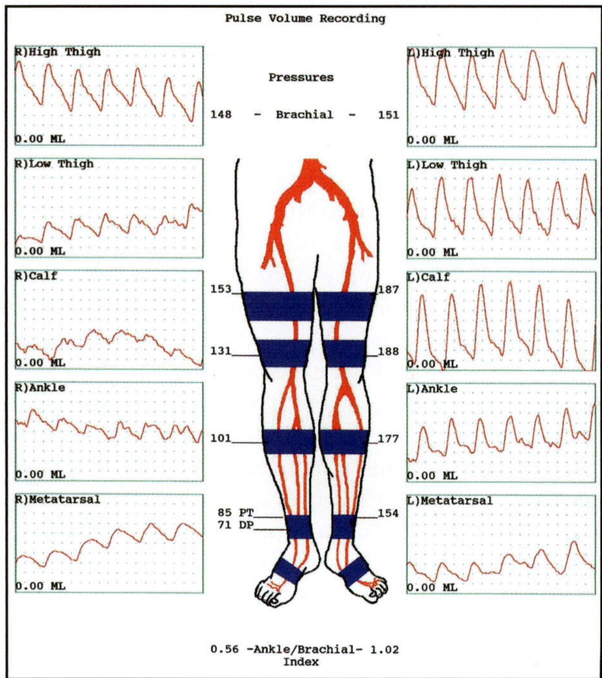

Figure 4. Comprehensive Lower Extremity Arterial Study Showing Segmental Systolic Pressure Measurements and Segmental Pulse Volume Recording. Right Leg Shows Femoral-Popliteal Occlusion. Left Leg is Normal.

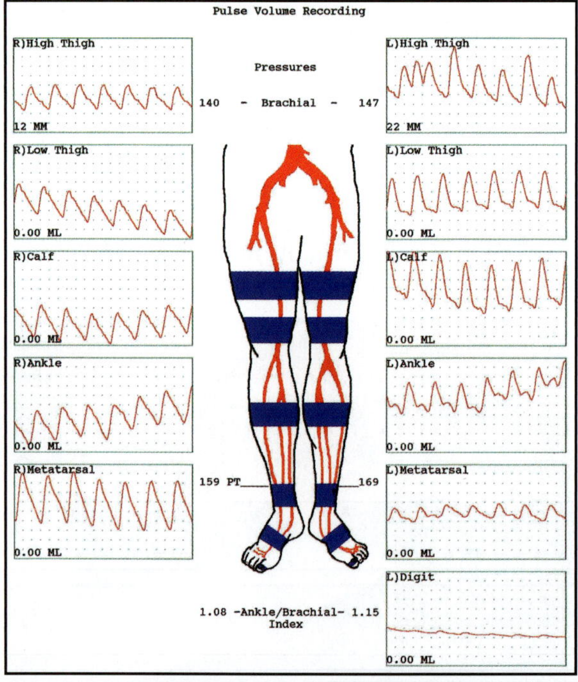

Figure 5. Comprehensive Lower Extremity Vascular Study Showing Mild Iliac Occlusive Disease In Right Leg with Loss of Dicrotic Notch. Left Leg is Normal.

Pulse-volume recorders have the advantages of being more sensitive than segmental systolic pressure measurements, are not particularly operator dependent and detect occlusive disease in the presence of heavily calcified vessels. The heavy vessel calcification does not affect volume changes in the extremities with systole and diastole and the PVR is not dependent on compression of these calcified vessels. It has been used to serially evaluate patients with very acceptable reproducibility. It also easily identifies disease progression and improvement from intervention. Pulse-volume recording has been reported by Kempezinski (15) and others to have a 90–95% accuracy for disease localization compared to arteriography.

There are limitations to the PVR. It is sensitive to changes in cardiac output. Therefore, the interpretation of serial studies in a patient who receives new medication (beta blocker) or has a myocardial event which adversely affects cardiac output may have PVR changes suggesting progression of arterial occlusive disease which are artifactual. Additionally, the data generated by PVR is qualitative and not quantitative with respect to segmental limb blood flow and there is some variation in results generated from machines produced by different manufacturers. Pulse-volume recorders are moderately expensive—approximately $25,000–$30,000 and the cost of an individual test ranges from $175.00–$400.00. It always includes segmental systolic pressure measurements along with segmental plethysmography.

Exercise Testing

Patients with advanced arterial occlusive disease in their lower extremities can usually be adequately evaluated by segmental systolic pressure measurements and segmental pulse-volume recordings obtained at rest. However, some patients will have segmental stenoses which do not affect blood flow in an extremity in a resting or non-stressed state. When demand for increased blood flow occurs, these stenoses become hemodynamically significant and flow limiting. Exercise lowers resistance in the vascular bed of an extremity and specifically the muscle mass. The decreased vascular resistance facilitates increased blood flow or perfusion. As previously discussed, the demand for increased flow changes a non-hemodynamically significant stenosis at rest to one which is flow limiting during exercise. Exercise testing is most useful for evaluating complaints of claudication, documenting reproducibility of symptoms and defining exercise tolerance. It can also be used to demonstrate to patients with poorly healing soft tissue wounds on feet or toes that perfusion to the wound is impaired by diverting blood flow away from the wound to an exercising muscle mass. In patients with normal arterial circulation this is of little consequence. However, patients with significant arterial disease proximal to the soft tissue wound will have impaired perfusion to the wound while they are working the muscle mass of the extremity, i.e., walking (5, 7).

Exercise testing is usually accomplished using either foot pump (heel-toe) or motorized treadmill exercise. Foot pump testing is used for patients limited by advanced cardiac or pulmonary disease or who have soft tissue wounds on the feet or toes which impede their ability to walk because of pain. The duration of foot-pump exercise is usually two minutes.

Treadmill testing is done for patients who are able to ambulate without significant compromise from other comorbidities. Two treadmill stress exercise programs are usually offered. The low speed program is run to a maximum of five minutes of ambulation on a treadmill operating at 1.5 or 1.7 mph in a fixed 10–12% grade elevation. The high speed program is used primarily for claudicants and is five minutes of ambulation at 2.25–2.5 mph and fixed 10–12% grade elevation.

Patients who cannot ambulate or foot pump effectively can have the effects of exercise on lowering limb vascular resistance simulated by creating a state of reactive hyperemia. This is done by inflating a thigh blood pressure cuff well above systolic pressure and maintaining that inflation for 3 to five minutes. The cuff is then rapidly deflated and changes in distal systolic pressure measurements and PVR wave forms are noted. A lesion which is hemodynamically insignificant in the resting state may become manifest during the effects of reactive hyperemia. Finally, most exercise testing has ankle systolic pressure measurements and pulse-volume recordings obtained immediately at completion of the exercise stress and then at one minute intervals during the recovery phase up to five or ten minutes post exercise. Mild occlusive disease or disease which is well collateralized will show rapid recovery to baseline following exercise. Patients with severe occlusive disease may not reach baseline even after ten minutes of recovery.

The limitations of exercise testing are that the exercise programs tend to vary from laboratory to laboratory and therefore, the exercise stress for an individual patient done during serial exams at different labs may be variable. Exercise testing adds $35.00–$100.00 additional charge to the previous described arterial tests.

Color Flow Duplex Ultrasound Imaging

Color flow duplex imaging of lower extremity arteries has been useful in accurately localizing and categorizing arterial lesions identified by segmental systolic pressure measurements and segmental plethysmography. Several published series have suggested it is equal in accuracy to that of arteriography. It is this author's (Buckley) opinion that color flow Duplex imaging is more appropriate for localizing focal, short segment lesions rather than mapping the entire aorto/ilio/femoral/popliteal/tibial arterial system. Interpretation of color flow duplex ultrasound images is dependent on the quality of the study. Skilled ultrasonographers equipped with the more sophisticated imaging units will produce highly accurate evaluations (Figure 6). In addition to visualizing the arterial lesion directly, 100% peak systolic velocity increases in an area of stenosis (velocity ratios $\geq$ 2) compared with a normal segment of artery proximal to the stenosis indicates a hemodynamically significant stenosis of 50% diameter reduction or greater. Color flow duplex imaging will usually describe the artery being evaluated as either being patent without significant stenosis, patent with stenosis $\geq$ 50%, or segmentally occluded.

Color flow duplex ultrasound imaging is especially valuable for evaluating suspected arteriovenous fistula, pseudoaneurysms vs. hematomas and peripheral aneurysms. It is useful as a screening tool to identify patent target vessels for distal bypass purposes. Its sensitivity and specificity for identifying arterial occlusive lesions has been estimated at approximately 70–80% sensitivity and > 90% specificity.

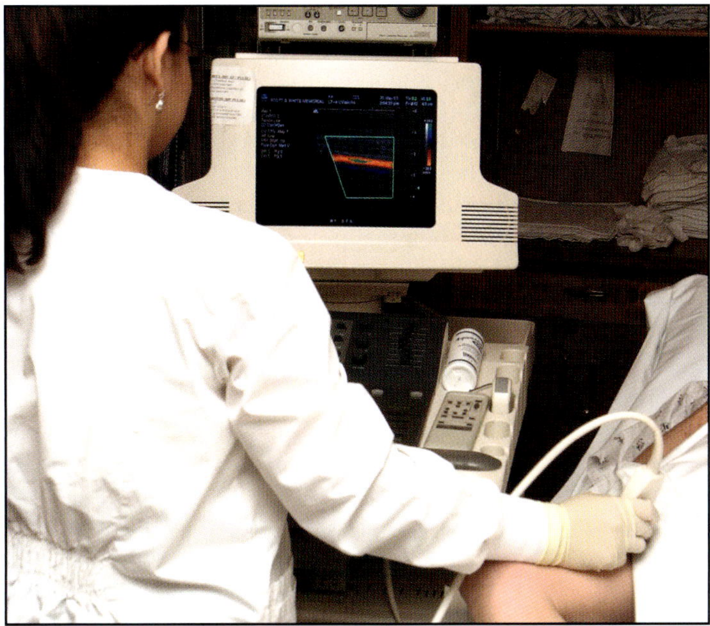

Figure 6. Color Flow Duplex Ultrasound Image of a Proximal Right Superficial Femoral Artery.

Bilateral arterial mapping of the lower extremity arterial tree requires a skilled technologist, a high quality color flow duplex imaging unit and is labor intensive and costly. This author rarely uses color flow duplex ultrasound imaging for this purpose. Color flow duplex ultrasound imaging is used in our vascular laboratory to localize arterial occlusive lesions identified by other non-invasive testing, especially when selecting patients for possible endovascular therapy. It is also used for surveillance of previously constructed lower extremity arterial bypass grafts and for evaluating the greater or lesser saphenous veins for use as a bypass conduit (8).

Equipment and technologist costs necessary to provide this service are substantial. High quality color flow duplex ultrasound imaging units cost $125,000–$200,000 and experienced technicians command salaries of $50,000–$60,000 or more per year. The cost to the patient for a color flow duplex imaging evaluation averages $250.00–$300.00 if the exam is used to define and localize a suspected specific arterial lesion. Bilateral full lower extremity arterial mapping procedures are usually billed at $850.00–$1,000.00 or more.

SUPPLEMENTAL OR NICHE EVALUATION TECHNIQUES
Transcutaneous Oxygen Tension (TcpO$_2$)

Transcutaneous oxygen tension reflects the metabolic state of target tissues and when used for assessment of lower extremity arterial perfusion relates primarily to the metabolic state of the skin. Measurement of TcpO$_2$ is affected by cutaneous blood flow, abnormal venous pressure, metabolic activity, oxyhemoglobin dissociation and oxygen diffusion through tissue. The best means for obtaining tissue pO$_2$ information is with devices which use sensors that are implanted into the tissue being studied. Unfortunately, there are a variety of reasons why the use of direct tissue penetrating devices are impractical—pain with application, potential for spreading contamination, and, in the USA, lack of an FDA approved device for human applications. More commonly, $TcpO_2$ measurements are obtained from sensors that are attached to the surface of the skin that has been appropriately degreased (Figure 7). The values for tissue oxygen tension are obtained from the area of the limb being evaluated for healing potential and can be compared to a standard reference measuring site (usually the skin on the chest wall just below the clavicle). As mentioned previously, numerous factors can artificially elevate or cover $TcpO_2$ values, i.e., studies with the feet in dependent position, infection, etc. When studied in the supine position, normal $TcpO_2$ values should be approximately $\geq$ 50–60 mm Hg on the dorsum of the feet with some increase in oxygen tension when measurements are made more proximally in the extremities. It is generally accepted that $TcpO_2$ measurements $\geq$ 35–40 mm Hg have a high probability for healing a soft tissue wound using local wound care measures. Transcutaneous oxygen tension values obtained which are $\leq$ 10–20 mm Hg suggest a poor potential for wound healing and identify a need for revascularization if these low values are the result of impaired arterial perfusion to the area studied. For more information about $TcpO_2$ values as an assessment tool for wounds see the chapter by Dietz and Sheffield titled "Noninvasive Wound Assessment Tools."

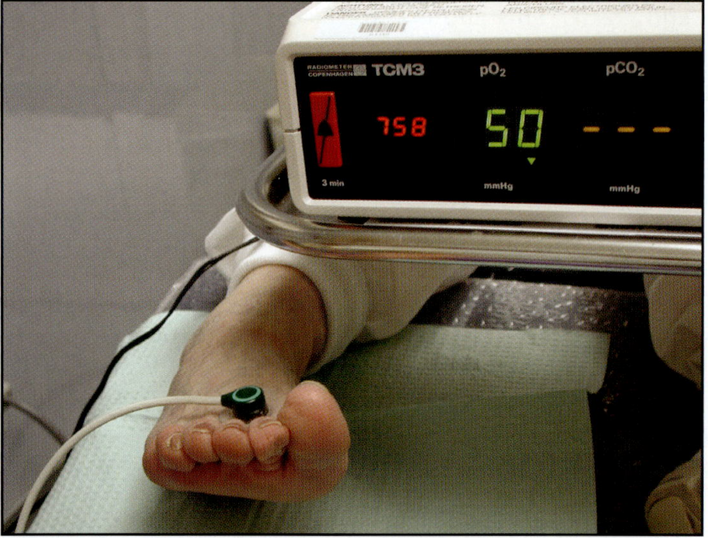

Figure 7. Transcutaneous Oxygen Tension Measurement Made Using Non-Penetrating Sensor.

Laser Doppler Velocimetry and Skin Blood Pressure Measurement

Laser Doppler velocimetry is recognized as a valid, physiologic means for detecting skin blood flow. It is used together with a pneumatic cuff to estimate skin blood pressure at various points on an extremity. In this circumstance, the laser Doppler velocimeter serves as a blood flow sensor placed under a pneumatic cuff. Skin blood pressure measurements on the plantar skin of the great toe and foot are normally approximately 75 mm Hg $\pm$ 10 mm Hg. As would be expected, much lower pressures are found when patients have significant arterial occlusive disease in the extremity being evaluated, i.e., 50–70 mm Hg pressures in claudicants and 10–40 mm Hg in limbs with rest pain or non-healing soft tissue wounds.

Laser Doppler velocimetry derived skin blood pressure measurements and $TcpO_2$ measurements are generally used in conjunction with other forms of lower extremity physiological vascular testing to predict wound healing using local wound care, define the level for successful amputation or identify need for revascularization.

For more information about laser Doppler flowmetry as an assessment tool for wounds see the chapter by Dietz and Sheffield titled "Noninvasive Wound Assessment Tools."

MINIMALLY INVASIVE AND INVASIVE LOWER EXTREMITY ARTERIAL STUDIES

Minimally invasive and invasive lower extremity arterial examinations should be used primarily when it has been determined that the patient is in need of an intervention to improve blood flow to an extremity. These diagnostic procedures may also be used to evaluate unusual arterial pathology which cannot be detected using non-invasive examination techniques. In general, these diagnostic procedures provide accurate anatomic localization of arterial lesions and assess the overall severity of the extent of the occlusive process. They should not be used as "first line" screening procedures to determine the presence or absence of arterial pathology. Each of these procedures has some morbidity and/or mortality. They are all expensive and, in general, do not lend themselves to repetitive use in the same patient. They provide only limited physiologic information and are most useful to the Vascular Surgeon or Endovascular Therapist for purposes of planning invasive treatment. The cost of these studies ranges from $1200.00–$3500.00.

MINIMALLY INVASIVE LOWER EXTREMITY STUDIES
Magnetic Resonance Angiography (MRA)

Magnetic resonance imaging is derived from the reactions of various tissues to a magnetic field stimulated by a radiofrequency radiation pulse. The signal, which is generated by this action, is related to the proton density of each specific tissue. Magnetic resonance angiography is a physiologic method for vascular imaging which distinguishes it from contrast angiography which is a pure anatomic imaging modality. Magnetic resonance angiography images are formed by using the effect related to the flow of blood relative to the surrounding stationary soft tissue. This effect can be enhanced through the use of an intravenous or intra-arterially administered contrast agent. MR angiography has the advantage of having large fields of view, can obtain images with and without the use of contrast, avoids the need for arterial puncture with its attendant complications, and uses a contrast agent with minimal nephrotoxicity (10).

The limitations of MRA are exclusion criteria for use of the technology in a particular patient—presence of a pacemaker, etc. Signal drop out or flow voids occur when arterial stenoses reach 70% or greater and, therefore, it is difficult to assess accurately a more severe degree of stenosis. Magnetic resonance angiography is more sensitive than conventional angiography in detecting target vessels for bypass purposes in extreme "low flow" perfusion situations. While this has been useful in many patients, MRA has sometimes identified target vessels which at the time of surgical exploration were unsuitable for bypass purposes because of severely limited outflow bed. In many centers, MRA of the lower extremities is replacing contrast angiography as the sole preoperative imaging technique. As this technology continues to improve through developments in hardware, software and contrast agents, its application will continue to expand. Magnetic resonance angiography is more cost effective than contrast angiography. Studies are typically $1200–$1500 cheaper than similar contrast arteriography costs and MR studies are performed as pure outpatient evaluations.

Spiral Computed Tomography Angiography

Spiral computed tomography angiography with 3-dimensional reconstructions of the acquired images has been extremely valuable in evaluating intra-abdominal and intra-pelvic arterial pathology. It has helped revolutionize the treatment of aortic, iliac and visceral aneurysm disease. At present, in the extremities its usefulness is confined to evaluating uncommon problems—peripheral aneurysms, adventitial cystic disease and arterial entrapment syndromes. The usefulness of this technique in evaluating infrapopliteal arterial pathology has been limited by the need to deliver sufficient quantities of intravenously administered contrast to these arteries without also enhancing the adjacent veins. At present, MRA is far superior to spiral computed tomography angiography for evaluating lower extremity arterial pathology (9).

INVASIVE LOWER EXTREMITY ARTERIAL STUDIES
Contrast Angiography

Contrast angiography, including digital subtraction image enhancing techniques, is still considered in most centers as the "gold standard" for evaluating lower extremity arterial occlusive disease. It is commonly employed when arterial reconstruction is contemplated. It accurately depicts arterial anatomy. Because it requires arterial puncture for intra-arterial access, direct intra-arterial pressure measurements can be made across a lesion for purposes of evaluating hemodynamic significance. Generally, pressure gradients of 15 mm Hg or greater indicate that the lesion produces a significant effect on blood flow (11).

A complete lower extremity arteriographic evaluation should include anterior-posterior and lateral views of the abdominal aorta showing branch arteries to include the celiac, mesenteric, renal and iliac arteries. It should also include oblique pelvic views to visualize common iliac lesions which are frequently located on the posterior wall of these vessels. These views are also necessary to visualize stenoses in the orifices of the hypogastric and profunda femoral arteries. Infrainguinal run-off studies should visualize the superficial femoral and popliteal arteries in their entirety including the trifurcation and all three tibial vessels. Foot views should show the dorsalis pedis, distal posterior tibial and their major branch arteries including the plantar arch and digital vessels (Figure 8). All of these described views are absolutely essential when planning limb salvage revascularization procedures. Missing a significant

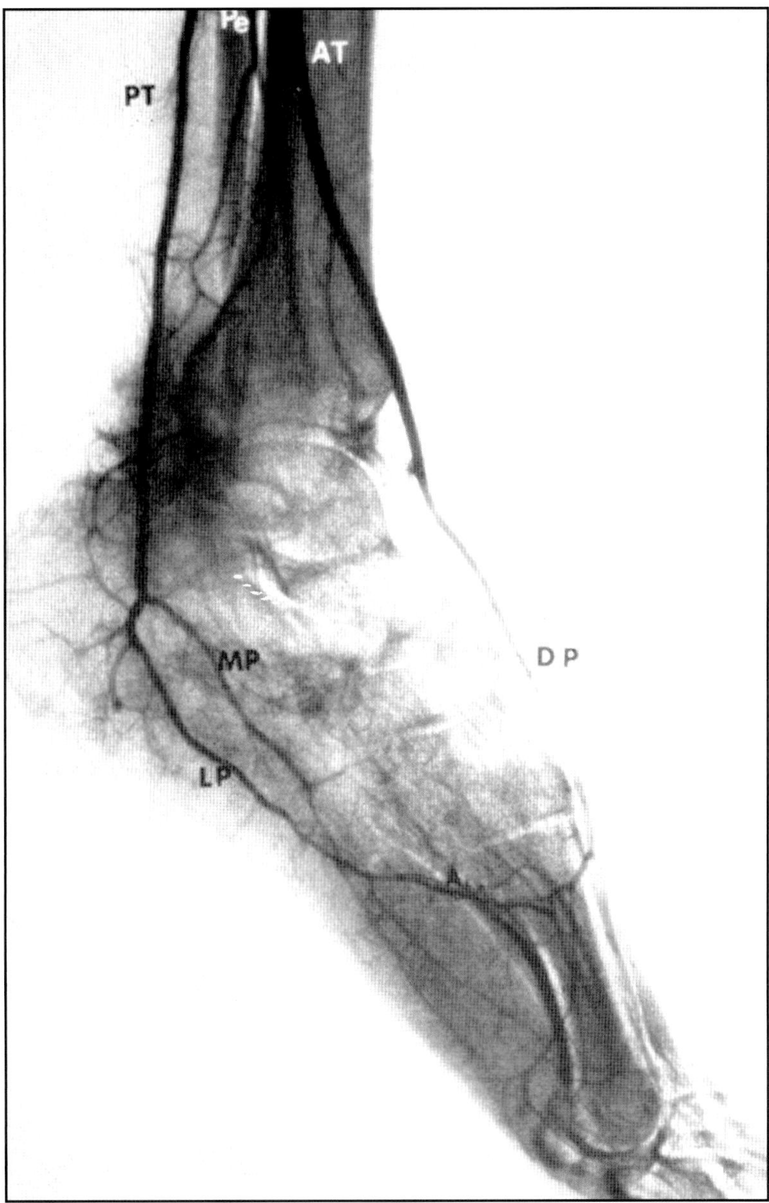

Figure 8. Digital Subtraction Arteriogram Showing Arterial Visualization Essential for Planning Infrapopliteal or More Distal Revascularization Procedure.

inflow lesion will predispose a reconstruction to early failure. Similarly, revascularizing a vascular bed that has no branches going to the area of a poorly healing soft tissue wound can result in a patent bypass but continued poor wound healing and ultimate need for amputation.

The limitations of arteriography are that it has definite morbidity and mortality. Arterial access is associated with local hematoma, pseudoaneurysm and traumatic A-V fistula formation. It can also result in local arterial injury with thrombosis or distal embolization. The contrast agents used for vessel opacification have potential nephrotoxicity and have an incidence of allergic reactivity including anaphylaxis. In general, these studies provide only anatomic information and are not helpful in assessing the physiologic effects on limb perfusion produced by the underlying arterial occlusive process.

SUMMARY

The information provided in this chapter should serve as a general guideline for the evaluation of patients with lower extremity arterial occlusive disease. The reader is directed to the attached reference list for more specific and detailed information relevant to the diagnostic procedures described in this text.

REFERENCES

1. Weale FE. *An Introduction to Surgical Haemodynamics.* Chicago, IL: Year Book Medical Publishers, 1967.

2. Raines J, Darling RC, Buth J, et al. Vascular Laboratory Criteria for the Management of Peripheral Vascular Disease of the Lower Extremities. *Surgery* 1976; 79:21-29.

3. Buckley CJ, Darling RC, Raines J. *Equipment and Examination Techniques Important in the Management of Peripheral Vascular Diseases. Clinical Vascular Laboratory Manual,* Vascular Surgery Unit, Wilford Hall USAF Medical Center, Vascular Laboratory, Massachusetts General Hospital and Department of Surgery, Harvard Medical School.

4. Bernstein EF. *Noninvasive Diagnostic Techniques in Vascular Disease.* St Louis, MO: CV Mosby Co: 1985.

5. Sumner DS. Essential Hemodynamic Principles. In *Rutherford Vascular Surgery, 5th edition* (2000). Philadelphia, PA: WB Saunders: 73-119.

6. Baker JD. The Vascular Laboratory. In *Rutherford Vascular Surgery, 5th edition* (2000). Philadelphia, PA: WB Saunders: 127-139.

7. Zierler RE, Sumner DS. Physiologic Assessment of Peripheral Arterial Occlusive Disease. In *Rutherford Vascular Surgery, 5th edition* (2000). Philadelphia, PA: WB Saunders: 140-164.

8. Zwolak RM. Arterial Duplex Scanning. In *Rutherford Vascular Surgery, 5th edition* (2000). Philadelphia, PA: WB Saunders: 192-213.

9. Fillinger MF. Computed Tomography and Three-Dimensional Reconstruction in Evaluation of Vascular Disease. In *Rutherford Vascular Surgery, 5th edition (2000).* Philadelphia, PA: WB Saunders: 230-268.

10. Velazquez OC, Baum RA, Carpenter JP. Magnetic Resonance Imaging and Angiography. In *Rutherford Vascular Surgery, 5th edition* (2000). Philadelphia, PA: WB Saunders: 269-285.

11. Hodgson KJ. Principles of Arteriography. In *Rutherford Vascular Surgery, 5th edition* (2000). Philadelphia, PA: WB Saunders: 286-302.

12. Baker JD. The Vascular Laboratory. In *Vascular Surgery: A Comprehensive Review, 6th edition,* W.Moore (ed) (2002). Philadelphia, PA: WB Saunders: 248-263.

13. Winsor T. Infuuence of Arterial Disease on the Systolic Blood Pressure Gradients of the Extremity. *Am J Med Sci* 1959; 220:117-126.

14. Strandness DE, Schultz RD, Sumner, et al. Ultrasonic Flow Detection–Useful Technique in the Evaluation of Peripheral Vascular Disease. *Am J Surgery* 1967; 113:311-320.

15. Kempezinski RK. Segmental Volume Plethysmography in the Diagnosis of Lower Extremity Arterial Occlusive Disease. *J Cardiovasc Surg 1982; 23:125-129.*

REVIEW QUESTIONS

1.) In evaluating adequacy of lower extremity arterial perfusion an ankle-brachial index (ABI) of less than 0.4 indicates:
   a. Normal circulation
   b. Intermittent claudication
   c. Severe lower extremity ischemia
   d. None of the above

2.) Plethysmography used to evaluate segmental limb blood flow during the cardiac cycle is based on a principal that during systole there is an increase in the total volume of the extremity and during diastole the limb volume returns to base line.
   a. True
   b. False

3.) Exercise testing is most useful for:
   a. Evaluating complaints of claudication
   b. Documenting reproducibility of symptoms
   c. Defining exercise tolerance
   d. A and b, but not c
   e. A, b, and c are correct

4.) Transcutaneous oxygen tension values obtained which are $\leq$ 10–20 mm Hg suggest a poor potential for wound healing and identify a need for revascularization if these low values are the result of impaired arterial perfusion to the area studied.
   a. True
   b. False

5.) The "gold standard" for evaluating lower extremity arterial occlusive disease that is commonly used when arterial reconstruction is contemplated because it accurately depicts arterial anatomy is:
   a. Contrast angiography
   b. Magnetic resonance angiography
   c. Spiral Computed Tomography Angiography
   d. Laser Doppler Velocimetry

Answers 1c, 2a, 3e, 4a, 5a

CHAPTER 5

NON-INVASIVE WOUND ASSESSMENT TOOLS

CHAPTER FIVE OVERVIEW

NON-INVASIVE WOUND ASSESSMENT TOOLS

Duane A. Dietz, Paul J. Sheffield

INTRODUCTION

Prior to initiating the wound management plan, it is important for the wound care practitioner to assure that the wound has enough blood supply and oxygen to heal. Transcutaneous oximetry (TCOM) and laser Doppler flowmetry (LDF) are common non-invasive tools used by wound treatment centers for assessing problem wounds.

To avoid confusion in terminology, in this chapter TCOM refers to the equipment (transcutaneous oxygen monitoring) or the procedure (transcutaneous oximetry) used for obtaining tissue oxygen values in the skin. $P_{tc}O_2$ or $TcpO_2$ (transcutaneous oxygen tension) refers to the tissue pO_2 data obtained by TCOM, and is expressed in mm Hg. Although $P_{tc}O_2$ is technically correct, $TcpO_2$ is the more common term used by wound centers, government agencies and insurance carriers, and therefore used in this chapter.

TRANSCUTANEOUS OXIMETRY AS A WOUND ASSESSMENT TOOL

Transcutaneous oximetry and perfusion data have been used by physicians in many specialties to make decisions about the treatment of their patients. For example, TCOM is used by neonatologists to assess the quality of pulmonary function in neonates thereby avoiding invasive arterial blood gas testing. TCOM and LDF are routinely used as aids to choose a course of treatment. Physicians in wound treatment centers use transcutaneous oxygen ($TcpO_2$) values for evaluating degrees of hypoxia, determining wound healing potential, determining treatment options for a particular wound, determining appropriate amputation levels, selecting patients for hyperbaric oxygen (HBO) treatment, and predicting non-responders to various treatment modalities including HBO. Determining the tissue oxygen status of a wound area is important because severely hypoxic wound beds render ineffective certain treatments such as skin grafting, growth factor treatments, or living tissue replacements, e.g., fibroblasts, keratinocytes, and dermal composites. A severely hypoxic wound bed also indicates that treatment options to correct the hypoxia (revascularization and HBO) should be employed.

Transcutaneous oximetry is routinely used in wound treatment centers that are equipped with hyperbaric chambers to select patients for hyperbaric oxygen therapy by identifying hypoxic wounds. It is also used to determine which hypoxic wounds might respond to hyperoxia. For patients that receive HBO, TCOM can be used to determine when HBO can be discontinued.

To understand the information obtained from TCOM, it is important to differentiate it from pulse oximetry. Pulse oximetry is a colormetric measure of hemoglobin oxygen saturation and is more of an indicator of pulmonary oxygen exchange. Pulse oximetry does not necessarily correlate to arterial pO_2. Transcutaneous oximetry has been shown to correlate to arterial pO_2 and thereby can be used to determine the amount of oxygen that is available for tissue metabolism.

The following sections include a discussion of the technical aspect of TCOM, values that are obtained for normal and ischemic tissues in both normobaric and hyperbaric conditions and methods for obtaining reliable and reproducible results. There is also a discussion of the $TcpO_2$ assessment protocol used at the Nix Wound Care and Hyperbaric Medicine Center in San Antonio, Texas (1).

HOW TRANSCUTANEOUS OXIMETRY WORKS

A transcutaneous oximeter (Figure 1) uses a large Clark polarographic electrode that is modified to contain a heating element and thermister. The heating element maintains a preset temperature of 42–45°C, and is continuously monitored by the thermister. A phosphate buffer and potassium chloride solution is contained between the electrode surface and an oxygen permeable membrane. Typically, the electrode is attached to the skin by an adhesive fixation device that is filled with contact solution so as to maintain a continuous liquid pathway for the oxygen to diffuse from the skin to the electrode. A constant polarizing voltage is applied to the cathode within the sensor. The polarized oxygen electrode provides electrons to reduce molecular oxygen as it arrives at the electrode surface. Independent of the polarizing voltage, an extra current is derived from the reduction of oxygen at the electrode surface, as in the presence of water, oxygen is converted to hydroxyl ion. The current generated is directly proportional to the number of oxygen molecules in solution and to the pO_2 of the solution (per Henry's Law). In this manner, the oxygen sensor can be used to determine the oxygen tension in the skin capillaries.

Baumberger and Goodfriend (2) first demonstrated that oxygen diffused through the skin by immersing a subject's finger in a phosphate buffer solution that was heated to 45°C for about 60 minutes to show that the pO_2 in the buffer solution approximated the subject's arterial oxygen tension. Huch and associates (3) developed the TCOM technology for use in neonates. In order for the oxygen to diffuse to the skin surface where it can be analyzed, the non-invasive sensor must cause physiological changes in the underlying tissue. The primary effects are changes in local perfusion, skin lipid structure, oxygen solubility, and the oxyhemoglobin dissociation curve. Heating the sensor to 42–45°C transfers heat to the skin surface directly beneath the electrode that dilates capillaries, opens skin pores, decreases oxygen solubility, and shifts the oxyhemoglobin curve to the right for a more ready release of oxygen (4). In the absence of heat, diffusion of oxygen from tissue to skin surface contributes less than 3.5 mm Hg to the PO_2 at that location (5). In contrast, when the skin surface is heated to 44–45°C, the resultant physiological responses produce oxygen tensions at the skin surface that closely approximates arterial oxygen tension derived from the capillary bed beneath the sensor (3). The best correlation between $TcpO_2$ and arterial pO_2 appears to occur in newborn infants, presumably due to their thin skin and the absence of barriers that would prevent oxygen from diffusing through the skin to reach the sensor.

As an assessment tool for potential HBO candidates, $TcpO_2$ indicates if the tissue near the wound is hypoxic, and if it responds to respired oxygen. Low $TcpO_2$ values are sometimes difficult to interpret, as it could be due to poor perfusion or other factors such as vasoconstriction or edema. In those cases, additional vascular assessment is necessary. One of the methods gaining popularity in the wound center is laser Doppler flowmetry (LDF) (6), which is discussed later in this chapter.

Since TCOM is a non-invasive evaluation, it is generally not painful and tolerated by most patients. Most of the problems associated with $TcpO_2$ assessment actually stem from the devices used for oxygen delivery. Patients who are prone to confinement anxiety or true claustrophobia sometimes have difficulty keeping the oxygen hood or mask in place for the time required to adequately complete the test. Accommodations need to be made for these patients and it should be noted that if a patient cannot tolerate a surface TCOM test then they will be unlikely to tolerate the confinement that is involved with hyperbaric oxygen treatments.

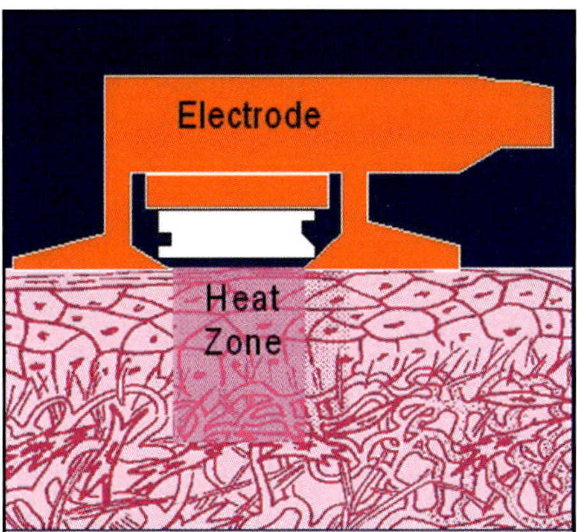

Figure 1. Schematic of Transcutaneous Oximeter. Heating the skin to 42–45°C beneath the electrode (heated zone) opens skin pores, dilates capillaries, decreases oxygen solubility, and causes oxyhemoglobin to release oxygen.

NORMAL TCPO₂ VALUES

Table 1 contains "normal" $TcpO_2$ values of Dooley et al. (1997) (7) obtained in 72 healthy subjects (53 males, 19 females) for chest, calf, and midfoot. Data were obtained at 1.0 ATA (air), 1.0 ATA (oxygen) and 2.4 ATA (oxygen), and reveals a significant gender difference only at the calf. In the authors' experience, normal values at 1 ATA range from 55–70 mm Hg when breathing air and 250–450 when breathing oxygen. Hyperbaric oxygen values at 2.0 ATA range from 700–900 mm Hg, and at 2.4 ATA range from 900–1300 mm Hg. From the data obtained, a regional perfusion index can be calculated. The regional perfusion index (RPI) is the ratio of the limb $TcpO_2$ to the chest $TcpO_2$ while breathing room air at 1 ATA. If the value on the mid foot is 55 mm Hg and at the chest is 70 mm Hg, the RPI would be 55/70, or 0.8. From Table 1 it can be seen that a normal RPI is about 0.75 -0.9.

TABLE 1. NORMAL TCPO$_2$ VALUES IN HEALTHY SUBJECTS

	21% O$_2$/1 ATA	100% O$_2$/1ATA	100% O$_2$/2.0 ATA	100% O$_2$/2.4 ATA
Chest[a]	67±12	450±54	——	1312±112
Calf (male)[a]	49±14	281±78	596±146[b]	1027±164
Calf (female)[a]	59±12	367±59	720±216[b]	1174±127
Midfoot[a]	63±13	280±82	457±195[b]	919±214

[a] *Dooley J, King G, and Slade B, 1997(7).*
[b] *Fife CE, Unpublished data.*

USES OF TRANSCUTANEOUS OXIMETRY
Evaluation of Tissue Hypoxia

A literature review by Sheffield (1) confirmed that transcutaneous oximetry is commonly used to evaluate tissue hypoxia in pediatric ICU, plastic surgery, vascular surgery, anesthesiology, orthopedics, wound care, and hyperbaric medicine. $TcpO_2$ assessment was clinically useful in determining healing potential, selecting amputation level, evaluating revascularization procedures, and assessing severity and progression of peripheral vascular disease.

Determination of Wound Healing Potentials

Patients who breathe room air and who have $TcpO_2$ values above 40 mm Hg or a RPI above 0.6 should have sufficient tissue oxygenation to heal wounds using conventional wound care, skin grafting, application of topical growth factors, or application of living tissue replacements, such as fibroblasts, keratinocytes, and dermal composites. Conversely, patients who have $TcpO_2$ values below 40 mm Hg or a RPI below 0.6 are considered to have significant tissue hypoxia that will negatively impact wound healing. These patients would be considered candidates for revascularization or aggressive HBO treatment to avoid amputation. Tissue oxygen tension is not the only factor in determining the potential for a wound to heal or not to heal. Other factors such as blood glucose levels, nutrition, infections, renal failure, smoking and unrelieved pressure on the wound, can have a negative impact on wound healing. Since persistent smoking has been shown to have a negative effect on wound healing, wound patients should be discouraged from smoking. Otto and associates (8) retrospectively reviewed outcomes from 180 diabetic patients with lower extremity wounds and reported that the average patient with a history of smoking who benefited from HBO needed between 8 and 14 more treatments for the same outcome as a nonsmoker. This translated into an added cost of $4,000–$7,000 for the average patient who smoked. Considering the multi-factorial nature of wound healing, it is difficult to predict a positive outcome based on adequate $TcpO_2$ values alone. Wound healing potentials based on $TcpO_2$ values should be considered and reported as a failure to heal potential. In this way, one can avoid giving an implied guarantee of success to the patient and/or family.

Gorman (9) conducted a review of diabetic foot wounds in which he used relative $TcpO_2$ (% of chest control) and ankle pressure to predict treatment outcome. He concluded that patients, who have relative $TcpO_2$ values greater than 85% and ankle pressure greater than 90 mm Hg, will heal without supplemental oxygen. Conversely, those with relative $TcpO_2$ values less than 20% and ankle pressure less than 75 mm Hg are unlikely to heal. Using Gorman's criteria, candidates for HBO should be those patients whose relative $TcpO_2$ values were 20–85% and ankle pressure of 75–90 mm Hg.

Selection of Amputation Site

Normal wound healing of an amputation site requires a $TcpO_2$ value of at least 40 mm Hg or regional perfusion index of about 0.6. White & Klein (10) reviewed transcutaneous oximetry studies involving 260 amputees who did not receive HBO2 and concluded that a $TcpO_2$ value of 40 mm Hg or greater was predictive of spontaneous healing while values below 35 mm Hg were associated with failure. Hauser (11) prospectively assessed 159 wounds (93 local debridements and 66 amputations) in 113 high-risk diabetic patients with peripheral vascular disease. He reported excellent outcome when RPI was greater than 0.6 and poor outcome when RPI was less than 0.4. It is common to receive a request for a TCOM evaluation to determine an amputation level. As discussed above, wound healing is multifactorial and a full evaluation of the patient is required to make appropriate treatment recommendations and decisions.

Selection of Patients for HBO2 Treatment

Fife (12) described the TCOM testing procedures and selection criteria of wound patients who were candidates for HBO2 treatment in Fife's and Warriner's chapter entitled "Hyperbaric Oxygen Therapy Applications in Wound Care." The patients received at least two of the following tests: 1) Baseline measurement breathing air at 1 ATA; 2) oxygen response measurement breathing 100% O_2 at 1 ATA, and 3) HBO2 response breathing 100% O_2 at 2–2.5 ATA. Fife et al. (8) also conducted a retrospective analysis of outcomes for over 1100 diabetic foot ulcer patients seen in five wound treatment centers. Fife (2002) reported that when oxygen-breathing $TcpO_2$ values increased to above 35 mm Hg at sea level, the likelihood of benefiting from HBO2 was 77% and the test was 69% accurate. Pecoraro et al. (19) found $TcpO_2$ values to be useful as predictors of healing in diabetic patients and in selecting patients for adjunctive HBO2 to correct underlying tissue hypoxia either alone or in combination with revascularization. In a study of predictors for non-healing in diabetic foot wounds Pecoraro concluded that periwound cutaneous perfusion is the critical physiological determinant of diabetic ulcer healing, indicating a 39 fold increased risk of early healing failure when the average periwound $TcPO_2$ is <20 mm Hg. Sheffield (1) retrospectively found that diabetic patients with forefoot wounds (n = 84) had an 8-fold increase in likelihood of successful outcome with HBO2 when baseline transmetatarsal $TcpO_2$ values were greater than 30 mm Hg as compared to $TcpO_2$ values less than 30 mm Hg (p < .05).

Evaluation of Response to HBO2 Treatment

There is controversy as to the predictive wound healing value of $TcpO_2$ studies done at sea level versus studies done while the patient is pressurized inside the hyperbaric chamber. A number of investigators have suggested that the best predictor of wound healing success would be a $TcpO_2$ study that is conducted under hyperbaric conditions at 2.0–2.4 ATA, but the suggested absolute values vary widely. The reports have focused on diabetic patients because that is the subgroup of HBO2 patients whose numbers are large enough for their outcome data to become statistically significant. Myers and Emhoff (15) reported that diabetic patients (n = 11), with below-knee $TcpO_2$ values less than 20 mm Hg, would heal if 900–1100 mm Hg could be achieved on the initial HBO2 exposure. Wattel et al. (16) concluded that $TcpO_2$ values above 500 mm Hg during HBO2 were predictive of healing in diabetic patients with plantar ulcers. Mathieu et al. (17) reported that $TcpO_2$ values during HBO2 must be above 600 mm Hg for healing of lower extremity ulcers secondary to arterial insufficiency. Campagnoli et al. (18) reported that diabetic patients (n = 28) healed if $TcpO_2$ values were above 400 mm Hg during HBO2, and observed that the faster the rise, the greater likelihood of an efficient support microcirculation, thereby improving the patient's chances of a favorable outcome. Strauss et al. (19) reported that 98% of patients with foot wounds (n = 87) healed when $TcpO_2$ exceeded 200 mm Hg during HBO2 (100% oxygen for 90 minutes at 2 ATA, 202 kPa). In a retrospective analysis of outcomes for over 1100 diabetic foot ulcer patients, Fife et al. (13) reported that when in-chamber $TcpO_2$ increased to 200 mm Hg or better, the likelihood of benefiting from HBO2 was 94% and the test was 75% accurate. Despite the fact that this study lacked a control group of patients denied HBO2 therapy, the predicted outcome was impressive for diabetic foot ulcer patients for whom $TcpO_2$ values were above 200 mm Hg. The Authors postulate that after some, yet-to-be-determined threshold value is achieved raising $TcpO_2$ above that value confers no added benefit (13). Sheffield and Workman (20) reported improved $TcpO_2$ baseline at the wound site taken at seven-day intervals while the patients received HBO2 therapy indicating that hyper-oxygenation enhanced angiogenesis in human wounds. Thus, when a wound can be healed with HBO2 treatment, there is a better chance of it remaining healed when the treatment is complete. At the author's hyperbaric facility, HBO2 treatments are considered to be therapeutic if $TcpO_2$ values of 200 mm Hg can be achieved during HBO2 treatments. In the case of compromised flaps or grafts, the desired value is at least 50 mm Hg.

STEPS NEEDED TO ATTAIN REPRODUCIBLE TCPO$_2$ DATA IN THE CLINICAL SETTING

Obtaining Formal Training

Transcutaneous oximetry is as much an art as a science. In order to obtain reproducible results, it is important to standardize the data collection technique. Data collection requires a skilled technologist using rigorous and consistent protocol. Interpretation of data requires a complete understanding of the limits of the technology. The Undersea and Hyperbaric Medical Society

(UHMS), which is an international professional society for hyperbaricists, acknowledges this need and requires transcutaneous oximetry instruction for physicians who attend any UHMS Designated Introductory Course in Hyperbaric Medicine (21). The National Board of Diving and Hyperbaric Medical Technology (NBDHMT), which is the certifying board for hyperbaric registered nurses (CHRN) and hyperbaric technologists (CHT), requires transcutaneous oximetry instruction for nurses and technologists who attend any NBDHMT Designated Introductory Course in Hyperbaric Medicine. In the United States, some Medicare Intermediaries have imposed specific certification requirements on those who desire to bill Medicare, and have limited those who could perform the TCOM test to physicians, certified vascular technologists, certified hyperbaric technologists (CHTs), or certified hyperbaric registered nurses (CHRNs). It would be prudent to check with the Medicare fiscal intermediaries and third party payers on their certification requirements before billing them for services.

Selecting the Monitor

Several manufacturers produce transcutaneous oximeters that have been used for TCOM studies of HBO2 candidates (22). The most common transcutaneous monitors are: SensorMedics "MicroGas" (formerly Kontron), Novametrics, Perimed, and Radiometer. In 1983, Sheffield and Workman (23, 24) reported the first $TcpO_2$ data recorded under hyperbaric conditions (100% oxygen at 2.4 ATA, 238 kPa). Using a Radiometer TCM1 oximeter, they reported values exceeding 1,000 mm Hg in both healthy subjects and in patients. As of this writing, the Radiometer TINA sensor used in the TCM3, TCM30, and TCM400 series of monitors (Radiometer, Copenhagen, Denmark) are the only sensors that have been tested and shown to be compatible with operation in a hyperbaric chamber filled with pure oxygen (22). Since the Perimed monitor (Perimed, Stockholm, Sweden) is equipped with the Radiometer TINA sensor, their sensor is also approved for use in a pure oxygen environment. Fire safety considerations require the monitor to remain outside the chamber, thus requiring the sensor to be installed with leads that pass through the metal portion of the chamber hull.

Calibrating the Sensor

It is advisable to install a new membrane on the sensor every two weeks and to follow the manufacturer's instructions for calibration. If the time between $TcpO_2$ evaluations is greater than two weeks, new membranes can be installed when a $TcpO_2$ test is planned. Modern TCOMs use a two-point calibration where the low calibration point is zero and the high calibration point is the pO_2 in room air. In order to have an accurate calibration, the barometric pressure in the room must be measured then 20.9% of that value (the fraction of oxygen in air) is used as the high calibration point. The oximeter will set the low calibration point automatically and might be capable of setting the high calibration point automatically if equipped with an internal barometer.

Selecting the Sensor Temperature

Transcutaneous sensors measure the approximate arterial oxygen values in the capillary bed beneath the chosen site. Heating the skin 42–45°C causes physiological changes beneath the sensor that opens pores, dilates capillaries, increases skin perfusion, increases metabolism, reduces oxygen solubility, and causes hemoglobin to release oxygen. Tolerance of the skin to 44–45°C heat is limited. The heat causes erythematous marks that are often seen after removal of the TCOM sensors (Figure 2), which typically fade after a few hours. A temperature setting of 45°C gives the best arterial value, but it also increases the risk of causing a blister on the skin. Figure 3 shows a blister wound on the dorsum of the foot following a 2-hour exposure with the TCOM sensor set at 45°C. The diameter of the blister wound matches the size of the TCOM sensor. Temperatures above 45°C should not be used.

To avoid burning the patient, the authors use a 44°C sensor temperature and limit the heat applied at one site to no more than 1 hour. Thus, $TcpO_2$ values reported by these authors will be about 2% lower than at other laboratories that collect $TcpO_2$ values at 45°C. For whatever sensor temperature setting is chosen, it is important to be consistent, and to report the temperature setting in scientific reports.

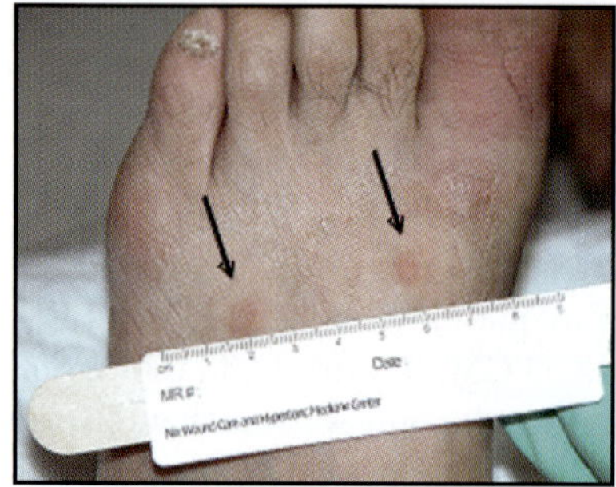

Figure 2. After removal of the TCOM electrode an erythematous mark is often seen which typically fades after a few hours.

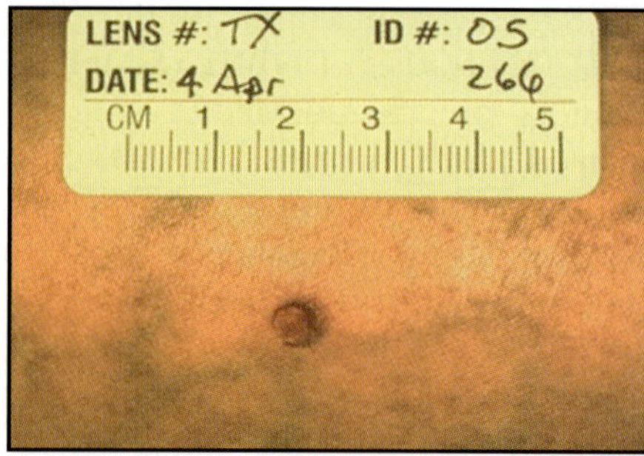

Figure 3. Prolonged application of TCOM sensor (2 hours at 2.4 ATA) set at 45°C produced a blister on the dorsum of the foot. The diabetic patient with acute arterial insufficiency had presented for evaluation post surgery for osteomyelitis. The diameter of the blister matched the size of the TCOM electrode.

Preparing the Site for Electrode Placement

The sensor site should be shaved, cleaned with alcohol, and exfoliated with adhesive tape to remove superficial layers of dry, loose skin cells. The site should not overlie a bony prominence, tendon or callous (25). Flat or slightly convex areas provide the most reliable sensor contact. The fixation ring should be checked for tightness of seal from the surrounding air. If multiple sites are to be measured, the fixation rings should be affixed so that the electrode wires will all be positioned in the same direction. This reduces movement artifacts and risk of electrode displacement should the patient move. A measurement taken in the web space between the toes is least reliable because the sensor is prone to leak at the curvature. Applying Skin Prep to the adhesive site will sometimes help adhere the sensor to the skin, but it must not be applied beneath the sensor's membrane, as it will interfere with oxygen diffusion though the skin, prevent oxygen from reaching the sensor, and give a falsely low $TcpO_2$ value.

Choosing a Method of Assessment

A number of methods have been used to assess healing potential. These include: 1) a single $TcpO_2$ value adjacent to the wound; 2) a map of multiple sites around the wound; 3) a map of several sites on the affected limb; 4) a comparison of periwound or amputation site values expressed as a percentage of control values at the chest, or Regional Perfusion Index (RPI); and 5) a comparison of the mean values of two or more sites near the wound. The method chosen will depend on the number of electrodes available. But regardless of the assessment method, it is important to be consistent. Considering normal circulation to the limb, there should be a standard approach to positioning the sensor. This will provide more consistent data and allow a means of comparing data among a subgroup of patients. Figure 4 is an example of standardized sites at which $TcpO_2$ data are collected at the authors' assessment laboratories. At the author's laboratories nine sensors are typically used: two are placed at the mid calf level, two at the mid foot level, two at the anterior foot, one at wound level on the opposite limb, and one is placed at the second intercostal space on the left chest (designated as control). If a pacemaker or other implanted device is located at the control site, the right second intercostal space may be used. The remaining electrode can be placed wherever additional information is desired. Adjustments in the standard lead placement sites will need to be made based on the number of leads available at a particular facility.

Allowing Adequate Time for Electrode Equilibration and TCOM Evaluation

Acquiring a $TcpO_2$ baseline value of the supine patient takes twenty minutes. As the sensor heats the skin, equilibration of the electrode occurs within 10–15 minutes for subjects with normal circulation, but requires about 15–20 minutes for patients with compromised circulation (1).

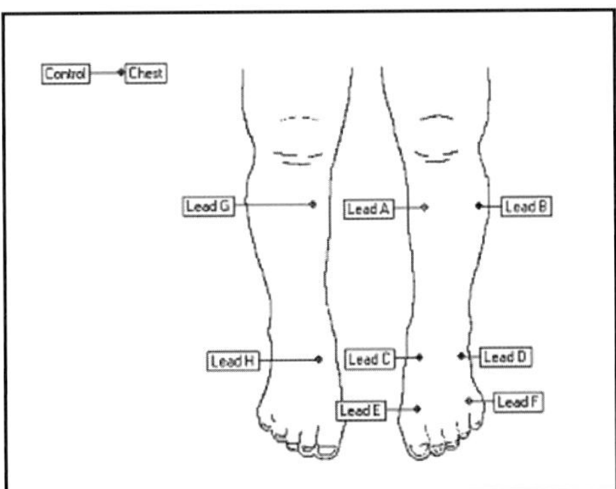

Figure 4. Author's (DD) Standard TCOM Lead Placement. The sequence is typically medial to lateral, proximal to distal on the extremity with the wound in question.

Standardizing the Testing Procedure

A standard testing procedure is important to produce reliable data. The procedure used at the author's (DD) wound assessment laboratories is a 45-minutes assessment as shown in Table 2 which identifies three tests. Test 1 is the baseline $TcpO_2$ (air) value that identifies whether the tissue surrounding the wound is normoxic or hypoxic. This test identifies periwound nutritive pO_2 values in the normal resting state of the patient. There are two physiological challenges: elevated limb and oxygen challenge. Test 2 is a five minute elevated limb challenge that consists of the leg being elevated 30° to identify the presence of large or small vessel disease that would cause pO_2 to fall until the patient is returned to the normal supine position. This test identifies whether there is adequate vascular reserve for normal oxygenation to be sustained during leg elevation. Test 3 is a ten minute oxygen challenge that identifies the wound area's response to oxygen. This test identifies the periwound nutritive oxygen value attained during oxygen breathing. The sensor is allowed to return to baseline after each physiological challenge in order to check for electrode drift, malfunction or dislodgement. Some would argue that this assessment takes too much time, and would be satisfied with a 30-minute assessment that includes only $TcpO_2$ baseline on air (20 minutes) and an oxygen challenge (10 minutes). However, the leg elevation phase is important to test for critical limb ischemia which would warrant further investigation for a correctable cause. To save time, some technicians allow only 10 minutes for the electrode to equilibrate. However, a 20-minute equilibration period is better for reproducible results.

TABLE 2. $TCPO_2$ ASSESSMENT PROCEDURE FOR MAPPING THE SKIN SURFACE OF LOWER LIMB

Test	Assessment	Time Required (Min)	Lapsed Time (Min)
	Electrode equilibration (air)	15	15
Test 1	**Baseline TcpO$_2$ (air)**	**5**	**20**
Test 2	**Elevated limb (air) challenge**	**5**	**25**
	Baseline TcpO$_2$ with leg level (check for electrode drift)	5	30
Test 3	**100% oxygen challenge**	**10**	**40**
	Baseline TcpO$_2$ on room air (check for electrode drift)	5	45
	Total evaluation time	**45**	**45**

INTERPRETING THE DATA

Some physicians predict wound healing by interpreting the raw $TcpO_2$ values. Others calculate a "relative value," or a limb to chest ratio, called a "regional perfusion index" (RPI = limb $TcpO_2$/chest $TcpO_2$). Others calculate the mean of data from two or more sites near the wound. There is no consensus on the best method for collecting or interpreting the data. However, it is clear that interpretation demands careful assessment of the tissue on which the sensor is placed, so the interpreter should observe the wound and choose the location of the sensors. If it is not possible for the interpreter to observe the sensor placement, then good quality photos should be taken to show the interpreter the quality of the skin and locations on which the sensors are placed. Interpretation of the TCOM results should not be made using the $TcpO_2$ data alone. An appropriate history and physical will add valuable information to the interpretation. History such as ischemic symptoms, claudication, previous wounds and their outcome, chronic diseases such as diabetes mellitus, coronary artery disease, pulmonary disease, strokes, renal failure and mobility all weigh in the final interpretation of the $TcpO_2$ results, determination of healing potentials and treatment recommendations. For accuracy in interpretation, the quality of the $TcpO_2$ data is very important and observing the tracings is useful in determining the quality of the data collected. Figure 5 shows tracings with high variability indicating poor quality data. Figure 6C shows the $TcpO_2$ tracings from a typical TCOM evaluation. In this particular recording, the trace lines are smooth indicating good quality data. [All tracings in this chapter were obtained using PeriSoft for Windows, Perimed AB, Stockholm, Sweden, *www.perimed.se*.]

One important note is that the TCOM evaluation in Figure 6C was done by a highly experienced technician and the TCOM evaluation in Figure 5 was done by a technician with less experience.

Basic $TcpO_2$ Interpretation

In the testing procedure outlined in Table 2, there are three tests performed in the evaluation. The first test is the baseline oxygenation while breathing room air. A reading is taken at the 20 minute mark for each of the electrode sites and this gives an impression of the normal capillary oxygen levels available to the tissues for that patient. This can be used to estimate the failure to heal potential for the current wound if it is given standard wound care.

The second test is the leg elevation challenge. This is a test for critical limb ischemia. In this test, the leg is elevated 30° to 45° for five minutes. Normally

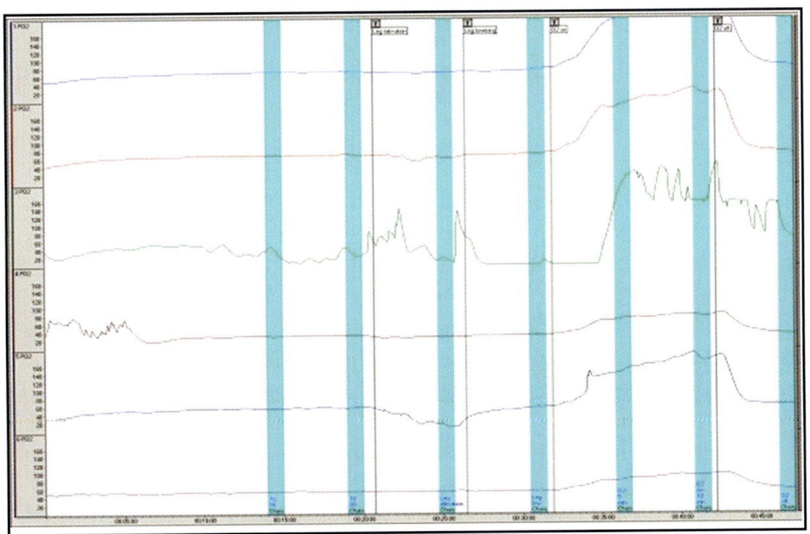

Figure 5. *TcpO₂ Tracings From A Substandard TCOM Evaluation Using Six Sensors. High variability in lines indicate poor quality tracing. Artifacts at tracings 3, 4 and 5 were caused by patient movement and leaks under the sensor fixation ring.*

there is an initial decrease in oxygen tensions. In the non-ischemic extremity, the oxygen tensions should recover to the previous baseline. This will not occur in an ischemic extremity. A decrease of more than 10% is considered significant. Often patients will complain of pain when they elevate their legs, which is relieved when the legs are in a dependent position. The suspected ischemia will be confirmed with this test. When the legs are dependent, perfusion can be increased by increasing the hydrostatic pressure in the vascular system. Since the reflexive response by many health care providers is to elevate any extremity with a problem, you can be the patient's best friend when you tell them that they can dangle their legs.

The third test is the oxygen challenge. During this test, the patient breathes 100% oxygen via an oxygen hood or a tightly fitting face mask. Nasal cannula or non-rebreather masks do not provide 100% oxygen and should not be used. While the patient is breathing oxygen, there should be an elevation in oxygen tensions measured by the electrode and the range of expected values is listed in Table 1. In the ischemic and hypoxic extremity, those values would not be achieved. For hypoxia to be considered reversible and the patient to be considered a possible candidate for HBO2 treatments, oxygen tensions should reach at least 40 mm Hg and the percent change from baseline should be at least 50%. If either of these conditions is not met, then the probability of success with HBO2 is low. The third test is sometimes repeated under HBO2 conditions with a goal of achieving $TcpO_2$ values above 200 mm Hg.

Case 1 (Figures 6A-D & Table 3) describes a TMA that failed to heal despite standard wound care. TCOM assessment was conducted to help clarify the treatment options. The case illustrates how the three tests outlined in Table 2 are used.

Case 1

Patient FSG-327 is a 54-year-old male who had developed an ulcer on his right foot in early June. The ulcer became infected and he underwent a third ray resection on 17 June. Following surgery, he was determined to have osteomyelitis and he underwent a right transmetatarsal amputation (TMA) on 2 July. The TMA failed to heal despite routine wound care and he was referred to the Wound Healing Center on 16 July for evaluation and treatment. He had a 10 year history of non-insulin dependent diabetes which was complicated by retinopathy and neuropathy. There was no history of previous wounds or peripheral vascular disease.

The right foot had a non-healed TMA (Figure 6A). The open wound measured 67 x 32 x 2 mm. The wound bed consisted of fibrotic and necrotic tissue with some exposed adipose tissue. There was minimal granulation tissue present. There was no exposed bone identified. There was no drainage or odor detected. The surrounding skin was not erythematous or warm to touch. Pedal pulses were palpable.

TCOM Assessment: Figure 6B shows the placement of the 9 sensors (control and leads A–H) used for the TCOM assessment. The $TcpO_2$ tracings for the data are seen in Figure 6C. Table 3 shows the numeric list of $TcpO_2$ values for baseline (air), leg elevation challenge, and oxygen challenge.

$TcpO_2$ Interpretation: The $TcpO_2$ values of the right mid foot (leads C and D) indicates moderate to severe baseline hypoxia with values ranging from 5 to 33 mm Hg. There was a significant decrease (greater than 10%

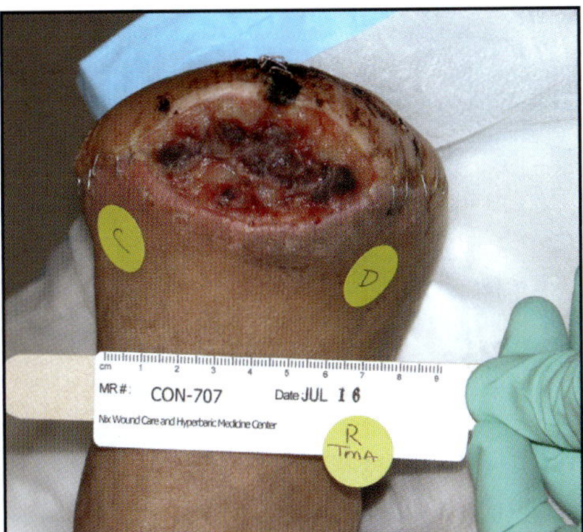

Figure 6A. Case 1—Patient FSG-327 / CON 707. (Figures 6A through 6D) Failing right TMA at initial consultation).

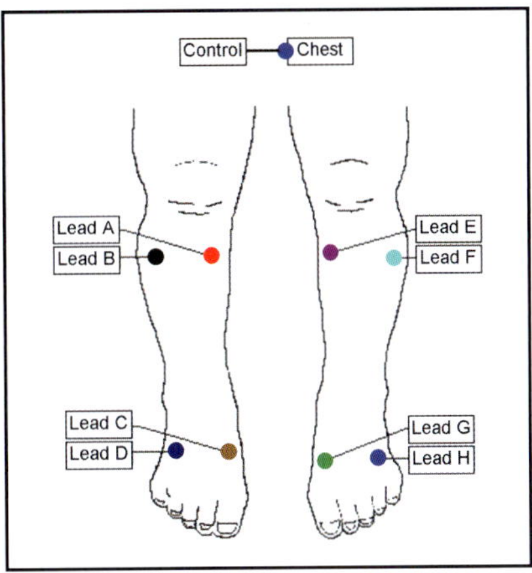

Figure 6B. TCOM sensor placement for Patient FSG-327. The 9th sensor is at chest control site.

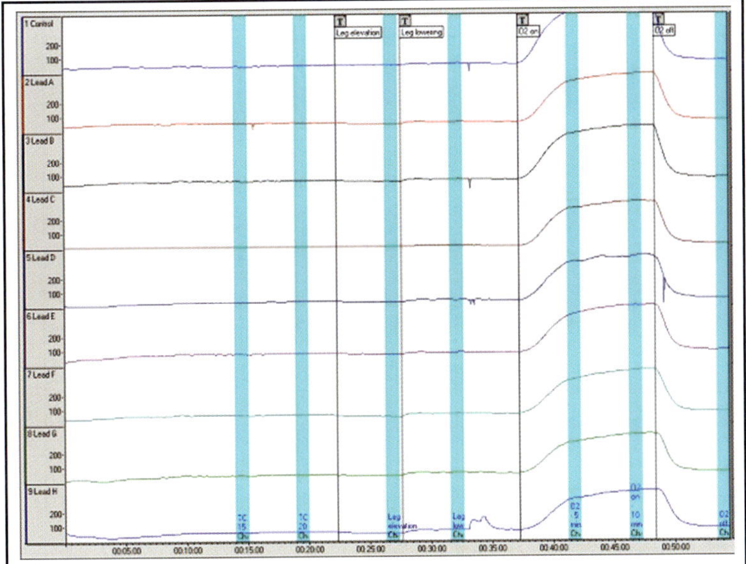

Figure 6C. Patient FSG 327. TcpO2 tracings from a typical TCOM evaluation using nine sensors. Smooth lines indicate good quality tracing. Numerical data are at Table 3.

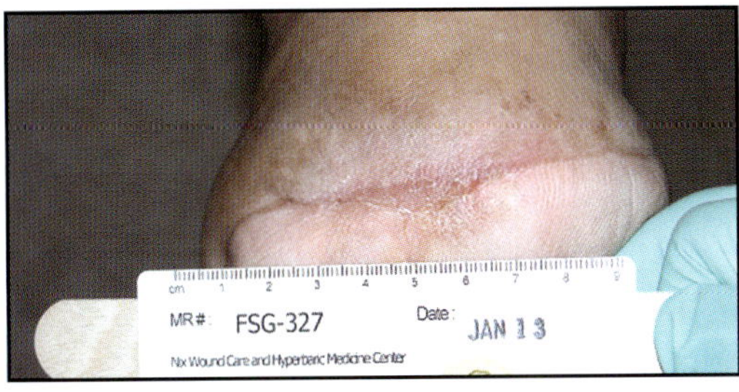

Figure 6D. Six-month follow-up after successful treatment with HBO2 and wound care.

TABLE 3. TCPO2 VALUES FOR FSG 327 (CASE 1)

Item	Air 15 min	Air 20 min	Leg elevation	% Change Air 20 to Elevation	Leg lowered	O_2–5 min	O_2–10 min	% Change Air 20 to O_2 10	O_2 off
Control	41	45	48	6%	56	417	467	937%	72
Lead A	51	52	44	-15%	57	343	393	659%	67
Lead B	57	59	52	-12%	65	385	438	646%	73
Mean A, B	54	55	48	-13%	61	364	415	652%	70
Lead C	5	5	3	-46%	9	271	319	5826%	16
Lead D	28	33	28	-16%	42	306	345	930%	49
Mean C, D	17	19	16	-20%	26	289	332	1607%	32
Lead E	73	75	70	-8%	82	350	412	447%	93
Lead F	58	59	47	-21%	66	302	365	519%	74
Mean E, F	66	67	58	-13%	74	326	389	479%	83
Lead G	43	47	40	-14%	58	273	329	602%	61
Lead H	57	60	50	-17%	68	285	337	463%	77
Mean G, H	50	53	45	-15%	63	279	333	524%	69

The shaded regions indicate the data which was used for interpretation.

decrease) in tissue oxygen tensions with elevation of the leg indicating decreased vascular reserve. There was an adequate response to inspired 100% oxygen at the right mid foot and all other levels tested. The failure to heal potential on standard wound care for the right foot wound was considered high. HBO2 was recommended to correct the underlying hypoxia, prevent spread of necrosis, and aid wound healing.

Outcome: After informed consent was obtained, Patient FSG-327 received a total of 26 daily HBO2 treatments over a course of 31 days. A 2.4 ATA treatment table was used which included three 30-minute oxygen breathing periods interrupted by two 10-minute air breaks. Hyperbaric oxygen treatments were discontinued when the wound appeared to be adequately granulated. The patient continued to receive weekly wound care only treatments and was healed 13 weeks after completing HBO2 treatment. Figure 6D is the 6-month follow-up after successful treatment with HBO2 and wound care.

PRECAUTIONS FOR INTERPRETING TCPO$_2$ RESULTS

There are a number of physical and pathological conditions that can cause a false impression of the local capillary (nutritive) oxygenation.

Conditions that Cause High Values

Transcutaneous oximetry values can be elevated if there is a leak under the fixation device. An air leak under the fixation device is a common problem and requires that the operator monitor the machines for indications of an air leak, especially when the limb is repositioned. A large air leak will be read by the sensor as approximately 159 mm Hg at sea level (760 mm Hg x 0.209=159 mm Hg) or 20.9% of the ambient barometric pressure. A smaller air leak may read somewhat less as the oxygen is consumed by the electrode. If the values read by the electrode are not congruent with neighboring electrodes or higher than what would normally be expected, be suspicious of an air leak. Figure 7 shows a TCOM tracing with an air leak in Leads D and E. Air leaks are usually seen as a sudden increase in the TcpO$_2$ value and appear as a squared wave on the tracing. These particular leaks occurred when the leg was elevated and the TcpO$_2$ values went from near 0 to 160 mm Hg in about 10 seconds. The leaks were corrected by reaffixing the sensor and the remainder of the tracings showed good data.

Conditions that Cause Low Values

Transcutaneous oximetry values can be reduced if the sensor is positioned over bone, tendon, or callus. Transcutaneous oximetry

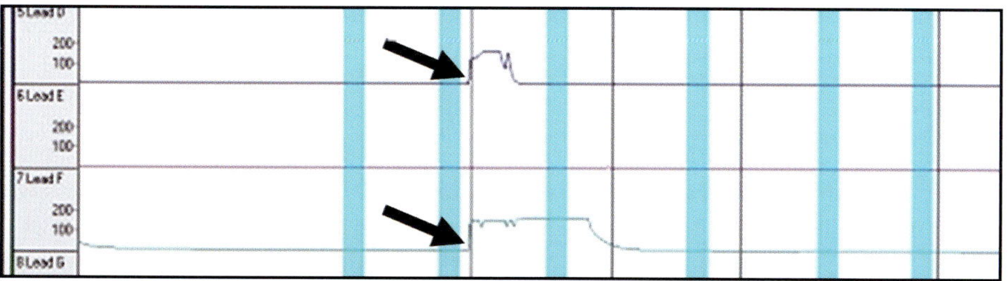

Figure 7. Air leaks in leads D and F as indicated by arrows.

electrodes should not be placed on the soles of the feet due to thickness of the pad or callus that is typically present as this will produce unreliable and misleading data. The $TcpO_2$ values may also be reduced by several pathological conditions, such as edema, active infection, inflammation, thick or sclerotic skin, occluded vessels, severed vessels as in a flap, and irradiated tissue. Tobacco products also cause $TcpO_2$ values in smokers to be about 10% below nonsmokers (23) and remain significantly reduced for about an hour after smoking (26) as a result of vasoconstriction by nicotine. But there is some evidence of improved tissue oxygenation after a few days of smoking cessation (27).

Values Vary by Body Location

Knowing where the electrode is placed will help the interpreter explain the data obtained, since $TcpO_2$ varies at different locations of the body. Refer to Table 1 to see the variance in values obtained at the chest, calf, and mid foot.

Sensors Consume Oxygen while Measuring it

A recording of near zero sometimes occurs even though the tissue is viable. The carotid body reacts to elevated pO_2 by causing vasoconstriction. If the $TcpO_2$ value is less on oxygen than on air, it is suggestive of a proximal occlusion or severe arterial disease (13).

The interpreter must be aware that the sensor consumes oxygen in the process of measuring it. Thus, there must be continuous resupply of oxygen to the tissues beneath the sensor or the $TcpO_2$ values will diminish to near zero. Severed vessels, as in a flap, will cause the electrode readings to diminish to near zero, since there is no resupply of oxygen. Measurements over inadequately perfused tissue (i.e., dry gangrene, or distal end of a flap) may continue to decrease despite the patient breathing oxygen.

Case 2 (Figures 8A-G) describes a compromised flap on the scalp in which $TcpO_2$ values were obtained at the proximal, medial, and distal portions of the failing flap. As time lapsed during oxygen breathing, $TcpO_2$ values increased at the proximal and medial portions of the flap, but diminished at the distal portion due to oxygen consumption by the electrode. There were simply no functioning blood vessels beneath the distal electrode to resupply the oxygen that was being consumed. This phenomenon has led some reporters to presume that there is a reduction in $TcpO_2$ due to vasoconstriction, when, in fact, there were no vessels available to constrict. Similarly, values taken on the plantar surface of the foot are unreliable because the footpad is too thick for timely, adequate oxygen resupply at the sensor.

Case 2

Patient FSG458MN is a 46 YOF who had a large arteriovenous malformation removed from the left retromastoid/ suboccipital area. The area was covered with a large skin flap originating at the neck level. The entire distal aspect of the flap became dusky and dark purple due to venous occlusion prior to presentation. Patient was referred to the Wound Care and

Hyperbaric Medicine Center for assistance in salvaging the skin flap. Discoloration was consistent with flap failure. Table 4 shows the values obtained at the proximal, medial, and distal portions of the flap on the TCOM assessment that was performed at atmospheric pressure (1 ATA) and a hyperbaric oxygen challenge at 2.4 ATA. $TcpO_2$ evaluation at 1 ATA (Figure 8A1) revealed that the entire flap had significant hypoxia. Values shown are air/oxygen. Baseline air recording (lapsed time = 20 minutes) was followed by 10 minutes of oxygen breathing (lapsed time = 30 minutes). The proximal area responded well to 100% oxygen challenge (air/O_2 = 28/186), but the distal portion did not respond so well (air/O_2 = 19/11). $TcpO_2$ assessment at 2.4 ATA (Figure 8A2) revealed significant improvement of tissue oxygenation at the proximal portion (air/HBO2 = 58/836) but did not improve at the distal portion (air/HBO2 = 18/8).

Because of the devastating nature of the loss of the flap, the wound care physician felt that a trial of HBO2 therapy was warranted to stop the spread of the flap failure and to develop a granulation base for future grafting. After informed consent was obtained, the patient received a total of 29 HBO2 treatments. After 1 week, the failed portion was demarcated (Figure 8B). After the 25th HBO2 treatment (3 weeks) the flap was resected and was necrotic. The patient returned to surgery for another flap procedure, which revealed a rich granulation base (Figure 8C). A muscle flap was applied (Figure 8D) and covered by mesh graft (Figure 8E). The patient received additional 4 HBO2 treatments, which concluded with 29 treatments at week 4 (Figure 8F). Follow-up photo at week 8 (Figure 8G) revealed that the new flap/graft was viable and results were excellent.

TABLE 4. PATIENT FSG458MN TCOM ASSESSMENT OF COMPROMISED FLAP

Breathing Gas	Time	$TcpO_2$ at 1 ATA			$TcpO_2$ at 2.4 ATA		
		Control	Proximal A	Distal B	Proximal A	Medial B	Distal C
Air	20 minutes (Baseline)	27	28	19	58	18	18
Oxygen	5 minutes	302	136	14	610	28	12
Oxygen	10 minutes	325	186	11	654	44	10
Oxygen	15 minutes				806	44	08
Oxygen	20 minutes				836	48	08

$TcpO_2$ values were obtained at the proximal, medial, and distal portions of the flap at atmospheric pressure (1 ATA) and a hyperbaric oxygen challenge at 2.4 ATA. (TCOM sensor temperature set at 44°C).

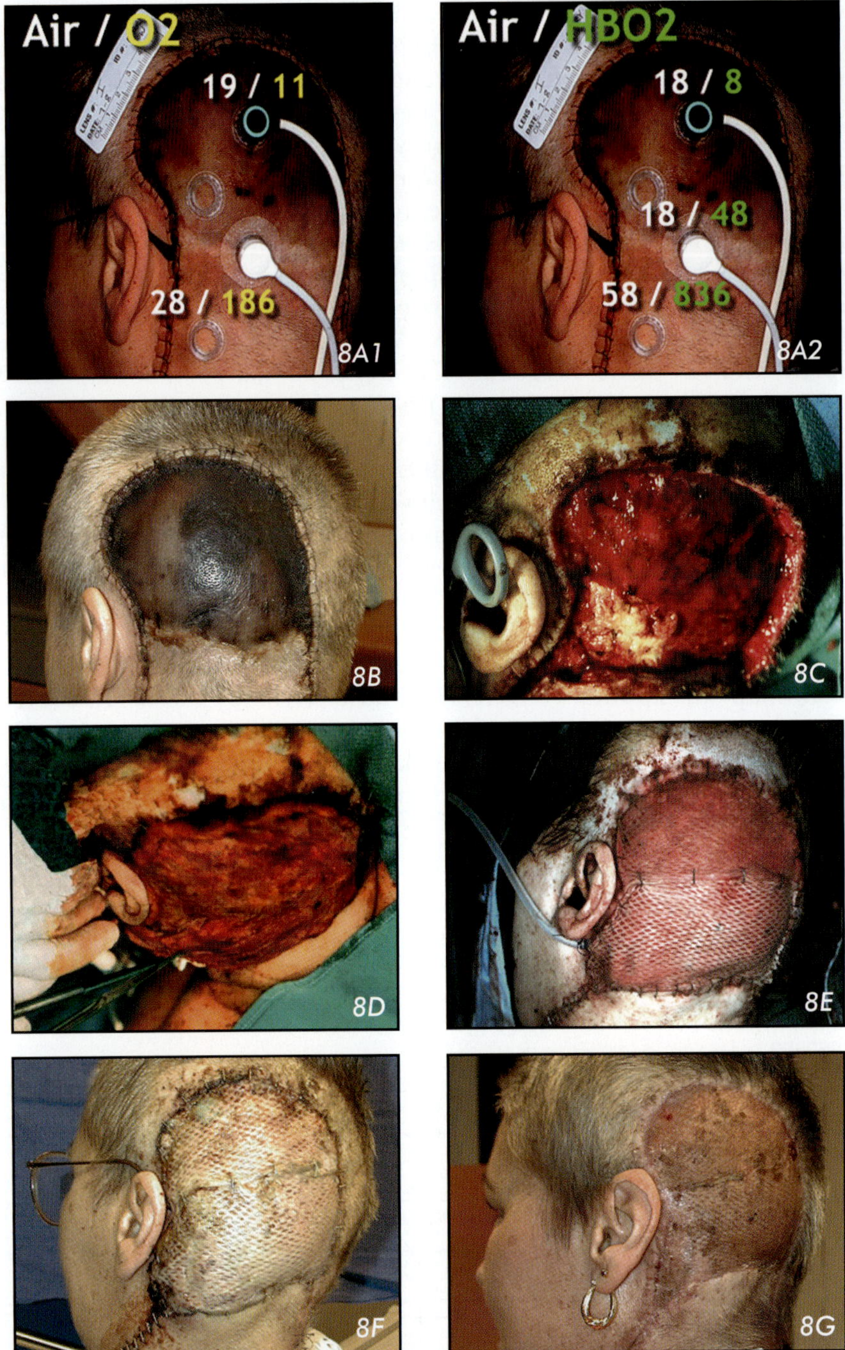

Figure 8. Patient FSG458MN–Case 2 (Photos A–G).
(A1 and A2) TcpO2 values were obtained at the proximal, medial, and distal portion of a failing compromised flap of the scalp on initial assessment at 1 ATA and at 2.4 ATA.
(B) After one week of adjunctive HBO2, the failed portion of flap was clearly demarcated.
(C) After three weeks of HBO2, the excised flap shows rich red granulation base.
(D) A muscle flap is placed and E, covered with mesh graft.
(F) At week 4, HBO2 ends.
(G) Follow-up at week 8 shows full take of graft.

A SUGGESTED PROTOCOL FOR TcpO$_2$ ASSESSMENT OF HBO2 CANDIDATES

Assessment Protocol

TcpO$_2$ assessment of potential HBO2 candidates may consist of 5 tests that answer 5 basic questions about whether the wound: 1) is severely hypoxic, 2) is complicated by large or small vessel disease, 3) will respond to oxygen, 4) will respond to HBO2, and 5) is to the point that it will heal without further HBO2 treatment. The 5 tests are as follows:

Test 1

TcpO$_2$ baseline air value at 1 atm abs. Affix the electrode to skin and allow equilibrating 20 min before recording the TcpO$_2$ baseline (air) values. Hypoxia exists if TcpO$_2$ <40 mm Hg.

Test 2

Leg elevation (30°). Elevate the leg for 5 min. As the leg is elevated, perfusion decreases in the leg. Healthy subjects immediately return to near normal due to autoregulation. In patients, however, presence of large or small vessel disease causes perfusion to remain diminished while the leg is elevated. A decrease of more than 10% is considred significant.

Test 3

Oxygen challenge at 1 atm abs. Administer pure oxygen via a tightly fitted oxygen mask or hood with neckdam for 10 min before recording TcpO$_2$ (oxygen) value. Values on O$_2$ should be at least 50% rise above air values and reach at least 40 mm Hg.

Test 4

Oxygen challenge at 2–2.5 atm abs. Administer pure oxygen inside the chamber via a tightly fitted oxygen mask or hood with neckdam for 10 min before recording TcpO$_2$ (oxygen) value. A mask or hood is not necessary for delivery of oxygen inside a monoplace chamber that is filled with pure oxygen. Values on O$_2$ should be at least 200 mm Hg (50 mm Hg for flaps and grafts).

Test 5

Repeat TcpO$_2$ baseline air value at 1 atm abs. Affix the electrode to skin and allow for equilibrating 20 min before recording the TcpO$_2$ baseline (air) value. Normalization of baseline values to >40 mm Hg would indicate the healing process is in place. The questions and their respective tests are shown in Table 5.

At the Nix Wound Care and Hyperbaric Medicine Center in San Antonio, Texas, HBO2 candidates each receive a TcpO$_2$ assessment. If the overall evaluation identifies the patient as an HBO2 candidate, the patient is selected for treatment based on the following TcpO$_2$ criteria:

1. TcpO$_2$ of 1–40 mm Hg with significant rise on 1 atm abs O$_2$ challenge (at least 50% rise to exceed a minimum value of 40 mm Hg).
2. HBO2 candidates with borderline 1 atm abs data are given an oxygen challenge at 2.4 atm abs. A course of HBO2 treatment is started if the TcpO$_2$ values are equal to or exceed 200 mm Hg (50 mm Hg for flaps and grafts).

TABLE 5. A PROTOCOL FOR TCPO2 ASSESSMENT OF PATIENTS WHO ARE CANDIDATES FOR HBO2

QUESTION	TEST	TEST CRITERIA
Is wound healing complicated by severe hypoxia?	1. TcpO$_2$ baseline air value at 1 atm abs.	1. Hypoxia exists if TcpO$_2$ is < 40 mm Hg
Is wound healing complicated by large or small vessel disease?	2. Leg elevation (30°)	2. Disease is present if TcpO$_2$ remains diminished while leg is elevated
Does the wound site respond to oxygen breathing?	3. Oxygen challenge at 1 atm abs.	3. Values on O$_2$ should be at least 50% rise and reach at least 40 mm Hg
Does the wound site respond to hyperbaric oxygen?	4. Oxygen challenge at 2-2.5 atm abs.	4. Values on O$_2$ should be at least 200 mm Hg (50 mm Hg for flaps and grafts).
Is the wound at the point where it will heal without further HBO2 treatment?	5 .Repeat TcpO$_2$ baseline air evaluation at 1 atm abs in 3-4 wk intervals.	5. Normalization of baseline values >40 mm Hg would indicate the healing process is in place

This protocol was also used to evaluate the application of laser Doppler flowmetry in selected patients, which is reported below.

LASER DOPPLER FLOWMETRY AS A WOUND ASSESSMENT TOOL

Laser Doppler flowmetry (LDF), is used along with other tests to predict wound healing using local wound care, to define the level for successful amputation, or to identify need for revascularization. Buckley and Lee described the methodology in their chapter "Non-invasive and Invasive Evaluations For Lower Extremity Arterial Occlusive Disease" (28).

The focus of this section is the basic LDF operating principles and the procedures for assessing skin blood flow and skin perfusion pressure. Also included is a protocol that combines LDF (with heat provocation) with TCOM for assessing wound patients as potential candidates for HBO2 therapy. The proposed protocol was developed at the Nix Wound Care and Hyperbaric Medicine Center, Nix Medical Center, San Antonio, Texas and has been previously reported (6).

In wound centers, TCOM and LDF are routinely used to help choose a course of treatment. Transcutaneous oximetry measures the local tissue oxygen tension derived from the local capillary (nutritive) blood perfusion. It indicates if the tissue is hypoxic, and if it responds to inspired oxygen. Laser Doppler flowmetry with heat provocation (44°C) measures the total blood perfusion in local tissue, including capillaries, arterioles, venules and shunts. Local heat provocation causes vasodilatation, enabling LDF to be used for assessment of the tissue reserve capacity and severity of ischemia. Additionally, use of occlusion as a provocative test can determine skin perfusion pressure (SPP). Combining LDF and TCOM provides additional information for predicting healing.

The section concludes with a suggested classification system for degrees of ischemia and hypoxia based on LDF and TCOM assessment.

APPLICATIONS OF LASER DOPPLER FLOWMETRY

The first use of LDF is attributed to Riva and associates who measured blood flow in the retinal artery in 1972 (29). In 1975, Stern (30) was the first to use LDF for assessing skin blood flow. Laser Doppler Imaging became possible in 1991 when two groups, Nilsson and associates (31) as well as Essex and associates (32) independent of each other developed a continuous scanning laser beam technique in which a low intensity laser light beam was projected on the skin surface by a moving mirror. In 1992, Dwars and van den Broek used a pressure cuff and laser Doppler to test the reactive hyperemic state of the capillary bed in response to pressure, and proposed criteria for selecting lowest level of amputation (33).

LDF is commonly used to determine cutaneous blood flow, (34) evaluate blood flow in free flaps, (35) to assess burn depth and area, (36) to suggest amputation levels (37), and to diagnose ischemic tissue disorders, such as peripheral vascular disease (38). It is becoming increasingly important in wound care and hyperbaric medicine centers (6).

LASER DOPPLER FLOWMETRY INSTRUMENTS

Laser Doppler Flowmetry (LDF) is a non-invasive method of using laser light to detect blood movement in a small tissue sample. There are two basic types of laser Doppler flowmetry instruments that assess blood movement in the microvasculature of the skin: Laser Doppler Perfusion Monitoring (LDPM) and Laser Doppler Perfusion Imaging (LDPI). LDPM requires contact with the skin through a fiber optic probe whereas LDPI uses a laser beam to scan the tissue and present a two-dimensional picture of the perfusion. Discussion of LDPI is outside the scope of this chapter, as it is not commonly used in wound centers and the authors have no experience with it.

There are a number of LDPM instruments available on the market. Two LDPM models have been evaluated in the authors' wound assessment laboratories and will be specifically referenced herein. One model (Vasamed, Eden Prairie, Minnesota) was used with occlusion to determine skin perfusion pressure (SPP) and another model (Perimed AB, Stockholm, Sweden) was used with heat provocation to determine microcirculatory blood flow. The LDF monitoring devices discussed herein require contact with the skin.

HOW LASER DOPPLER FLOWMETRY WORKS

Doppler Effect

Laser Doppler Flowmetry uses the Doppler Effect to assess blood movement within the microvasculature of the skin. A probe that contains two optic fibers is placed on the skin as illustrated at Figure 9. One is the transmitter and one is the receiver. The transmitter emits a beam of light of a specific wavelength that enters the tissue and becomes scattered. Blood cells moving within the region that is illuminated by the beam cause the light to change frequency, which is called a Doppler shift. Within the tissue is a mixture of Doppler shifted light and non-Doppler shifted light. The proportion of shifted to non-shifted light is related to the number of moving objects (blood cells) within the path of the light and the magnitude of the frequency shift is related to the velocity of the moving objects. Part of the light within the tissue is scattered back to the receiver in the probe where it is returned by optic fiber to the instrument's photo detector, which converts it to electrical signals. These signals are separated into different groups that represent the various parameters such as blood perfusion, concentration of moving blood cells, and velocity. Nilsson et al. (39) and Ahn et al. (40) have described the technical aspects of signal processing.

Parameters

The concentration of moving blood cells (CMBC) is proportional to the number of moving cells that causes Doppler shifts within the tissue volume being measured. This parameter is sometimes used to study blood cell defects, such as sickle cells. Velocity represents the relative average velocity of the blood cells moving in the measured tissue volume. The velocity parameter might be used to study the effect of drugs and effect of provocation. Blood perfusion is a dimensionless value, expressed as Perfusion Units (PU), which is a product of the relative number of moving blood cells that causes Doppler shifts and the mean velocity at which these cells move through the measured volume.

Blood Perfusion (PU) = CMBC x Mean Velocity of the Cells

Depth of Measurement

Laser Doppler flowmetry identifies the total blood perfusion in the measured volume; typically the capillaries, arterioles, venules, and shunts. The measured volume is the region under the probe to which the laser light is transmitted and returned (See Figure 9). The measuring depth depends on the tissue properties, the probe configuration, and the wavelength of the light source. Instruments are available with a variety of wavelengths, but each laser Doppler typically has a fixed wavelength. For example, Perimed laser Doppler instruments (Perimed AB, Stockholm, Sweden) are equipped with a light wavelength of 780 nm and their standard probes have a fiber separation of 0.25 mm. The measuring depth in normal skin is about 0.5–1.0 mm. This depth of measurement is only an estimate since several factors influence the degree of absorption of light by the tissue. The most important factor is the blood content, but pigmentation may also influence the measuring depth. The degree of oxygenation will also influence the measuring depth if the light source has a wavelength strongly deviating from the Isobestic Point (about 800 nm). The Isobestic Point is the wavelength at which the absorption by the two forms of the hemoglobin molecule (Hb and HbO_2) is the same). Light sources with shorter wavelengths have less penetration depth (see Figure 9). A light source with wavelength 543 nm (visual green) has less penetration depth than 633 nm (visual red), which has less penetration depth than 780 nm (nonvisual, near infrared) (41). The measuring depth also increases with greater fiber separation (distance between the transmitting and receiving optic fibers).

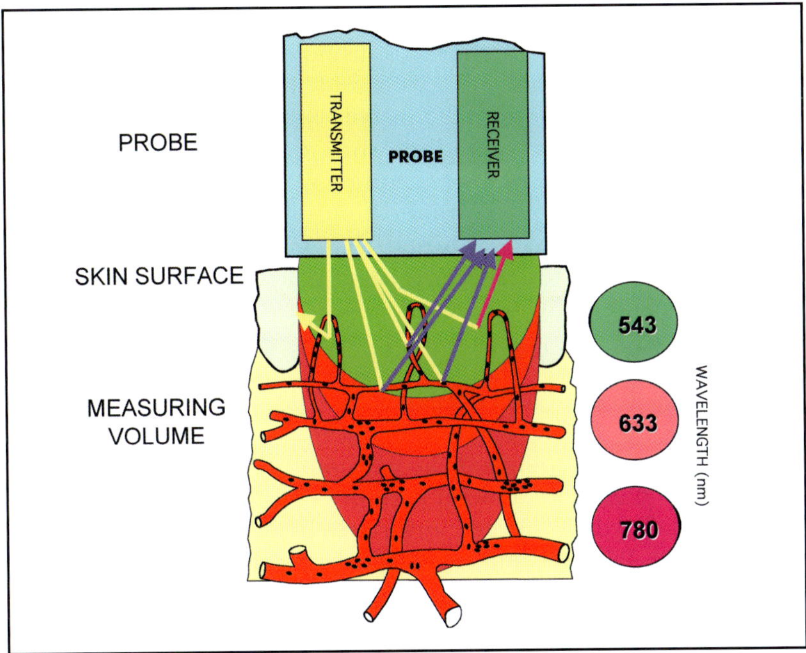

Figure 9. LDF measures blood flow in skin. A transmitter emits light of a specific wavelength. Moving objects in the light path causes a change in frequency, or Doppler shift. Some light is scattered back to a receiver that transmits it back to the instrument for analysis. The region under the probe to which light is transmitted and reflected identifies the measuring volume. Laser light sources with longer wavelengths have more penetration depth. Measuring depth in normal skin is usually about 0.5–1.0 mm.

USES OF LASER DOPPLER FLOWMETRY

LDF is used along with other tests to predict wound healing using local wound care, to define the level for successful amputation, or to identify need for revascularization. An SPP value less than 30 mm Hg is usually considered a reliable indicator of amputation. However, HBO2 treatment has been used to salvage limbs when SPP is below 30 mm Hg. Laser Doppler with heat provocation has promise as an assessment tool for predicting outcome in HBO2 candidates, particularly when combined with $TcpO_2$ assessment.

Evaluation of Skin Perfusion

Buckley and Lee (28) described in their chapter "Non-Invasive and Invasive Evaluations for Lower Extremity Arterial Occlusive Disease" the application of laser Doppler for determining skin blood flow. Depending upon the provocative test that is applied, this technology can be used for obtaining values for digital systolic blood pressure, skin perfusion pressure, or microcirculatory blood flow. Three commonly used provocative tests are occlusion, heat, and posture (elevating or lowering the limb). Without a provocative test, the laser Doppler simply identifies the presence of microcirculatory blood flow, and this can vary dramatically depending on the degree of microcirculatory vasodilatation and constriction. This makes LDF difficult to use as a predictor of wound healing, since the large natural variation in microcirculatory blood flow makes it difficult to distinguish between normal and diseased tissue without provoking the tissue.

Vasomotion

In an unprovoked tissue there are usually large oscillatory variations in the local blood flow that are associated with small vessel rhythmical diameter changes (vasomotion). Stansberry et al. (42) observed that the patterns of peripheral vasomotion were disordered in diabetes and suggested that the loss of low-frequency oscillations was due to a peripheral vascular abnormality that extends past the capillary network to arterial vessels. Stansberry proposed that measurement of vasomotion might prove useful as a test for peripheral neurovascular function.

PROVOCATIVE TESTS

Occlusion as a Provocative Test

Laser Doppler is used together with a pneumatic cuff to estimate skin blood pressure at various points on an extremity. Occlusion of the area being measured can be done with a blood pressure cuff. Pressure cuffs of different sizes are available for digits (for toe/finger pressure), feet, and the limbs (ankle/brachial pressure). Pressure units are available that can standardize the test by monitoring the cuff pressure and regulating its deflation linearly.

Digital Systolic Blood Pressure (Toe Pressure)

Digital systolic blood pressure is measured at the toe by placing a cuff on the toe and attaching the laser Doppler probe distal to the cuff. The cuff is inflated to a pressure well above systolic blood pressure and then the pressure is slowly and linearly released until the laser Doppler probe detects return of blood flow. The digital systolic blood pressure (toe pressure) is the pressure at which perfusion returns. The pressure taken on the toe is more reliable than ankle pressure for patients with hardened or calcified vessels. Ankle pressure is routinely measured to determine the ankle-brachial index. According to Second European Consensus document on chronic critical leg ischemia (43),"An ankle systolic pressure of 50 mm Hg or less or a toe systolic pressure of 30 mm Hg or less suggests the presence of critical limb ischemia." Perimed (Perimed AB, Stockholm, Sweden) manufactures a device that obtains toe pressures by incorporating laser Doppler with an air pressure unit that monitors the cuff pressure and regulates the cuff deflation linearly.

Buckley and Lee discuss the use of laser Doppler in determining skin systolic blood pressure for patients with arterial occlusive disease in their chapter "Non-Invasive and Invasive Evaluations for Lower Extremity Arterial Occlusive Disease." They report skin blood pressure values of 75 ± 10 mm Hg in normal foot, 50–70 mm Hg in limbs with claudication, and 10–40 mm Hg in limbs with rest pain or non-healing soft tissue wounds.

According to Ubbink, a toe pressure lower than the ankle pressure generally indicates very distal obstruction. When ankle blood pressures cannot be measured, toe pressures (< 30 mm Hg) are only used to assess critical ischemia. A toe pressure below 60–70 mm Hg is sometimes associated with poor wound healing. No clearly defined toe pressure cut-off value exists to discern normal from moderate ischemia (44).

Post Occlusive Reactive Hyperemia (PORH)

Post occlusive reactive hyperemia, also known as post-ischemic reactive hyperemia, is a clinical test to screen patients with arterial occlusive disease. PORH is induced by release of a 3–5 minute arterial occlusion, typically by a cuff at ankle level with the laser Doppler probe placed dorsally on the foot or on the first toe. After release of the cuff, the perfusion level increases dramatically, usually many hundred percent above basal levels. Different parameters are being used to evaluate the PORH and some commonly used are the time to peak, peak value, and increase from basal level to peak level. Ijzerman et al. (45) used this method to determine that cigarette smoking causes an acute impairment of microvascular function in humans. Wahlberg et al. (46) used the method to detect circulatory changes caused by arterial reconstruction.

Skin Perfusion Pressure (SPP) or "Capillary Pressure"

Skin perfusion pressure is obtained by inflating a blood pressure cuff with the laser Doppler probe beneath the cuff. The laser Doppler detects the occlusion and the pressure at return of perfusion, which is the SPP. Both Vasamed [Vasamed, Eden Prairie, Minnesota] and Perimed [Perimed AB, Stockholm, Sweden] manufacture a device that obtains SPP by incorporating laser Doppler with an air pressure unit that monitors the cuff pressure and regulates its deflation linearly. Skin perfusion pressure is a quantitative measurement of blood pressure within the capillaries of the skin, which is given in mm Hg. There is a role in wound healing for SPP since it quantitatively determines the level of chronic ischemia for patients with chronic foot ulcers and identifies candidates for amputation. Edema, anemia, or calcification of vessels does not affect the SPP test. The interpreter uses SPP data to diagnose critical ischemia, identify regional ischemia, determine the risk of ulcer formation, predict wound healing potential, and determine amputation level. Castronuovo and associates (47) reported that the probability of healing without amputation or revascularization was 85% when SPP was 30 mm Hg or higher, but the probability declined to only 8% when SPP was 15 mm Hg, making healing very unlikely (Table 6). Thus, healing is compromised when the SPP is too low. Fischer et al. (48) created a device that combined two laser Doppler probes with a pressure cuff at the base of the toe to conduct simultaneous measurements of digital artery pressure and skin perfusion pressure.

TABLE 6. SKIN PERFUSION PRESSURE AS A PREDICTOR OF HEALING (47)

SPP Values in mm Hg	Probability of Healing w/o Amputation or Revascularization	Likelihood of Healing
At 30 mm Hg	85%	Very Likely
At 25 mm Hg	55%	Possible
At 20 mm Hg	23%	Unlikely
At 15 mm Hg	8%	Very Unlikely

Heat as a Provocative Test

Perfusion increases when skin temperature rises. Heat provocation is initiated by applying heat locally at the probe. Vasodilatation occurs when the skin beneath the sensor is heated to 42–44°C, causing perfusion in the region to increase. The reactive hyperemia (i.e., the increase in perfusion after local heating following the heat provocation) indicates the tissue reserve capacity and severity of ischemia. Such measurements may be used to determine the viability of tissues with impaired microcirculation, the degree of microcirculatory impairment, the likelihood of healing, and the level of amputation. The temperature of choice by the authors is 44°C since it matches the temperature setting chosen for the TCOM electrode (6). In response to heat provocation, perfusion is considered normal if the LDF % increase is >500 %. If tissue reserve capacity is too low, healing is compromised.

Posture (Leg Elevation) as a Provocative Test

As the leg is elevated 30° from the normal (supine) position, perfusion decreases in the leg. In a healthy subject, due to autoregulation, perfusion returns almost immediately to near normal. However, presence of large or small vessel disease causes perfusion to remain diminished until the patient is returned to the normal (supine) position. This provocative test for assessing problem wounds is sometimes performed for simultaneous measurements of laser Doppler and TCOM (6). The LDF values are most helpful when the $TcpO_2$ values are falsely low because of inflammation or acute edema. When LDF values are too low, healing is compromised. The range of LDF values for healthy subjects and wound patients are outlined in Tables 7 and 8.

Posture (Leg Lowering) as a Provocative Test (Veno-Arteriolar Reflex)

Venous pressure increases in the lower limb on dependency, stimulating a local sympathetic axon reflex that triggers precapillary and arteriolar vasoconstriction of the distal vascular bed. The resulting decrease in arterial calf inflow, known as the veno-arteriolar response (VAR), is a mechanism that prevents blood from pooling in the feet. This reflex is important for preventing edema and sustaining an adequate blood supply to the brain while a person is standing. The VAR is impaired in critical leg ischemia (49).

TABLE 7. MEAN LDF AND TCPO$_2$ VALUES FOR HEALTHY SUBJECTS AND WOUND PATIENTS (HEALED AND NOT HEALED) (6)

Subjects	LDF			TcpO$_2$		
	LDF Baseline (PU)	LDF after heating (PU)	LDF% Increase	TC Baseline (mm Hg)	TC O$_2$ Challenge (mm Hg)	TC % Increase (mm Hg)
Healthy Controls n=22	11	121	1217	73	381	417
Patients Healed n=35	22	85	362	37	193	947
Patients Not Healed n=11	17	28	69	12	17	79

TABLE 8. SUGGESTED CLASSIFICATION SYSTEM FOR DEGREES OF ISCHEMIA AND HYPOXIA BASED ON LDF AND TCPO$_2$ DATA

Degrees of Ischemia				Degrees of Hypoxia	
Assessment	LDF (% change)	SPP[a] (mm Hg)	Toe Pressure[b] (mm Hg)	Assessment	TcpO$_2$ (mm Hg)
Normal	>500	>40		Normal	>40
Moderate Ischemia	150–500	30–40	<60–70	Moderate Hypoxia	20–40
Severe Ischemia	<150	<30	<30	Severe Hypoxia	<20

Sheffield PJ et al. 2001, (16), [a]Castronuovo JJ et al., (47), [b]Second European Consensus document on chronic critical leg ischemia (43) and DT Ubbink (A personal communication, August 2003).

USE OF LDF IN COMBINATION WITH TCOM

Ubbink and associates (44) investigated the usefulness of skin microcirculatory studies as a predictor of imminent major amputation in 111 patients with non-reconstructible critical limb ischemia. The studies included nailfold capillary microscopy (CM; big toe, sitting), transcutaneous oximetry (TcpO$_2$; forefoot, supine; 44°C), and laser Doppler perfusion measurements (LD; pulp of big toe, supine). Microcirculation responses were assigned as "good," "intermediate," or "poor" as shown at Table 9. Patients that were included had chronic rest pain or small ulcers and an ankle blood pressure of 50 mm Hg or less or an ankle-to-brachial pressure index (ABI) of 0.35 or less. Limb survival at 12 months was 17% in the "poor" microcirculatory group, 63% in the "intermediate" microcirculatory group, and 88% in the "good" microcirculatory group (P < 0.0001). The investigators concluded that microcirculatory screening and classification was useful in detecting non-reconstructible critical ischemia that requires amputation. Most of the "poor" patient group required amputation, whereas in the "intermediate" and "good" groups, non-surgical treatment was sufficient for limb salvage.

Scheffler et al. (50) evaluated the influence of positional maneuvers and systolic ankle arterial pressure on TcpO$_2$ in peripheral arterial disease and published TcpO$_2$ criteria for diagnosis of critical limb ischemia: Ankle Systolic Pressure less than 60 mm Hg; Supine TcpO$_2$ less than 10–15 mm Hg; Dependent TcpO$_2$ less than 40-45 mm Hg.

Franzeck and associates (51) used a special combined electrode incorporating both TCOM and laser Doppler in the same probe head to assess cutaneous reactive hyperemia in short-term and long-term type I diabetes. Fife

TABLE 9. MICROCIRCULATORY SCREENING AND LIMB SURVIVAL

Response	CM (Capillary density/mm)	TcpO2 (mm Hg)	LDF (Reactive Hyperemia)	Limb Survial 6 months	Limb Survial 12 months
Good	>20	>30	present	88%	88%
Intermediate		10–30		80%	63%
Poor	<20	<10	absent	42%	17%

and associates (52) used TCOM and skin perfusion pressure (SPP) to evaluate 23 patients who underwent HBO2 treatment for lower extremity wounds and compared them to controls. Measurements were recorded over the dorsal foot while the patient breathed air at sea level, oxygen at sea level, and hyperbaric oxygen at 2 ATA. Outcome was classified as healed, improved, not improved, or amputated. Wound patients had significantly lower SPP than controls. In this small series, statistical correlations between $TcpO_2$, SPP, and outcome were disappointing. However, Fife reported that the most promising method was the combination of in-chamber TCOM and SPP. Some of the patients improved or healed despite their SPP being below 30 mm Hg. Previously, an SPP less than 30 mm Hg had been accepted by those authors as a reliable indicator of amputation. The authors suggested that HBO2 alters the previously demonstrated relationship between SPP and outcome, but the new relationship was not defined by their study.

As of this writing, an ongoing prospective, comparative study at the Loma Linda University Medical Center is evaluating the efficacy and outcome of chronic extremity wounds using SPP as compared to $TcpO_2$. Concurrent room-air measurements on corresponding sites were done with SPP and TCOM on 100 patients (mean age 63.1 years) with chronic extremity wounds. SPP and $TcpO_2$ values above 30mm Hg were used to predict a positive outcome. Follow-up was conducted at either 6 or 12 months. Preliminary results show that 89 of the 100 patients (89%) had wound healing. SPP correctly predicted healing in 82 of the 89 patients (92%) versus $TcpO_2$ that predicted healing in 60 of the 89 patients (67%) [p < 0.01] The authors concluded that in their study-in-progress of 100 patients, SPP had a significantly higher accuracy than TCOM in predicting healing outcome of chronic extremity wounds (53). However, the authors suggest using a combination of the two procedures because they are measuring separate physiological parameters: perfusion and nutritive oxygen. (Samples, R. A personal communication. September 2006).

Combining LDF and TCOM as a Predictor of Wound Healing

Transcutaneous oximetry is a standard technique for qualifying patients for HBO2 treatment by assessing their wounds for complications of hypoxia and ability to respond to oxygen (1). Transcutaneous oximetry measures the local tissue oxygen tension that is derived from the local capillary (nutritive) blood perfusion. Transcutaneous oximetry indicates if the tissue is hypoxic and if it will respond to inspired oxygen. Low $TcpO_2$ values are sometimes difficult to interpret, since the cause may be due to lack of blood perfusion, capillary malfunction, or several other factors. Combining LDF and TCOM has been shown to provide additional information for selecting the appropriate treatment to enhance wound healing (6). The LDF values are most useful when the $TcpO_2$ values are falsely low because of inflammation or acute edema.

Laser Doppler flowmetry measures the total blood perfusion in local tissue, including capillaries, arterioles, venules and shunts. Laser Doppler flowmetry with local heat provocation (44°C) causes maximum vasodilatation, enabling the use of LDF to assess the tissue reserve capacity and severity of ischemia.

In a prospective outcome study, Sheffield and associates (6) compared the predictive value of $TcpO_2$ and LDF with heat provocation in 22 healthy subjects and 46 randomly selected patients with problem wounds who presented for assessment as potential HBO2 candidates. The LDF and TCOM test procedures are described in the next section below.

Laser Doppler flowmetry perfusion baseline was determined before heat was applied to the LDF probe. The probe was then heated to 44°C to create maximum dilatation. The values were reported in perfusion units (PU). From these data, the percent change in mean perfusion before and after heat provocation was calculated (LDF % increase). Both baseline $TcpO_2$ on air at 1 ATA (TC Baseline) and maximum $TcpO_2$ on oxygen at 1 ATA (TC O_2) were measured. Two separate physiological challenges were administered: elevated legs and oxygen challenge. Each subject had two LDF and two $TcpO_2$ recordings made simultaneously on a lower extremity. For patients, the TCOM electrodes were placed approximately 1 cm from the edge of the wound and the LDF probes were placed 1 cm proximally to the TCOM sensor.

The mean LDF and $TcpO_2$ values for each experimental condition are at Table 7. Statistically significant differences were shown between healthy controls and patients for both LDF (p < 0.0001) and $TcpO_2$ (p < 0.0001); and between healed and non-healed patients for both LDF (p < 0.0001) and $TcpO_2$ (p < 0.0002). In both healed and non-healed patients, presence of inflammation caused LDF values to be elevated above healthy controls, whereas the $TcpO_2$ values were lowered.

SUGGESTED CLASSIFICATION SYSTEM FOR DEGREES OF ISCHEMIA AND HYPOXIA

Table 8 is a suggested classification system for degrees of ischemia and hypoxia. Perfusion of the local tissue when 44°C heat was applied was considered normal with an LDF % increase of greater than 500%, moderately ischemic with values between 150 and 500%, and severely ischemic with values below 150%. In the study described above (6), LDF parameters for healing were LDF max > 20 PU and LDF % increase > 150%. Similarly, $TcpO_2$ was considered to be normal at values of greater than 40 mm Hg, moderately hypoxic with values between 20 and 40 mm Hg, and severely hypoxic with values below 20 mm Hg. Transcutaneous oximetry values taken during air breathing (TC Air) and oxygen challenge (TC O_2) were used to determine the course of treatment. Transcutaneous oximetry parameters for healing were TC Air > 1, and TC O_2 > 35, plus TC % increase > 50%. The authors concluded that LDF with local heat provocation (44°C) appeared to be a useful complement to $TcpO_2$ for assessing problem wound patients as a prediction of wound healing, especially at low $TcpO_2$ values. For completeness of Table 8, SPP values are added from the 1997 data of Castronuovo and associates (47) and toe pressure values are added from the Second European Consensus document on critical limb ischemia (43).

Case 3

Patient AAI-624 is a 66-year-old female who was referred for evaluation of gangrene of her toes. She stated that she began to develop pain in her feet three months previously. This pain occurred at rest and was relieved by walking. She was initially treated by her primary physician for arthritis without relief. She was evaluated by a vascular surgeon three weeks prior to presentation and was found to have decreased circulation below the ankles and was not considered to be a candidate for revascularization. She began to develop gangrene of the toes about two weeks prior to presentation.

TCOM Assessment: The $TcpO_2$ baseline values indicated severe hypoxia in the right foot and normal values to mild hypoxia in the left foot. There was a moderate decrease in oxygen tensions with elevation of the legs indicating a decreased vascular reserve. There was an adequate response to inspired 100% oxygen in the left forefoot. There is no response to inspired 100% oxygen in the right foot. Based on these results, the failure to heal potential for wounds of the left foot (Figure 10A) was considered moderate. The failure to heal potential for wounds of the right foot (Figure 10B) was high.

LDF Assessment: A laser Doppler study was performed with heat provocation using the Center's standard testing procedure described below. The results are at Table 10 and the values are reported in percent change of perfusion units. Laser Doppler flowmetry indicates moderate ischemia in the left foot based on mean value of 216 (Moderate ischemia is defined in the

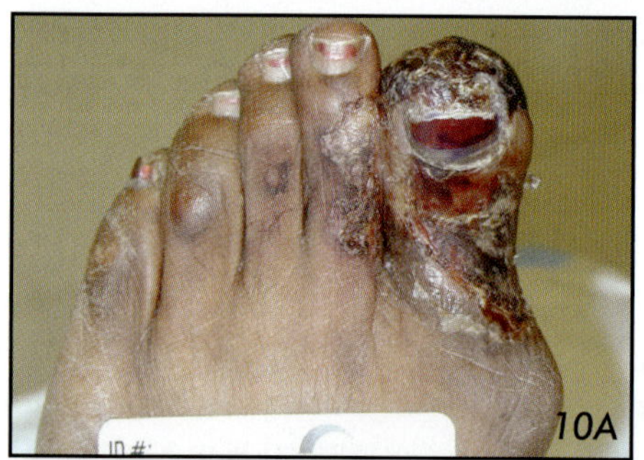

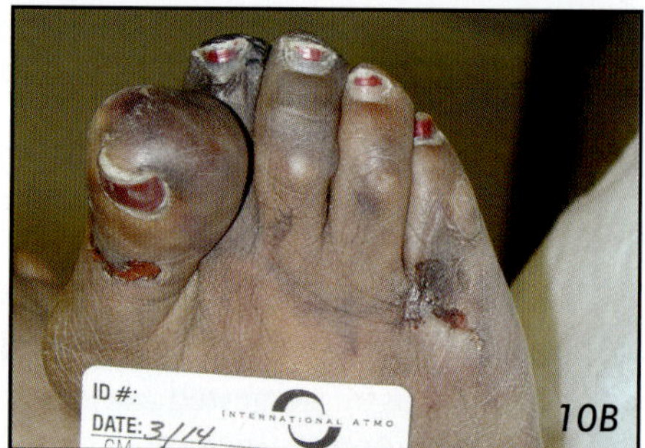

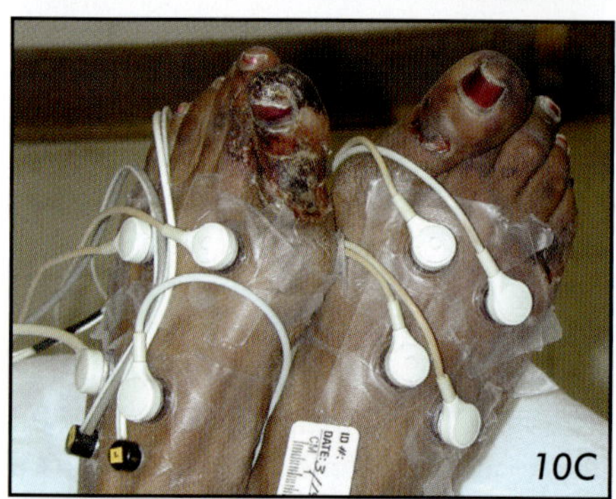

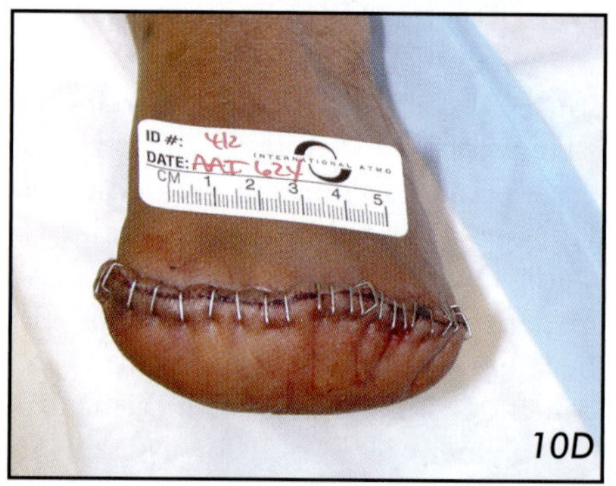

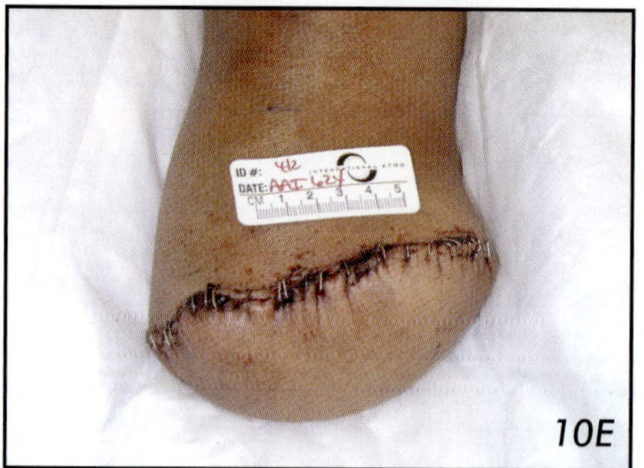

Figure 10. Patient AAI-624. (Photos A - E). Assessment and Outcome.
(A and B) On initial assessment, gangrenous toes are similar in appearance on both the left foot and right foot.
(C) TCOM and Laser Doppler assessment reveal major differences in degree of tissue hypoxia and ischemia, and failure to heal potential of the two limbs.
(D) The left limb is salvaged with a TMA.
(E) A BKA is required on the right.

range of 150–500% change in PU per column 2 of Table 8). There is a decrease in flow with elevation indicating poor vascular reserve.

Wound Care Physician's Recommendation: Based on the history and evaluation, the treatment recommendations were to begin HBO2 therapy to better demarcate the extent of the gangrene and minimize the amount of tissue lost from the left foot. There was no perceived benefit from HBO2 for the right foot and a below the knee amputation was recommended after the initial HBO2 treatments.

Outcome: After four HBO2 treatments, the level of ischemia had sufficiently demarcated and she underwent a left TMA and a right BKA. Hyperbaric oxygen treatments were continued following surgery and the wounds were, acceptably healed after 21 treatments.

TABLE 10. PATIENT AAI 624. RESULTS OF LASER DOPPLER STUDY WITH HEAT PROVOCATION

	Heat (PU % change)	Legs Elevated (PU % change)	Legs level (PU % change)
Left medial midfoot	324	-36	-2
Left lateral midfoot	109	-23	7
Mean	216		

COMBINED LDF AND TCOM TEST PROCEDURE FOR EVALUATING THE WOUND PATIENT

The following test procedure combines LDF and TCOM as assessment tools. It was developed at the Nix Wound Care and Hyperbaric Medicine Center, Nix Medical Center, San Antonio, Texas, with technical support from Perimed (Perimed AB, Stockholm, Sweden). The procedure has been previously reported (6). The test procedure was developed to ensure that laser Doppler studies were performed in a consistent manner for data to be used in diagnostic studies. The procedure uses local heat as the provocative test.

Equipment used in the study included:

- Two Radiometer TCM3 Transcutaneous Oxygen Monitors (Radiometer, Copenhagen, Denmark);
- A two-channel laser Doppler System comprised of a PeriFlux System 5000, Perimed AB, Sweden with 2 PF 5010 LDPM Units, one PF 5020 Heat unit, and two PROBE 457 Small Thermostatic Probes (Perimed AB, Stockholm, Sweden);
- A laptop computer;
- Data collection was performed using PeriSoft for Windows 1.30 (Perimed AB, Stockholm, Sweden);
- Two leads applied at each anatomical region in order for mean values to be computed for the simultaneous recordings.

Set Up Procedures Before Starting the Test:
1. Turn on the TCOM monitors and calibrate them at a preset temperature of 44°C.

2. Turn on laser Doppler (Perimed PeriFlux System 5000) at least 20 minutes prior to beginning the study.
3. If present, turn on 8 channel A/D converter to collect data from additional TCOM monitors of other makes.
4. Turn on computer:
    a. Log onto the computer.
    b. Start the PeriSoft for Windows program.
5. Enter patient information.
6. Prepare the patient for the test.
    a. Brief the patient on purpose and procedures of the test.
    b. Obtain informed consent.
    c. Place the patient in a comfortable supine position.
    d. Select the anatomical sites to be tested. Choose two sensor sites in each anatomical region to be tested so as to acquire the mean of two values in that region.

Starting the Test:

1. For TCOM: Place the TCOM fixation rings on the selected sites. Wait until baseline LDF data has been collected for 3 minutes into the study before placing the TCOM sensors into the fixation rings. This avoids any possibility that heat from the TCOM electrode will interfere with the LDF baseline values.
2. For LDF: Apply double-sided adhesive tape proximal to the TCOM fixation rings. Place one laser Doppler lead a distance of 1 cm proximal to each of the two TCOM fixation rings.

Conducting the Test:

Procedures for conducting the test are at Table 10. Graphical representation of the combined LDF and TCOM test procedures are at Figure 11.

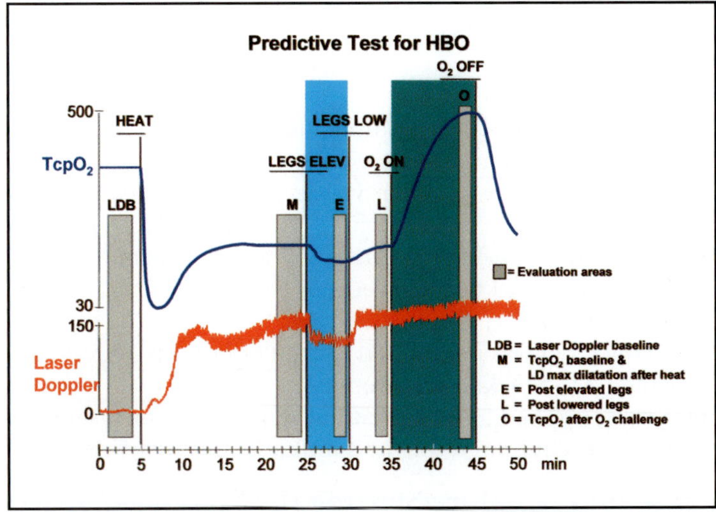

Figure 11. Graphical Representation of Combined LDF and TCOM Test Procedures.

TABLE 11. CONDUCTING THE TEST

Lapse Time	LDF Study	TCOM Study
	Baseline Test: Supine Position	
0–2 minutes	1. Prepare sites to be measured. Place unheated LD probes.	1. Prepare sites to be measured. Place TCOM fixation rings.
2 minutes	2. Start LDF baseline test.	
2–5 minutes	3. Record LDF baseline value (average of 3 minutes).	2. Affix TCOM electrodes.
5 minutes	**LDF Provocative Test: Heat**	**TCOM Baseline Test**
5 minutes	4. Start LDF (with heat) test. Heat LD probes (44°C).	3. Start TCOM baseline test (air).
5–25 minutes	5. Equilibrate LDF with heat. Wait 20 minutes.	4. Equilibrate TCOM electrodes (air). Wait 20 minutes.
24–25 minutes	6. Record LDF max after heat (average of last minute).	5. Record $TcpO_2$ baseline (air) (average of last minute).
25 minutes	**LDF & TCOM Provocative Test: Elevate Legs (30°)**	
25–30 minutes	7. Equilibrate LDF (elevated legs). Wait 5 minutes.	6. Equilibrate TCOM (elevated legs). Wait 5 minutes.
29–30 minutes	8. Record LDF leg elevation value (average last minute).	7. Record $TcpO_2$ leg elevation value (average last minute).
30 minutes	**Lower Legs to Normal Position**	
30–35 minutes	9. Equilibrate to supine position. Wait 5 minutes.	8. Equilibrate to supine position. Wait 5 minutes.
34–35 minutes	10. Record LDF post lowered legs (average of last minute).	9. Record $TcpO_2$ post lowered legs (average of last minute).
35 minutes		**TCOM Provocative Test: Oxygen Challenge (Start 100% Oxygen Breathing)**
35–45 minutes	11. Remove the LD Probes.	10. Equilibrate TCOM electrodes (oxygen). Wait 10 minutes
44–45 minutes		11. Record $TcpO_2$ oxygen value (average of last minute).
45 minutes		**Remove Oxygen Breathing**
45–50 minutes		12. Equilibrate TCOM electrodes (air). Wait 5 minutes.
49–50 minutes		13. Record $TcpO_2$ air value (average of last minute).
50 minutes		14. Remove TCOM electrodes.

Processing the Data:

In the Perimed PeriSoft for Windows software, the following parameters are used to select appropriate LDF and $TcpO_2$ data points collected during the test.

For LDF:

1. LDF baseline (without heat) is computed as the average of the first three minutes of the LDF values recorded after affixing the sensor (lapse time of 3–5 minutes).
2. LDF provocative test (after heat) is computed as the average of the last minute of the LDF values recorded 20 minutes after heat is applied (lapse time of 24–25 minutes).
3. LDF provocative test (leg elevation) is computed as the average of the last minute of the LDF values recorded 5 minutes after legs are elevated (lapse time of 29–30 minutes).
4. LDF completion of provocative test (leg elevation) is computed as the average of the last minute of the LDF values recorded 5 minutes after legs are lowered to normal (supine) position (lapse time of 34–35 minutes).
5. An oxygen challenge is not used for LDF because previous studies in the authors' laboratory showed no significant change in LDF when oxygen was breathed.

For TCOM:

1. $TcpO_2$ baseline is computed as the average of last minute of the $TcpO_2$ equilibration values recorded 20 minutes after affixing the TCOM electrode (lapse time of 24–25 minutes).
2. TCOM leg elevation provocative test is computed as the average of the last minute of $TcpO_2$ values recorded 5 minutes after legs are elevated (lapse time of 29–30 minutes).
3. TCOM completion of leg elevation provocative test is computed as the average of the last minute of $TcpO_2$ values recorded 5 minutes after legs are lowered to normal (supine) position (lapse time of 34–35 minutes).
4. TCOM oxygen challenge provocative test is computed as the average of the last minute of $TcpO_2$ values recorded ten minutes after oxygen breathing begins (lapse time of 44–45 minutes).
5. After the oxygen challenge, the Remove Oxygen Breathing test is computed as the average of the last minute of $TcpO_2$ values recorded five minutes after oxygen breathing stops (lapse time of 49–50 minutes).

Using Mean Values:

In this protocol, simultaneous measurements in the same anatomical region are performed using two TCOM electrodes and two laser Doppler probes. When multiple sensors are used, the mean value of the measurements is used for statistics and NOT each individual value. The reason for this is that since both measurements are performed simultaneously on the same anatomical region of the limb, they are not independent of each other and should not be treated statistically as independent.

This is easiest understood by use of an example. If one patient has a low value for the first measurement, there is a very high likelihood that the second measurement simultaneously recorded in the same anatomical region will also be low. Statistically this is very different from making one measurement on one patient, and then making one measurement on a second patient. In the latter case the likelihood that the second measurement is high or low does NOT depend on the value obtained from the previous patient.

Precautions During LDF Setup and Testing:

1. Ensure that the patient is comfortable before starting the test.
2. Choose the site to place the probe, keeping in mind that selection of the assessment location is crucial. The LDF probe may be placed either near the wound or at a standardized site on the limb.
3. When used in conjunction with TCOM, the LDF probe should be placed about 1 cm proximal to the TCOM electrode to avoid interference by the heated electrode. Collect baseline (unheated) LDF values before heating the TCOM electrode.
4. Several sites may be monitored simultaneously. When two probes are placed close together the laser Doppler signals may interfere with each other (cross talk) since additional light may be picked up by the receiving fiber. On the skin, probes should be separated by at least 9 mm distance (Operators Manual, Perimed AB, Stockholm).
5. Since skin perfusion is temperature dependent, skin temperature should be controlled. For reproducible skin perfusion measurements, repeat measurements should be done under standard conditions of room temperature, allowing the patient to adapt to the room temperature for about 30 minutes before starting the test (54).
6. Successive studies should be done under the same conditions at the same time of day. The patient should be encouraged to avoid hot drinks and tobacco (55).
7. The skin must be prepared by cleansing with alcohol. However, it is important not to perform tape stripping or shaving at the LDF probe site, as this will create a hyperemic response.
8. The LDF probe is affixed with double-sided tape or a fixation ring. Position the probe without pressure where the tip touches the tissue to be studied. Applying pressure to the top of the probe will restrict the capillary perfusion beneath it, and must be avoided or the readings will be incorrect.
9. Movement artifacts occur when the patient moves or the optical fibers are moved during measurements. Movement artifacts cause a false positive addition to the signal. Making the patient comfortable before starting the test and briefing the patient on the need to avoid movement can minimize movement artifacts. Positioning the probe leads parallel with the limb and taping them in place will also reduce movement artifact. Do not apply tape over the top of the sensor to avoid applying pressure to the skin that restricts flow.

10. The fiber optic cable should be positioned so that it curves gently without kinks. The cable should also be secured in such a way that it does not pull at the tissue or move freely, as that will cause artifacts.

11. After completing the study, carefully remove the probes, taking care not to tear fragile skin. Observe and report unusual findings where the probe was placed on the skin. In the short duration (< 1 hr) of the test with heat provocation temperature of 44°C, there is usually no problem. However, temperatures over 40°C may cause burns in babies and there are time limits to heat provocation in young children and the elderly.

12. Each manufacturer provides a list of precautions that the technologist must follow when using their equipment.

Case 4

Patient AAI 618 JL is a 53 YOM who developed a blister over the 5th toe 7 months prior to presentation at the Wound Healing Center (Figures 12A-D). The blister ruptured to produce an ulcer for which he received a long course of oral antibiotics and dressing changes without resolution. Within 2 weeks after the antibiotics were halted, the foot became red and swollen, and there was a foul-smelling drainage from the wound. He was hospitalized with a fever, at which time cultures revealed *Group B streptococcal* and *Staphylococcus aureus*. Radiographs revealed osteomyelitis in the distal end of the 5th metatarsal. Calcification of the arteries was noted. A previous angiogram did not indicate any large vessel disease. Examination revealed a 1 x 1.2 cm wound at the lateral aspect of the base of the 5th toe that was covered by thick eschar. The surrounding skin was erythematous and warm to touch. The toe appeared ischemic. LDF, ABI, and TCOM assessments were requested to assist in surgical planning for a partial 5th ray amputation. Figure 12A shows the positioning of the LDF and TCOM sensors for concurrent evaluations of perfusion and oxygenation of the lower leg and foot.

TCOM Assessment: A transcutaneous oximetry study was conducted while the patient was breathing room air and 100% oxygen at 1 atm abs following the Center's standard testing procedure as described above. The strip chart recording of results is shown at Figure 12B and the pertinent values (reported in mm Hg) are shown at Table 12. Seven electrodes were used for the test. The values assessed were the mean percent change between two measured sites taken: 1) 15 cm below the knee, 2) at the metatarsals, and 3) at the toes. No difficulties were encountered during the test.

Interpretation: Baseline (air) $TcpO_2$ values indicate moderate hypoxia below the knee and at the metatarsals, and severe hypoxia at the toes. There is a significant decrease in oxygen tension with leg elevation, indicating poor vascular reserve. There is an adequate response to inspired oxygen.

Explanation: TCOM measures the local tissue oxygen tension that is derived from the local capillary (nutritive) blood perfusion. $TcpO_2$ indicates if the tissue is hypoxic and if it will respond to respired oxygen. $TcpO_2$ values above 40 mm Hg are considered normal, 20–40 mm Hg are considered moderately hypoxic, and below 20 mm Hg are considered severely hypoxic. Based on these results, the failure to heal potential with standard wound care for this wound is high.

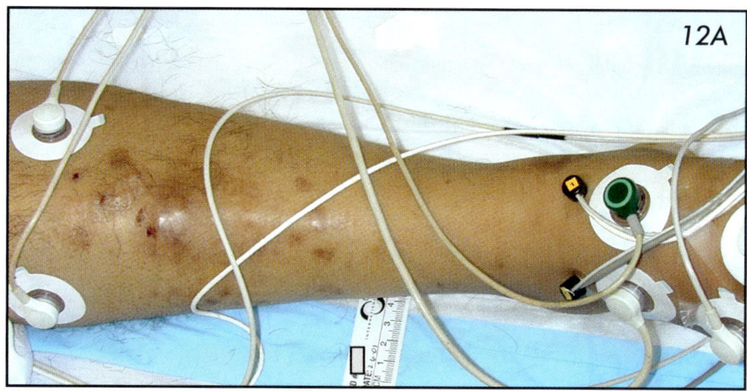

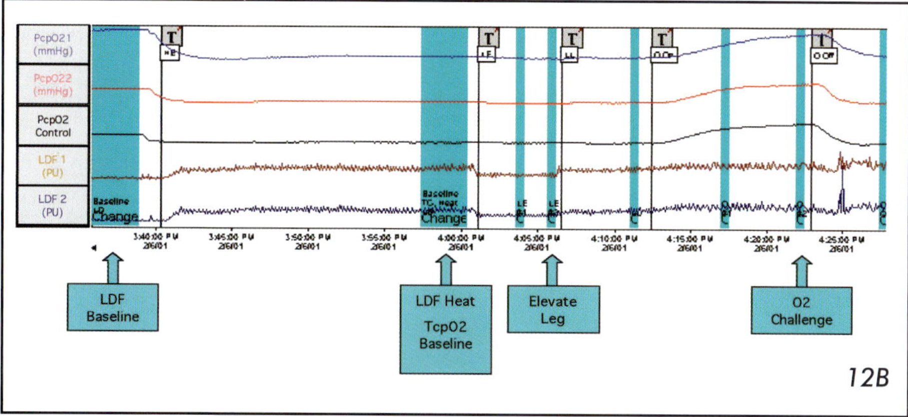

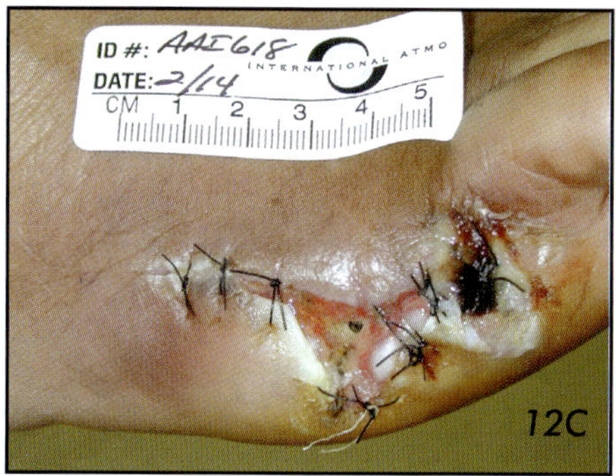

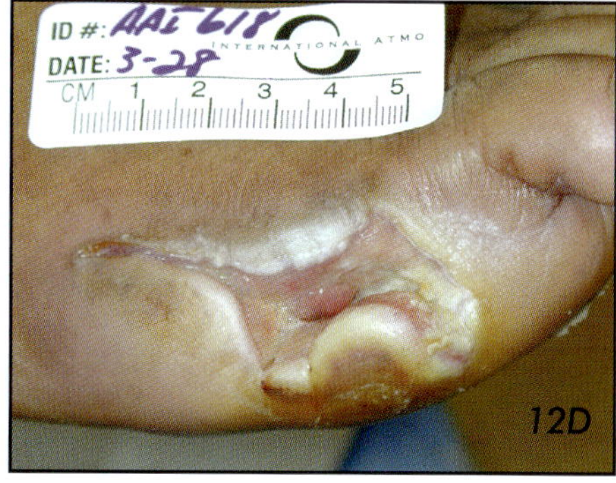

Figure 12 (A through D). Patient AAI 618 JL with foot wound.
(A) Day 1: LDF (2 probes) and TCOM (6 electrodes) are used for non-invasive evaluation of the lower limb.
(B) LDF and TcpO2 tracings show baseline data and responses to leg elevation and oxygen challenge.
(C) Day 6: Non-healing wound following 5th Ray amputation.
(D) Day 40: Successful outcome after 30 HBO2 and aggressive wound care.

LDF Assessment: A laser Doppler study was performed with heat provocation following the Center's standard testing procedure. The strip chart recording of results is shown at Figure 12B and the pertinent values (in perfusion units) are shown at Table 12. The values are reported in perfusion units and percent change in perfusion units following heat provocation. The mean percent change between two measured metatarsal sites is the value assessed. No difficulties were encountered during the test.

Interpretation: LDF shows moderate ischemia at the metatarsal region of the foot as indicated by the 307% rise in perfusion units in response to heat provocation.

Explanation: LDF measures the total blood perfusion in local tissue and indicates if the tissue is ischemic. With local heat provocation, vasodilatation is maximized, enabling the use of LDF to assess the tissue reserve capacity and severity of ischemia. Percent change in values greater than 500% is considered normal, 150–500% is considered moderately ischemic, and below 150% is considered severely ischemic.

Wound Care Physician's Recommendation: Following surgery, the treatment plan should include daily wound care and HBO2 to help control infection and prevent spread of necrosis. The surgeon, who would provide continued surgical management, will need to make periodic reassessments.

Outcome: Following 5th ray amputation, the wound had dehisced (Figure 12C). Over the course of 6 weeks, the patient received daily wound care and 30 HBO2 treatments, after which, the wound appeared to have reached maximum benefit of HBO2 (Figure 12D). During the next 2 weeks, the patient received additional wound care and on the third office visit, the wound was acceptably healed. For a discussion of the therapeutic options for hypoxia and ischemia see the chapter by GR Weir and FJ Cronje entitled, "Ischemia and Hypoxia: The Therapeutic Options."

TABLE 12. PATIENT AAI 618 JL. LDF AND TCOM ASSESSMENT OF FOOT WOUND AT 1 ATA.

		Mean TcpO$_2$ (mm Hg)				Mean LDF (PU)	
Test	Time (min)	Control	Below Knee	Metatarsal	Toe	Metatarsal	% Rise
LD Baseline	3					15	
LD Heat	20					46	307
TCOM Baseline	20	37	26	29	19		
Elevated Leg	5	37	18	17	9		
100% O$_2$	10	367	227	186	214		

Temperature settings for TCOM sensor and LDF heat provocation were 44°C.

CONCLUSION

Tissue oxygenation and perfusion data are used by physicians in many specialties to make medical decisions about the treatment of their patients. In wound centers, transcutaneous oximetry and laser Doppler flowmetry are used to evaluate hypoxia and ischemia, to determine wound healing potential, to determine appropriate amputation levels, to select patients for hyperbaric oxygen treatments, and to evaluate responses to treatment. Determining the tissue oxygenation and perfusion status of a wound area is important because moderately hypoxic or ischemic wound beds render ineffective certain standard treatments such as skin grafting, growth factor treatments, or living tissue replacements. These wound assessment tools can identify severely hypoxic or ischemic wound beds that may require revascularization or aggressive HBO2 treatment to avoid amputation.

ACKNOWLEDGMENTS

The authors thank Kjell Bakken and Bjorn Bakken for their assistance in developing the LDF and $TcpO_2$ protocol that is published herein. Thanks to Perimed AB (Stockholm, Sweden) and Vasamed (Eden Prairie, Minnesota) for providing the laser Doppler equipment needed for the evaluations. We are also grateful to Phil Lazzara and Robert B. Sheffield for providing technical expertise with the TCOM equipment. Also acknowledged are the technical expertise of Kevin I. Posey in collecting the data, the administrative skill of Suzanne Pack, and the dedication of the men and women of International ATMO, Inc. for participating as subjects in the evaluations.

REFERENCES

1. Sheffield PJ. Measuring tissue oxygen tension: a review. *J Undersea Hyperb Med* 1998:179-188.

2. Baumberger JP, Goodfriend RB. Determination of arterial oxygen tension in man by equilibration through intact skin. *Fed Proc* 1951; 10:10-11.

3. Huch R, Lubbers DW, Huch A. Quantitative continuous measurement of partial oxygen pressure on the skin of adults and newborn babies. *Pflugers Arch* 1972; 337:185-198.

4. Lubbers DW. Theoretical basis of the transcutaneous blood gas measurements. *Critical Care Med* 1981; 9:721-733.

5. Evans NTS, Naylor PFD. The systemic oxygen supply to the surface of the human skin. *Resp Physiol* 1967; 3:21-37.

6. Sheffield PJ, Dietz D, Posey KI, et al. Use of transcutaneous oximetry and laser Doppler with local heat provocation to assess patients with problem wounds. In: NM Petri, D Andric, D Ropac (eds), *Book of Proceedings, 1st Congress of the Alps-Adria Working Community on Maritime, Undersea, and Hyperbaric Medicine.* Split, Croatia: Croatian Maritime, Undersea and Hyperbaric Medical Society of Croatian Medical Association, 2001:341-344.

7. Dooley J, King G, Slade B. Establishment of reference pressure of transcutaneous oxygen for the comparative evaluation of problem wounds. *Undersea & Hyperb Med* 1997, 24(4): 235-244.

8. Otto GH, Buyukcakir C, Fife CE. The effect of smoking history on treatment regimen and cost in diabetic patients undergoing hyperbaric oxygen therapy (HBO2) (abstract). *Undersea Hyperb Med* 1999; 26 (Suppl): 55.

9. Gorman DF. Oxygen therapy in the diabetic foot. In: Frykberg RG (ed). *The High Risk Foot in Diabetes Mellitus,* New York, NY: Churchill Livingstone, 1991; pp 441-447.

10. White RA, Klein SR. Amputation level selection by transcutaneous oxygen pressure determination. In: Moore WS and Malone JM (ed). *Lower Extremity Amputation* Philadelphia, PA: WB Saunders, 1989; pp 44-49.

11. Hauser CJ. Tissue salvage by mapping of skin surface transcutaneous oxygen tension index. *Arch Surg* 1987; 22: 1128-1130.

12. Fife CE. Hyperbaric oxygen therapy applications in wound care. In: Sheffield PJ, Fife CE, Smith APS (Eds). *Wound Care Practice* Flagstaff, AZ: Best Publishing, 2004; 661-684.

13. Fife CE, Buyukcakir C, Otto GH, et al. The predictive value of transcutaneous oxygen tension measurement in diabetic lower extremity ulcers treated with hyperbaric oxygen therapy: A retrospective analysis of 1144 patients. *Wound Rep Reg* 2002; 10:198-207.

14. Pecoraro RE, Ahroni JH, Boydo EJ, et al. Chronology and determinants of tissue repair in diabetic lower-extremity ulcers. *Diabetes* 1991; 40:1305-1312.

15. Myers RAM, Emhoff TA. Transcutaneous oxygen measurements in the non-healing diabetic wound. In: Program and abstracts. Eight International Congress on Hyperbaric Medicine, Bethesda, MD: *Undersea Medical Society* 1984; pp 185-186.

16. Wattel FE, Mathieu MD, Fossati P, et al. Hyperbaric oxygen in the treatment of diabetic foot lesions. Search for healing predictive factors. *J Hyperb Med* 1991; 6(4):263-268.

17. Mathieu DM, Wattel FE, Bouachour G. Post traumatic limb ischemia: Prediction of final outcome by transcutaneous oxygen measurements in hyperbaric oxygen, *J Trauma* 1990; 30: 307-314.

18. Campagnoli P, Oriani G, Sala G, et al. Prognostic value of PtcO2 during hyperbaric oxygen therapy. *J Hyperb Med* 1992; 7(4):223-227.

19. Strauss MJ, Breedlove JW, Hart GB. Use of transcutaneous oxygen measurements to predict healing in foot wounds (abstract). *Undersea Hyperb Med* 1997; 24 (suppl): 15.

20. Sheffield PJ, Workman WT. Non invasive tissue oxygen measurements in patients administered normobaric and hyperbaric oxygen by mask. *Hyperb Oxyg Rev* 1985; 6(1):47-62.

21. Sheffield PJ. UHMS designated introductory course in hyperbaric medicine, *Pressure* 1998; 27(6): 1-2,5.

22. Marotte S, Larson-Lohr V, Weaver LK. Performance evaluation of transcutaneous oxygen ($TcpO_2$) monitors (abstract). *Undersea Hyperb Med* 1993; 20(Suppl): 28

23. Workman WT, Sheffield PJ. Continuous transcutaneous oxygen monitoring in smokers under normobaric and hyperbaric oxygen conditions. In: Huch R, Huch A (eds), *Continuous Transcutaneous Blood Gas Monitoring*, New York: Marcel Dekker, 1983; pp 649-656.

24. Sheffield PJ, Workman WT. Transcutaneous tissue oxygen monitoring in patients undergoing hyperbaric oxygen therapy. In Huch R, Huch A (eds): *Continuous Transcutaneous Blood Gas Monitoring*, New York: Marcel Dekker, 1983; pp 655-660.

25. Clarke D. Transcutaneous monitoring of pO_2 in hyperbaric medicine, *Patient Focus Circle*, Copenhagen, Denmark: Radiometer Medical A/S, 1997.

26. Jensen JA, Goodson WH, Hopf HW, et al. Cigarette smoking decreases tissue oxygen. *Arch Sur*, 1991; 126:1131-1134.

27. Strauss AG, Hart GB, Strauss MB. Effect of smoking cessation on transcutaneous oxygen measurements - a case report and review (abstract). *Undersea Hyperb Med* 1997; 24 (suppl): 36.

28. Buckley CJ, Lee SD. Non-invasive and invasive evaluations for lower extremity arterial occlusive disease. In: Sheffield PJ, Fife CE, Smith APS (eds), *Wound Care Practice* Flagstaff, AZ: Best Publishing, 2004; 101-116.

29. Riva C, Ross B, Benedek GB. Laser Doppler measurements in capillary tubes and retinal arteries. *Invest Opthalmol* 11:936-944, 1972.

30. Stern MD. In vivo evaluation of microcirculation by coherent light scattering. *Nature* 254:56-58, 1975.

31. Nilsson G, Jakobsson A, Wardell K. Tissue perfusion monitoring and imaging by coherent light scattering. SPIE Vol. 1524. *Bioptics: Optics in Biomedicine and Environmental Sciences* 1991.

32. Essex TJH, Byrne PO. A laser Doppler scanner for imaging blood flow in skin. J Biomedical Eng 1991; 13 (May), 189-194.

33. Dwars TA, Van den Broek. Criteria for reliable selection of the lowest level of amputation in peripheral vascular disease. *J Vasc Surg* 1992 (15) 536-542.

34. Choi CM, Bennett RG, Laser Doppler to determine cutaneous blood flow. *Dermatol Surg* 2003; Mar 29(3): 272-80.

35. Yuen JC, Feng Z. Monitoring free flaps using the laser Doppler flowmeter: five-year experience. *Plast Reconstr Surg* 2000;105: 55-61.

36. Jeng JC, Bridgeman A, Shivnan L, et al. Laser Doppler imaging determines need for excision and grafting in advance of clinical judgment: a prospective blinded trial. *Burns* 2003 Nov;29(7):665-70.

37. Gebuhr P, Jorgensen JP, Vollmer-Larsen B, et al. Estimation of amputation level with a laser Doppler flowmeter. *J Bone Joint Surg Br* 1989 May; 71(3):514-517.

38. Van den Brande P, Welch W. Diagnosis of arterial occlusive disease of the lower extremities by laser Doppler flowmetry. *Int Angiol* 1988 Jul-Sep;7(3):224-230.

39. Nilsson GF Signal processor for laser Doppler tissue flowmeters. *Med & Biol Eng & Compu* 1984;22: 343-348.

40. Ahn H, Johansson K, Lundgren O, et al. In vivo evaluations of signal processors for laser Doppler tissue velocity. *Med & Biol Eng & Compu* 1987;25: 207-211.

41. Bonner R, Nossal R. Principles of laser Doppler flowmetry, In: Shepherd & Öberg eds., *Laser Doppler Blood Flowmetry*. Dordrecht, The Netherlands: Kluwer Academic Publishers, 1990; 17-45.

42. Stansberry KB, Shapiro SA, Hill MA, et al. Impaired peripheral vasomotion in diabetes. *Diabetes Care* 1996;19(7): 715-721.

43. Second European Consensus. Second European Consensus document on chronic critical leg ischemia. *Circulation* 1991;84:1-26.

44. Ubbink DT, Spincemaille GH, Reneman RS, et al. Prediction of imminent amputation in patients with non-reconstructible leg ischemia by means of microcirculatory investigations. *J Vasc Surg* 1999; 30(1):114-121.

45. Ijzerman RG, Serne EH, Van Weissenbruch MM, et al. Cigarette smoking is associated with an acute impairment of microvascular function in humans. *Clinical Science* 2003; 104, 247–252.

46. Wahlberg E, Olofsson P, Swendenborg J, et al. Changes in postocclusive reactive hyperaemic values as measured with laser Doppler fluxmetry after infrainguinal arterial reconstruction. *Eur J Vasc Endovasc Surg* 1995; 9(2): 197-203.

47. Castronuovo, JJ, HM Adera, JM Smiell, et al. Skin perfusion pressure measurement is valuable in the diagnosis of critical limb ischemia. *J Vasc Surg* 1997; 26: 629-37.

48. Fischer M, Hoffmann U, Oomen P, et al. Simultaneous measurement of digital artery and skin perfusion pressure by the laser Doppler technique in healthy controls and patients with peripheral arterial occlusive disease. *Eur J Vasc Endovasc Surg* 1995; 10(2):231-236.

49. Wahlberg E, Jorneskog G, Olofsson P, et al. The influence of reactive hyperemia and leg dependency on skin microcirculation in patients with peripheral arterial occlusive disease (PAOD) with and without diabetes. *Vasa* 1990; 19(4): 301-306.

50. Scheffler A, Eggert S, Rieger H. Influence of clinical findings, positional maneuvers and systolic ankle arterial pressure on $TcpO_2$ in PAD, *Eur J F Clin inv* 1992; 22:420-26.

51. Franzeck UK, Stengele B, Panradi U, et al. Cutaneous reactive hyperaemia in short-term and long-term type 1 diabetes – Continuous monitoring by combined laser Doppler and transcutaneous oxygen probe. *Vasa* 1990; 19:8-15.

52. Fife CE, O'Malley E, Hildreth S, et al. Skin perfusion pressure and transcutaneous oximetry as a predictor of outcome in wound healing (abstract). *UHM* 1999; 26 (Suppl): 36

53. Lo T, Sample R, Prins R, et al. Prediction of wound healing outcome in 100 patients using Skin Perfusion Pressure and transcutaneous PO_2. *UHM* 2004; 31(3): 329 (Abstract)]

54. Michaels J, Alsbjorn B, Sorenson B. Clinical use of laser Doppler flowmetry in a burns unit. *Scand J Plast Reconstr Surg* 1984; 18: 65-73.

55. Ziemba AL. Laser Doppler Flowmetry (LDF). In: Larson-Lohr V, Norvell HC (eds), *Hyperbaric Nursing* Flagstaff AZ: Best Publishing 2002; 315-321.

REVIEW QUESTIONS

TCOM

1.) Transcutaneous oximetry data are used in medical decision making to:
    a. Choose successful amputation sites
    b. Determine wound healing potential
    c. Select candidates for hyperbaric oxygen therapy
    d. Predict nonresponders to treatment
    e. Any of the above

2.) Transcutaneous oxygen sensors can be used to determine the oxygen tension in
    a. Skin capillaries
    b. Bone marrow
    c. Muscle
    d. Cerebral circulation
    e. Tendons

3.) Air-breathing patients whose $TcpO_2$ values are above 40 mm Hg should have sufficient tissue oxygenation to heal with:
    a. Standard wound care
    b. Grafting
    c. Application of living tissue replacements such as fibroblasts, keratinocytes, and dermal component
    d. Application of growth factors
    e. Any of the above

4.) When measuring the $TcpO_2$ for a wound of the toe, the TCOM sensor site should be:
    a. On an unshaved area
    b. On the dorsum of the foot where it is flat or slightly concave
    c. On the plantar region of the foot
    d. Completely covered with Skin Prep
    e. Over a bone

5.) Conditions that cause $TcpO_2$ values to be elevated above normal include:
    a. Leak under the fixation ring
    b. Acute edema
    c. Active infection
    d. Thick or sclerotic skin
    e. Irradiated tissue

Laser Dopler

6.) Laser Doppler flowmetry data are used in medical decision making to:
    a. Define the level of successful amputation
    b. Predict wound healing using local wound care
    c. Identify need for revascularization
    d. Assess blood flow and skin perfusion pressure
    e. Any of the above

7.) When applied to the skin, laser Doppler flowmetry measures the total blood perfusion in:
   a. Skin capillaries, arterioles, venules, and shunts
   b. Bone marrow
   c. Muscle
   d. Cerebral circulation
   e. Tendons

8.) The measured depth of the laser Doppler in tissue depends on all of the following EXCEPT:
   a. Wavelength of the probe
   b. Blood content
   c. Pigmentation
   d. Distance between the transmitting and receiving optic fiber
   e. Blood flow

9.) Commonly used provocative tests for laser Doppler flowmetry to evaluate skin perfusion include all of the following EXCEPT:
   a. Occlusion
   b. Heat
   c. Posture (raised or lowered limb)
   d. Oxygen

10.) In the absence of a provocative test, laser Doppler flowmetry is difficult to use as a predictor of wound healing because:
   a. The large natural variation in microcirculatory blood flow makes it difficult to distinguish between normal and diseased tissue
   b. Laser Doppler cannot identify presence of blood flow without the provocation
   c. The measured depth changes based on the provocative test
   d. The test is too painful to the patient

Answers: 1e, 2a, 3e, 4b, 5a, 6e, 7a, 8e, 9d, 10a

EVIDENCE–BASED WOUND CARE

CHAPTER SIX OVERVIEW

NOTES

EVIDENCE–BASED WOUND CARE

Robert A. Warriner III

WHAT IS EVIDENCE–BASED MEDICINE?

Evidence–based medicine had it origins at McMaster University in Canada in the early 1990s and was initially defined as an approach to health care practice in which the clinician is aware of the evidence in support of his or her clinical practice and the strength of that evidence. The definition put forth by David L. Sackett in 1996 (1) is perhaps the most useful and states that "evidence–based medicine is the conscientious, explicit, and judicious use of current best evidence in making decisions about the care of individual patients. The practice of evidence–based medicine means integrating *individual clinical expertise* with the *best available external clinical evidence* from systematic research. By individual clinical expertise we mean the proficiency and judgment that individual clinicians acquire through clinical experience and clinical practice." He defines the italicized critical values identified above as follows: Individual clinical expertise is "more effective and efficient diagnosis" and "more thoughtful identification and compassionate use of individual patients' predicaments, rights, and preferences in making clinical decisions about their care." Best available external clinical evidence is "clinical research into the accuracy and precision of diagnostic tests (including the clinical examination), the power of prognostic markers, and the efficacy and safety of therapeutic, rehabilitative, and preventive regiments" which "invalidates previously accepted diagnostic tests and treatments and replaces them with new ones that are more powerful, more accurate, more efficacious, and safer."

For any practice of evidence–based medicine to be effective, the clinician must be able to accurately define the patient's clinical condition as well as contributing circumstances (social, cultural, and financial) that will impact any treatment application, identify knowledge gaps and frame questions to fill those gaps, conduct an efficient literature search for primary source documents or peer reviewed clinical practice guidelines that best match the individual patient's condition, critically appraise the research evidence and guideline recommendations, and apply that evidence to this specific patient's care. Two fundamental principles underlie this process (2): 1) appropriate application of a hierarchy of evidence to guide clinical decision making and 2) appropriate application of the evidence obtained from a benefit and risk perspective that also considers such issues as inconvenience, costs, alternative management strategies, and patient values.

Table 1 gives one example of a hierarchy of strength of evidence for treatment decisions where systematic reviews of multiple randomized trials of sufficient quality of trial design and number of patients included as the "gold" standard for defining evidence in support clinical decision making. Unfortunately, randomized clinical trial design can be subject to a number of effects that can lead to misinterpretation of the reported findings including natural history of the disease under study, placebo effects, patient and clinician compliance with defined protocols (particularly problematic in wound care trials reported to date), patient and clinician expectations producing bias, and patients' desire to please. An interesting alternative to the conventional randomized multi patient clinical trial is the N of 1 RCT in which a patient or patients undertake pairs of treatment periods in which they receive a target treatment in 1 period of each pair and a placebo or alternative treatment in the other with both patients and clinicians blinded to the allocation of the study intervention and placebo control. Such studies, while potentially useful in some circumstances, are probably unsuited to the typical wound treatment effectiveness questions that we address due to the impact of time and treatment or non treatment on the inherent response of the wound.

TABLE 1. HIERARCHY OF STRENGTH OF EVIDENCE FOR TREATMENT DECISIONS (2)

N of 1 randomized trial
Systematic reviews of randomized trials
Single randomized trial
Systematic review of observational studies addressing patient-important outcomes
Single observational study addressing patient-important outcomes
Physiologic studies
Unsystematic clinical observations

Further complicating this process is the application of the conclusions drawn from clinical trials completed on other patients to a specific, individual patient. Randomized, controlled trials only provide us with information about groups, not individuals (3). Individual patients may differ from those included in the clinical trial in terms of basic characteristics (age, sex, pregnancy), the presence of different patterns of co-morbidities or confounding factors, occurrence of side effects of the intended treatment, and personality, social, cultural, and financial factors affecting the individual patient not addressed in the clinical trial. Finally, and critically, the randomized trial may have compared a treatment intervention against an acceptable standard or alternative treatment but not all possibly effective alternative treatments (particularly problematic in wound care clinical trials).

The hierarchy must not be considered to be absolute. If treatment effects are sufficiently large and consistently demonstrated, observational or cohort studies may provide acceptable evidence. However, observational studies are characterized by their own set of potential biases unless the numbers of patients included are significant (2). Sackett (1) would also agree that some questions about therapy do not require randomized trials (i.e., successful interventions for rare or otherwise fatal conditions), or where appropriate randomized trials likely cannot be completed with any reasonable degree of effort applied (disease or injury statues that occur in very diverse populations or where important co-morbid conditions cannot be adequately assessed or addressed in the trial design), or when it is not possible to wait for trials to be conducted. In such cases the next best level of external evidence must be identified.

A couple of cautions regarding applying traditional evidence–based medicine to individual patient care: 1) the highest level of evidence, the meta-analysis or systematic review of multiple randomized clinical trials, does not take into account unpublished, possibly non-significant results (3), 2) the effectiveness of the application of an evidence–based treatment in a specific patient by a specific clinician, and 3) the potential to oversimplify the complex nature of clinical care.

The following additional resources are helpful in developing a greater understanding of the application of evidence–based medicine regardless of the setting.

- Guyatt G, Rennie D (eds). *Users' Guides to the Medical Literature: Essentials of Evidence–Based Clinical Practice*. AMA Press, Chicago, 2002, 442 pages (includes CD ROM).
- Jenicek M, Hitchcock DL. *Evidence–Based Practice: Logic and Critical Thinking in Medicine*. AMA Press, Chicago, 2005, 302 pages.
- Brown MM, Brown GC, Sharma S. *Evidence–Based to Value-Based Medicine*. AMA Press, Chicago, 2005, 339 pages.
- Straus SE, Richardson WS, Glasziou P, Haynes RB. *Evidence–Based Medicine: How to Practice and Teach EBM, 3rd ed.* Elsevier Churchill Livingstone, Edinburgh, 2005, 299 pages (includes CD ROM and web access to CQ Log and EBM Tables).

In addition, a number of websites are also available and are particularly useful and include:

- The Cochrane Collaboration and the Cochrane Library located at *http://www.cochrane.org*
- The Centre for Health Evidence at *http://www.cche.net*
- Users' Guides Interactive at *http://www.userguides.org*
- The Centre for Evidence–Based Medicine, Oxford-Centre for Evidence–Based Medicine, Oxford, England at *http://www.cebm.net*
- PubMed at *http://www.ncbi.nlm.nih.gov/entrez/query.fcgi?DB=pubmed* and *http://www.pubmedcentral.nih.gov*
- CINAHL (nursing database) at *http://www.cinahl.com*
- The National Guidelines Clearinghouse at *http://www.guideline.gov*
- The Agency for Healthcare Research and Quality at *http://www.ahcpr.gov/clinic/epcix.htm*
- Patient Oriented Evidence that Matters (POEM) at *http://www.infopoems.com/*

Finally, a number of review articles have discussed literature searching strategies for the effective practice of evidence–based medicine. Doig and Simpson (4) have outlined a three step process to improve the value of returns on literature searches in answering evidence–based questions. These steps briefly summarized include:

1. Focusing the clinical question in such a way that phrasing facilitates the literature searching process producing more precise answers (going from general to specific in layered searches with proper use of MeSH terms).
2. Take advantage of PubMed clinical queries including the systematic review filter and research methodology filters,
3. Refining search terms using appropriate MeSH primary and alternate terms by using the "Details" button on the search screen to assess the actual searching strategy used by PubMed in deriving the results obtained and displayed, using the MeSH database to refine the search terms, and using the display citation feature of the search to find MeSH categories applied to any individual article identified.

There are limitations to this methodology. Some valuable lower level of evidence reports may be missed (5) unless the initial broad based search is not scanned prior to applying the systematic review filter. Ryan, et al. (6) has outlined alternative strategies for primary literature identification which are also quite useful.

EVIDENCE–BASED MEDICINE: IMPACT ON MEDICINE AND WOUND CARE

While no doubt exists in the minds of proponents of evidence–based medicine that efforts to establish such practices have been beneficial, there is little direct evidence that physicians who practice evidence–based medicine have consistently better outcomes than those who do not. Nevertheless, it would seem appropriate that properly applied evidence–based medicine concepts should improve patient care and patient outcomes. Furthermore, there is recognition amongst epidemiologists, clinicians, regulatory and clinical/scientific bodies, and payers that 1) much geographic variation in the frequency of application of medical and surgical procedures exists with significant differences in patient outcomes and costs of care which cannot be explained by differences in patient demographics or clinical characteristics, 2) "strong evidence" that much of the care being provided may be inappropriate, 3) many patients may not be receiving beneficial services, and 4) health care costs continue to rise (7). No where is this more likely to be true than in wound care.

Many of our procedures, methods, materials, and technologies used in wound management may not fulfill the rigorous requirements to qualify as supported by higher level evidence (8). Much of our core clinical research suffers from inadequate sample sizes, poor trial design with nonrandom allocation of patients to treatment and control arms, non-blinded assessment of outcomes, poor descriptions of control and concurrent interventions, and short follow up periods. Additionally, the baseline standard background therapies may not be consistently applied within and among treatment and control arms, or, treatment may be compared to "standard" but not "optimal" therapeutic alternatives. Trial design in wound care studies may be hampered by inappropriate requirements placed by regulatory bodies such as the FDA on control arms or outcomes measured (9).

A few examples from our own literature serve to highlight some of these difficulties. The 1994 AHCPR Clinical Practice Guideline Number 15: Treatment of Pressure Ulcers (AHCPR #95-0652, December 1994) contained 81 specific recommendations based on a review of 45,000 abstracts from which 17,000 manuscripts were selected. Of those manuscripts selected, only 40 percent were research based. Specific recommendations were graded as class A (based on good science), class B (based on poor science), and class C (expert panel consensus). Of the 81 specific recommendations, only two were class A and nine were class B with the remaining 70 recommendations being class C level of evidence.

In the clinical trials for recombinant human platelet-derived growth factor (rhPDGF), Steed (10) identified the significant impact of debridement frequency on outcomes in the rhPDGF treatment group. Healing outcomes varied from 20–83 per cent between sites in the multicenter clinical trial with lowest frequency of debridement sites yielding the lowest healing percentages. Inconsistency in applying the clinical trial protocol can clearly alter the significance of the effect of the treatment intervention.

Boulton and Armstrong (11) in an editorial on clinical trials in neuropathic diabetic foot ulceration pointed out the inconsistency in offloading prescribed and utilized as a major potential contributor to variability in outcomes reported in various clinical trials of dressings and interventions in support of diabetic foot ulcer healing.

Gottrup (8) rightly points out that another feature that may impact the quality of evidence generated in wound care is the fact that the majority of products used in wound care are classified by the FDA as medical devices which may be deemed safe for use after successful investigations for safety based on Phase 1 and 2 trials yielding satisfactory outcomes or on the basis of 510k approval because of substantial equivalence to already approved products or technologies. In this circumstance there is little incentive for the manufacturers to fund more substantial Phase 3 or 4 clinical trials. That this is likely true is demonstrated in the recent review by Bouza, et al. (12) in which a systematic review of the efficacy of modern dressings in the treatment of venous leg ulcers failed to show any difference in healing frequency between gauze and modern wound dressings.

Increasingly federal agencies (Center for Medicare and Medicaid Services) and third party payers are applying evidence–based standards to the development of payment policies (7,13). Unfortunately, in many cases, only meta-analysis and systematic reviews of multiple randomized clinical trials, or in some cases significantly positive single well-designed randomized clinical trials are used to set coverage policies for existing and new technologies and interventions. Other forms of evidence are frequently overlooked or discounted. This is particularly true in the area of wound care related technology. Such policy decision processes are even being applied to long-standing technology interventions where the sense of clinicians is that there is overwhelming experiential evidence to justify continued use and to argue against, from an ethical perspective, the performance of randomized trials at this time.

In wound care particularly, we need to more aggressively explore the other types of evidence available to answer our most critical clinical questions. Patient data sets where uniform baseline care has been provided may provide extremely useful information with validity when sample sizes are enough. Prospective cohort series may be useful when cost assessments of apparently equally effective technologies are employed. Cooperative relationships amongst wound care providers are likely needed to collect such data or to provide sufficient patient enrollment numbers to perform appropriate multicenter randomized clinical trials when those are deemed appropriate or essential. Finally, we need to address endpoints other than total wound closure as valid markers of product and technology effectiveness and achieve a better understanding of the impact of co-morbidities on wound healing and the effectiveness of treatment interventions.

This author agrees with others that we have a responsibility to collect data prospectively and support randomized controlled clinical trials of proper design and quality for some existing and all new technologies. However, this author feels that the existing literature, while flawed and incomplete, likely provides us with sufficient information if consistently and systematically applied to produce significant improvements in wound healing outcomes today.

EVIDENCE IN WOUND CARE
Systematic Reviews and Clinical Practice Guidelines

Table 2 describes the hierarchy of preprocessed or analyzed evidence and is useful in identifying the types of evidence–based publications that are available to the clinician. While the clinician frequently goes to the primary literature to answer a specific question, more often than not we look to summaries, synopses, and systems as described in the table. Some recent examples of each type of preprocessed or analyzed evidence are given below.

Primary studies:
- Katz IA, Harlan A, Miranda-Palma B, et al. A radnomized trial of two irremovable off-loading devices in the management of plantar neuropathic diabetic foot ulcers. *Diabetes Care* 2005; 28:555-559
- Armstrong DG, Lavery LA, Wu S, Boulton AJM. Evaluation of removable and irremovable cast walkers in the healing of diabetic foot wounds. *Diabetes Care* 2005; 28:551-554.

Summaries:
- Mason J, O'Keeffet C, McIntosh A, et al. A systematic review of foot ulcer in patients with Type 2 diabetes mellitus. I: prevention. *Diabetic Medicine* 1999; 16:801-812.

- Mason J. O'Keeffet C. Hutchinson A, et al. A systematic review of foot ulcer in patients with Type 2 diabetes mellitus. II: treatment. *Diabetic Medicine* 1999; 16: 889-909.

Synopses:
- Eldor R, Raz I, Ben Yehuda A, Boulton AJM. New and experimental approaches to treatment of diabetic foot ulcers: a comprehensive review of emerging treatment strategies. *Diabetic Medicine* 2004; 21:1161-1173.
- Sharp CA. McLaws M. Estimating the risk of pressure ulcer development: is it truly evidence–based? *Int Wound J* 2006; 3:344-353.

Systems:
- Wraight PR, Lawrence SM, Campbell DA, Colman PG. Creation of a multidisciplinary, evidence–based, clinical guideline for the assessment, investigation, and management of acute diabetes related foot complications. *Diabetic Medicine* 2005; 22:127-136.

TABLE 2. HIERARCHY OF PREPROCESSED EVIDENCE (2)

Primary studies
Preprocessing involves selecting only studies that are both highly relevant and with study designs that minimize bias and thus permit a high strength of inference
Summaries
Systematic reviews providing clinicians with an overview of all the evidence addressing a focused clinical question
Synopses
Synopses of individual studies or of systematic reviews encapsulating the key methodologic details and results required to apply the evidence to individual patient care
Systems
Practice guidelines, clinical pathways, or evidence–based textbook summaries of a clinical area providing the clinician with information needed to guide the care of individual patients

Summaries and synopses are the type of analyses provided by organizations such as the Cochrane Collaboration and the Cochrane Library (accessible on the web at *http://www.cochrane.org*). The Cochrane Collaboration is an international evidence–based review group that includes two panels that consider topics of interest to wound care clinicians, a skin group and a wound group. Cochrane Reviews consider only randomized controlled clinical trials that must meet minimum inclusion standards. There are over 30 different Cochrane Reviews addressing skin and wound care issues. Some of the pertinent Cochrane Reviews are listed in Table 3. Notice that Cochrane Reviews are frequently negative or non committal with respect to the question addressed based on the limitation of the review process to randomized controlled clinical trials only.

TABLE 3. SELECTED RECENT COCHRANE REVIEWS IN SKIN AND WOUND CARE

Subject	Title	Authors' Conclusions
Therapeutic ultrasound for pressure ulcers	Cochrane Database Syst Rev. 2006 Jul 19;3:CD001275	There is no evidence of benefit of ultrasound therapy in the treatment of pressure ulcers. However, the possibility of beneficial or harmful effect cannot be ruled out due to the small number of trials, some with methodological limitations and small numbers of participants. Further research is needed.
Dressings for healing venous leg ulcers	Cochrane Database Syst Rev. 2006 Jul 19;3:CD001103	The type of dressing applied beneath compression has not been shown to affect ulcer healing. For the majority of dressing types there was insufficient data to allow us to draw strong conclusions except for hydrocolloid compared with a low adherent dressing. The result of the meta-analysis indicate no significant difference in healing rates between hydrocolloid dressings and simple, low-adherent dressings when used beneath compression. Decisions regarding which dressing to apply should be based on local costs of dressings and practitioner or patient preferences.
Electromagnetic therapy for treating venous leg ulcers	Cochrane Database Syst Rev. 2006 Apr 19;2:CD002933	There is currently no reliable evidence of benefit of electromagnetic therapy in the healing of venous leg ulcers. Further research is needed.
Electromagnetic therapy for treating pressure ulcers	Cochrane Database Syst Rev. 2006 Apr 19;2:CD002930	The results provide no evidence of benefit in using electromagnetic therapy to treat pressure ulcers. However, the possibility of a beneficial or harmful effect cannot be ruled out, due to the fact there were only two included trials both with methodological limitations and small numbers of participants. Further research is recommended.
Silver based wound dressings and topical agents for treating diabetic foot ulcers	Cochrane Database Syst Rev. 2006 Jan 25;1:CD005082	Despite the widespread use of dressings and topical agents containing silver for the treatment of diabetic foot ulcers, no randomized trials or controlled clinical trials exist that evaluate their clinical effectiveness. Trials are needed to determine clinical and cost-effectiveness and long term outcomes including adverse events.
Wound cleansing for pressure ulcers	Cochrane Database Syst Rev. 2005 Oct 19;4:CD004983	We identified only three studies addressing cleansing of pressure ulcers. One noted a statistically significant improvement in pressure ulcer healing for wounds cleansed with saline spray containing Aloe vera, silver chloride and decyl glucoside when compared with isotonic saline solution. Overall, there is no good trial evidence to support use of any particular wound cleansing solution or technique for pressure ulcers.
Skin grafting for venous leg ulcers	Cochrane Database Syst Rev. 2005 Jan 25;1:CD001737	There is evidence that a bilayer artificial skin, used in conjunction with compression bandaging, increases the chance of healing a venous ulcer compared with compression and a simple dressing. Further research is needed to assess whether other forms of skin grafts increase ulcer healing.
Hyperbaric oxygen therapy for chronic wounds	Cochrane Database Syst Rev. 2004;2:CD004123	In people with foot ulcers due to diabetes, HBO2 significantly reduced the risk of major amputation and may improve the chance of healing at one year. The application of HBO2 to these patients may be justified where HBO2 facilities are available, however, economic evaluations should be undertaken.
Support surfaces for pressure ulcer prevention	Cochrane Database Syst Rev. 2004;3:CD001735	In people at high risk of pressure ulcer development, consideration should be given to the use of higher specification foam mattresses rather than standard hospital foam mattresses. The relative merits of higher-tech constant low pressure and alternating pressure for prevention are unclear. Organizations might consider the use of pressure relief for high risk patients in the operating theater, as this is associated with a reduction in post-operative incidence of pressure ulcers.
Dressing and topical agents for arterial leg ulcers	Cochrane Database Syst Rev. 2003;3:CD001836	There is insufficient evidence to determine whether the choice of topical agent or dressing affects the healing of arterial leg ulcers. Inadequate description of the people in the one included trial means that the results cannot be easily applied to other clinical populations.

TABLE 4. GUIDELINES FOR GRADING EVIDENCE IN CLINICAL GUIDELINES (AMERICAN COLLEGE OF CHEST PHYSICIANS)

Grade of Recommendation/ Description	Methodological Quality of Supporting Evidence	Implications
1A/strong recommendation, high-quality evidence	RCTs without important limitations or overwhelming evidence from observational studies	Strong recommendation, can apply to most patients in most circumstances without reservation
1B/strong recommendation, moderate quality evidence	RCTs with important limitations (inconsistent results, methodological flaws, indirect or imprecise) or exceptionally strong evidence from observational studies	Strong recommendation, can apply to most patients in most circumstances without reservation
1C/strong recommendation, low-quality or very low-quality evidence	Observations studies or case series	Strong recommendation, but may change when higher quality evidence becomes available
2A/weak recommendation, high-quality evidence	RCTs without important limitations or overwhelming evidence from observational studies	Weak recommendation, best action may differ depending on circumstances or patients' or societal values
2B/weak recommendation, moderate-quality evidence	RCTs with important limitations (inconsistent results, methodological flaws, indirect or imprecise) or exceptionally strong evidence from observational studies	Weak recommendation, best action may differ depending on circumstances or patients' or societal values
2C/weak recommendation, low-quality or very low-quality evidence	Observational studies or case series	Very weak recommendations; other alternatives may be equally reasonable

TABLE 5. CLASSIFICATION OF CLASS AND LEVEL OF EVIDENCE IN CLINICAL PRACTICE GUIDELINES

Class I	Conditions for which there is evidence and/or general agreement that the procedure or treatment is useful and effective.
Class II	Conditions for which there is conflicting evidence and/or a divergence of opinion about the usefulness/efficacy of a procedure or treatment.
Class IIa	Weight of evidence/opinion is in favor of usefulness/efficacy.
Class IIb	Usefulness/efficacy is less well established by evidence/opinion.
Class III	Conditions for which there is evidence and/or general agreement that the procedure/treatment is not useful/effective and in some cases may be harmful.
Level of Evidence A: Highest Rank	Data derived from multiple randomized clinical trials that involved large numbers of patients.
Level of Evidence B: Intermediate Rank	Data derived from a limited number of randomized trials that involved small numbers of patients or from careful analyses of nonrandomized studies or observational registries.
Level of Evidence C: Lower Rank	Expert consensus was the primary basis for recommendation.

American College of Cardiology/American Heart Association

Systems as a type of preprocessed evidence brings us to the challenge of identifying quality **clinical practice guidelines**. Clinical practice guidelines typically present a synthesis of available evidence. All guidelines are derived more or less from scientific evidence although the rating of that evidence may vary as well as the quality of evidence sources utilized to develop the guideline. Realizing that "expert opinion" is a form of evidence requires the application of a formal consensus development methods to assure that the final opinions are valid, reproducible, and valid (14). The methods used to achieve consensus should be defined in the final guideline document. Rating quality of evidence in clinical practice guidelines has been thoroughly discussed elsewhere (15, 16). International standards in are development (AGREE Collaboration, on the web at *http://agreecollaboration.org/*). Two such schemes are included in Tables 4 and 5.

The National Guidelines Clearinghouse (NGC) on the web at *http://www.guideline.gov* was created as a public resource for evidence–based clinical practice guidelines as part of the Agency for Healthcare Research and Quality (AHRQ). The collection includes both U.S. and international guidelines. To date over 20 skin and wound care related guidelines are accessible on this website. In addition to individual guidelines, various guideline syntheses, the most recent of which are pressure ulcer prevention and pressure ulcer management. The site also provides access to AHRQ technology assessments. Table 6 lists some of the more recent and relevant guidelines available through the NGC. Table 7 lists additional evidence–based guidelines not currently included on the NGC website at this time. In all cases it is important to know the guideline author, the process by which evidence is graded or classified, and the potential influence of any external sponsoring agent (pharmaceutical or wound care technology provider).

TABLE 6. SOME RELEVANT SKIN AND WOUND CARE CLINICAL PRACTICE GUIDELINES LISTED ON THE NGC WEBSITE

Guideline	Source	Date	Identifier
Diabetic foot disorders a clinical practice guideline	American College of Foot and Ankle Surgeons, 66 pages	2007	pending
Guideline for management of wounds in patients with lower-extremity venous disease	Wound, Ostomy, and Continence Nurses Society, 42 pages	2005	NGC:004431
Summary algorithm for venous ulcer care with annotations of available evidence	Association for the Advancement of Wound Care, 25 pages	2005	NGC:004280
Guideline for management of wounds in patients with lower-extremity neuropathic disease	Wound, Ostomy, and Continence Nurses Society, 57 pages	2004	NGC:003898
Diagnosis and treatment of diabetic foot infections	Infectious Disease Society of America, 26 pages	2004	NGC:003874
Clinical guidelines for type 2 diabetes. Prevention and management of foot problems	National Collaborating Centre for Primary Care (non-US), 103 pages	2004	NGC:003546
SOLUTIONS® wound care algorithm	ConvaTec, 8 pages	2004	NGC:004749
Guideline for prevention and management of pressure ulcers	Wound, Ostomy, and Continence Nurses Society, 52 pages	2003	NGC:003071
Guideline for management of wounds in patients with lower-extremity arterial disease	Wound, Ostomy, and Continence Nurses Society, 44 pages	2002	NGC:002516

TABLE 7. ADDITIONAL EVIDENCE–BASED CLINICAL PRACTICE GUIDELINES OR PROTOCOLS OF IMPORTANCE

Diabetic Foot Ulcer
Steed DL, Attinger C, Colaizzi T, Crossland M, Franz, M, Harkless L, Johnson A, Moosa H, Robson M, Serena T, Sheehan P, Veves A, Wiersma-Bryant L. Wound Rep Reg. 2006; 14(6) 680-692. (professional society, recommendations are provided an evidence score)
Frykberg RG, Zgonis T, Armstrong DG, Driver VR, Giurini JM, Kravitz SR, Landsman AS, Lavery LA, Moore JC, Schuberth JM, Wukich DK, Andersen C, Vanore JV. Diabetic foot disorders: a clinical practice guideline. J Foot Ankle Surg. 2006; 45(5)(Supplement): S1-S66. (professional society, well referenced but recommendations are not provided an evidence score, guideline developed with industry support)
Wraight PR, Lawrence SM, Campbell DA, Colman PG. Creation of a multidisciplinary, evidence–based, clinical guideline for the assessment, investigation and management of acute diabetes related foot complications. Diabet Med. 2005; 22(2):127-136. (recommendations are provided an evidence score)
Brem H, Sheehan, P, Boulton AJM. Protocol for treatment of diabetic foot ulcers. Am J Surgery 2004; 187(Suppl to May): 1S-10S. (review article, recommendations are not provided an evidence score)
Venous Leg Ulcer
Robson MC, Cooper DM, Aslam R, Gould LJ, Harding KG, Margolis DJ, Ochs DE, Serena TE, Snyder RJ, Steed DL, Thomas DR, Wiersma-Bryant L. Guidelines for the treatment of venous ulcers. Wound Rep Reg. 2006; 14(6):649-662. (professional society, recommendations are provided an evidence score)
Brem H, Kirsner RS, Falanga V. Protocol for the successful treatment of venous ulcers. Am J Surgery. 2004; 188(Suppl to July): 1S-8S. (review article, recommendations are not provided an evidence score)
Pressure Ulcer
Whitney, J, Phillips L, Aslam R, Barbul A, Gottrup F, Gould L, Robson MC, Rodeheaver G, Thomas D, Stotts N. Guidelines for the treatment of pressure ulcers. Wound Rep Reg. 2006; 14(6):663-679. (professional society, recommendations are provided an evidence score)
Brem H, Lyder C. Protocol for the successful treatment of pressure ulcers. Am J Surgery. 2004; 188(Suppl to July): 9S-17S. (review article, recommendations are not provided an evidence score)
Arterial Insufficiency Ulcer
Hopf HW, Ueno C, Aslam R, Burnand K, Fife C, Grant L, Holloway A, Iafrati MD, Mani R, Misare B, Rosen N, Shapshak D, Slade JB, West J, Barbul A. Guidelines for the treatment of arterial insufficiency ulcers. Wound Rep Reg. 2006; 14(6): 693-712. (professional society, recommendations are provided an evidence score)

Wound care would benefit from an independent clinical trial review website such as is provided for the use of hyperbaric oxygen treatment by *www.hboevidence.com* that addresses the quality of trial design and the analysis of the data from all clinical trials of hyperbaric oxygen treatment.

PUTTING THE PROCESS TO WORK: AN EXAMPLE

A 57-year old male smoker with no history of diabetes, peripheral vascular disease (claudication), or collagen vascular inflammatory disease presents with a recurrent left lower extremity ulceration. Your initial evaluation leads you to a diagnosis of venous leg ulcer. You know that compression is the logical and appropriate primary intervention for this lower extremity ulcer. Should you use a multi four-layer compression wrap or a short stretch compression bandage to control edema and treat the ulcer?

- *Step 1.* Phrase the clinical question as specifically as possible and with greatest reference to the patient in question. Is short stretch compression superior to multi four-layer compression in the treatment of venous leg ulcers? Are there contraindications to short stretch compression that would limit its application in my patient?

- *Step 2.* Do evidence–based clinical practice guidelines exist that address this question? A trip to the National Guideline Clearinghouse at *www.guideline.gov* reveals three guidelines addressing venous leg ulcer management:

  1. Smith & Nephew Ltd. Grace P, editor. Guidelines for the management of leg ulcers in Ireland. Dublin (Ireland): Smith & Nephew Ltd; 2002. 44p.
  2. Wound, Ostomy, and Continence Nurses Society (WOCN). Guideline for management of wounds in patients with lower-extremity venous disease. Glenview (IL): Wound, Ostomy, and Continence Nurses Society (WOCN); 2005. 42 p. (WOCN clinical practice guideline; no. 4). [86 references]
  3. Association for the Advancement of Wound Care (AAWC). Summary algorithm for venous ulcer care with annotations of available evidence. Malvern (PA): Association for the Advancement of Wound Care (AAWC); 2005. 25 p. [147 references]

The following information on short stretch compression was obtained from the evidence–based clinical practice guidelines. Smith & Nephew… "The first line management of venous leg ulcer patients following assessment with ABPI 0.8 to 1.2 is graduated high compression bandaging, including short stretch bandage regimes…Short stretch bandaging is a suitable treatment for ambulant patients who find multi-layer bandage system a problem at night." (No evidence weighting). WOCN… "Treatment with short stretch compression bandaging may reduce pain . (level of evidence = A)." AAWC… "Short stretch bandage given level of evidence rating A." This information indicates that short stretch compression is effective and may reduce pain but does not clearly define any possible difference in effectiveness.

- *Step 3.* Do a literature search using appropriate MeSH terms and keywords. A search using the terms "short stretch compression" and "multilayer compression" and "venous leg ulcer" identified multiple hits that included one systematic review (Cochrane Database, 2001) and three randomized, prospective, controlled clinical trials. The systematic review was completed prior to the publication of the three randomized trials and was therefore discounted. The largest trial involving 387 adult patients randomized to either four-layer or short-stretch bandages (VenUS I trial Br J Surg 2004;91(10):1292-1299, 1300-06). In this trial healing time was longer in the short-stretch group but not statistically significantly different unless prognostic factors were included in a Cox proportional hazards regression model which demonstrated a lower probability of healing with short stretch compared to the four-layer bandage. An economic analysis revealed significant cost savings in favor of four-layer over the short stretch bandaging. A second study (Wound Rep Reg 2004;12(12):157-162) involving 156 patients demonstrated no statistically different closure rates between the short stretch and four-layer bandaging groups. A third study involving 89 patients (J

Wound Care 2003;12(4):139-143) demonstrated a statistically significant difference in healing in favor of the four-layer over the short-stretch bandaging system. As in the VenUS I trial, costs were also lower in the four-layer bandaging group.

- *Step 4.* Develop a recommendation that is applicable to the patient in question. In this case the preponderance of evidence supports four-layer bandaging for compression over short stretch bandaging in terms of both clinical effectiveness and cost effectiveness. The one caveat noted in the Smith & Nephew guideline is that the short stretch bandage may be more comfortable at night in some patients. As frequently happens, unanticipated information of potential importance emerged in this literature search. Several articles appeared using these search criteria comparing compression with and without vein ablation surgical procedures and supporting the value of surgical treatment in combination with compression in improving venous leg ulcer healing.

EVIDENCE–BASED WOUND CARE: THE FUTURE

Evidence–based medicine is here to stay. That is probably a good thing provided we adhere to its original intent as stated by Sackett and quoted at the beginning of this chapter. In wound care we have a great deal of work to do to establish a sufficiently credible evidence base for much of what we do. That being said, most of our current poor outcomes are probably related to failure to do what we know rather than not knowing what to do. It is also important to remember that there may be interventions where no evidence is currently available. While "it is a short step from without substantial evidence to with substantial value" (18), the absence of evidence of effectiveness is not the same as absence of effectiveness. As wound care clinicians we need to commit ourselves and our resources to strengthening the evidence basis for what we do, especially when new, costly, or potentially harmful technologies are involved.

REFERENCES

1. Sackett DL, Rosenberg WMC, Gray JAM, et al. Evidence–based medicine: what is and what isn't. *BMJ* 1996; 312:71-72.

2. Guyatt GH, Haynes RB, Jaeschke RZ, et al. Users' guides to the medical literature XXV. Evidence–based medicine: Principles for applying the users' guides to patient care. *JAMA* 2000; 284(10):1290-1296.

3. Williams DDR, Garner J. The case against 'the evidence': a different perspective on evidence–based medicine. *Brit J Psychiatry* 2002; 180:8-12.

4. Doig GS, Simpson F. Efficient literature searching: a core skill for the practice of evidence–based medicine. *Intensive Care Med* 2003; 29:2119-2127.

5. Brochard L, Mancebo J, Tobin M. Searching for evidence: don't forget the foundations. *Intensive Care Med* 2003; 29:2109-2111.

6. Ryan S, Perrioer L, Sibbald RG. Searching for evidence–based medicine in wound care: an introduction. *Ostomy/Wound Management* 2003; 49(11):67-75.

7. Steinberg EP, Luce BR. Evidence–based? Caveat Emptor! *Health Affairs* 2005; 24(1):80-92.

8. Gottrup F. Guest Editorial: Evidence is a challenge in wound management. *Lower Extremity Wounds* 2006; 5(2):74-75.

9. FDA Wound Healing Clinical Focus Group. Guidance for industry: Chronic cutaneous ulcer and burn wounds—developing products for treatment (Draft—Not for Implementation). *Wound Rep Regen* 2001; 9(4): 258-268.

10. Steed DL, Donohoe D, Webster MW, et al. Effect of extensive debridement and treatment on the healing of diabetic foot ulcers. *J Am Cool Surg* 1996; 183:61-64.

11. Boulton AJM, Armstrong DG. Editorial: Trials in neuropathic diabetic foot ulceration. Time for a paradigm shift? *Diabetes Care* 2003; 26(9):2689-2690.

12. Bouza C, Munoz, A, Amata JM. Efficacy of modern dressings in the treatment of leg ulcers: a systemait creview. *Wound Rep Reg* 2005; 13:218-229.

13. Tunis SR. Perspective: A clinical research strategy to support shared decision making. *Health Affairs* 2005; 24(1):180-184.

14. Heffner JE. Does evidence–based medicine help the development of clinical practice guidelines? *Chest* 1998; 113:172S-178S.

15. Guyatt GH, Gutterman D, Baumann MH, et al. Grading strength of recommendations and quality of evidence in clinical guidelines. Report from American College of Chest Physicians Task Force. *Chest* 2006; 129:174-181.

16. Hadorn DC, Baker D, Hodges JS, et al. Rating the quality of evidence for clinical practice guidelines. *J Clin Epidemiol* 1996; 49(7):749-754.

17. AHA. Manual for ACC/AHA Guideline Writing Committees, Section II: Tools and Methods for Creating Guidelines, Step Six: Assign Classification of Recommendations and Level of Evidence. from Methodologies and Policies from the ACC/AHA Task Force on Practice Guidelines on the web at *http://circ.ahajournals.org/manual/manual_IIstep6.shtml*

18. Bradley F, Field J. Letter: Evidence–based medicine. *Lancet* 1995; 346:838-839.

REVIEW QUESTIONS

1.) Evidence–based medicine is the conscientious, explicit, and judicious use of current best evidence in making decisions about the care of:
   a. Individual patients
   b. Selected categories of patients
   c. Selected classes of wounds
   d. None of the above

2.) The hierarchy of strength of evidence for treatment decisions includes which of the following?
   a. Systematic reviews of randomized clinical trials
   b. Single randomized clinical trial
   c. Physiologic studies
   d. All of the above
   e. A and b, but not c

3.) In an N of 1 randomized clinical trial, a patient or patients undertake pairs of treatment periods in which they receive a target treatment in 1 period of each pair and a placebo or alternative treatment in the other with both patients and clinicians blinded to the allocation of the study intervention and placebo control.
   a. True
   b. False

4.) Which of the following about the strength of evidence hierarchy is FALSE?
   a. The highest level of evidence is meta-analysis, or systematic review of multiple randomized clinical trials.
   b. The meta-analysis does not take into account unpublished, possibly non-significant results.
   c. If treatment effects are sufficiently large and consistently demonstrated, observational or cohort studies may provide acceptable evidence.
   d. The hierarchy must be considered to be absolute.

5.) Physicians who practice evidence–based medicine have consistently better outcomes than those who do not.
   a. True
   b. False

Answers: 1a, 2d, 3a, 4d, 5b.

NOTES

Section 3
Principles of Wound Management

CHAPTER **7**

GENERAL PRINCIPLES OF WOUND CARE

CHAPTER SEVEN OVERVIEW

NOTES

GENERAL PRINCIPLES OF WOUND CARE

Liza Ovington

INTRODUCTION

Management of nonhealing wounds has progressed significantly in the past decade. The tools and technologies in the wound care clinician's armamentarium have burgeoned with advances in diagnostics, disease management, topical devices and drugs, and bioengineering. While these tools have provided important incremental advances in healing rates and outcomes for chronic wounds, the basic underlying principles of wound management must not be overshadowed by technology. We will review these basic principles of wound management in this chapter. These principles include diagnosis, topical management of microorganisms, optimization of systemic and local factors affecting wound healing, and accurate measurement of wound status.

IMPORTANCE OF PROPER DIAGNOSIS OF NONHEALING WOUNDS

Chronic wounds are commonly described as falling into the major categories of leg ulcers due to venous or arterial insufficiency, diabetic foot ulcers, and pressure ulcers. However, there are many potential causes of chronic ulcers and it is likely that any one ulcer has multiple contributing factors, all of which must be addressed in order for sustained wound closure to occur. Successful management of chronic wounds depends not so much on topical products as on the ability of the clinician to identify the underlying causes of the ulcer and address them. This identification process should incorporate a detailed physical examination and history focusing on precipitating factors along with close attention to clinical clues from the appearance of the ulcer and the surrounding skin. Laboratory tests from blood samples or tissue biopsy may also be required for a complete diagnosis (1).

Many nonhealing wounds may masquerade as a common etiology such as a venous ulcer and if treated as such without recognition of the true cause, may not heal. For example, a lower extremity ulcer may be caused by an autoimmune disorder such as pyoderma gangrenosum and may occur in a patient who also suffers from venous hypertension. If the ulcer is treated only as if it were due to venous hypertension (a contributing factor) and not recognized as pyoderma gangrenosum (the root cause), it may not heal and may even be treated inappropriately and become worse. It has been suggested that all nonhealing wounds of certain duration should be biopsied for cancer.

Once an accurate diagnosis has been made, treatment of the chronic wound should focus on disease management principles. Disease management is an approach to healthcare based on the premise that complex, chronic disorders are characterized by specific symptoms, co-morbidities and complications that are often preventable and manageable. Effective chronic disease management stresses risk identification, interventions for prevention and treatment, and patient education.

Chronic wound care is an especially appropriate area for a disease management approach. Often, the clinician and patient focus on the major symptom—the wound—without paying enough attention to the underlying causes (i.e., pressure, venous insufficiency, uncontrolled diabetes) and contributing factors (nutrition, local wound environment, etc.).

Of particular importance in disease management is the aspect of patient education. Patients should be provided one-on-one education and written materials regarding their specific disease process. It should include what they can do to manage their disease and prevent complications as well as information about their treatment, signs and symptoms of infection and when to call the physician office. Patients and family members who feel knowledgeable about their care are likely to be more compliant with treatment recommendations, leading to improved healing outcomes.

For more on wound etiology see the chapter by APS Smith entitled "Etiology of a Problem Wound."

IMPORTANCE OF LOCAL BIOBURDEN MANAGEMENT/INFECTION CONTROL

Local infection impairs the healing process of any wound in a variety of ways. The bacteria causing the infection will be in competition with the local cells of the wound for oxygen and nutrients. The local host cells, such as the fibroblasts, macrophages, and endothelial cells will then not be able to efficiently carry out their role in the tissue repair process. Also, high levels of superficial bacteria will stimulate the prolonged release of inflammatory mediators such as cytokines and proteolytic enzymes by host cells, which actively work to degrade the bacteria, but also degrade local cells and granulation tissue protein components. The bacteria themselves also release toxins into the wound tissue that can degrade it and further stimulate or prolong the inflammatory process.

Wound etiology is an important factor in terms of a particular wound's susceptibility to infection. In large part, the most common types of chronic wounds—pressure ulcers, venous leg ulcers, arterial ulcers, diabetic foot ulcers—are caused by impairment of blood flow to the affected area. Acute wounds—surgical incision sites, burn wounds, and skin graft donor sites— usually possess adequate circulation. This feature of blood supply alone plays perhaps the single largest role in a wound's susceptibility to infection by pathogenic organisms. With an adequate blood supply, the wound can be accessed by endogenous phagocytic cells that fight the infective process and receive adequate oxygen for these cells to function.

For complete discussion of biofilm see the chapter by R Wolcott entitled "Biofilm-Based Wound Care."

WOUND DEBRIDEMENT

Perhaps the most effective action that can be undertaken to control local bioburden and to prevent wound infection is to keep the wound free of devitalized, necrotic tissue that serves as the nutritional source for bacterial proliferation. Any devitalized tissue will present a physical impediment to granulation and epithelialization. New tissue will not be able to "burrow" under eschar to fill a wound. The necrotic material also provides an ideal medium for bacterial growth. To optimize the wound environment and promote healing, some form of debridement must remove it. A variety of wound debridement techniques—surgical or sharp, mechanical, chemical or enzymatic, and autolytic—are available depending on the nature and extent of the devitalized tissue. If necrotic tissue is adequately removed through appropriate debridement methods there will be less of an opportunity for bacteria to colonize the wound and progress to infection.

Surgical or Sharp Debridement

The most efficient and aggressive method of debridement is sharp or surgical debridement, in which the necrotic tissue is removed with sterile instruments such as scalpels, scissors, and forceps. This method requires a practitioner who has had specific education and training in tissue anatomy and assessment as well as in the instrumental procedures. While very efficient, this aggressive procedure is not always possible because a qualified practitioner may not be available or because of specific patient conditions (dry gangrene, ischemic wound, unknown vascular status, etc.).

Mechanical Debridement

Mechanical debridement involves the use of an external force to remove devitalized tissue. Wet-to-dry dressings are a traditional method of mechanical debridement. To debride by this method, dressings need to be allowed to dry so that necrotic material adheres to the dressings and is removed as the dressings are removed. Wet-to-dry dressings are nonselective, and are very difficult to remove without tearing out new, healthy tissue. This procedure is different from packing a wound with saline-moistened gauze to provide a moist wound environment. In this case, the gauze should not be allowed to dry, and a wet-to-moist or wet-to-damp dressing technique is used. Another form of mechanical debridement that is gaining popularity is the use of pulsed lavage devices that deliver saline to the wound surface at high pressures followed by suction (2). This method will dislodge not only foreign materials but also devitalized tissue.

Chemical or Enzymatic Debridement

The most common chemical agents for debridement are proteolytic enzymes. Enzymes are indicated for debridement of necrotic tissue and for liquefaction of slough in acute and chronic wounds. Manufacturer's directions must be carefully followed to avoid deactivation of the debriding agent with inappropriate wound cleansers. Care should be taken not to expose the periwound skin to the enzyme agent because some of them may irritate intact tissues. If enzyme debriding agents are used on eschar, it is recommended to crosshatch the eschar with a scalpel before application. As with any debriding method, these agents should be used only for a limited period. When the wound is clear of debris, a reassessment must be done and another wound management plan should be implemented.

Autolytic Debridement

With this debridement method, the body uses its own endogenous enzymes and phagocytic cells to break down necrotic debris under a moisture-retentive dressing. Transparent film, hydrocolloid, or hydrogel dressings are sometimes used to initiate this process. These dressings provide and maintain a moist environment, which keeps phagocytic cells viable and also allows the enzymes in the wound fluid to liquefy necrotic tissue. This is the most selective, although sometimes the slowest way to debride. Autolytic debridement is not recommended for infected wounds, since occlusion could increase the already high bacterial counts in the wound bed.

Debridement techniques are described in depth by TA Emhoff and SA Ferro in their chapter entitled "Wound Debridement."

TOPICAL ANTIMICROBIALS FOR LOCAL BIOBURDEN CONTROL

Some clinicians advocate using only systemic antibiotics to treat wound infections, however it has been pointed out that many chronic wounds have impaired blood flow which can compromise the delivery of the systemic antibiotic to the wound. Antibiotics must get to the site of the wound infection in appropriate concentrations. This means that the therapeutic plan must consider management of collateral issues, such as whether the patient has edema at the wound site or decreased perfusion. Systemic antibiotics alone are believed by many to be inadequate for treatment of local wound infection, and topical treatment of the wound tissues is a helpful adjunct.

Topical antibiotics are commonly used to manage local wound infections either alone or in combination with systemic treatment. While the topical formulation may indeed have a better chance of reaching the involved wound tissues than systemic antibiotics—there is concern that long-term usage may promote colonization of the wound by resistant bacteria. If topical antibiotics are used it is suggested that they be used only for a limited period of time—two weeks has been suggested (3).

Topical antiseptics are simple chemicals such as iodine, acetic acid, and sodium hypochlorite (Dakin's solution) that destroy bacteria by lysing their cell walls. Unlike antibiotics, which are specific to particular types of bacteria, chemical antiseptics usually have a broad range of antimicrobial activity against both Gram positive and Gram negative species as well as many fungi and viruses. Antiseptics could therefore be valuable tools in controlling bacterial levels in non-healing chronic wounds, which often have polymicrobial colonization.

Antiseptics have often been the subject of derision in wound care based on claims that they may also be toxic to other types of cells in addition to bacteria. Many antiseptics have shown toxicity not only to bacteria but also to human cells such as fibroblasts and white blood cells. Most of these reports of toxicity are from in vitro studies which may not accurately represent the situation of using the antiseptic in an open wound. Much of the data to support allegations of cytotoxicity of antiseptics has come from in vitro studies where isolated cells were immersed in antiseptics for 15 or 30 minutes (4,5,6).

It may be true that the use of antiseptic agents in contaminated wounds may harm some of the superficial wound cells as well as bacteria, and potentially slow the healing process. However, in the case of wound colonization, the limited use of antiseptics may have a net benefit in bringing the wound back into bacterial balance to enable healing to progress. Another benefit of antiseptics is that they have not been known to promote clinically relevant bacterial resistance despite centuries of use.

An in vivo study evaluated the effects of five different antiseptic solutions on the healing of partial thickness wounds in a pig model (7,8,9). Various parameters of wound healing were analyzed. It was interesting that for the parameter of wound re-epithelialization—the point at which we judge wounds to be clinically healed—none of the antiseptic agents had any detrimental effect as compared to control (saline).

When a wound is infected or critically colonized, it means there is an overabundance of bacteria relative to the host immune system and the wound is stuck in an inflammatory or tissue destructive phase—there is little or no tissue building activity going on from the tissue cells anyway. At this point, the bacteria and their secreted chemicals may be more toxic to the wound cells than the topical antiseptic.

For more information about topical antimicrobials for bioburden control see the chapter by R Wolcott entitled "Biofilm-Based Wound Care." For discussion of infection control in skin and muscle infections see the chapter by JL LeFrock and JT Mader entitled "Skin, Skin Structure, and Muscle Infections." For discussion of infection control in post operative wound infections see the chapter by JL LeFrock entitled "Post-operative Surgical Site Infections and Non-necrotizing Skin and Soft Tissue Infections."

IMPORTANCE OF SYSTEMIC OPTIMIZATION

For better chance of a successful healing outcome, it is important that the patient be in the best possible systemic condition to mount and support the healing process. A critical systemic parameter for successful healing is nutritional status. There is also a growing body of evidence that pain and patient emotional status have significant effects on healing (7,8,9).

Nutrition

Adequate nutrition plays a critical role in generating new tissue for healing. When a wound is sustained, a patient's metabolism and nutritional needs increase significantly. The average energy expenditure for a non-wounded adult is 20–25 calories per kg of weight. Average energy expenditure for an adult with a wound is 35–40 calories per kg of weight (10).

Synthesis of new tissue requires proteins, carbohydrates, fats, vitamins, minerals, trace elements and water. Even after the wound is healed, adequate nutrition is important to maintain tissue integrity and prevent recurrence of the wound. The healing of a wound requires the de novo synthesis of connective tissue and epithelial tissue. Proteins such as collagen, elastin and keratin must be assembled from amino acids by cells such as the fibroblast. The cells themselves must replicate and move throughout the wound bed. Macrophages scour the wound for foreign materials and necrotic tissues, fibroblasts build scaffolds of collagen and fibrin, and epithelial cells replicate and migrate to close the wound. Even after wound closure, various enzymes are active in remodeling the collagen fibers to achieve greater tensile strength. There are tremendous metabolic energy demands for all this cellular migration and activity.

There are multiple options for nutritional assessment of the wound patient. There are physical methods such as skin fold analysis at different anatomical sites which are traditional anthropometric methods but which suffer from not incorporating gender differences, bone mass or body build as well as not being highly reproducible. Height-weight ratios such as the body mass index are preferred because they address some of these issues and correlate well to body fat. There are also chemical or laboratory methods of nutritional analysis, primarily reflecting protein levels. These lab values are usually objective and easily obtained but they may be influenced by medical conditions such as stress or infection.

Proteins

Protein is critical for the synthesis of new connective tissue components, including collagen. Proteins and their constituent amino acids are also vital to the synthesis of antibodies and enzymes. Daily protein requirements for a healthy, non-wounded adult average about 0.8 grams of protein per kilogram of body weight. Having a partial thickness wound almost doubles the protein requirement. Deeper or multiple wounds will drive the requirement up even further. Protein deficiency during wound healing can manifest as reduced elasticity of the scar and as a weakened immune defense. A common indicator of protein levels is the serum albumin level. Normal serum albumin levels fall between 3.5–5.0 g/dl. Serum albumin levels below 3.5 g/dl are considered inadequate for wound healing. However since the half life of albumin is on the order of three weeks, serum albumin levels may appear adequate for some time even though an inadequacy exists. A more sensitive indicator of protein levels is the serum pre-albumin level. Pre-albumin has a half-life of about three days.

Carbohydrates and Fats

Carbohydrates supply energy (via ATP production) for all of the cellular chemical reactions that are taking place during the wound healing process. Without adequate carbohydrates, the body will break down proteins for energy and contribute to protein deficiency. Fats are a well-known source of stored energy that is accessed only after carbohydrates and proteins are depleted.

Fat metabolism generates prostaglandins and other substances involved in the inflammatory response. Fats are also important to the synthesis of the lipid layers of cell membranes.

Vitamins and Trace Elements

Various vitamins have critical roles as co-enzymes in wound healing processes. Vitamin C is involved in the synthesis of collagen and vascular membranes. The B vitamins are also involved in collagen synthesis and antibody production. Vitamin A is important in the cross-linking of collagen fibers, in the process of epithelialization, and in inflammatory processes. Vitamin K is crucial to the coagulation cascade and vitamin E is an antioxidant, which ultimately protects cell walls from oxidative damage. Zinc is a cofactor in more than 100 enzyme reactions. It is a vital constituent for protein synthesis and cell proliferation as it plays an essential role in the structure of enzymes involved in the synthesis of nucleic acids of DNA and RNA. Zinc is also thought to have a role in cellular movement. Iron is necessary for oxygen transport in the body. Both iron and copper are involved in collagen cross-linking and the production of erythrocytes. Vitamin supplements of up to 20 times the RDA may be appropriate for a wound patient (11). Dosing should be examined in relation to the specific vitamin.

For complete discussion of nutrition see chapter by A Dennis Wauters entitled "Nutrition and Hydration."

ISSUES OF WOUND PAIN

Pain management for patients with chronic wounds is gaining more and more attention among health care professionals. Patients who are in constant pain are less likely to be compliant and may become depressed, anxious or stressed. There is a growing body of literature suggesting that stress and depression may influence endogenous corticosteroid levels and have a potential impact on healing. Patients should be questioned about their pain levels during the history and throughout treatment.

Importance of Local Optimization of Wound Microenvironment

Not all systemic factors that impair healing are amenable to change or optimization. However local factors are now more easily addressed with the wide variety of currently existing topical wound care products and technologies. For example, tissue hydration status is affected by selecting an appropriate wound dressing. It has long been recognized that tissues heal optimally in an environment that preserves their inherent moisture levels for which a wide variety of wound dressings are available that create, maintain, or restore such an environment. While gauze has been a traditional wound dressing for many years, it does not effectively maintain hydration (even when moistened with saline) and may allow healing tissues to dry out, adhere to the gauze fibers and be traumatically removed upon changing the gauze dressing. Newer wound dressings are composed of polymeric materials such as plastic films and foams, gels and gelling fibers, and colloidal materials, which balance moisture tissue levels and facilitate the healing progress. These moisture retentive dressings also stabilize wound temperature by preventing evaporative moisture loss from the tissues, which occurs with a subsequent temperature drop. Wounds treated with such dressings have repeatedly been shown to reach epithelialization in one-half the time of wounds treated with saline and gauze.

A more recent area of therapeutic intervention for wounds with impaired healing is that of local biochemical optimization. Research studies have shown consistent differences in the array and levels of chemicals found locally in the tissues and fluids of normally healing wounds as compared to those found in wounds with slow healing or no healing. Specifically, the levels of growth factors, cytokines, and proteolytic enzymes are found to be different in healing versus nonhealing wounds of many etiologies. Some of the biochemicals may be managed locally with newer interactive topical dressings. In severely hypoxic wounds, the hypoxia must be corrected within the wound microenvironment before certain products can be effective.

For in depth discussion of wound dressings see the chapter by V Larson Lohr and CA Fleck entitled "Modern Wound Dressings - Principles, Form and Function." For information about the goals of advanced therapeutics see the chapter by APS Smith and TA Bozzuto entitled "Advanced Therapeutics: The Biochemical and Biophysical Basis of Wound Care Products."

Importance of Wound Assessment

Accurate and ongoing wound assessment is an important task in wound management. There are many reasons to do it and to do it thoroughly and consistently. By assessing the wound on a regular basis, the clinician will be able to gauge the progress or lack of healing as well as the success or failure of a particular therapy or product. Wound assessment may also guide the clinician to a particular topical treatment based on the local wound conditions.

A lack of healing progress may indicate a need to change the therapy or product being used. Depending on the specific healthcare system, assessment and documentation of the wound's progress may be used to justify continued use of a product and, alternatively, a lack of progress with conventional therapy may be used to justify a new approach.

Importantly, because wound management is a multidisciplinary effort, accurate wound assessment and documentation of that assessment is of great benefit in fostering communication between the various healthcare professionals that may be involved in the patient's care. Documentation of wound progress or deterioration provides a written history of the wound and its responses to treatment.

Wound assessment techniques are presented in depth by RA Warriner in two chapters entitled: "Wound Assessment," and "Evidence-Based Wound Care." The tools used for vascular assessment are discussed by CJ Buckley and SD Lee in their chapter, "Non-Invasive and Invasive Evaluations for Lower Extremity Arterial Occlusive Disease." The noninvasive tools used in wound assessment are discussed by D Dietz and PJ Sheffield in their chapter, "Non-Invasive Wound Assessment Tools."

MEASURING WOUNDS

Carrying out a wound assessment will involve making both qualitative and quantitative measurements. Common qualitative measures include descriptions of tissue type and color, descriptions of exudate color and consistency, and descriptions of any odors.

Specific quantitative assessments include linear measures of the wound dimensions (using centimeter units) and relative amounts of different tissue types visible in the wound (i.e., 50% granulation and 50% slough tissue).

The dimensions of length and width of the wound are the most common measurements carried out to monitor wound-healing progress. Measuring length and width of a wound to calculate its area sounds simple except that very few chronic wounds are perfect rectangles (skin graft donor sites are the closest). Most wounds are irregular in shape and it may be confusing to determine what to call the length and what the width. The general convention in measuring wounds is to locate the longest axis or diameter of the wound and assign this axis as the length—some references suggest measuring the longest axis in the head- to-toe direction; however this can be confusing depending on the location of the wound and may also lead to inconsistencies. This method may also lead to "widths" that are larger than the "lengths" which is not standard. Therefore, selecting the longest axis as the length of the wound, regardless of its orientation is the current standard. Once the length has been identified, the width is determined by then locating the longest wound axis, which is perpendicular to the length.

Discussion of wound measurement techniques and the documentation thereof is at the chapter by EP Rios and V Larson Lohr entitled, "Documentation: Telling the Story of Care."

CONCLUSION

More and more new products and therapies are appearing in the wound care marketplace and many offer intriguing approaches to the management of chronic wounds. It is important however, not to be distracted from the foundations of good wound care by the novelty of a new item. The wound healing process is a complex cascade of overlapping biological events characterized by a variety of cell types and chemicals and impacted by a variety of systemic and local conditions. Optimization of these local and systemic factors that affect the overall healing process is the key to achieving healing. In other words, there are some basic principles of good wound care that should be addressed long before deciding on a topical or adjunctive treatment for the wound.

It is advised to adopt a stepwise approach to wound management that begins with the basic principles and advances to topical treatment options in order of their complexity. Many of the newer therapies such as growth factors and bioengineered tissue have a high purchase cost although they prove quite cost effective in use. However, if the conditions for healing are not optimized through attention to basic wound care principles, these newer therapies are not likely to perform well and may even fail.

REFERENCES

1. Seaman S. Considerations for the global assessment and treatment of patients with recalcitrant wounds. *Ostomy Wound Manage* 2000 Jan; 46(1A Suppl):10S-29S; quiz 30S-31S.

2. Morgan D, Hoelscher J. Pulsed lavage: promoting comfort and healing in home care. *Ostomy Wound Manage* 2000 Apr; 46(4):44-9.

3. Agency for Health Care Policy and Research (AHCPR). Treatment of pressure ulcers. Rockville (MD): U.S. Department of Health and Human Services, Public Health Service, AHCPR; 1994 Dec. 154 p. (Clinical practice guideline; no. 15).

4. Hellewell TB, Major DA, Foresman PA, et al. A cytotoxicity evaluation of antimicrobial and non-antimicrobial wound cleansers. *Wounds* 1997; 9(1):15-20.

5. Foresman PA, Payne DS, Becker D, et al. A relative toxicity index for wound cleansers. *Wounds* 1993; 5:226-231.

6. Doughty D. A rational approach to the use of topical antiseptics. *JWOCN* 1994; 21(6):223-231

7. Kiecolt-Glaser JK, Marucha PT, Malarkey WB, et al. Slowing of wound healing by psychological stress. *Lancet* 1995 Nov 4; 346(8984):1194-6.

8. Marucha PT, Kiecolt-Glaser JK, Favagehi M. Mucosal wound healing is impaired by examination stress. *Psychosom Med* 1998 May-Jun; 60(3):362-5.

9. Cole-King A, Harding KG. Psychological factors and delayed healing in chronic wounds. *Psychosomatic Medicine* 63:216-220 2001.

10. Pinchcofsky DG. Nutritional assessment and intervention, in Chronic Wound Care: (2nd Edition), Krasner and Kane, Health Management Publications, Wayne PA, 73-83; 1997.

11. Mazzotta MY. Nutrition and wound healing. *J of the American Podiatric Med Assoc*, September 1994; 84(9):456-462.

REVIEW QUESTIONS

1.) Effective chronic disease management stresses:
   a. Risk identification
   b. Interventions for prevention
   c. Interventions for treatment
   d. Patient education
   e. All of the above

2.) Chronic wounds caused by impairment of blood flow to the affected area commonly include all of the following types EXCEPT:
   a. Pressure ulcers
   b. Venous leg ulcers
   c. Arterial ulcers
   d. Diabetic foot ulcers
   e. Burn wounds

3.) Acute wounds usually possess adequate circulation and include all of the following EXCEPT:
   a. Surgical incision sites
   b. Skin graft donor sites
   c. Burn wounds
   d. Radiation injury

4.) The most effective action that can be undertaken to control local bioburden and to prevent wound infection is:
   a. Debridement
   b. Topical antibiotics
   c. Systemic antibiotics
   d. Sufficient diet
   e. Pain control

5.) When the daily protein requirement for a healthy, non-wounded adult averages about 0.8 grams of protein per kilogram of body weight, the protein requirement for a patient having a partial thickness wound is about
   a. Halved
   b. The same
   c. Doubled
   d. Tripled
   e. Quadrupled

Answers: 1e, 2e, 3d, 4a, 5c

NOTES

ISCHEMIA AND HYPOXIA: THE THERAPEUTIC OPTIONS

CHAPTER EIGHT OVERVIEW

NOTES

Ischemia and Hypoxia: The Therapeutic Options

Gregory R.Weir, Frans J. Cronje

"For the life of the flesh is in the blood." (Leviticus 17:11)

Adequate delivery of blood and oxygen is essential to sustain life. This truth was already recognized in 1727 BC in the Code of Hammurabi of Mesopotamia that contains a phrase: "to pour out his life-blood like water." In the Enuma Elish, blood was considered the essential ingredient in the creation of mankind. Ugaritic and Egyptian sources also recognised the importance of blood as a life source (1). Indeed, not only life, but also wound healing, depends on it.

The transport and delivery of oxygen to tissue is a function of blood flow. Under normal physiological conditions blood flow and blood oxygen content are matched to ensure normal function of body tissues. In the event of injury, increased oxygen demands may be met by an increase in the extraction of oxygen from hemoglobin as well as by increases in perfusion. These mechanisms offer limited physiological reserve, however. Importantly, both mechanisms depend on a patent conduit whereby the oxygen can be transported from the alveoli to the affected tissue.

Ischemia (*isch*-restriction; *-hema*-blood) is a restriction in blood supply, generally due to factors related to blood vessels such as stenoses or occlusions, leading to damage or dysfunction of tissue (2).

Hypoxia (*hyp*-low; *-oxia*-oxygen) is a condition in which tissues are deprived of oxygen, irrespective of the cause. This distinguishes it from hypoxemia, which is a reduction in blood oxygen content specifically (2). Whether due to ischemia or hypoxemia, hypoxia is a final common pathway in many causes of wound healing failure.

Unfortunately, methods for reversing hypoxia in chronic wounds are often complex and costly. Essentially there are two strategies: (a) improving circulation and (b) improving oxygenation. The reason why many of these interventions work is that intact skin requires very low quantities of oxygen to survive, but 30 to 40 mm Hg pO_2 at tissue level to heal. So, if oxygen delivery can be maintained to the point of healing, a subsequent return to a lower baseline may not be detrimental. Importantly, this also emphasizes the importance of preventing primary wounding of ischemic tissues.

The aim of this chapter is to list and describe the various therapeutic options for treating ischemia and/or hypoxia that are available to clinicians.

It emphasises the important elements that may favour the use of one modality above another as well as indicating where a combination may be helpful.

PERFUSION STRATEGIES

Perfusion strategies are aimed at reversing ischemia. They usually fall within the clinical disciplines of vascular surgery, intervention radiology and cardiology. Optimal medical perfusion strategies are advocated for all patients with arterial disease[†] (3, 4). These may even be adequate for mild arterial disease. They include smoking cessation (5); lipid, hypertension and diabetes control; and anti-platelet therapy. Even if surgery is indicated, anti-platelet therapy should be started preoperatively and be continued as adjuvant pharmacotherapy after the endovascular or surgical procedure. Co-existing morbidities such as coronary—and renal artery stenosis or cerebrovascular disease should also be addressed when indicated (3,4).

If a patient has evidence of critical limb ischemia[♣] (4), the use of endovascular or surgical perfusion strategies is justified in an attempt to save the extremity. The choice of endovascular vs. open surgical alternatives is not always easy. However, the Inter-Society Consensus for the Management of Peripheral Arterial Disease (TASC II) offers some guidance by stratifying vascular lesions in the following way: So-called "A" lesions represent those where endovascular interventions offer good resolution; "B" lesions offer adequate results using endovascular methods, so that this approach is the preferred option, unless open revascularization is indicated for other associated lesions in the same anatomical area; "C" lesions have superior long-term outcomes using open revascularization, so that endovascular methods are used only in the case of patients with a high operative risk; and "D" lesions where endovascular methods do not yield adequate results, thus excluding them as a primary treatment.

Endovascular Perfusion Strategies
Angioplasty

This is arguably the least invasive intervention to restore circulation. A percutaneous Seldinger technique is used to insert a cannula into a large artery, either proximal or distal to the lesion, under local anaesthetic. Usually the common femoral artery is the point of access or, in selected cases, the brachial artery. A guide wire is placed through the cannula into the artery under fluoroscopic guidance. An arterial sheath is then placed over the guide wire to protect the punctured artery. Intra-arterial contrast is administered to identify lesions within the arterial lumen. These lesions can then be crossed using the guide wire (Figure 1). An angioplasty balloon is inserted over the guide wire, whereupon the diseased section of the artery is dilated by inflation of the balloon. In selected cases, a stent can be placed into the artery to

---

† Recent trials do not support the value of prostanoids in promoting amputation free survival. There is also no other pharmacotherapy that can be recommended for the treatment of critical limb ischemia. Gene therapy has shown promising early efficacy but further trials are warranted (4).

♣ The Inter-Society Consensus for the Management of Peripheral Arterial Disease (TASC 11), recommends that the term critical limb ischemia be used for all patients with a.) chronic ischemic rest pain; and/or b.) ulcers or gangrene, attributable to objectively proven arterial occlusive disease. The term implies chronicity and is to be distinguished from acute limb ischemia.

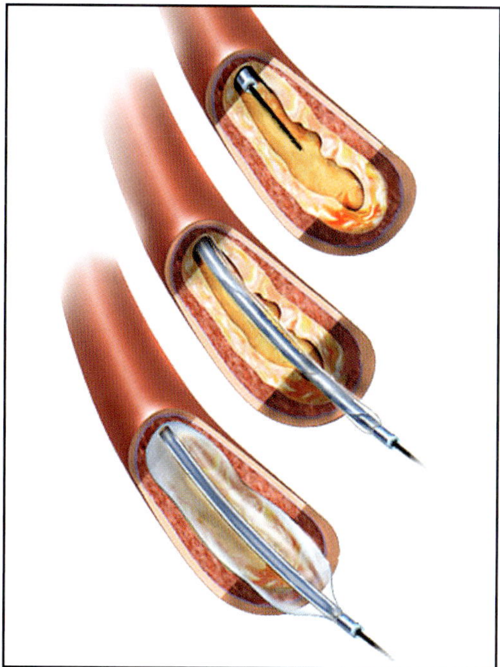

Figure 1. Percutaneous transluminal angioplasty.

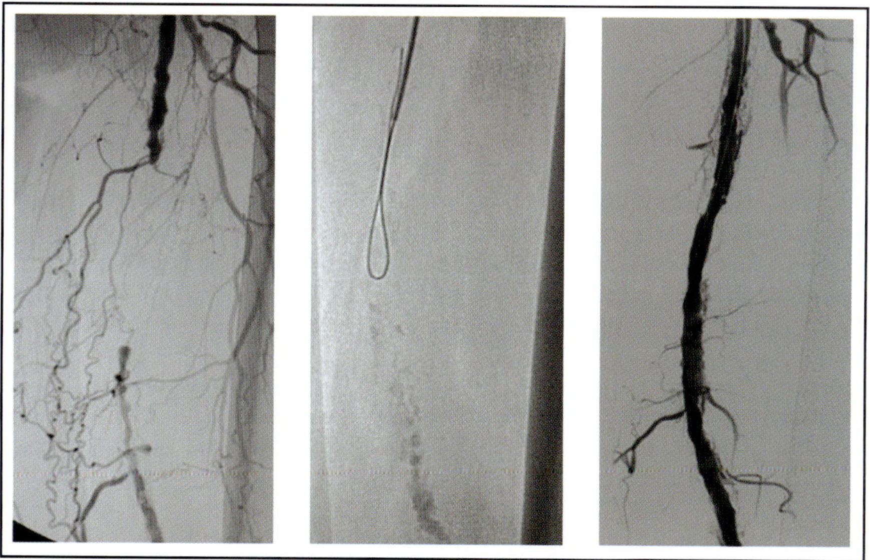

Figure 2. Percutaneous sub-intimal angioplasty.

maintain the lumen. The success of the procedure is dependent on the length of the stenosis or occlusion, the quality of inflow proximally and the quality of run-off distally.

Even very long occluded segments can be crossed with a sub-intimal angioplasty technique that tunnels between the tunica intima and tunica media of the artery rather than through the stenosis (Figure 2).

Potential complications associated with endovascular procedures include hemorrhage, thrombosis, re-stenosis and occlusion. Although the patency rates for some of these procedures may only be measured in months, they may allow wounds to heal during that time. It also affords the patient the opportunity to form a more extensive network of collateral vessels. Risk factor modification and optimal medical therapy contribute significantly towards a favourable outcome.

Recommendation 35 of the Inter-Society Consensus for the Management of Peripheral Arterial Disease (TASC II) states that, in situations where the outcome of endovascular revascularization vs. open repair/bypass are considered equivocal (in terms of short-term and long-term symptomatic improvement), endovascular techniques should be used first (4).

Catheter Directed Thrombolytic Therapy

Thrombolysis has become increasingly common in emergency, medical and surgical practice. It is the standard of care for most myocardial infarctions and it is used extensively in hyperacute thrombotic stroke. Within the context of acute thrombotic events involving limb arteries, catheter directed thrombolysis is used to dissolve thrombus, exposing the underlying stenosis. The stenosis can then be addressed by means of an angioplasty or bypass surgery, if required.

Surgical Perfusion Strategies

Endarterectomy

This is an open surgical procedure, requiring limited access, during which the endothelial lining and subjacent atheromatous lesions are removed from the vessel. It is performed quite frequently for carotid artery stenosis. For ischemia of the lower extremity, femoral artery endarterectomies can be performed in patients with isolated occlusions of that artery. The limited access makes this procedure appropriate for higher surgical risk patients. It can even be performed under local anaesthesia.

Arterial bypass

Extensive vascular pathology sometimes requires the use of vascular bypass procedures. The objective is to create a natural (i.e., autogenous) or artificial (i.e., prosthetic) conduit able to bypass the obstruction. The proximal anastomosis is made in a relatively disease-free segment of the artery. The distal anastomosis is done beyond the most distal occlusion. The success of bypass procedure depends on good arterial inflow (i.e., proximal arterial circulation), good arterial outflow (i.e., distal arterial circulation) and an adequate conduit. As a rule the conduit of choice is an autogenous vein. Reversed saphenous vein, when used for a femoro-popliteal bypass, has superior patency when compared to prosthetic conduits (i.e., polyester or PTFE) (4, 6) (Figure 3). This becomes both clinically and statistically significant when the bypass is performed distal to the knee joint. If an autogenous conduit is not available, the use of a prosthetic conduit is justified. Prosthetic conduits are used as a matter of routine in bypass procedures of larger diameter vessels, e.g., aorta-bifemoral bypass with a bifurcated prosthesis for aorta-iliac occlusive disease and abdominal aortic aneurisms. The use of prosthetic graft material is associated with a higher risk of sepsis, which carries high morbidity and mortality. Notwithstanding the risks, durable salvage can be obtained in 85 to 89% of cases of critical limb ischemia (7).

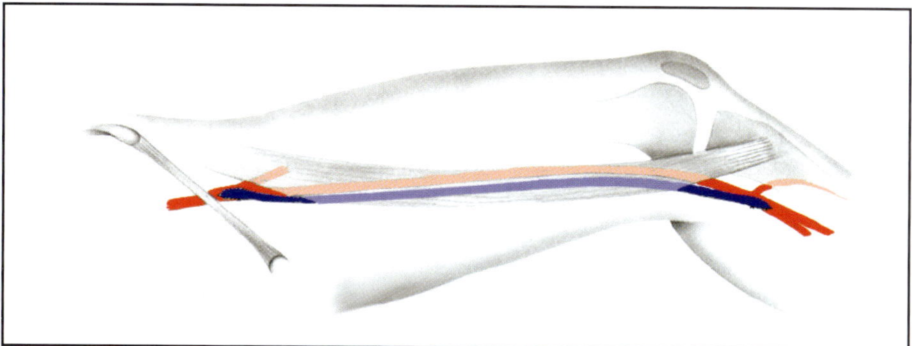

Figure 3. Percutaneous sub-intimal angioplasty.

Diabetic patients with skin ulceration present unique challenges. Typically they have extensive pathology of the infra-popliteal arteries. Although some of the lesions can be addressed with balloon angioplasty, a large proportion cannot be managed using endovascular techniques. Femoro-pedal bypasses have been used quite frequently with surprisingly good results. In spite of the fact that the long-term patency rates of these bypasses are low, they still improve overall limb salvage rates. This may be because bypass procedures afford enough time for wounds to heal; they palliate rest pain; and they allow time for new collateral vessels to form. Average patency rates are listed in Figure 4. Primary amputation is only considered in those patients where retaining the limb will directly contribute to an increased risk of mortality.

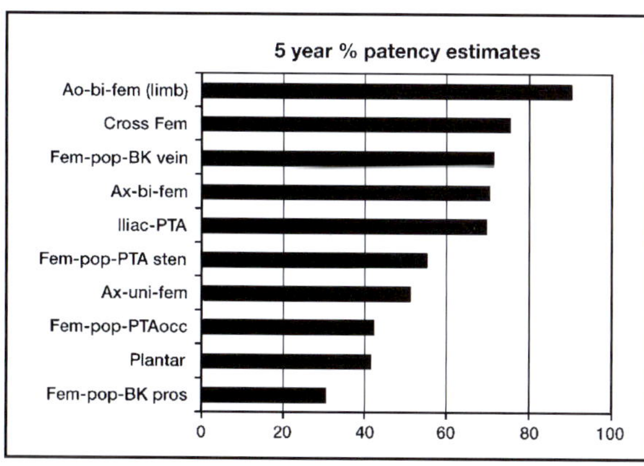

Figure 4. Average results for surgical treatment: Ao-bi-fem-Aorto-bifemoral bypass; Fem-pop-femoro-popliteal; BK-below knee; Ax-bi-fem Axillo-bifemoral; PTA-Percutaneous Transluminal Angioplasty; Ax-uni-fem-Axillo-unifemoral bypass; pros-prosthetic (4).

OXYGENATION STRATEGIES

For patients with incomplete arterial obstruction, adequate oxygenation may be achieved by increasing dissolved blood oxygen content using either normobaric (i.e., O_2 delivered to the patient at 1 ATA) or hyperbaric (i.e., O_2 delivered to the patient at 2 to 3 ATA) oxygen therapy (8).

Normobaric Oxygen

This is used every day in surgical theatres and in hospital wards. It is generally underutilised, given the wealth of scientific support confirming its value in wound healing and its ability to prevent wound sepsis and dehiscence, particularly following abdominal surgery (9).

Oxygen delivery systems range in terms of the route, volume and concentration of oxygen they provide. Venturi masks can offer 24–60% oxygen. They deliberately mix the oxygen with air, thereby delivering a high volume of oxygen enriched air able to keep up with a patient's inspiratory flow rate, without being unduly wasteful of the oxygen supply. For lower concentrations of oxygen, this is the most reliable system. Simple oronasal masks and nasal cannulas are not ideal. Oronasal masks rarely fit properly and patients frequently dislodge them or have them hanging around their necks or blowing in their ears. Nasal cannulas deliver 24–40% oxygen within a tolerable flow rates, but they require nasal breathing. It is not uncommon to see patients snoring through the mouth as the nasal cannula fizzes gently in the background. Tight fitting non-rebreather masks are the best way to deliver high concentrations of oxygen, i.e. 80–90%.

Breathing high concentrations of normobaric oxygen can increase plasma dissolved oxygen by up to 2 ml/oxygen/dl—which is approximately 40% of the average quantity of oxygen extracted from hemoglobin by body tissues (8). More important than blood oxygen content, however, is the ability of this increased oxygen concentration in plasma to diffuse further into tissues. This concept is often difficult to convey to medical professionals who consider, quite erroneously, that hemoglobin saturation is a definitive measure of tissue oxygenation.

There are no limits or restrictions on the use of normobaric oxygen at inspired fractions of < 0.5 (i.e., < 50%). The continuous delivery of 80 to 100 % oxygen should be limited to 24-36 hours.

Hyperbaric oxygen (HBO2)

By delivering oxygen to patients at increased ambient pressure, HBO2 is able to extend the beneficial effects of oxygen supplementation. However, even though HBO2 therapy can increase dissolved blood oxygen by up to 6 ml/oxygen/dl (enough to sustain life without blood), it still requires a conduit to transport the oxygen to the affected tissue.

The application of HBO2 therapy, being less familiar, frequently has to compete with a number of other medical and surgical therapies that have already established themselves through common practice and/or modern evidence-based medical processes. To secure more general acceptance and to ensure its appropriate use, HBO2 has to meet the same standards and should be applied judiciously (8).

At a consensus meeting in Lille, France, in December 2004, the evidence supporting the use of HBO2 was evaluated using modern evidence-based medicine criteria (10). From a wound care perspective the accepted indications for HBO2 treatment are rated. Readers are referred to the relevant chapters in this book for more details by R A Warriner entitled "Wound Assessment," and "Evidence–Based Wound Care."

A recent Cochrane review concluded that hyperbaric therapy significantly reduces the risk of major amputation in patients with diabetic ulcers (11). The results have been criticised due to methodological shortcomings. Nevertheless, the TASC II document suggests that HBO2 may be considered in selected patients with ischemic ulcers who have not responded to, or are not candidates for, revascularization (4). There is no clinical evidence to justify the use of topical oxygen therapy (12).

DISCUSSION

The availability of perfusion and oxygenation strategies offers a unique spectrum of potential solutions and risk-benefit choices for patients with ischemic/ hypoxic wounds. Therefore, the respective specialists should be included in the multi-disciplinary teams serving these patients. Ultimately, the goal is to offer patients a holistic approach to their problems; a cost-effective solution to effectively heal their wounds; a sound method for removing or attenuating the underlying causes; and the opportunity to improve the quality of their lives. A multidisciplinary approach also protects patients against possible maverick enthusiasts who favour one specific treatment modality.

Although one cannot overstate the importance of involving the patient in the decision making process, direct communication between the members of the team managing the patient is equally important. If it is thought that more advanced and costly strategies should be implemented, a multidisciplinary meeting is appropriate to consider the alternatives and then present them to the patient. Baseline clinical and special investigations that should be available for discussion include the following:

- Patient demographics
- Patient history (Medical, Surgical, Wound Care)
- Current medication
- Vital signs (Blood pressure, Pulse)
- Clinical examination
- Serum Glucose
- Ankle-brachial pressure indices (ABPI)♥

♥ Ankle-brachial pressure measurement is absolutely essential in the examination of a patient with a wound of his lower extremity. An ankle-brachial pressure index (ABPI) is determined by dividing the highest Doppler pressure of a limb at the level of the ankle by the highest Doppler pressure of either upper limb at the level of fossa cubiti. An ABPI of less than 0.9 or higher than 1.3, is considered abnormal. Higher indices (>1.3) might indicate severe sclerosis with poor compressibility of the arteries. Diabetes should then be excluded. Lower indices (<0.9) are indicative of occlusive arterial disease. An ABPI of less than 0.5 should be followed by an urgent referral to a vascular surgeon, especially in the presence of an ulcer. The presence of an abnormal ABPI is also associated with an increased risk of cardiovascular morbidity and mortality. Standard ankle-brachial pressures are not always accurate in diabetics. False high values are often obtained due to arterial sclerosis. Toe pressures are more sensitive in this group of patients.

Following initial assessment of the patient, the next step is to determine the need for, and selection of, appropriate special investigations and interventions depending on the clinical situation. The relevance and value of any special investigation should be based on whether it will influence the management of the patient. These may include transcutaneous oximetry; magnetic resonance angiography—regarded as superior to digital subtraction angiography and CT-angiography (13); X-rays; wound biopsy; and wound or tissue microbiology.

All patients with critical limb ischemia should undergo comprehensive vascular workup (4). If any doubts exist on the interpretation of preliminary vascular assessments, patients should be offered the benefit of further vascular investigations. This is particularly important in diabetic patients. A delayed diagnosis of significant peripheral vascular disease may have disastrous complications. The American College of Cardiology and American Heart Association's guidelines on the management of patients with peripheral arterial disease include the recommendation, based on Class I Level B evidence, that patients with critical limb ischemia and skin breakdown should be referred to healthcare providers with specialized expertise in wound management (3). See RA Warriner's chapter "Evidence–Based Wound Care" for a discussion of levels of evidence.

Diagnostic evaluation of patients with critical limb ischemia should provide: (a) objective confirmation of the diagnosis; (b) localization of the responsible lesion(s) with an assessment of relative severity; (c) assessment of the hemodynamic requirements for successful revascularization (i.e., proximal vs. combined revascularization of multilevel disease); and (d) assessment of the individual patient's endovascular or operative risk (14).

Patients with complex ischemic/hypoxic wounds, who either do not have clinically significant arterial disease (i.e., they have microvascular disease) or are not candidates for endovascular or surgical perfusion strategies, should be considered for HBO2 therapy. Transcutaneous oximetry offers an objective method for determining which patients are most likely to benefit from HBO2 (15). Patients, who have had successful revascularization procedures, should also be reconsidered for oxygen therapy if their wounds do not respond adequately following the vascular intervention.

Not surprisingly, a grey area exists between the choice of perfusion strategies and oxygenation strategies. The following flow chart has been used at our centre and offers a structured way to evaluate and manage patients with complex wounds (Figure 5).

The presence of macrovascular arterial insufficiency per se is not a contra-indication to HBO2 (16). In our clinical experience, a $PtcO_2 > 40$ mm Hg on air or during 100% normobaric oxygen inhalation has been the tipping point for the decision of whether patients with acceptable ABPI's should preferentially receive HBO2 rather than vascular surgery as the primary intervention. However, to continue HBO2, transcutaneous oximetry must confirm that the minimum therapeutic value (i.e., $PtcO_2 > 200$ mm Hg) can be achieved under hyperbaric conditions (15).

If there is no improvement in $PtcO_2$ levels with the patient breathing oxygen and hyperbaric oxygen, revascularization should be reconsidered. Age is not considered a contraindication to revascularization procedures. A study by

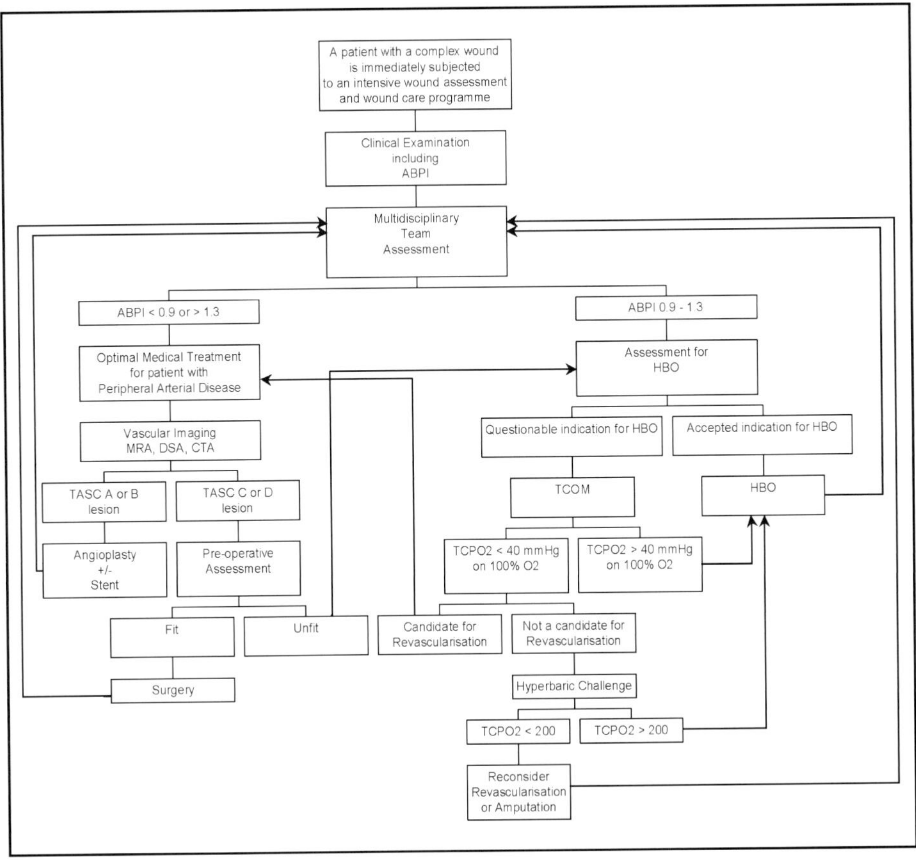

Figure 5. Flowchart for the management of hypoxic/ischemic wounds.

Ouriel has even demonstrated statistically significant benefit in terms of morbidity and mortality, when comparing bypass procedures to amputations (17). However, if perfusion strategies remain inappropriate, amputation may need to be considered.

In some situations, however, multidisciplinary teams should exercise self-restraint. If the patient is considered high risk for intervention, or if HBO2 is contraindicated, a conservative approach may be appropriate. If so, the patient should be reassessed frequently to ensure appropriate control of the patient's pain and risk factors and to monitor the wound. If the conservative approach fails due to propagating sepsis or intractable pain, or if it becomes unacceptable to the patient, intervention becomes unavoidable.

For patients with advanced disease and functional impairment, an early amputation and rehabilitation might be more appropriate than a prolonged, expensive and labour intensive attempt to salvage a dysfunctional limb that will continue to reduce the patient's quality of life. Psychological support and rehabilitation are then imperative. The decision to amputate and the choice of the level of amputation should be considered carefully. It should weigh up the patient's chances of healing, rehabilitation potential and overall quality of life (4). Accordingly, an orthopaedic surgeon is a vital member of the wound care team. They should be involved early in the overall assessment of the patient, irrespective of the prognosis or the perfusion and oxygenation strategies that may be available.

Finally, there are patients who will present with unsalvageable ischemia who also have a negligible chance of survival or quality of life after amputation. The most appropriate, humanitarian decision may then be to opt for effective pain management and palliative wound care (18).

CONCLUSION

The perfusion and oxygenation strategies described in this chapter can help the clinician to improve the delivery of oxygen and essential nutrients to a compromised wound. If these strategies are available at your facility—involve and consider them. If not, consider timely referral for the benefit of your patient.

REFERENCES

1. Morris HM. *Science and the Bible*. Chicago: Moody Press; 1986.

2. Stedman's Medical Dictionary. 28th ed: Lippincott Williams & Wilkins; 2005.

3. Hirsch AT. ACC/AHA 2005 Guidelines for the Management of Patients with Peripheral Arterial Disease. *Journal of the American College of Cardiology* 2006;47(6).

4. Norgren L. Inter-Society Consensus for the Management of Peripheral Arterial Disease (TASC II). *Eur J Vasc Endovasc Surg* 2007;33(Supplement 1).

5. Ameli FM. The effect of post-operative smoking on femoro-popliteal bypass grafts. *Ann Vasc Surg* 1989;3:20-5.

6. Kreienberg PB. Early results of a prospective randomized trial of spliced vein versus polytetrafluoroethylene graft with a distal vein cuff for limb-threatening ischemia. *J Vasc Surg* 2002;35:299-306.

7. Taylor LM. Limb salvage and amputation for critical ischemia: the role of vascular surgery. *Ann Surg* 1991;126:1251-8.

8. Handbook of Hyperbaric Medicine. London: Springer-Verlag; 2005.

9. Hopf HW. Development of subcutaneous wound oxygen measurement in humans: contributions of Thomas K Hunt, MD. *Wound Repair Regen* 2003;11(6):424-30.

10. European Committee for Hyperbaric Medicine. Recommendations of the 7th European Consensus Conference on Hyperbaric Medicine. *Underwater Hyp Med* 2005;6:29-40.

11. Kranke P. Cochrane Database Syst Rev 2004;CD004123.

12. Cronje FJ. Oxygen therapy and wound healing - topical oxygen is not hyperbaric oxygen therapy. *South African Medical Journal* 2005;95(11).

13. Owen RS. Magnetic resonance imaging of angiographically occult runoff vessels in peripheral arterial occlusive disease. *N Engl J Med* 1992;326:1577-81.

14. Dormandy JA, Rutherford RB. Management of peripheral arterial disease. 2000;31:S1-S296.

15. Fife CE, Buyukcakir C, Otto GH, et al. The predictive value of transcutaneous oxygen tension measurement in diabetic lower extremity ulcers treated with hyperbaric oxygen therapy: a retrospective analysis of 1,144 patients. *Wound Repair Regen* 2002;10(4):198-207.

16. Hopf HW, Ueno C, Aslam R, et al. Guidelines for the treatment of arterial insufficiency ulcers. *Wound Repair Regen* 2006;14(6):693-710.

17. Ouriel K. Limb threatening ischemia in the medically compromised patient: amputation or revascularization. *Surgery* 1998;104:667-72.

18. Campbell WB. Non-intervention and palliative care in vascular patients. *British Journal of Surgery* 2000;87:1601-2.

REVIEW QUESTIONS

Illustrative Case Presentation

A 78 year old, non insulin dependent diabetic patient presents with an ulcer on the dorsum of her left foot extending to the first toe. This ulcer is secondary to a thermal injury (hot water bottle). Her diabetes is well controlled, but she has significant peripheral neuropathy. She has previously had coronary artery disease requiring bilateral saphenous vein harvesting for coronary artery bypass grafting. On clinical examination she has no palpable foot pulses and ABPI's of 0.8 bilaterally. The wound is 5 mm deep with, what appears to be superficial necrosis. Surrounding cellulitis suggests the presence of more extensive underlying and adjacent infection. Magnetic resonance angiography shows extensive atherosclerosis of the superficial femoral artery without significant stenoses. The fibular artery is patent up to the level just above the ankle. Both the anterior and posterior tibial arteries are completely occluded. The posterior tibial artery is visible just above the level of the ankle. No surgical or endovascular options are available to improve her peripheral circulation, other than an extensive bypass procedure. As the ulcer and associated infection are becoming a problem, intervention is required.

1.) What is the most important priority in managing a septic diabetic foot?
    a. Revascularization
    b. Surgical management of the infection
    c. Intravenous antibiotics
    d. Conservative management
    e. Immediate proximal amputation

2.) What would favour the use of HBO2 in this patient?
    a. Lack of vascular alternatives
    b. History of diabetes
    c. History of neuropathy
    d. The ABPI of 0.8
    e. Positive results of transcutaneous oximetry

3.) When would primary proximal amputation be a preferred choice?
    a. When propagating infection, intractable pain or functional impairment related to the limb do not justify salvage
    b. If no perfusion strategies exist and conservative management is unacceptable or fails
    c. If the patient requests it
    d. If transcutaneous oximetry does not support the use of HBO2
    e. All of the above

4.) Why would a patient with no palpable pulses have an ABPI of 0.8?
    a. Technical error
    b. Diabetic patients often have calcified arteries resulting in artificially higher ABPI's
    c. Diabetic neuropathy
    d. All of the above
    e. None of the above

5.) Using the flowchart for managing hypoxia vs. ischemia – Figure 5. What would be the appropriate management of this patient if HBO2 is not indicated (i.e., $PtcO_2$ <200 mm Hg)?

    a. Conservative management
    b. Reconsider revascularization or amputation
    c. Amputation
    d. Trial of HBO2
    e. None of the above

For this particular patient, transcutaneous oxygen measurement was done on selected sites on her foot, in proximity to the wound. Measurements were done on room air, as well as on oxygen administered via a non-rebreather mask. The initial $PtcO_2$ of 24 mm Hg on room air rose to 83 mm Hg after 10 minutes on 100% O_2. Following local debridement of the necrotic and infected tissue and appropriate antibiotics, the patient was referred for HBO2. The $PtcO_2$ values were 250 mm Hg in the hyperbaric chamber. The patient continued with a course of HBO2 and had uncomplicated healing of the wound.

Answers: 1e, 2e, 3e, 4b, 5b

NOTES

WOUND DEBRIDEMENT

CHAPTER NINE OVERVIEW

NOTES

WOUND DEBRIDEMENT

Timothy A. Emhoff, Sherry A. Ferro

INTRODUCTION

Historically, a clean wound was associated with a healing wound, prompting the use of such agents as honey (to osmotically control bacteria), maggots (to debride dead tissue) and various dressings to absorb the odors and debris, which were associated with a poorly healing wound. Although it seems perfectly obvious that debris, slough, exudate and avascular tissue all degrade a wound's ability to heal, we are only now starting to identify those factors associated with non-viable tissue that degrade and slow the healing process. Studies on chronic wound effluent have shown that these wounds have reduced mitogenic activity, a substantially increased amount of protease activity, and a cytokine environment that is substantially more pro-inflammatory. Changing this environment to one that promotes cellular activity and healing is part of the reason why debridement is important in chronic wound care. Debriding a wound of necrotic tissue, slough, bacteria and devitalized tissue enhances a wound's ability to get back on a healthy healing trajectory, converting a "chronic" wound to an "acute" wound.

RATIONALE

Presently, we know that most clean wounds do heal and the addition of expensive topical wound care products, whether tissue, creams, absorbents, moisturizers, antimicrobials or collagens, should come only after a clean bed of tissue is exposed. We also know that bacteria, harbored in dead tissue, can be harmful: that a quantity of 10^5 organisms per gram of tissue or fluid risks a systemic infection whether it be in skin, bone, muscle, urine or bile. Bacteria-laden wounds do not heal and do not accept skin grafts. Bacteria produce wound-healing inhibiting enzymes (metalloproteases) and also consume local wound resources such as oxygen and amino acids that are not then available to promote wound healing. Non-debrided soft tissue wounds are also known to be associated with a higher rate of clinical infection, sepsis and non-healing. This has been accepted for many years and is reinforced in the 1976 study of sacral decubitus wounds by Galpin, Chow, Bayer, and Guze (3).

Surgically, "draining pus" is the mainstay of infection control: antibiotics and local wound care only supplement the treatment. However, the decision to debride a patient with fever, high white blood cell count and local signs of infection (erythema, pain, fluctuance, fever) is easy when compared to the decision for debridement in a chronic wound which is not painful, has little or no erythema, the patient has no fever, and a normal white cell count. These wounds are best assessed for problematic bacterial burden (causing poor or non-healing) using criteria such as increased pain, increased friability of the granulation tissue, foul odor and wound regression. Debridement in this latter situation can be just as important in returning the wound to a healing trajectory as it is in the first situation in controlling the systemic infection.

The concept of wound "bioburden" has recently been introduced to help understand the significance of certain wound characteristics, which lead to a persistently non-healing wound. This bioburden can be reduced or eliminated through the use of debridement. The problem lies in deciding which technique to use. Taking the most extreme strategy of excising the whole wound and then dealing with a "new" wound with no bioburden is excessive as well as costly, and may not solve the problem. If the bioburden is the result of chronic systemic factors, then all that is created with an aggressive excision is a new, bigger wound, which will soon have the same characteristics of the first. Also, aggressive debridement may not be possible or advisable over large vessels, vascular grafts, bone/tendon or around the face. Changing this wound "milieu" to reduce the bioburden then becomes the first priority in reestablishing a healing wound.

Controlling the bioburden should involve a strategy to reduce inflammation, remove dead tissue and control exudate. This exudate may be the source of problematic enzymes or the result of uncontrolled bacterial overgrowth. Thus, debridement should be considered first in the strategy to achieve a "healing environment" in an otherwise non-healing wound.

CHOICE OF DEBRIDEMENT

Like all other procedures done in medicine, patient selection is an extremely important process, both to choose the correct procedure and to choose the correct patient on whom to perform the procedure. Non-surgical or "less aggressive" debridement methods are inappropriate for a wound that is the source of systemic infection or is causing edema, erythema or pain in the surrounding tissue. Here, wide extirpation is necessary to avoid sepsis and bacteremia and must be done with full knowledge of the risks of major tissue loss and usually involves general anesthesia. Less aggressive means will only prolong the problem and lead to further debilitation and ultimately critical illness. On the other hand, a chronic, indolent wound in an otherwise clean environment may be dealt with in a much more gentle way, sparing the patient the pain and the risk of surgery while reestablishing a clean wound environment. Here, autolytic, enzymatic, blunt or biosurgical means can be used to clean the wound bed without the risks involved when exposing deeper structures (vessels, tendons, joint capsules, etc.) as one would with surgical excision. Also, these debridement methods can be instituted in a non-acute care setting, thereby eliminating all that is involved with a surgical procedure and an inpatient setting.

To help make this decision on proper debridement choice, the following mnemonic is helpful: *P A C U*:

P - Patient selection: which patient needs debridement.

There are numerous reasons for debridement which include the removal of devitalized tissue to expose the "healing epithelial edge" of tissue to a healthy wound bed, to remove tissue harboring bacteria, to reduce exudate production, to remove callous (non-viable tissue), to remove overhanging edges of wounds which are not in contact with a healthy wound bed or to remove coagulum from an otherwise vascular wound bed. When assessing a wound it is important to remember where healthy skin originates in order to cover an open wound. New skin comes from the edges via contraction and epithelialization, neither of which happens in an environment of calloused, dry or otherwise non-viable tissue. The barriers that each patient's wound presents to epithelialization and contraction must then be dealt with, the type of debridement then determined by urgency and mass of tissue to be removed. Urgent debridement to remove tissue that is infected and causing systemic infection, local pain and high exudates should be removed sharply/surgically. Inert tissue which is not infected (grossly), not highly exudative and relatively thin may be dealt with occlusively as long as the tissue is a mere barrier to healing and not a threat to health. Making this choice is not always easy since patient tolerance, pain, preferences, living situation, home health needs and resources all play a role in deciding how best to proceed. The question sometimes is asked: "Doesn't surgically debriding all wounds yield the cleanest environment in the quickest time?" The answer is that surgical debridement may not fit the patient: a general anesthetic may be necessary, but not appropriate for the patient's physiology. The patient may not have the resources (psychological or otherwise) to go though a formal procedure and may request to only be treated in a home setting. Extirpating a wound in an area with poor local tissue conditions may only compound the problem: a larger wound is made in a "hostile" healing environment of unrelieved pressure, malnutrition, poor hygiene, renal failure or anemia. It is sometimes best to work at controlling the local environment while debriding the wound with measures that remove only the non-viable tissues.

A - Analgesia: pain control during the debridement.

Surgical debridement requires at least local/regional analgesia. Even in an otherwise insensate area, analgesia is necessary to block nerve impulses that may cause hypertension, tachycardia and vasoconstriction: a "pain" response despite the patient's ability to report so. Holding the patient down while chanting, "It's OK, we're almost done," is not only inappropriate but is also inhumane and should never be done. Appropriate analgesia allows a procedure to be done in as humane a way as possible. Certain topical debriding agents can also be painful. This pain should be addressed as well, and may be treated with a variety of topical agents such as EMLA or lidocaine. Providing adequate analgesia increases patient satisfaction and the likelihood of continued cooperation with the debridement strategy. If adequate analgesia cannot be provided, then another type of debridement may be more appropriate.

> *C* - Capabilities of the caregiver: the armamentarium for
> debridement of the caregiver may be limited, but this should
> not change what is appropriate for the patient.

Non-surgeons may need to employ the capabilities of their surgical colleagues and surgeons may need to avail themselves to topical debridement and learn about ways other than cutting to remove tissue. Home health care providers must know when a wound is in trouble and when to refer for an urgent assessment and possible surgical debridement. An individual's capabilities must not limit the patient to only those interventions with which that provider is comfortable. It is necessary to be knowledgeable about what treatments are available and appropriate and then assist the patient in accessing the most beneficial treatment even if it's outside that individual's capabilities. An advantage of a comprehensive wound care program is that it offers all possible strategies and does not shoehorn patients into the product-of-the-month or the caregiver-of-the-day. Each of us does what he/she does best, but this should not blind our assessments of wounds to those few things we do best when in our best judgment something else is needed. We have to do what is best for our patients.

> *U* - Urgency: how quickly/completely does the wound need debridement?

This factor may supercede all others: a wound with necrotic tissue jeopardizing the health and possibly the life of a patient needs immediate removal of debris, despite risks of anesthesia, poor physiology and change of environment. At the other end of the spectrum, a wound with inert debris but in an otherwise healthy environment can be dealt with occlusively, on a gradual basis while not disrupting the patient's usual life style as long as progress is being made. A decision needs to be made at each wound assessment as to whether the current debridement strategy should continue, or whether a more aggressive approach is warranted. Is progress being made? Failure to progress should prompt another debridement strategy just as an acutely infected wound should prompt the consideration for extirpation.

METHODS
Wet-to-Dry

Historically, wet-to-dry has been the "gold standard" in dressings. This is the type every new doctor first hears about and rarely forgets (unfortunately). Usually when asked, "What kind of dressing do you want on that wound?" whether it be a new, clean, open wound or an older, dry, necrotic wound, the answer invariably is "wet-to-dry." Rarely does the ordering physician actually understand the purpose and the proper technique for this type of dressing as a debridement method. The technique requires frequent changes, since it is during the dressing change itself that the actual debridement occurs. A layer of moistened, woven gauze, applied to the wound bed, becomes adherent to the underlying tissue as it desiccates. When the dried dressing is removed, the adherent tissue is also removed. The result is a debridement that is traumatic and non-selective. The photo at Figure 1 illustrates a decubitus ulcer being debrided with moisten gauze which has been allowed to dry onto the wound bed. Its removal then pulls off the adherent eschar. This is repeated until the wound bed is clean. The materials themselves are usually cheap: a simple woven gauze, saline solution, a dressing cover and tape to hold everything in place: each component costing pennies. However, the true cost of this dressing technique can be many times the cost of the materials when you take into account the following:

1. The dressing must be left in place to dry, allowing tissue in contact with the gauze to incorporate into the interstices of the gauze, a process of hours.
2. The dressing must be done often: 3–4 times per day to debride and also maintain a healthy wound surface which must not be allowed to dry too much, which will only cause more damage to otherwise healthy tissue.
3. If the dressing is unable to be done by the patient, it will require the assistance of another, multiple times per day; and if that person is a home health nurse, this is not a free service!
4. The dressing, which is allowed to adhere to the wound surface to attach to the tissue to be removed, is often painful to remove, and may require pre-medication with an analgesic.
5. The dressing must be held in place, firmly in contact with the wound bed. If the patient is at all mobile, this could require a second dressing system to be put in place over the basic wet dressing.

Having said this, this technique still may be appropriate in the appropriate setting. An acute wound, in a hospitalized patient, which needs frequent monitoring before it can be deemed safe to cover, the "wet-to-dry" technique is quick, simple and by its nature, allows the wound to be assessed multiple times throughout the day. Pain control, materials and personnel are already in place. Patients may not be very mobile, making it sometimes simple to keep a dressing in place with an adhesive. Once the necessary debridement has been accomplished, then the dressing can be converted to one of moist occlusion, usually with a gel or antimicrobial cream/ointment, depending on drainage. The "wet-to-dry" aspect should be discontinued as soon the wound bed is clean: further adherence of the dressing will only harm vascular buds and newly marginating epithelial cells. In an acute wound, with a bed made clean and vascular with this technique, loosely approximating the skin edges while maintaining a moist wound environment will speed closure and protect the wound bed from desiccation. Containing drainage will help to monitor the amount of exudate, which is an indicator of increasing bioburden that will compromise further epithelial healing, but not cause deepening infection or harm to healthy tissue.

Once the wound is clean, non-infected, free of debris and new granulation tissue is forming, a useful strategy to significantly shorten wound healing time is the use of "tertiary closure," or closing a wound that has been treated open, expecting secondary contracture and epithelialization. These wounds are not allowed to enter into the "chronic" stage: the edges are instead coapted, usually with steristrips or skin sutures, which loosely bring the edges of the wound together and allows the wound to drain. This significantly shortens wound-healing time since the "contracture" phase has been accomplished by the sutures or tape. One such case of tertiary closure in a thigh wound illustrated in Figure 2A-C. The patient had a lateral thigh abscess drained, which subsequently was treated open, with gauze antimicrobial packing. Once the wound became healthy and was clearly on a

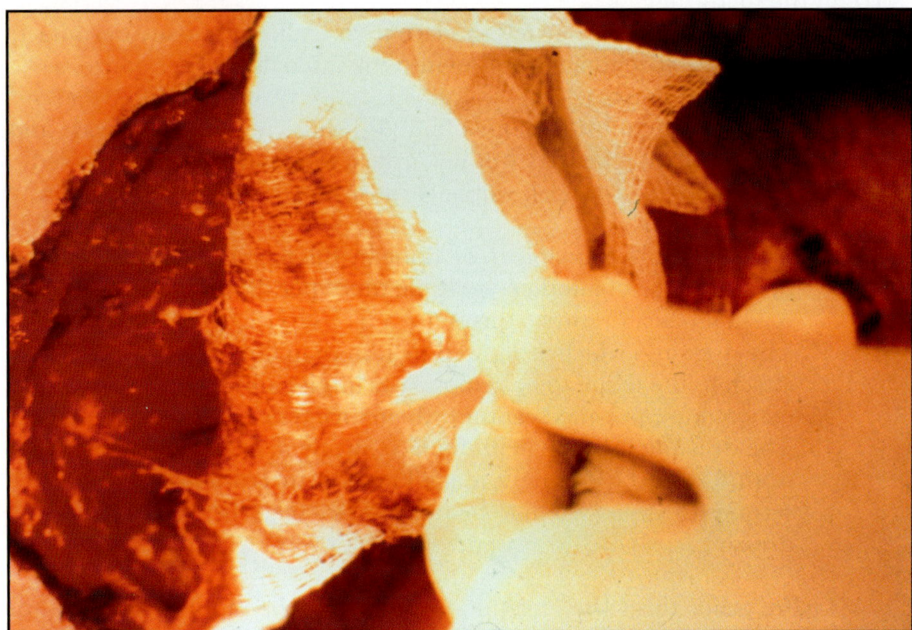

Figure 1. "Wet-to-Dry" moistened gauze allowed to dry onto a decubitus ulcer, then peeled off, removing adherent eschar.

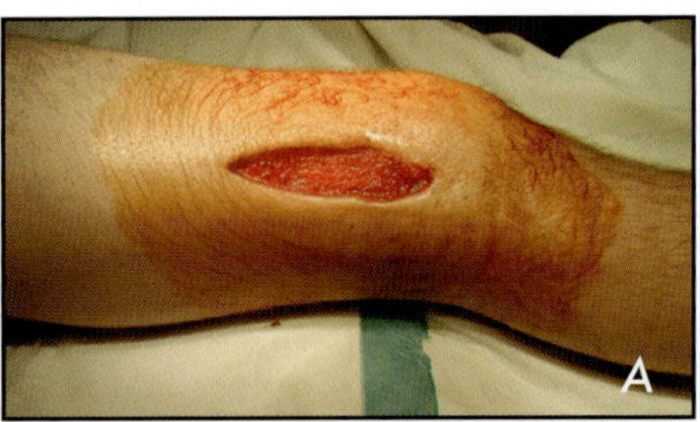

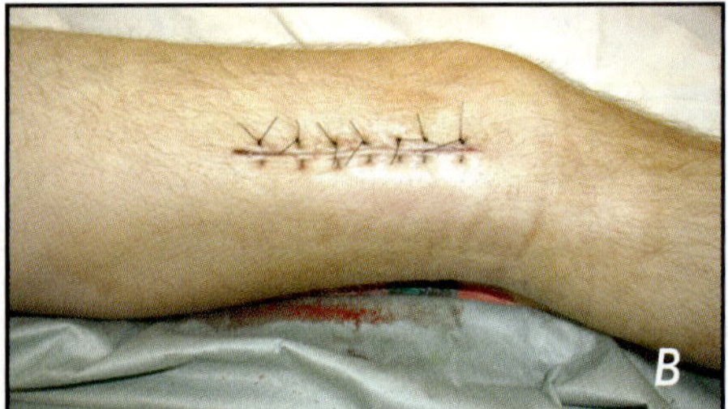

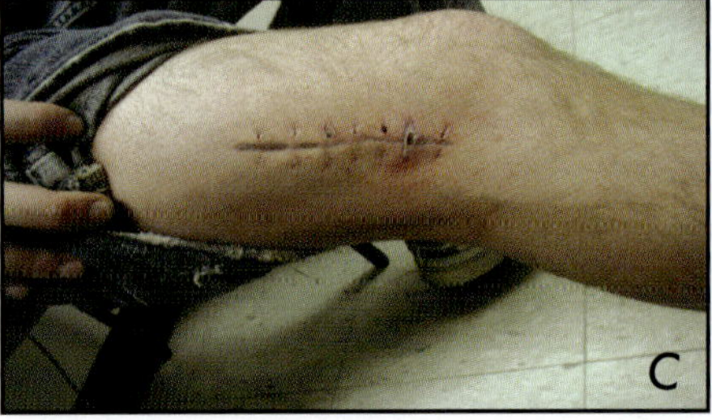

Figure 2. (A) Thigh wound, abscess drainage after antimicrobial packing.
(B) Wound loosely closed: "tertiary closure."
(C) Tertiary closure: two weeks later: sutures out, wound closed.

trajectory of contracting/healing, the edges were brought together with 2–0 nylon skin sutures and allowed to epithelialize and fuse. The sutures were removed two weeks later, with a healed wound, significantly reducing healing time and dressing changes.

Autolytic

Autolytic debridement is the most selective type of debridement. Only those tissues that are dead or devitalized (slough) are removed, leaving behind a healthy wound bed and edges. However, this can also be the slowest debridement method because separation of tissue planes occurs only over days/weeks as dead/devitalized tissues separate under a moist environment. This moist environment is provided by occlusive dressings or, if the wound is left uncovered, under a desiccated eschar. Moist healing, under an occlusive dressing was shown more than 40 years ago to be more rapid than under a dry, adherent eschar. An advantage to letting the eschar "slough" in the absence of infection or pus under the eschar "cover," is that the underlying structures are not allowed to desiccate during this process. This is illustrated in the following two photos of a patient with an injury to the anterior leg. A dry eschar had formed before she presented for therapy (Figure 3A). If the eschar had been sharply debrided, the underlying tibial periosteum may have been violated, making this very prone to desiccation and ultimately exposing the bone: a very difficult and time-consuming wound to heal. Instead, because there were no signs of infection, the eschar was left in place and hydrated with an occlusive sheet of hydrocolloid that was changed every three days. After one week (Figure 3B) the eschar began to separate and in another two weeks the wound totally epithelialized, all quite painlessly.

Providing a moist, occlusive environment then has several advantages. However, these advantages may not be appreciated by some clinicians who fear that occluding a wound that is not totally clean and healthy will somehow cause the wound to become infected or to deteriorate. This is a false concept. Occluding a wound in a moist environment accomplishes the following:

- Provides pain relief: dry, desiccated tissues contract and are painful
- Provides a means to control wound exudate
- Provides an environment for the enzymatic process to cleave the tissue planes between the dead and viable tissues
- Provides continuous wound treatment: the autolytic process is continuous as long as the environment is in place
- Maintains moisture which accelerates the autolytic process when compared to a desiccated environment
- Enhances epithelialization once a healthy wound bed is exposed to the healing edge of healthy tissue

These principles are depicted in this case illustration of a patient with a painful lateral leg ulcer (Figures 4A-C). Hydrocolloid was used to occlude the wound (which alleviated the pain) and provide a moist environment. Thick, dry eschar was softened; a "hydrated" wound bed then resulted in advancing the epithelial edges.

Choosing the dressing that provides this moist environment is a decision that is based on wound characteristics:

- Size
- Amount of wound exudate/transudate
- Amount of moisture present: maceration vs desiccation
- Depth
- Bioburden: bacterial overgrowth
- Length of time between dressing changes

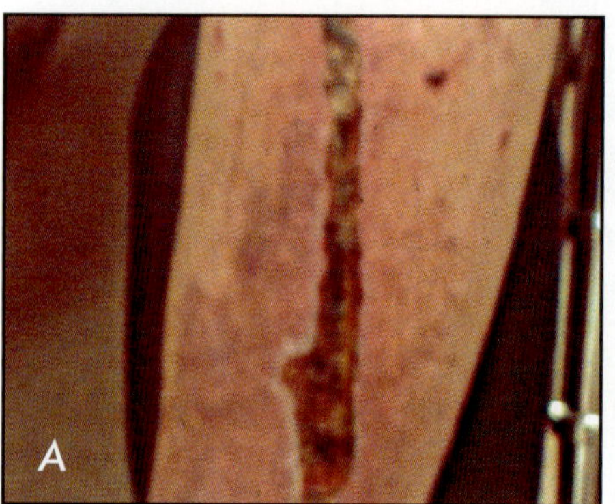
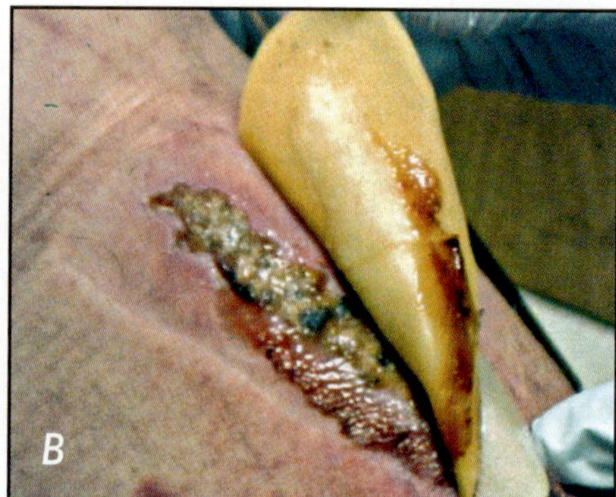

Figure 3. "Autolytic" (A) Anterior tibial wound with dry eschar.
(B) Anterior tibial wound one week after autolytically debrided with use of hydrocolloid

The goal of the autolytic process is to provide a comfortable wound environment under which the wound eschar/slough is separated from a presumably healthy wound bed. Dry, desiccated wounds require hydration, which can be accomplished with a gel or hydrocolloid. Very moist, highly exudative wounds require absorptive dressings to wick away fluids to prevent wound maceration. These wounds may also benefit from an antimicrobial product to treat bacteria (the source of the exudate) while absorbing the fluid. Deeper wounds or those which tunnel may require a foam or alginate to fill the cavity until wound contracture progresses.

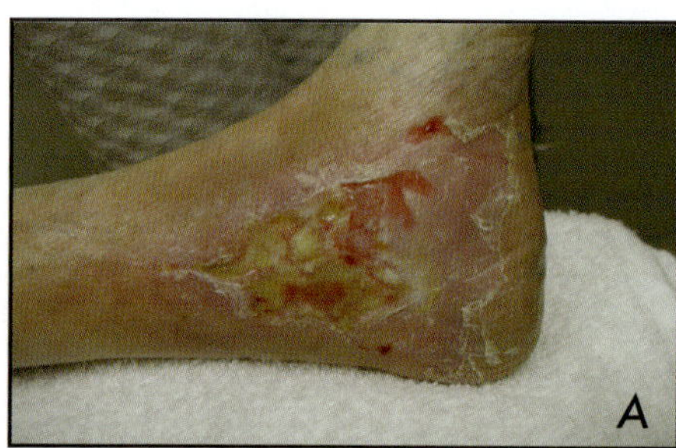
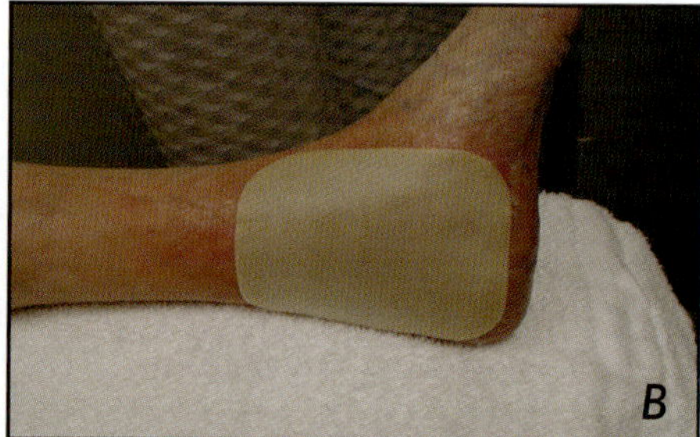
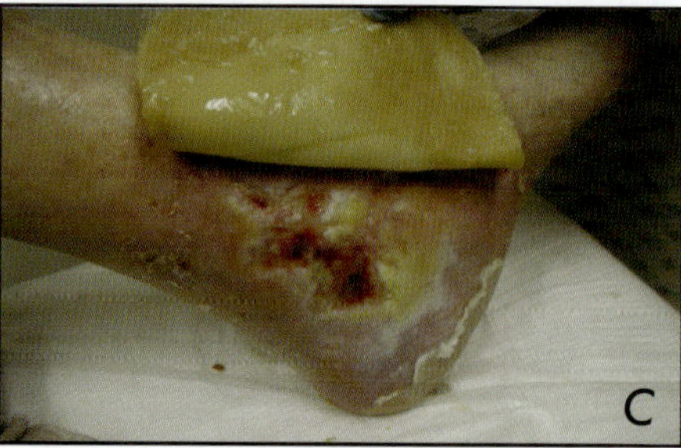

Figure 4. (A) Patient PC: before autolytic debridement.
(B) Patient PC: hydrocolloid applied.
(C) Patient PC: moist, autolytic debridement

At each dressing change the wound should be carefully inspected for signs that the slough or eschar is separating and that a tissue plane is forming over a healthy wound bed. Once this process begins it can be accelerated with the use of judicious sharp debridement by cleaning and removing the dead tissue with scissors or scalpel. Five minutes of sharp debridement are worth two weeks of moist, occlusive autolytic debridement. One must be careful in doing this not to enter the plane of healthy tissue: this is an area which is usually somewhat hyperemic and bleeding may be profuse and difficult to control without some type of cautery, either chemical or electrical. This hyperemic zone does not vasoconstrict well, probably due to local environmental factors, such as inflammatory mediators, tissue factors, cytokines and bacterial breakdown products. Blood loss may be significant!

Enzymatic

Enzymatic wound debridement is more specific than autolytic debridement although the principles are the same. The wound is treated in an occlusive environment to regain/maintain moisture while an enzymatic product is added to the wound bed to hasten the separation of slough/debris from the wound bed. The autolytic process itself occurs because of enzymes in the wound environment, byproducts of inflammatory cells and bacteria. In fact, the presence of bacteria actually aids this process: wounds without bacteria fail to heal, ostensibly because of the lack of these byproducts.

The added enzyme needs a secondary dressing, one that is chosen based again upon wound bed characteristics of amount of moisture, depth, exudate, and surrounding skin integrity. Size also matters. It is impractical to enzymatically treat a large wound requiring large amounts of an enzyme over many days. An initial bulk debridement may be necessary to remove the majority of dead tissue, followed by treating the slough/ wound bed interface with an enzyme.

Proteolytic enzymes are already present in a wound characterized by adherent slough or devitalized tissue, the products of bacteria and inflammatory cells. Why, then add more enzyme? The answer probably lies in the fact that the chronic wound environment is also characterized by proteolysis in addition to angiogenesis and epithelialization. This proteolysis may "overpower" certain proteins: cytokines, growth factors, protein matrixes etc., making their clinical effects seem less than what should be appropriate. By adding enzyme, the wound healing balance may then be restored, the wound progressing to a clean stage, and consequently, epithelialization. Some wounds, even after the slough has been removed, "stall" and do not epithelialize. When the enzyme is added back to the moist, occlusive environment, it breaks down certain proteins, promotes healthy wound healing, and epithelialization again progresses. These breakdown products may also serve as the needed chemoattractants, which then stimulate epithelialization and cellular migration.

Two general types of enzymes are available commercially: collagenase (Santyl®) and papain/urea (Panafil®, Accuzyme®, Gladase™), the first being a by-product of the bacteria clostridium histolyticum, the second an enzyme derived from the fruit carica papaya.

Collagenase cleaves glycine in helical regions of native collagen, but is not active against keratin, fat or fibrin. Theoretically, this activity aids in wound debridement by digesting collagen bundles that bind nonviable tissue to the wound bed surface, thus accelerating the process of ridding the wound surface of slough. No other product makes the claim of being active against this native collagen. Small studies have shown that the addition of this enzyme does enhance the process of slough removal. A more enticing use of this product, however, entails its use to restore an epithelialization-friendly environment: something that is seen occasionally clinically, but heretofore not specifically studied.

Papain/urea, on the other hand, helps separate slough from the wound bed by liquefying fibrinous debris. This is a less selective process than collagenase and one which is active over a wider range of pH, from 3–12. The addition of urea to the enzyme papain is necessary for two reasons. First, the papain must be "activated," which the urea does by exposing substances in the necrotic debris, and, second, it also denatures nonviable protein matter, making it more susceptible to proteolysis.

The patient who is to have enzymatic therapy should first be counseled as to what to expect. Often they hear "enzyme" and immediately have visions of an agent eating into their skin and digesting normal tissues, which of course is not true. Neither papain, nor collagenase has any appreciable effect on normal tissues, other than the moisture they provide. Pain, however, may be a real issue. The addition of urea sometimes causes significant pain making the product unusable in certain patients. The first time it is applied to a wound, one should have the patient wait a few minutes with the dressing in place to monitor the level of pain. Sometimes, although painful on application, the pain significantly subsides over a few minutes. However, the amount of pain some patients experience is so great that it precludes the use of urea altogether. Collagenase is rarely associated with pain on application, although an occasional patient will complain of enough pain to render it unusable.

The next two photos (Figures 5A–B) show wound debridement with enzymes in a patient who had failed multiple surgical debridements because of tissue ischemia. After each sharp debridement session (requiring general anesthesia) the tissue edge dried and necrosed, creating a larger, more painful wound. The patient refused further surgical debridement (appropriately) and amputation (not necessary). While she underwent daily hyperbaric oxygen treatment to treat her tissue ischemia, which was confirmed with $TcpO_2$ monitoring (Figure 5A), she had daily application of collagenase that, over a period of weeks, yielded a clean wound bed (Figure 5B). The process was relatively painless except for the dressing changes themselves. No further tissue was lost and the wound could be closed with the further use of hyperbaric oxygen therapy.

As with most other topical therapies, the use of an enzyme requires a secondary dressing that is chosen based on wound size, depth, exudate and condition of the surrounding skin. The enzyme is applied in a thin layer, covered with a moist dressing (if not highly exudative), and then changed daily or twice daily depending on the nature of the wound. Most second-degree burn wounds, characterized with a thin layer of slough, may be changed once daily as long as the wound bed remains well hydrated.

Bluntly removing the old enzyme with a saline-moistened gauze or other wound cleanser is important, since this is the time that slough separation can be examined and the adequacy of the wound debridement judged. Failure of the process to progress with the use of one product should prompt the use of the other product: failure of one does not necessarily mean failure of the other. Why one would work and the other would not work may not always be clear, but a strategy that clinically has stalled should not be continued.

There are concerns at times of using an enzyme in an environment that seems bacteria-rich or on a relatively new burn wound where infection may be a concern. Since neither enzyme has any appreciable antimicrobial properties, any bacterial/infectious concerns should be addressed separately. Polysporin powder is frequently added to collagenase as an antimicrobial agent where this is a concern, but there is no clear evidence that this practice is useful, or necessary. Studies have not shown that the use of an enzyme provided any benefit in reducing overall exudate which itself can be associated with bacterial overgrowth.

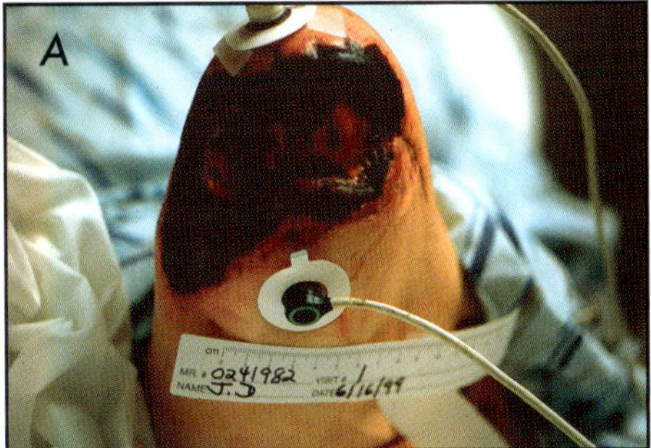

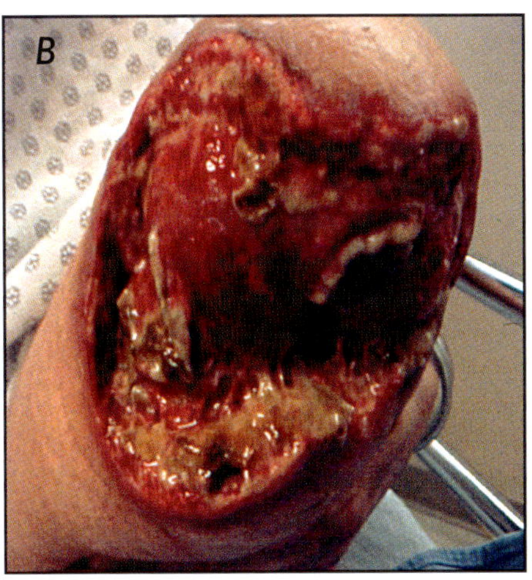

Figure 5. "Enzymatic." (A) Lower extremity wound, ischemic and painful. TcpO$_2$ electrodes in place.
(B) Lower extremity wound, enzymatically debrided with collagenase.

Blunt/Mechanical

Probably the most non-specific, "low-tech" form of debridement is blunt or mechanical debridement. It is also the most common form practiced. At each dressing change of a wound, some form of tissue/debris removal is accomplished by the mere act of removing the dressing and somehow cleansing the wound. It is during the wound cleansing that the debridement occurs, sometimes using water, saline, wound cleansers or moistened gauze to facilitate the process. It is non-specific however, what is not attached is removed, whether it is debris, exudate, slough, cellular byproducts, old topical ointments, antimicrobial agents, or healthy tissue. It is then that the surface and wound edges can be inspected and decisions on the next dressing made. This is an important issue for the wound care provider. Removal of the dressing, along with an appraisal of the wound base, the degree of hydration and the integrity/health of the surrounding skin are extremely important parts of the wound assessment that need to be made before the wound is cleaned and the next dressing applied. The dressing is the wound treatment, not just the wound cover, and the nature of that treatment, how it has performed, and over what period of time are all important factors to help decide on the next treatment (dressing). "Prepping" the patient by removing the old dressing and cleansing the wound bed before it is evaluated by the clinician should not be done. The dressing and the appearance of the uncleaned wound is a major part of the wound assessment and must be seen and assessed to make appropriate wound care decisions.

Cleaning the wound then is where "blunt debridement" is accomplished. A moist gauze rubbed over the surface may be painful, but is usually what is tried first. Pulling dead/dried tissue or callous from the wound bed or margin must be done towards the center of the wound, not outward, where healthy tissues may be damaged. Sometimes soaking the dressing off is necessary if the dressing has become too adherent, and merely pulling it off (the "wet-to-dry" technique) may cause bleeding and tissue damage. Once the dressing is off, cleansing the wound bed of debris may be done with gauze or a wound-cleansing agent, some containing surfactants which tend to break up adherent tissues. If too painful for blunt gauze debridement, wound irrigation may be tried, which is usually more comfortable. This technique entails the use of water (hydrotherapy), used in a tub or pulsed onto the wound, much as with a water pick. This latter technique is more physiologic, less cumbersome, uses less water and is more effective than simply immersing the area in a tub with circulating water (whirlpool). The "jet lavage" or "pulse lavage" technique usually is more effective and less damaging than the immersion technique, since only the wound bed is exposed to the water jet (Figure 6), rather than the entire limb or torso depending on the wound location with the whirlpool technique. The pulsating water should be controlled at a maximum pressure of 8–10 psi, higher pressures being associated with tissue damage. A controlled, pulsed stream of water is effective in breaking off slough, debris and cleansing the wound bed of creams and ointments left on from the previous dressing. This technique also avoids the potential harm of immersion therapy, which, if used over too long a period, can cause tissue edema and maceration. The pulsed lavage system can also be brought to the patient rather than the patient being transported to the tank, an obvious advantage with patients as critically ill as those with serious burns. The pulsed lavage system can be messy. The suction system linked to the lavage mechanism is not 100% effective in scavenging the effluent and some over spray usually has to be dealt with, but the total water used compared to an immersion tank is minuscule. As with any

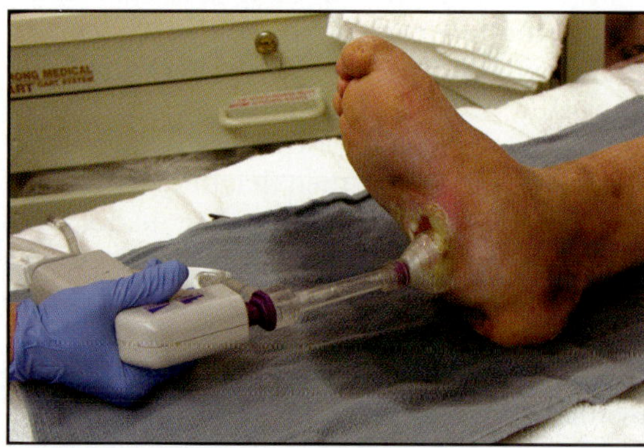

Figure 6. Pulsed lavage system used to bluntly debride neuropathic ulcer. Soft, rubber cone at the tip is used to control over spray and collect effluent through suction.

debridement technique, once the wound bed is clean, hydrotherapy should be stopped in order to avoid over-hydrating the wound and causing wound edge maceration, which will hamper epithelialization. It has been found, however, that some relatively clean wounds that continue to be highly exudative will benefit from the lavage on a two to three times per week basis, probably because the pulsed lavage dislodges a heavy bacterial bioburden on the wound surface. These wounds, when biopsied, may yield 10^5 organisms per gram of tissue and should be excised or continued on a topical antimicrobial with debridement, as long as progression continues.

Surgical/Sharp

Sharp debridement entails the use of scalpels and other sharp instruments such as curettes, scissors, blades and wire loops to sever tissue planes (see Figure 7). Sharp debridement may also require the concomitant use of some type of analgesia as well as strategies to control bleeding. Although the greatest amount of debris can be removed over the shortest period of time with sharp debridement, it also may cause the greatest harm over all other debridement techniques if used indiscriminately. Debriding tissues that cover vital structures such as tendons, major blood vessels/ grafts and joints may result in more damage to these deeper structures if they are left uncovered or are allowed to desiccate. Cutting into vessels which vasoconstrict poorly may cause significant bleeding problems that may not be controlled with pressure alone and may require special surgical tools/techniques to stop the hemorrhage (suture ligatures, cautery, etc.). Knowledge of anatomy and special training in surgical debridement is vital when using sharp debridement.

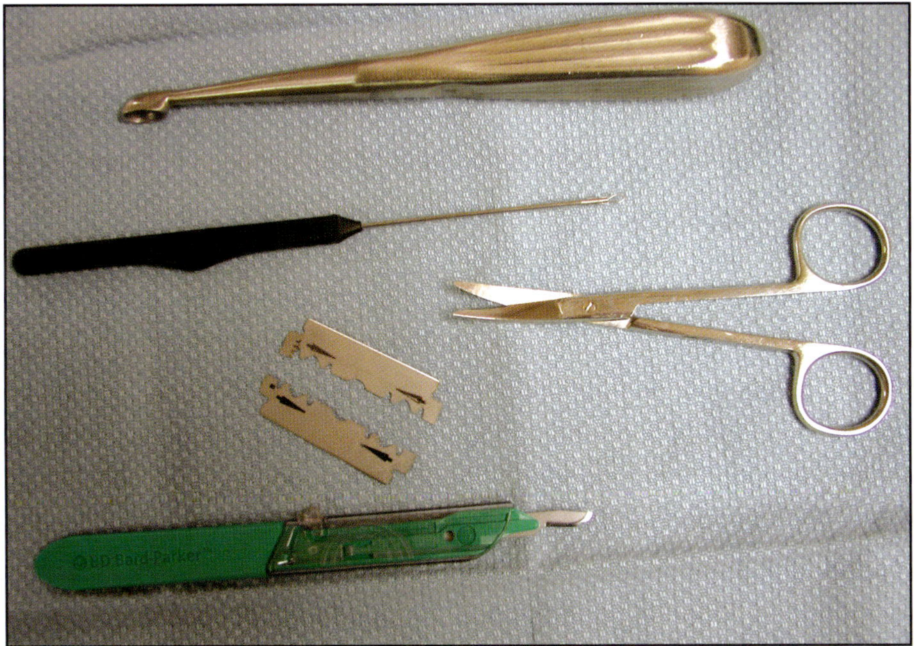

Figure 7. Sharp instruments used for surgical debridement (top to bottom): Bone curette, wire loop, curved, fine scissors, razor bade (cut in-half), #15 bladed scalpel.

Analgesia

Usually, neuropathic foot ulcers are the only wounds that do not require some form of analgesia before sharp debridement. These ulcers may be aggressively debrided without analgesia since, by definition, they are insensate. Steed and associates studied the effect of extensive debridement and treatment on the healing of diabetic foot ulcers (18). Their study showed the efficacy of the use of growth factors in neuropathic ulcers. The more aggressively debrided wounds derived the greatest benefit from the therapy, but debridement itself was also shown to be independently beneficial. To "saucerize" these foot ulcers a curved blade is fashioned from a double-edged razor blade, cut in half and sterilized (see Figure 7). This debridement tool is pinched into a "U" shape between the thumb and index finger and is used to carve out the edge of the ulcer to remove callous and debris in order to achieve a healthy edge and eliminate any undermining. This is illustrated in Figure 8, which shows a neuropathic ulcer being "saucerized" with a thin blade bent between thumb and index finger. This same technique can be used for any ulcer, but first analgesia must be established since the debridement will enter the healthy tissue interface, a sensitive area. EMLA (lidocaine 2.5%, prilocaine 2.5%) cream or gauze generously moistened with 4% lidocaine should be applied at least 30 minutes prior to the procedure. The EMLA is kept in place under a transparent film, the lidocaine-moistened gauze is held snugly in place with tape. Certain ulcers never seem to be able to be adequately anesthetized topically and consequently cannot be aggressively sharply debrided unless regional or general anesthesia is used. Here, clinical judgment must dictate the urgency or necessity of the sharp debridement.

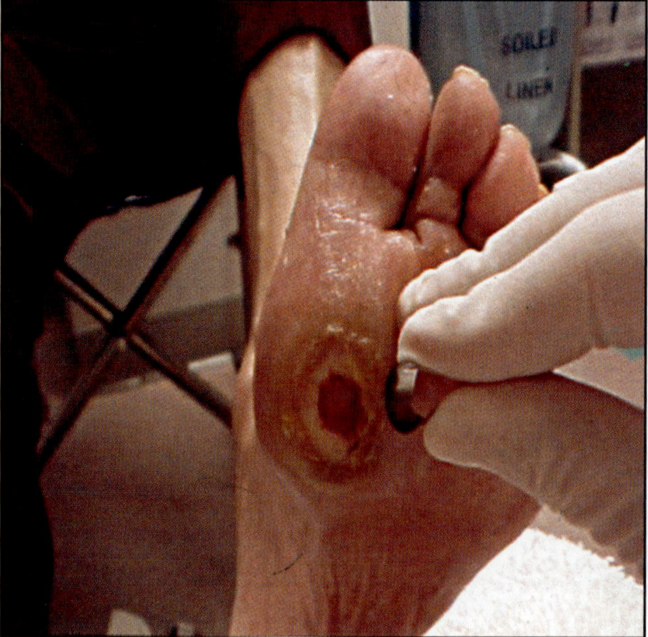

Figure 8. "Surgical/Sharp." Neuropathic ulcer being saucerized with the use of razor blade, sterilized and bent between thumb and index finger.

Can an alternative technique be used or does the situation warrant the added risks of regional/general anesthesia?

Injecting agents such as lidocaine or marcaine into the area to be debrided does not seem to work well. The area is usually hyperemic and may be acidotic, making these agents perform poorly. Also, in order to "block" the entire ulcer bed multiple injection sites are needed and one never seems to be able to block the bed itself, where the most aggressive debridement is needed.

Control of Bleeding

A drawback of sharp debridement is the risk of excessive bleeding. Control can sometimes be difficult since the blood vessels at the interface between hyperemic and devitalized tissue constrict poorly and bleeding can be profuse. Also, if tissues carry a large bioburden of bacteria, there may be a lush growth of neovascularization and bleeding may occur over wide, broad areas in addition to small individual vessels. Brisk bleeding from an otherwise healthy appearing wound bed may indicate a wound with greater than 10^5 bacteria, may require antimicrobial therapy and, if local factors (pain, hyperemia, wound regression) warrant, systemic antimicrobial therapy. Controlling a point of bleeding usually can be accomplished with point pressure and limb elevation if the wound is on a distal extremity. Chemical agents may also be used, but in addition to controlling bleeding, they also injure tissue. A point source may be controlled with a silver nitrate stick applied lightly to the source. This chemically denatures protein and seals the blood vessel. Diffuse bleeding from a surface may be much harder to control. Rolling silver nitrate sticks over the source sometimes works, but the rate of bleeding needs to be reduced first with elevation and pressure. Monsel's solution (ferric subsulfate), a chemical "styptic" agent is a better agent for diffuse surface bleeding or bleeding which is difficult to localize from a cavity or tunnel. The solution agglutinates surface proteins, sealing blood vessels with less heat than that generated from silver nitrate or electrical cautery (see Figure 9). The agent is simply applied to appropriately sized gauze or painted on with a Q-tip. The gauze can then be packed into the cavity or applied to the surface with light pressure applied for a few minutes. Significant bleeding can be brought under control with this method. The solution is relatively cheap and stores for months unrefrigerated. Since it comes in a multiple-use vial or container, there is concern that it may harbor bacteria, which may then be passed from patient to patient. However, microbiologic inoculation studies and contamination surveys indicate that Monsel's solution has properties that prohibit microbial growth. Both chemical agents (Monsel's and silver nitrate) cause tissue damage and discolor the wound bed: an important point to pass on to the next person who is to change the dressing since it may, on first inspection, look as if the wound has suddenly necrosed, taking on a gray-blackened appearance from the chemicals.

Electrical cautery (Bovie) can be used to control significant bleeding and is very effective. However, this requires special expertise, a costly cautery unit, and it will cause significant pain if the area is not deeply anesthetized or insensate.

With the appropriate analgesic and hemostatic agents on hand, sharp debridement then requires the appropriate instruments. Usually this is done with forceps to hold traction on the tissue to be removed (a "toothed" Addson's) and a fine, curved scissors or small scalpel (#15 blade). The curve in the scissors is an important feature used to keep the tips out of the tissue being debrided. The #15 blade scalpel also is small enough to control easily and the cutting surface is back from the tip, keeping the instrument from entering healthy tissue. Care must be taken to remove debris only in parallel with healthy tissue, thus avoiding creating tunnels, crevices and cutting into the hyperemic wound border, which can cause significant bleeding. This technique is illustrated at Figure 10, where a Stage III ulcer with adherent slough, moistened and separating after the use of enzymes, is being cut away with scalpel and forceps. Adherent slough may also be shaved from a wound bed with a sharp bone curette or wire loop, each being used to remove layers of devitalized tissue parallel to the wound bed or edge. Tunnels or undermined areas can also be effectively debrided with a curette (Figure 7).

Depending on the size of the wound, effectiveness of pain control, bleeding and overall goal of the debriding session, the wound may not be totally clean after only one procedure. Many small debriding sessions may be needed with frequent reassessments before the goal of a clean wound is reached. Once healthy tissue is exposed, topical occlusive wound care must be established to keep that tissue healthy and promote healing. Finding necrotic tissue at the next session may mean that the tissue was allowed to dry before angiogeneis could occur or that the tissue bed is overall ischemic and wider debridements will only create an enlarging wound. A different strategy must then be sought, as this is no longer an isolated wound problem.

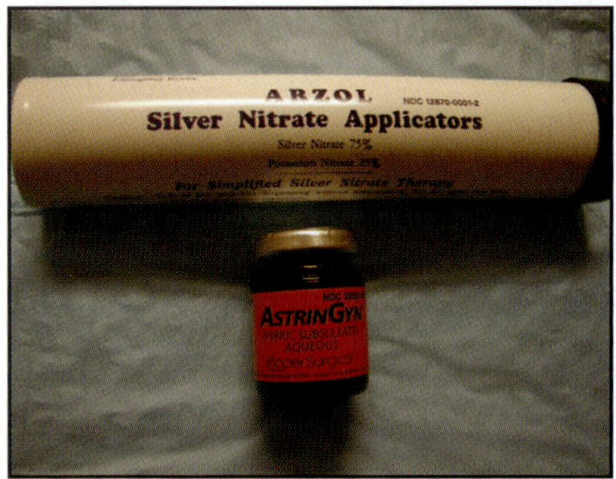

Figure 9. Silver nitrate and Monsel's solution: used for hemostasis.

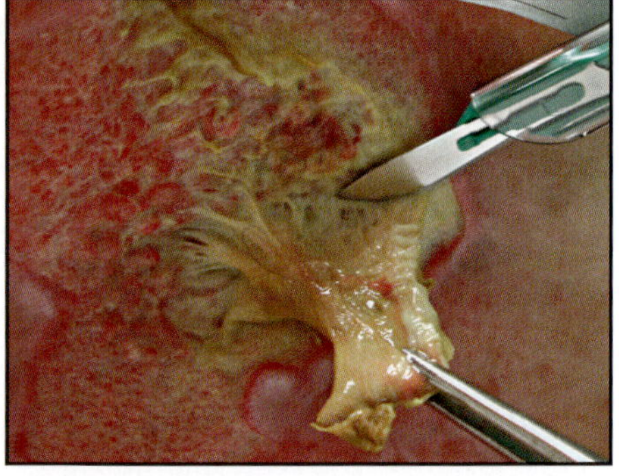

Figure 10. Decubitus ulcer being sharply debrided after eschar softened with collagenase. Note parallel angle of the blade, heel of the blade being used to cut, not the point.

Laser

Laser is certainly the "high tech" form of debridement and the most intriguing. There are relatively "low cost" (tens of thousands of dollars) diode lasers commercially available (Figure 11, CeramOptec; 515 Shaker Road East Longmeadow, MA) which are compact and easily suited for the outpatient setting. The low power beam, which is tunable from 1–50 watts, is easily controlled from a hand-held pencil-size device that can be focused on the wound bed and the tissue vaporized very precisely. There are some reports in

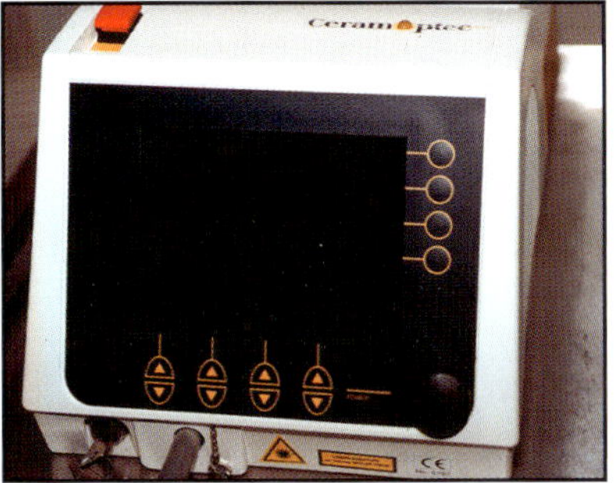

Figure 11. CeramOptec Diode Laser

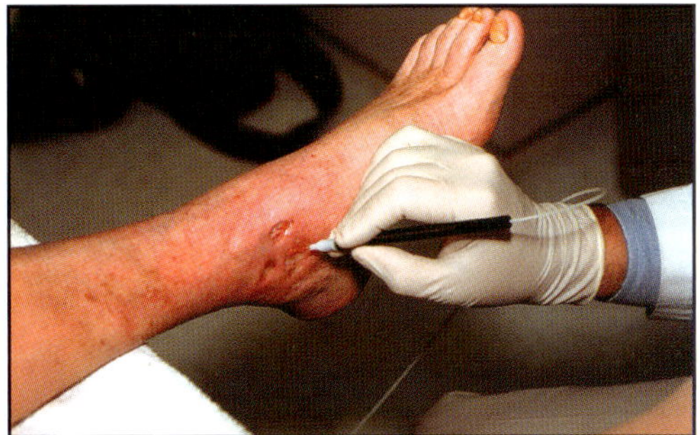

Figure 12. Diode laser being used to debride leg ulcer after being anesthetized with topical EMLA, and the tissue vaporized very precisely.

the literature using CO_2 lasers that this process is not only effective in debridement, but also "sterilizes" the wound bed since the beam is bactericidal (Figure 12).

Heating that vaporizes the tissue occurs over a very small area. Little "collateral" heating occurs and hence tissue not in direct contact with the beam remains unharmed. With the diode laser, the beam can be "pulsed" or "continuous." The "pulsed" mode is somewhat better tolerated with less heat build up over time. However, this is not "painless surgery" as the vaporizing beam can be painful and the same analgesic issues with sharp debridement apply to laser debridement. As with all medical lasers the unit and procedure needs its own space, apart from the flow of patients where eye protection is worn and only those participating are exposed. The glass electrode is disposable from patient to patient and is a cost concern.

An intriguing aspect of this form of debridement is that the energy used to vaporize tissue may also have an effect on the wound bed which may stimulate senescent cells, much as other forms of wound therapy (UV/C, electrical, thermal) may be "turning on" dormant processes. This is largely unproven, but small animal studies do show some promise. How this form of debridement fits into the overall armamentarium remains to be seen.

Ultrasound

One of the more exciting and promising tools of debridement, which also is nicely suited to the outpatient wound clinic, is low-frequency ultrasound. Like a laser, ultrasound can not only rid the wound of surface debris and necrotic tissue, but it also can provide a source of energy, which stimulates the wound bed, probably through a mechanism of low-level injury. The device allows for very selective debridement. The energy is directed through a small, hand held probe which is moved across the wound surface disrupting devitalized tissue while preserving healthy tissue. Figure 13A shows a venous stasis ulcer with adherent slough, and Figure 13B shows a venous stasis ulcer surface debridement with ultrasound. The equipment to provide this type of debridement (Soring Ultrasound Debrider (Figure 14A) and Soring Ultrasound Hand Piece (Figure 14B); *Soring Inc., 6646 Iron Horse Blvd. Suite D, North Richland Hills, TX 76180*) is fairly expensive: \$60,000.00–\$70,000.00, but the hand probes which actually perform the debridement are reusable over many times and are steam sterilized,

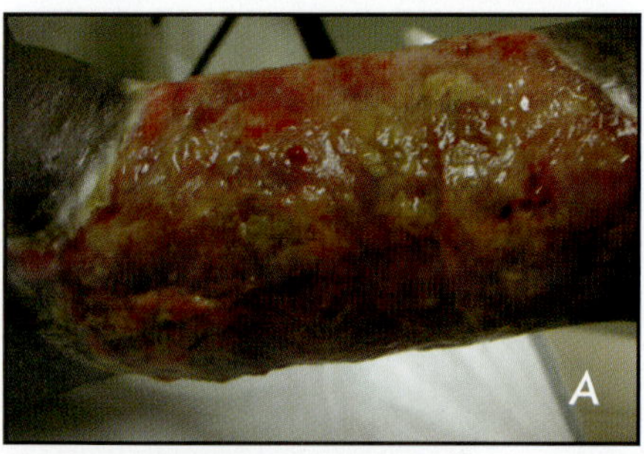
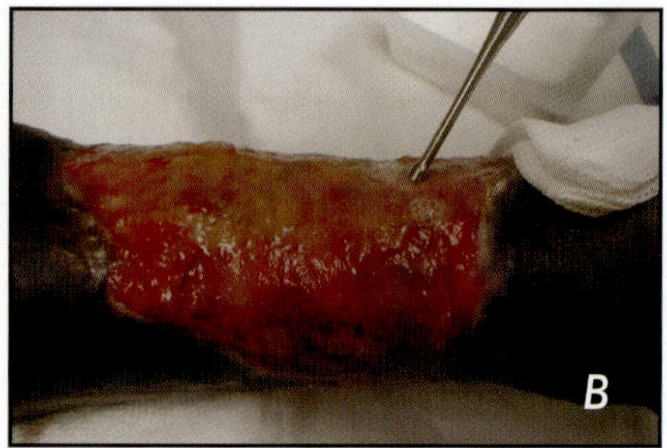

Figure 13. (A) Venous stasis wound: adherent slough.
(B) Venous stasis wound: surface debridement with ultrasound.

which can be done easily over a period of an hour. With two probes, then, four patients per AM or PM session can be treated.

In addition to debridement of surface eschar and debris, the following effects of low-frequency ultrasound have been claimed and reported on:

- Antimicrobial effect: directly bacterio/fungicidal to all (MRSA, VRE, etc)
- Disruption/removal of biofilms
- Enhancement of fibrinolysis
- Local vasodilatation

The antimicrobial effects are particularly interesting. Often the chronic wound fails to progress because of a heavy local bacterial tissue load which is harbored in the inert "biofilm" or eschar. By selectively ridding the wound of this layer healing cellular mechanisms may again proceed.

By coupling the delivery of the ultrasonic waves through a water-flush mechanism, debris is washed away, the wound is "cooled," avoiding local heating and coupling is enhanced. In addition, different hand piece tip configurations allow adjustment to different wound surfaces. The continuous stream of ultrasonic energy, coupled to a water spray provides custom, minimally invasive surface debridement to a 5 cm ulcer in as little as 5–10 minutes, beginning to end.

Like everything in medicine, nothing is without risk. The same is true for ultrasonic debridement. Initial cost is by far the most potent deterrent to its use. Not all wounds are candidates for ultrasonic debridement. The wounds most

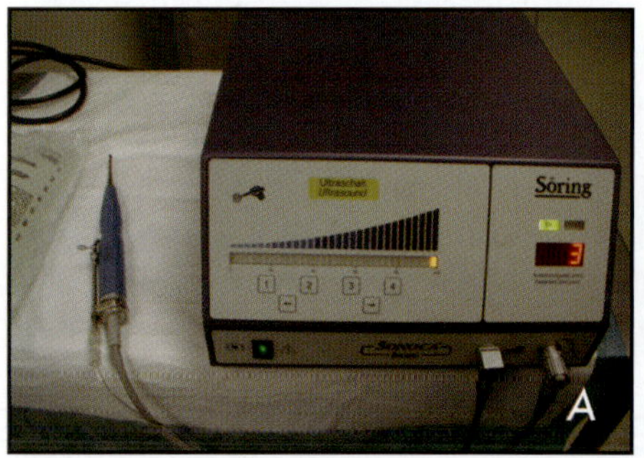
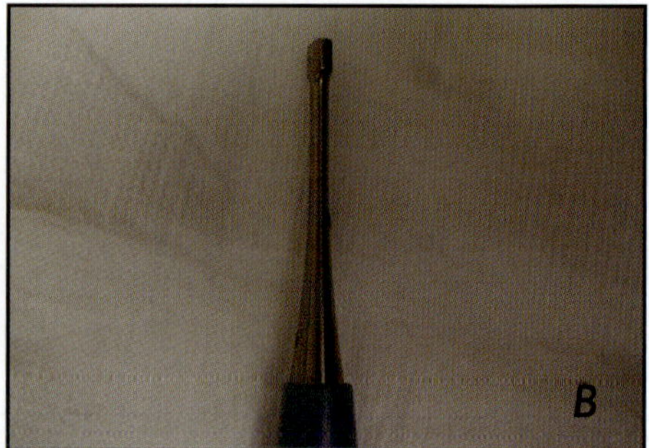

Figure 14. (A) Soring Ultrasonic Debrider. (B) Soring Ultrasonic Hand Piece.

likely to respond to this modality are those with flat surfaces with relatively shallow debris/eschar/biofilms. Pain can also be an issue. A patient with a painful wound will not tolerate the ultrasonic device without first some topical relief, usually with lidocaine or EMLA. Of course the asensate, neuropathic ulcer is perfectly suited for the process. Also, ulcers with deep, spreading infections or large/thick areas of necrotic tissue are not amenable to this modality. In such wounds a more extirpative, invasive process such as operative debridement should probably be used first to drain and remove the infective agents. The water spray that accompanies the delivery of the ultrasonic waves can also be a problem. Contamination outside the wound area may occur, and protective eyewear is vital.

Biosurgery

The blow fly larva, *Phaenicia sericata*, (maggots) has been used as a biosurgical debriding agent in the USA for over 70 years. First used as therapy in the 1930's, it fell out of favor when antibiotics became available, but now may be returning because of some unique characteristics. Maggots have been used successfully to debride pressure ulcers, venous stasis ulcers, diabetic foot ulcers and soft tissue wounds resulting from necrotizing soft tissue infections. Thirty larvae can consume 1 gram of tissue per day. They are radiation sterilized before they are used, so that they cannot convert from the larva to the pupae stage, thereby precluding flying insects from emanating from the wound! It is precise. Only necrotic debris is removed. After the larvae are applied, the wound is continually debrided until they are removed 2–3 days later. The larvae liquefy necrotic debris/tissue, kill bacteria (strept, staph, MRSA) by ingestion and digestion while secreting antibacterial secretions (ammonia) and in so doing stimulate the growth of healthy tissue. Usually, only one application of ten larvae per cm^2 is necessary to completely debride the wound, but further applications are possible if necessary to produce a clean wound.

With the advent of the Internet, the availability of the larvae (shipped through overnight mail) is but a few mouse clicks away at: *www.ucihs.uci.edu/com/pathology/sherman/home_pg.htm*.

The larvae are specially grown for this use and are sterile: they do not reproduce in the wound. After being placed into the wound the larvae immediately ingest debris/bacteria and become many times their initial size some days later, when they are removed. The process is painless and very effective especially in debriding wounds associated with interstices, tunnels, crevices, and difficult to access areas such as in the perineum and base of the skull. The larva will not burrow under skin, ingest healthy tissue nor will they "breed" in the wound. In a sensate area, however, the patient may feel movement from the larvae. A custom multi-layered dressing needs to used with this therapy, both to keep the maggots in place and to provide air/oxygen ingress while wicking away effluent which if heavy may be harmful to the maggots. Usually some sort of netting over which an absorbent dressing is used, the absorbent outer dressing changed as frequently as necessary so as to not allow fluid buildup in the wound cavity. Since even the least squeamish patient does not want to see maggots crawling in their tissue, some opaque covering also is used. (*http://www.ucihs.uci.edu/som/pathology/sherman/home_pg.htm*)

REFERENCES

1. Root-Bernstein R, Root-Bernstein M. Honey, Mud, Maggots and Other Medical Marvels: The Science Behind Folk Remedies and Old Wives Tales; Mariner Books, 1997.

2. Agren MS, Stromberg HE. Topical treatment of pressure ulcers: a randomized comparative trial of Varidase and zinc oxide. *Scand J Plast Renconstr Surg* 1985; 19(1): 97-100.

3. Galpin JE, Chow AW, Bayer AS, et al. Sepsis associated with decubitus ulcers. *Am J Med* 1976, Sept; 61(3): 346-50.

4. Lydon MJ, et al. Dissolution of wound coagulum and promotion of granulation tissue under DuoDerm. *Wounds* 1989 Aug;1(2): 95-106.

5. Lyman IR, Tenery JH, Basson RP. Correlation between decrease in bacterial load and rate of wound healing. *Surg Gynecol Obstet* 1970 Apr;130(4):616-21.

6. Gardner S, Frantz R, Doebbeling B. The validity of the clinical signs and symptoms used to identify localized chronic wound infection. *Wound Repair and Regeneration* 2001May-June 9: 178-186.

7. Falabella A. Debridement of Wounds. *Wounds* 1998 10 supplement C:1C-9C.

8. Mast B, Schultz G. Interactions of cytokines, growth factors and proteases in acute and chronic wounds. *Wound Repair and Regeneration* 1996 Oct-Dec 4: 411-420.

9. Rodeheaver GT, Smith SL, Thacker JG, et al. Mechanical cleansing of contaminated wounds with a surfactant. *Am J Surg* 1975 Mar; 129(3):241-5.

10. Daltrey DC, Rhodes B, Chattwood JG. Investigation into the microbial flora of healing and non-healing decubitus ulcers. *J Clin Pathol* 1981 Jul; 34(7):701-5.

11. Robson MC. Plastic surgery in quantitative bacteriology: its role in the armamentarium of the surgeon. In: Heggers JP, Robson MC, editors. Boca Raton, FL: CRC Press: 1991;71-84.

12. Hulten L. Dressings for surgical wounds. *Am J Surg* 1994;167:521-4.

13. Hutchinson JJ. Prevalence of wound infection under occlusive dressings: a collected survey of reported research. *Wounds* 1989;1:123-33.

14. Shapira E, Giladi A, Neiman Z. Use of water insoluble papain for debridement of burn eschar and necrotic tissue. Plast Reconstruct Surg 1973;52(3): 279.

15. Boxer AM, Gottesman N, Bernstein H, et al. Debridement of dermal ulcers and decubiti with collagenase. *Geriatrics* 1969 Jul;24(7):75-86.

16. Lee LK, Ambrus JL. Collagenase therapy for decubitus ulcers. *Geriatrics* 1975 May;30(5):91-3, 97-8.

17. Mosher B, Cuddigan J, Thomas D, et al. Outcomes of 4 methods of debridement using a decision analysis methodology. *Advances in Wound Care* 1999 Mar 12(2): 81-8.

18. Steed DL, Donohoe D, Webster MW, et al. Effect of extensive debridement and treatment on the healing of diabetic foot ulcers. *J Am Coll Surg* 1996 183: 61-64.

19. Lok C, et al. EMLA cream as a topical anesthetic for the repeated mechanical debridement of venous leg ulcers: A double blind, placebo-controlled study. *Journal of the American Academy of Dermatology* 1999 Feb 40(2): 208-213.

20. Jetmore A, Heryer J, Conner W. Monsel's solution: a kinder, gentler hemostatic. *Dis Colon Rectum* 1993 36(9): 866-867.

21. Rodeheaver GT, Smith SL, Thacker JG, et al. Mechanical cleansing of contaminated wounds with a surfactant. *Am J Surg* 1975 Mar;129(3):241-5.

22. Marangoni O, Melato M. Surgical cleansing of varicose ulcers of the leg using a CO_2 laser with rotating mirror scanner. *Journal of Clinical Laser Medicine & Surgery* 1998;16(3): 181-184.

23. Lee J, Tarpley, K, Miller A. CO2 Laser sterilization in the surgical treatment of infected median sternotomy wounds. *Southern Medical Journal* 1999 Apr 92(4): 380-384.

24. Thomas S. Using larva in modern wound management. *Journal of Wound Care* 1996 5: 60-69.

25. Sherman R. Maggot therapy for venous stasis ulcers. *Archives of Dermatology* 1996 132(3): 254-256.

26. Sherman R. A new dressing design for use with maggot therapy. *Plastic and Reconstructive Surgery* 1997 100(2): 451-456.

27. Mustoe, T. Chronic wound pathogenesis and current treatment strategies: a unifying hypothesis. *Plastic and Reconstructive Surgery* 2006 June Supp: 35S-41S.

28. Robson, M. Wound infection: A failure of wound healing caused by an imbalance of bacteria. *Surgical Clinics of North America* 1997 77:637.

29. Rupp, M. Monsel's solution: a potential vector for nosocomial infection? *Infection Control and Hospital Epidemiology* 2003 24: 142-144.

30. Attinger, C. Clinical approach to wounds: debridement and wound bed preparation including the use of dressings and wound-healing adjuvants. *Plastic and Reconstructive Surgery*. 2006 117(7S): 72S-109S.

REVIEW QUESTIONS

1.) The principle reason to quantitatively culture a chronic wound is to:
   a. Define the number of organisms per gram of tissue
   b. Define the type of wound inoculum: bacteria, fungus or virus
   c. Define the sensitivity of the organisms to help guide antibiotic therapy
   d. Decide if the "bioburden" is principally biologic or non-biologic

2.) Choice of debridement is determined by:
   a. Type and amount of debris to be removed
   b. Urgency of the debridement
   c. Ability of the person doing the debridement
   d. All of the above

3.) Properly done, a "wet-to-dry" dressing:
   a. Adheres to the underlying wound bed, indiscriminately removing any adherent tissue
   b. Is left uncovered to facilitate drying the gauze to the wound bed
   c. Is done infrequently to ensure adequate drying an adherence to the wound bed
   d. Usually offers the advantage of being done with relatively cheap materials
   e. A and D

4.) A common component of ultrasound, electrical stimulation and laser debridement is that they:
   a. All require the user to be specially licensed
   b. All provide some type of energy to the wound bed which then may stimulate senescent cells
   c. All require protective eyewear for the patient and user
   d. All require the patient to be on an IRB approved protocol, since all are experimental

5.) Debriding a wound "autolytically" requires
   a. A moist environment
   b. High levels of topically applied enzymes
   c. Cooperative, knowledgeable patients, since they do their own debridement
   d. High bacterial counts, since the bacteria supply the autologous enzymes

Answers: 1a, 2d, 3e, 4b, 5d.

PRINCIPLES OF SURGICAL WOUND MANAGEMENT

CHAPTER TEN OVERVIEW

NOTES

Principles of Surgical Wound Management

Donald M. Greer, Jr., James Martin Smith, David L. McCorvey

INTRODUCTION

When dealing with illness or injury, the goal is to return the patient to his previous state of well-being as quickly as possible. Furthermore, we must strive to do so at the lowest possible cost, and with minimal discomfort or pain for the patient.

The goal of surgical wound management is to obtain the best possible scar, in the shortest possible time, at the least possible expense, and with minimum discomfort to the patient. The best possible scar will be soft and pliable. The scar will lie in Relaxed Skin Tension Lines, and be as narrow as possible so as to provide the best possible esthetic result. The scar, while pliable, will be durable, able to stand up to the stress of daily life.

These goals are often modified by the patient's circumstances. We must treat the whole patient, not just the hole in the patient. A high fashion model will react very differently to a wound on the forehead from an assailant than a construction worker with the same wound created by a flying piece of scrap metal. They both deserve to be returned to their previous state of life. The construction worker will want to return to work as quickly as possible, with as few trips to the surgeon's suite as possible since his livelihood is unaffected by a small alteration in physical appearance. The model, whose livelihood is dependent on her physical appearance, will shield her wound from the sun for months, keep pressure on the scar for months, spend countless hours agonizing over the esthetic result, and may well ask for repeated dermaplaning to minimize the scar.

People have different preexisting health conditions, some of which profoundly affect wound healing. These must be kept in mind. An open wound on the ankle of an elderly paraplegic patient with diabetes and congestive failure is a far different matter than the same wound on the ankle of a marathon runner. Optimum management of a patient with a complex wound is often best accomplished if a team approach is utilized involving primary physician, wound care specialist, plastic and reconstructive surgeon, nutritionist, and other specialists. Underlying health care issues must be tended to if the best result is to be obtained. The reader is reminded, "Trifles make perfection, but perfection is no trifle."

Some wounds are easy and straightforward to manage, while others require sophisticated techniques to close. Some wounds are difficult to close with one technique, while another technique will close that same wound with ease. The same wound may sometimes be appropriately handled in several different ways with significantly different but acceptable final results. Furthermore a complex wound may benefit from different techniques at different stages in its healing. For this reason the skilled wound care specialist will constantly monitor the wounds being cared for. The wound will be observed to make sure it is making appropriate progress on a regular basis.

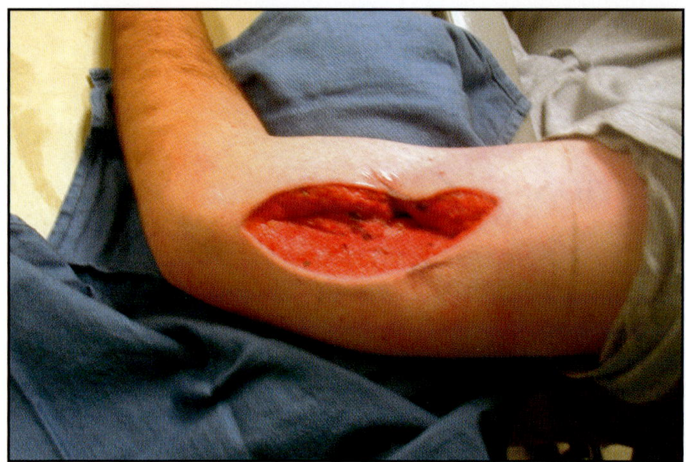

Figure 1. Clean granulating arm wound. The granulation tissue is uniform, and has a smooth rich red color.

Wounds do heal at a predictable rate. With experience the wound care specialist will learn the various stages of wound healing, and the rate at which they proceed. Deviation from this expected course should alert the wound care specialist that this wound is not progressing as expected. This must prompt a search for the reason healing is not progressing as expected. Correcting the problem will result in better results.

The process of wound healing is complex. Contraction and epithelialization are the two processes the wound care specialist deals with in managing wound healing. Careful and thoughtful observation of these two processes as wounds heal will bring greater understanding of the wound healing process, and better everyday care of patients with wounds.

Wound contraction results in a steady decrease in the size of the open defect, primarily due to the action of the myofibroblast. Contraction is a powerful force, which can be either beneficial or destructive to the patient. If a large open wound crossing a joint is allowed to heal by contraction, it may well produce a horrible deformity. The same size open wound on the buttock may contract to produce a quite acceptable scar. Wounds should never be allowed to heal by contraction if it will produce a deformity of adjacent anatomical structures. Not only is the anatomical location of the wound important, the age and condition of the patient will influence the wound healing process.

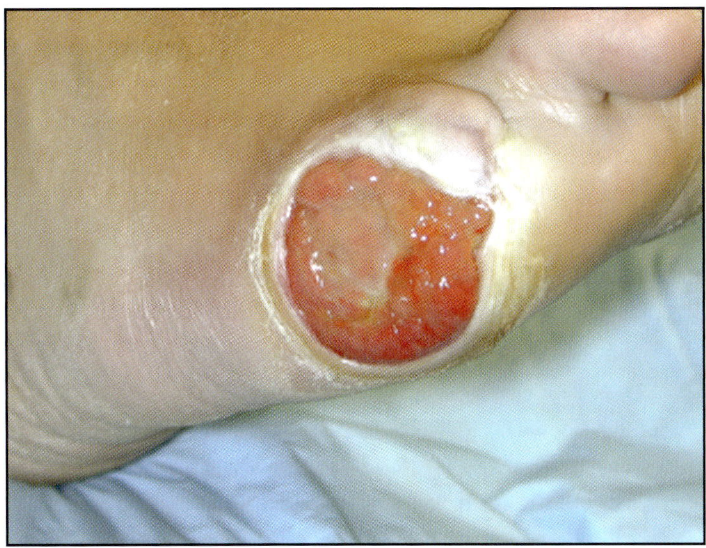

Figure 2. A chronic wound on the foot. This wound displays poor granulation tissue. Note the unevenness of the granulation tissue, and the glistening surface, which is indicative of edema in the tissue. The discerning observer will note a thin rim of pearly white tissue at the margin of the wound from 9 to 10 o'clock. This is typical of epithelial cells advancing across the wound. Note that the tissue in the bottom right part of the wound is hypertrophic granulation tissue.

Epithelialization is the process in which basal cells migrate across the wound surface to complete closure of a wound. Although individual cells cannot be seen, the advancing wave of cells can be seen as a thin border of pearly white creeping across the open surface. Seeing this pearly border is a sign the wound is doing well.

Knowing how wounds heal and at what rate also allows the wound care specialist to better evaluate new or different therapies. If it is proposed to treat an open wound which we know will heal in 11 days if treated in the usual way with the latest and greatest new development in wound dressing, which enables the wound to heal in ten days at triple the cost, the skilled wound care specialist will know whether the result is worth the added expense of the new therapy.

It is appropriate to consider the experience and technical skills of those caring for the wound. Some surgeons have better results with one technique than another. Obviously, if two possible operations will close the wound equally well, the surgeon should elect that procedure in which he personally has better results. If however, the wound clearly requires a procedure which the consulted surgeon is not comfortable doing, or does not routinely obtain good results with, further consultation is appropriate. Some wound care specialists have nearly universal success treating stasis ulcers with Unna Boots, while others rarely succeed. Either use a technique you know you will succeed with, or refer the patient to someone who usually does have success.

APPROACHES

Approaches to wound closure may be thought of in four groups:

1. Primary closure is usually the best alternative, and will customarily be chosen when possible.
2. Healing by secondary intention is the method to which most wound care specialists devote most of their efforts. It usually takes a prolonged time to complete. The wound care specialist dedicated to providing the best for his patients will ask whether another treatment modality would produce a healed wound sooner, or would produce a better result, and will guide treatment decisions accordingly.
3. Grafting refers to the process of *taking a block of tissue from one part of the body and placing it on another part of the body.* This means that the tissue being moved loses its blood supply, and therefore must acquire a blood supply from the area upon which it is placed (The bed). The area from which the tissue is taken (donor site) will have a wound as a result of taking the graft. If the donor site is small, it may be closed primarily. If it is large, then it will have to heal by other means. Because taking a graft always leaves a scar, the donor site must be chosen carefully. Grafts may be thin (split thickness skin grafts), or increasingly thicker. The thinner the graft, the more apt the graft will be able to successfully acquire a blood supply in the new site, and survive ("take"). Conversely, the thicker the graft, the greater the chance it will fail to acquire a blood supply sufficient to nourish it, and will fail. However thicker grafts which are successful will have greater durability, and have a better color match. Grafts which do not include dermis will contract significantly, while those grafts which contain dermis usually do not contract.
4. A flap is *a block of tissue taken from one part of the body and moved to another part of the body while maintaining its blood supply.* Because a flap keeps its blood supply, it will heal in wounds with very poor blood supply. Underlying anatomical structures which need to glide is another indication for a flap. Because a flap will keep it's color and consistency, and because it keeps the characteristics it had in the donor area, a flap may be used to reconstruct an esthetically import area, allowing the scars to be moved into less conspicuous places.

A flap may also be moved to a distant part of the body by reestablishing its blood supply with microvascular anastomoses. These are called "free flaps" or "neovascularised flaps."

There are almost always several different ways to close a wound. Balancing the advantages and disadvantages of the various approaches is important in selecting the best way to treat that particular patient. We want to obtain the best functional and aesthetic result possible, but we must bear in mind the financial and functional costs involved. The classical example of this dilemma is the carpenter who amputates his little finger at the mid-middle phalanx level. While reimplantation of the digit is technically possible, this would require prolonged and repeated hospitalizations, months of rehabilitation, and significant discomfort and pain. That carpenter is probably better off with closure of the amputation site, allowing a quick return to work. A classical pianist with the same injury represents a different set of parameters.

The KISS (Keep It Simple) principle should be remembered. More often than not it proves correct.

The choice of closure should progress from simple to complex. If a graft or flap is necessary, the choice should progress from the closest appropriate tissue to the more distant.

Any solution which produces a secondary problem equal to or greater than the original problem must never be chosen.

TECHNIQUES OF SURGICAL WOUND MANAGEMENT

Before proceeding to what seems the best way to close a wound, it is wise to review all the options in order to make sure the best choice has been considered. A list of possible techniques would include:

- Do nothing
- Primary closure
- Delayed wound closure
- Healing by secondary intention
- Grafts
    - Split Thickness Grafts
    - Full Thickness Grafts
    - Composite Grafts
- Flaps
    - Random Flaps
    - Axial Flaps
    - Musculocutaneous Flaps
    - Fasciocutaneous Flaps
    - Neovascularised Flaps

No Closure

Closing a wound does provide several advantages including accelerating the healing process, minimizing scar formation, reducing the risk of infection and contamination, and preventing fluid loss from an open wound. Wounds which do not breach the dermis will heal without a scar, and should be left to heal on their own. Prevention of infection, which would potentially breach the dermis is needed, nothing else.

The younger the patient the stronger the forces of wound contraction. A soft tissue only fingertip amputation in a very young patient which is allowed to heal by contraction will leave an almost imperceptible scar. An adult with the same wound will need operative management.

This is obviously the simplest way to manage a wound.

Primary Closure

Primary closure is the next simplest and best choice for uncomplicated wounds. However if the wound involves loss of so much tissue that significant tension is produced by primary closure, then other techniques need to be considered. Primary closure of a wound that results in deformation of an adjoining anatomical structure is unacceptable. In such cases, it is far better to apply a saline dressing and refer the patient to a reconstructive center even if it delays wound closure.

If the wound crosses relaxed skin tension lines, then the resulting scar will almost certainly be significant. A very experienced plastic surgeon might consider a flap or a z-plasty as part of the primary closure to produce a more flexible and better esthetic result. The planning of such procedures requires significant skill and experience, and should not be attempted by the inexperienced. These procedures can almost always be performed at a later date without compromising the final result.

Delayed Wound Closure

Delayed wound closure is indicated for wounds that are contaminated or contain devitalized tissue. In this technique, the wound is initially debrided as though it were to be closed at the time. Rather than being closed however, a dressing is placed in the wound. Some surgeons will then inspect the wound daily, but in the classical Delayed Wound Closure, the wound is covered with a dressing, which is left undisturbed for 3–4 days. At the end of that time the dressing is removed for the first time, and the wound carefully inspected for signs of infection or devitalized tissues. If the wound appears clean the wound is closed without further debridement. If signs of infection, or inadequate debridement appear, then the wound is treated as an infected wound. The wound healing process is not delayed using this technique.

Healing by Secondary Intention

A wound allowed to heal "on its own" is said to be "healing by secondary intention." Although this technique takes significantly longer than others, it avoids the problems of a trip to the operating room, and offers the ability to heal a wound which is grossly infected. The wound care specialist will see many cases of healing by secondary intention in the wound care center. The processes of wound contraction and epithelialization are responsible for the success of healing by secondary intention.

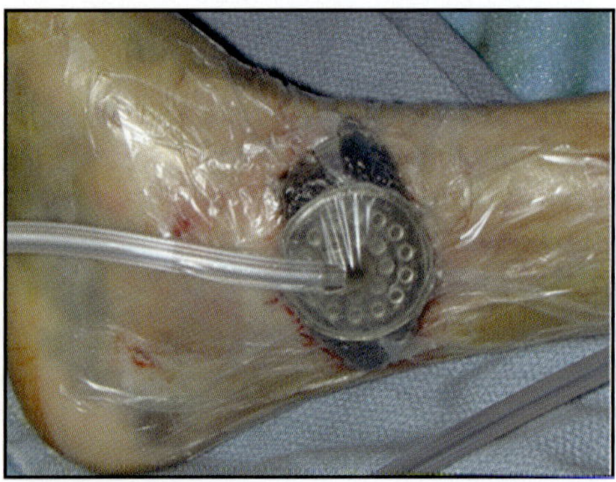

Figure 3. VAC device on the lower extremity.

Grafts

Although it is most common to move skin (i.e., split thickness skin graft), other types of tissue such as cartilage, bone, tendon, cornea, or fat can also be grafted. If the tissue comes from the patient, it is called an autograft. If the graft comes from another human, it is called an allograft. If the graft comes from another species, it is called a heterograft or xenograft. The most common heterografts for skin use are porcine, which are readily available commercially.

In general, skin grafts are used to close wounds when the area to be closed is greater than can be conveniently closed by either primary closure or by a flap. The goal of wound closure, in other words, is the restoration of the body's protective barrier.

In order to be successful the graft must come in close contact with the recipient bed and nothing must get between the graft and the bed. Immobilization is vital in order to ensure that no motion occurs between the graft and the host bed.

Temporary closure of a wound may be obtained with a variety of skin graft substitutes, which include amniotic grafts, allografts from cadaver donors, heterografts mostly from porcine donors, and synthetic skin substitute dressings. All of these grafts provide only a temporary closure of the wound. If they are left in place for a prolonged period, they will undergo rejection through the immune process. It is best to think of all of these aforementioned agents as biological dressings. Application of these dressings is quite simple and straightforward. It is a bedside technique. Anesthesia is not necessary. These grafts are often used to preparing a wound for subsequent split thickness skin autografting. If a heterograft successfully adheres to a wound bed and appears to "take," then a split thickness autograft is likely to be successful. If, however, the heterograft either floats off the bed or is dissolved in a sea of pus, the likelihood of success with a split thickness autograft is slim.

Heterografts do attach to the wound bed, and they do establish a vascular supply. This process can be useful in cleaning up a badly infected wound in preparation for autografting. If heterografts are applied as a dressing and changed regularly, they will gradually exclude pus from the graft/wound interface. This allows healthy granulation tissue to become established, which will result in a healthy bed on which to place an autograft. The heterograft should never be left in place for more than one week or else the rejection process may become initiated. Subsequent applications of heterografts that are left in place will be rejected with increasing speed. Though heterografts are costly, the expense is well worthwhile if they lead to successful takes of subsequent autografts.

Split graft

Split thickness skin grafts (autografts) provide permanent closure of a wound. Great variability exists among split thickness skin grafts in terms of thickness and the location in which they are placed. If all other things are equal, a thinner graft will usually be quicker to adhere, to become vascularized, and to heal. A thinner graft also means that the donor site will heal with less scarring. Thinner grafts are also more likely to take on a marginal host bed. However, thin grafts are significantly less durable than thicker grafts. The texture of thin grafts is not the same as that of the surrounding skin. They lack the subcutaneous glands of normal skin. Thus, they will not sweat and will not have the usual secretions necessary to lubricate the skin. Thin grafts almost always contract or shrink up in size. This can be an advantage if the wound is in the center of a large anatomical area. However, this can prove to be detrimental if the wound is near an anatomical feature or near a joint. The thinner a graft the more it will contract. Thin grafts are also usually lighter in color than either the donor site or the area surrounding the recipient site.

Split thickness skin grafts range in thickness from 0.004 inches (0.102 mm) to about 0.012 inches (0.305 mm). These grafts are best harvested using one of the various mechanical dermatomes. The thinnest practical grafts are 0.004 inches (0.102 mm) thick. These ultra thin grafts will have the structural strength and appearance of a single layer of wet toilet tissue. Thick partial thickness grafts will have considerable structural strength, and they will look like actual skin. Grafts that are significantly greater than 0.012 inches (0.305 mm) thick are closer to full thickness skin grafts.

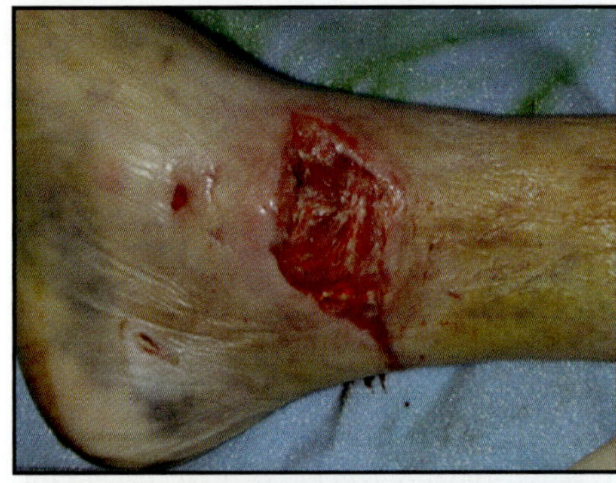

4A. Open wound on the ankle.

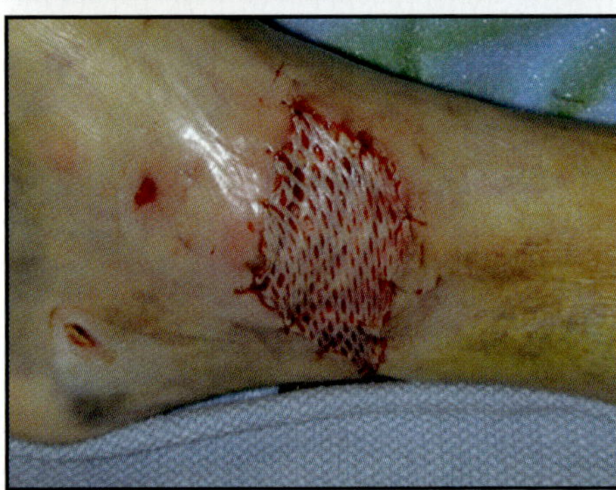

4B. The wound has been covered with a split thickness skin graft, which has been meshed and expanded. Mesh graft have two advantages. They allow a greater area to be covered with same size donor area. Meshing also allows secretions to escape out from under the graft, preventing it from being "floated" off the wound base.

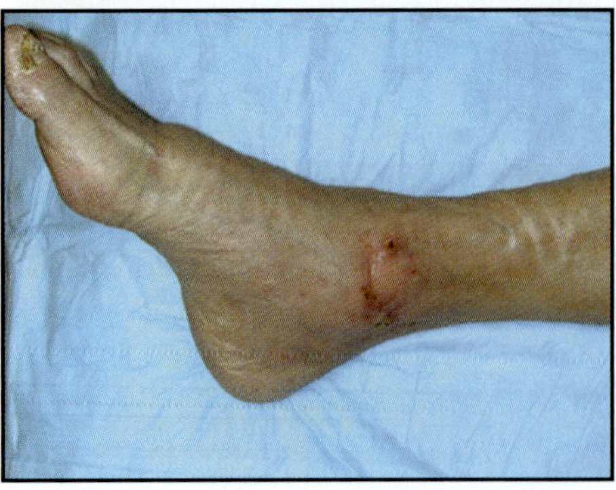

4C. The healed graft. Note the the mesh has filled in. Also note that the graft has contracted, making the wound smaller.

If a graft is taken from a site that has been previously used as a donor site for a split thickness skin graft, then the new graft will retain the color it had on the donor site after it has healed.

In summary, thin grafts generally have the advantage of being more likely to "take," although they are not as durable or aesthetic as the thicker grafts.

Full Thickness Grafts

If a more durable or more aesthetic closure is desired, thicker tissue than a split thickness skin graft must be used. The next thicker technique is a full thickness skin graft. Full thickness grafts usually retain their donor site color, texture, and appearance. They have good durability, but are not very resistant to sheer forces. Because full thickness skin grafts include much more tissue than split thickness grafts they require excellent vascular beds in order to take. Any active infection will almost certainly result in the loss of the full thickness graft. In addition, the donor site must be closed. The donor site closure is usually done by primary closure.

Full thickness grafts contract very little if any. If contraction does occur, it is usually due to an incomplete vascularity of the graft which results in death of part of the graft.

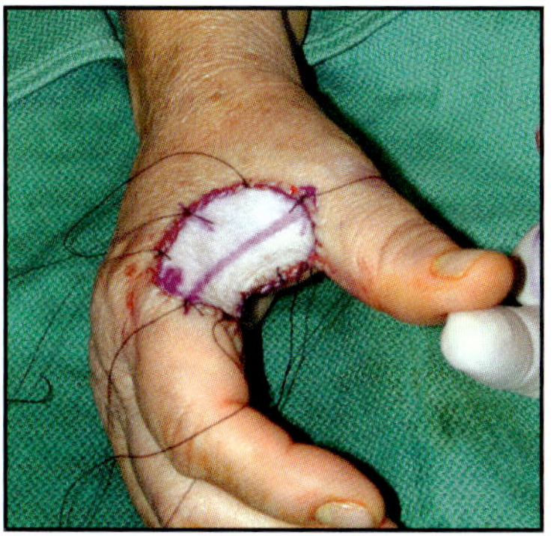

Figure 5. Full thickness skin graft to the right thumb web space.

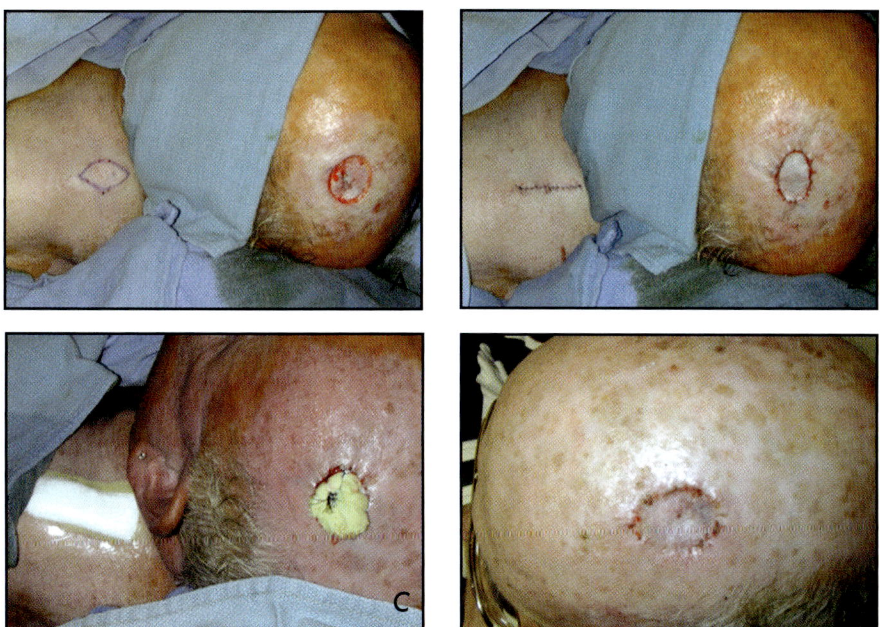

Figure 6 A–D. (A) A full thickness graft is planned from the supraclavicular area to the scalp. (B) The full thickness graft has been taken from the supraclavicular area, trimmed to fit the scalp defect, and sutured into the scalp defect. The supraclavicular donor site has been closed. (C) The full thickness graft has been covered with a tie-over pressure dressing (Stent) to apply pressure to keep the graft in close approximation to the wound base, and to prevent movement. (D) The graft after the stent and sutures are removed.

Because the donor site must be closed, the area available for full thickness grafts is limited. Typical donor sites for full thickness skin grafts include the retroauricular area, the groin, the heel of the hand, or the flexion crease of the wrist. The latter site is sometimes criticized because the resulting donor site scar may resemble a suicide attempt.

Composite Grafts

Composite grafts involve more than one organ system. One example is a graft taken from the helical rim of the ear which includes skin, subcutaneous fat, and sometimes cartilage. Such a graft can be harvested to reconstruct the alar rim of the nose. Choice of a composite graft is driven by the need for aesthetic results. Just as full thickness grafts require a better vascular bed than split thickness grafts, so do composite grafts require an even better blood supply than full thickness grafts. Any motion between the graft and the host bed will lead to graft failure.

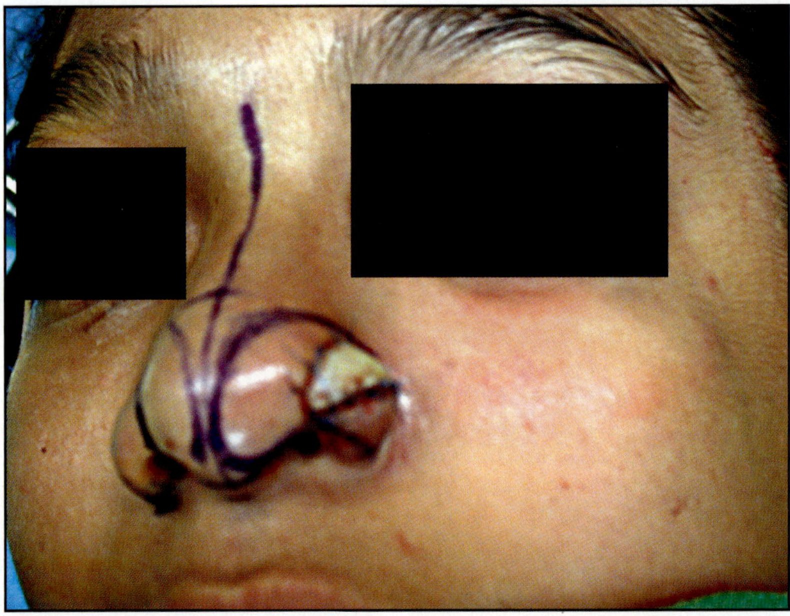

Figure 7. Composite graft reconstruction of left alar rim of the nose.

Flaps

In contrast to grafts, flaps take their own blood supply with them. Flaps will of necessity contain more than one organ system. For example, fasciocutaneous flaps contain skin, subcutaneous fat, blood vessels, lymphatic vessels, and fascia. Flaps may also be designed to contain or carry other organ systems such as bone or muscle. The tissue in flaps maintains its characteristic color, texture, flexibility, and hair pattern in the new location. This, of course, allows for an elegant reconstruction with closely matched tissue. On the other hand, it may lead to undesirable results. In a lip switch flap, for example, a block of tissue taken from the lower lip is rotated 180 degrees to fill a defect in the upper lip. The hair follicles in the flap will then produce a mustache growing up instead of the usual down.

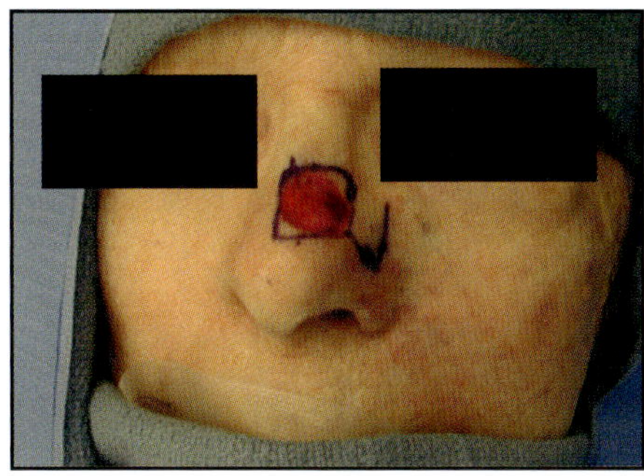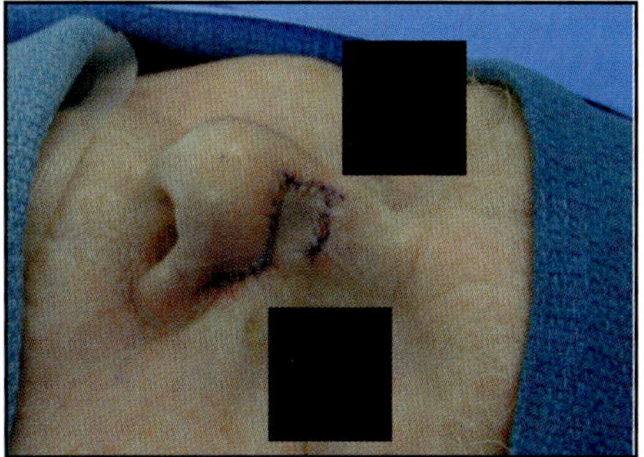

Figure 8 A–B. (A) A defect on the dorsum of the nose with the planning for a rhomboid flap. (B) The rhomboid flap has been advanced into the defect, and the donor site closed.

The design of flaps is too complex for this text, but flaps may be either "axial" or "random" in design. Flaps require expertise in planning and execution. They usually require more time in the operating room than grafts or primary closure. The flap which does well will require less post-operative care than a graft which does well. Flaps may provide excellent aesthetic results. They do require a donor scar in the immediate area. Because they carry subcutaneous tissue with them, they provide good durability and protection from sheer forces.

There are some absolute indications for a flap. If the recipient bed has poor or no blood supply, a graft will not heal, while a flap probably will. Therefore areas of radiation ischemia or exposed bone without viable periosteum need to be covered with a flap. Need for padding is another absolute indication for a flap. Grafts are not able to provide padding and will break down if exposed to pressure or sheer forces. Thus pressure sores or defects on the weight-bearing portion of the sole of the foot need a flap. Another absolute indication for a flap is the need for gliding motion underneath the healed wound. The subcutaneous tissue of a flap provides a milieu on which the tendons are able to glide quite nicely, while a graft will adhere to both tendon and surrounding tissue, and thus fix the tendon in place.

Relative indications for a flap include the need to fill a depression, the need to provide skin which is distensible, and the need to move a scar away from an area for either aesthetic reasons or increased durability.

Random Flaps

Random pattern flaps are skin flaps which rely on the dermal and subdermal vascular plexuses for survival. These are commonly used for reconstruction of small facial defects such as those arising from excision of skin cancers. Large random pattern flaps are sometimes used to close sacral pressure sores. As a general rule, the length of the random pattern flap must not exceed one and one-half times the width of the base or necrosis is likely to occur. One way to overcome the problem of inadequate flap length in a random flap is to perform a "delay" procedure in which the flap is elevated in stages allowing time for the dilatation of existing blood vessels in the flap to support the entire length of the flap. Random flaps are not based on a named vessel in the vascular pedicle.

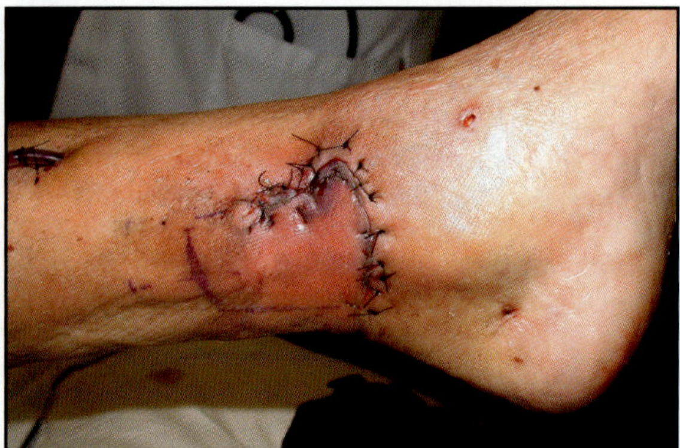

Figure 9. Random pattern flap to cover ankle wound.

Instead, the surgeon trusts to chance that there will be a vessel in the pedicle large enough to provide adequate vascularization to the entire flap. The pedicle of the flap may be left in place as a permanent bridge, or the pedicle may be divided after the flap has been in place long enough to heal and acquire a blood supply from it's new location.

Axial/Arterialized Flap

As knowledge of the circulation of flaps developed, it became apparent that the survival of flaps was dependent upon the presence of significant blood vessels within the pedicle of the flap. It was then recognized that certain flaps succeeded on a consistent basis due to a known vessel being present in the pedicle. Axial flaps are based on a named vessel in the vascular pedicle. The surgeon knows there is a vessel in the area of the flap, and will design the flap to include that particular vessel. Because axial pattern flaps are entirely dependent on one vascular pedicle, the base can be quite narrow and may even comprise only the vessels themselves. Examples of axial pattern flaps are forehead flaps based on the superficial temporal artery, or the supratrochlear artery, either of which can be used for nasal reconstruction. Other examples of an axial flap include the groin flap based on the superficial circumflex iliac artery, and the deltopectoral flap based on tributaries of the internal mammary artery.

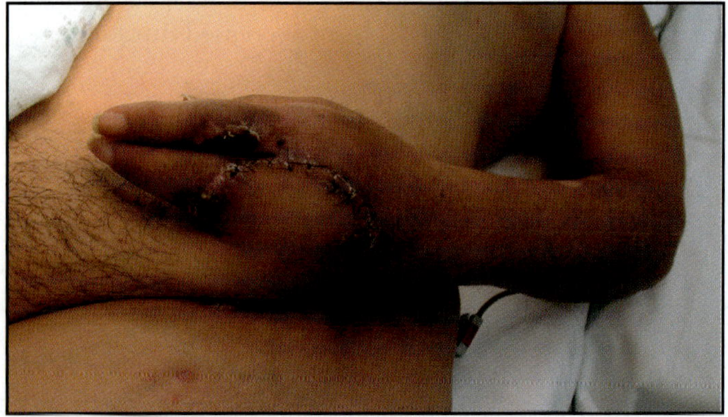

Figure 10. A groin axial pattern flap based on the superficial iliac vessel used to cover a hand defect.

Musculocutaneous Flaps

The next development in the knowledge of flaps was the recognition that a few muscles have a single or dominant vessel supplying vascularity to the muscle, and this vessel could be used as the vascular pedicle for a flap containing that muscle. The muscle can then carry the overlying skin, or attached bone. Some commonly used muscles for flaps include the temporalis, trapezius, pectoralis, latissimus dorsi, rectus abdominus, gluteus maximus, tensor fascia lata, gracilis, rectus femoris, gastrocnemius, and soleus muscles.

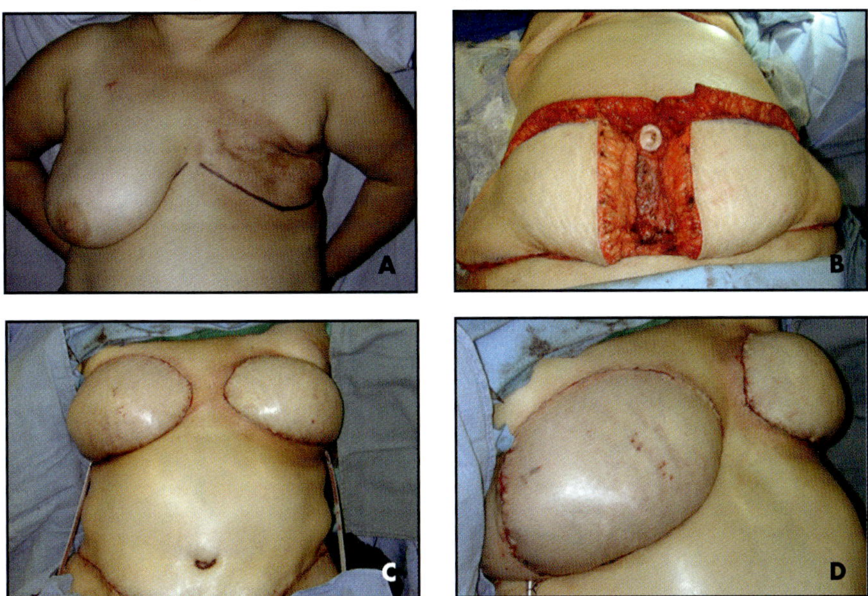

Figure 11 A–D. (A) A patient who has had a left mastectomy and radiation therapy. Note the radiation dermatitis. A bilateral breast reconstruction with TRAM flaps is planned.
(B) The bilateral flaps have been raised. These are axial flaps, using the blood supply within the rectus abdominis muscles to carry the skin and subcutaneous tissue.
(C) The flaps have been tunneled under the upper abdominal skin, placed on the chest wall, and shaped to form the breast mound.
(D) The subtle color changes in the right reconstructed breast mound are typical of color changes which must be noticed, and carefully followed. If this color tends toward normal, as happened in this case, nothing need be done. However if the color change progresses, intervention will be necessary if the flap is to be saved.

Fasciocutaneous Flaps

Fascial flaps utilize the perifascial plexuses—superficial or deep to the fascia and may include the fascia only, fascia and skin, or fascia, skin and bone. They provide a relatively thin flap and do not sacrifice muscle. Blood supply involves vessels which pass through intermuscular septa and give branches that perforate the fascia. Three types of fasciocutaneous flaps exist. The random pattern does not involve any distinct vessels through the flap. The second type is an axial pattern that is oriented and elevated on an axial artery that runs above or just beneath the fascia. Examples include the lateral arm flap based on the posterior radial collateral artery and the temporoparietal flap based on the temporal vessels. The third type involves a flap that is oriented over an axial artery which runs deep to the fascia. The radial forearm flap based on the radial artery is an example.

Free Flaps

Free flaps or neovascularized flaps are flaps with an identified axial blood supply which is completely detached from their blood supply and then re-attached to a blood supply at the recipient site with a microvascular anastomosis. The microvascular anastomoses required are technically challenging. Because all that is needed for a free flap to work are suitable donor and recipient vessels, flap transfer problems are greatly reduced. Free flaps can be transferred from distant donor sites as long as the blood supply can be reestablished. These flaps can include skin, fascia, muscle, and bone. Some of the more common free flaps include the free transverse rectus abdominus (TRAM), latissimus dorsi, and radial forearm flaps.

Historically plastic surgeons would develop a flap, and migrate it to a different part of the body in multiple stages. The development of free flaps has obviated the need for these complex, multiple staged procedures.

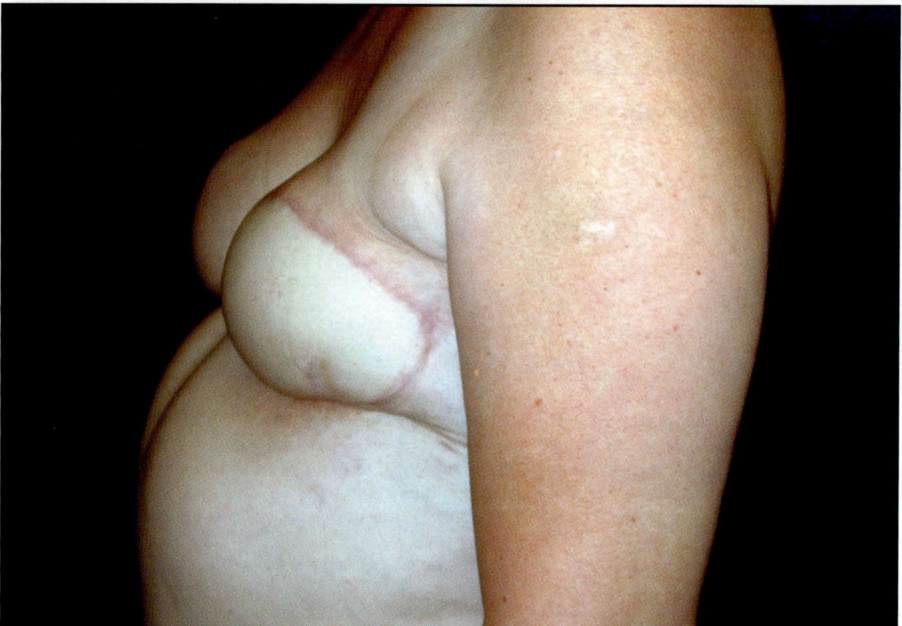

Figure 12. Left breast reconstruction with a free flap using the latissimus doris muscle and overlying tissues.

PREOPERATIVE CARE

One of the important roles of the wound care center is to prepare a wound bed for closure. This means removal of all non-vital material from the wound, development of a vascular bed for wound healing, and control of infection.

Debridement

Ambrose Pare, a noted surgeon in 16th century France, once said, "I dressed the wound, God healed it." Our role in healing wounds is often to get out of the way so that natural processes can heal the wound. In this regard, the first and most important duty of the wound care specialist is to accurately and repeatedly observe the wound. Careful observation will focus attention on what needs to be done. Wounds that are locally contaminated with necrotic material or infected tissue must be cleared of necrotic material. If there is a significant amount of necrotic tissue it is well to start with sharp debridement. A scalpel or scissors along with pickups are used to remove as much necrotic tissue as possible. It is important to not be too aggressive when performing sharp debridement. Most of the wounds that are referred to the wound care specialist will consist of "problem wounds." Frequently circulation in the wound will be marginal. If the debridement injures living tissue, it will further delay the healing process. A perfect debridement would remove every piece of necrotic tissue that was attached to the viable tissue, while not injuring a single living cell. In practice, a thin layer of marginally viable tissue is usually left behind. This thin rim of tissue will separate when the underlying bed becomes sufficiently vascularized, or it may be removed later. If underlying viable tissue is exposed to air, it will dry out and die. It will then become another layer that must be debrided. Of course, another option is to use moist wound care techniques. Debridement techniques are discussed in detail by TA Emhoff and SA Ferro in their chapter entitled "Wound Debridement" and will not be reiterated here.

A word about instruments is appropriate. Every physician will have his or her particular set of favorite instruments. Just as each of us has a slightly different shaped hand, there exists a different instrument to fit the hand in different ways. Finding the instrument that best fits your hand will enable you to do a more accurate and better job. This cannot be determined by looking at the pages of a catalog. One has to hold the instrument in his or her hand and see how it functions. In debriding a grossly necrotic wound, any pair of Mayo scissors will suffice. When doing the final finishing touches of fine debridement, more delicate instruments are in order. Many surgeons find Brown-Adson forceps are delicate enough to pick up small pieces of tissue, yet strong enough to hold on to resistant tissue. Delicate dissecting scissors such as Kaye dissecting scissors or tenotomy scissors, will allow for an accurate dissection. Such instruments manufactured by quality instrument makers will be expensive but will last many decades, making them a wise investment. See the Bangasser and Bozzuto chapter entitled "Coding, Charging, Billing, and Collecting" for details regarding the way in which debridement procedures are documented and billed.

When not to debride

Once the wound is free from necrotic and infectious tissue, further debridement is unnecessary and meddlesome.

In some situations it may be decided to allow tissue to auto amputate. In that circumstance no debridement should be done until the line of viable tissue has clearly declared itself. In cases of gangrene due to frostbite it is important to not debride the necrotic tissue. In frostbite there is a zone of injured tissue which will recover if left undisturbed, but which will die if the distal frankly necrotic tissue is debrided.

When there is underlying vascular disease with associated gangrene it is conventional to wait for a line of demarcation. The degree of underlying ischemia should be assessed and corrective vascular surgery must always be considered.

Dressings

After the great mass of necrotic tissue is debrided, the task of removing the remaining vestiges of necrotic tissue begins. This usually coincides with the appearance of the capillary bed so important for the success of the future graft. Traditionally, this debridement is done with dressing changes. There are a multitude of ways to do dressing changes, each with its advantages and disadvantages. The observant wound care specialist will choose the best technique for each specific wound, and probably will find different techniques more effective at different stages of each wound.

Wet to dry dressing changes were the original technique for debriding wounds and are still commonly used by surgeons. While this debridement method is inexpensive, it is painful and nonspecific in its debridement properties. Dressing principles are discussed in detail in Larson-Lohr and Fleck's chapter entitled "Modern Wound Dressings—Principles, Form and Function" and will not be reiterated here. Large wound defects may be best managed with negative pressure wound therapy ("the VAC"). This technology is discussed by Smith and Bozzuto in the chapter titled "Advanced Therapeutics: the Biochem and Biophy Bases of Wound Products." The VAC can be used to bring a wound to the point that healing by delayed secondary intention is possible. Alternatively, if surgical closure is necessary, treatment beforehand with the VAC may allow a much smaller flap to be performed.

Infection

Wounds need to be clean and free from infection before consideration for wound closure. Several techniques help determine whether or not a wound is clean enough for successful grafting. The use of heterografts to test the recipient bed has been discussed already.

Quantitative tissue culture may be helpful in revealing the amount of residual infection left in a wound. A biopsy or tissue specimen from the wound using aseptic technique may be performed to numerically quantify the amount of aerobic bacteria or yeast remaining in the wound. Preliminary results can be found after one day, and the final result is usually available within three days. This culture is particularly helpful for the management of wounds in burn patients. Colony counts higher than 10^5 colony forming units (CFU) per gram of tissue indicate the presence of infection sufficient to prevent successful wound closure.

Touch plates may be helpful to assess infection if other techniques have not helped. This technique is controversial. Most microbiologists believe that touch plates are unnecessary, but occasionally they provide valuable information not obtained by other means. This technique requires the preparation of a Petri dish filled to the brim with agar. The overfilled dish is pressed against the wound and then cultured in the standard fashion. The usefulness of this technique arises from the isolation of unusual bacteria. These bacteria are often overgrown or suppressed with the usual broth or swipe techniques of culturing wounds. These mixed infections have the ability to dissolve a graft quite rapidly. A detailed discussion of infection management in wound care is provided in the LeFrock chapter titled "Post-Operative Surgical Site Infections (SSIs) and Non-Necrotizing Skin and Soft Tissue Infections."

When Not to Close Wounds

The main contraindications to wound closure are an unclean wound, or inadequate blood supply. If there is residual infection, necrosis, or cancer, then the wound is better left open. Necrotic wounds may need several debridements before they are ready for closure. Margins of wounds that may contain cancer need to be assessed and any positive margins excised before undertaking wound closure. Some contaminated wounds with marginally viable edges can be left open but dressed appropriately to prevent desiccation to allow the wound to "declare itself." After demarcation, non viable tissue can be removed. When all tissues are viable, and infection is under control, the wound may be closed.

The goal is the establishment of a rich vascular network or bed of capillaries upon which to place the graft, free of infection. The ideal bed will look like rich and very expensive red velvet. A bed of pale or irregular velvet is a sign that the vascular bed is not fully developed. While a skin graft may take upon such an inferior bed, its success is less likely than that of a graft placed upon a richly vascularized bed. A glistening appearance on the surface of a bed of capillaries indicates the bed has edema, and will be less likely to support a graft. In such cases it is better to delay coverage until the capillary bed is in better condition.

When to Call for Plastic Surgery Consultation

Plastic surgery consultation can be sought both for help in preliminary assessment and therapy planning, and when wounds are ready for closure. The Wound Care Specialist or Wound Center that is fortunate enough to have access to a plastic surgeon interested in wound healing will find it useful to discuss cases early in their assessment. These informal (curbstone consultations) discussions benefit the patient by having his problem reviewed from different perspectives, and often will suggest innovative therapy options.

The Plastic Surgeon should be called:

- When the wound is clean and ready for operative closure
- When the wound cannot be expected to heal within 30 days
- When bone, joint, or tendon become exposed (promptly)
- When the required debridement is more extensive than that normally performed in the wound care clinic
- When the wound does not progress in healing as expected or regresses
- When the total wound care plan for the patient is uncertain
- When conservative wound treatment has failed
- After the underlying problems causing the wound have been addressed
- After the patient's nutritional status has been optimized
- After the patient is stable and medically cleared for surgery

Patients should be stable, and other factors that affect wound healing, such as malnutrition or diabetes, need to be under control. The type of wound may dictate the timing for wound closure. For instance, patients with stage III or IV pressure sores need to have clean wounds that are static or improving before wound closure can be considered. About 80% of venous stasis ulcers will heal with compression. If this is unsuccessful, then the remainder can usually be healed by split-thickness skin grafts with or without ligation of adjacent perforating veins. Peripheral vascular ulcers due to arterial insufficiency or other vasculitis syndromes are best treated by correcting the underlying disease and local wound care. (See Boccolandro's chapter titled "Chronic Critical Limb Ischema and Limb Salvage"). If the underlying problem cannot be treated it is unlikely that a stable healing wound can ever be achieved. With amputation stumps, the wound must be clean before attempting closure or coverage. Amputation stumps resulting from trauma are often contaminated and need proper debridement prior to stump closure. Foot ulcers such as from diabetes are often the result of pressure over bony prominences in the setting of neuropathy. Conservative measures such as pressure relief and diabetes control should be tried prior to consulting the surgeon.

There are some wounds which demand very early consultation for coverage. Exposed tendons and exposed bone will usually desiccate unless very promptly covered with viable tissue. If such a situation develops, Plastic Surgery Consultation must be obtained as an urgent matter.

Ionizing radiation, whether as a result of radiation therapy or the result of environmental and/or occupational hazards will result in an obliterating arteritis, which is progressive for the rest of the patient's life. This produces ischemia which is painful, and which may progress on to ulceration. Reconstruction of these wounds almost always requires a flap. Because the flap brings its own blood supply into the area the edges of the flap will have a good blood supply, and frequently will be able to supply oxygenated blood to the radiation damaged skin surrounding the flap. This halo of newly vascularised tissue will be clearly seen as the flap and wound heals.

In addition to the outlined medical therapies, the patient should receive medical clearance before undergoing surgery to ascertain whether the overall medical condition permits the occasionally lengthy reconstructive procedures required. For burn wounds, immediate grafting after early excision of necrotic tissue allows for rapid healing with optimal functional and cosmetic results. Early coverage also minimizes the immunosuppressive, infectious, and metabolic consequences of a large burn.

Summary

The wound care specialist must remember the multitude of ways in which a wound may be closed, review the patient's situation on a regular basis, and always be ready to alter therapy should a better alternative appear.

The wound care specialist will constantly build his or her knowledge of the ways in which wounds normally heal. If a wound fails to progress as expected, search for the reason will be undertaken. An overlooked factor in the patient or the wound is more likely to be the cause than a problem with the treatment protocol.

POST-OPERATIVE CARE
Seromas/Hematomas

A seroma or a hematoma in a closed wounds acts as a physical barrier to the healing process. They form a thicker scaffold for fibroblasts to migrate across, and thus make for a wider scar. They also place tension on the wound closure which may cause wound dehiscence. If a seroma or hematoma is detected following wound closure, prompt drainage or evacuation needs to be performed.

Skin Grafts

Since skin grafts do not have their own blood supply, they must acquire a vascular supply from the recipient bed. The process of acquiring this blood supply is a wonderful but delicate process, easily disturbed. The initial nourishment of the graft is by diffusion across the bed/graft interface. This process of diffusion can provide only a very limited supply of nutrients, not enough to nourish the graft for any great length of time. Any physical barrier such as a hematoma, edema fluid, a seroma, pus, necrotic tissue, or foreign bodies between a graft and the capillary bed will lead to failure of the graft, at least in the portion where there is a barrier. The ultimate success or "take" of a graft is dependent upon the graft's ability to acquire a blood supply from the underlying bed. The better the vascularity of the bed, the more likely the graft is to succeed. Furthermore, anything which disrupts the attachment of the graft after it is attached will lead to failure of the graft. This attachment is extremely fragile in the first few days, which means that the graft requires very meticulous care and diligent protection. This requires absolute immobilization of the grafted area for the first 3–5 days or until the bolster is taken down, if a bolster or stent is used. If an extremity is grafted, this may involve splinting of the extremity. Extremities should also be kept elevated to control edema and swelling. Obviously, the longer the cells of the graft are without nourishment, then the longer they are at risk. By the same token, a thicker graft makes it more difficult for the recipient bed to provide sufficient nourishment for all cells of the graft.

Stent or bolster dressings

There are two general ways in which grafts may be cared for in the immediate post-operative period. Most surgeons will fix the graft in place, and then cover it with an occlusive dressing. This dressing is designed to place pressure upon the graft in order to keep the graft in intimate contact with the bed. Often times the dressing is held in place with sutures which are tied over the dressing.

These dressings are called a "bolster" or "stent." The name "stent" comes from the name of a German dental supply company that manufactured a thermoplastic rubber-like dressing compound used as a dental wound dressing. Bolsters are usually left on for about five days to help the graft stay pressed down on the recipient bed and prevent potential spaces for hematoma or seroma formation. If an occlusive dressing is used, it must be inspected carefully every day. The dressing should be smelled during inspection. If any signs of bleeding or infection appear, then the dressing must be removed immediately and the problem addressed. An infection has the potential to totally destroy a thin graft in a matter of hours.

An exception to this rule applies when one utilizes the negative pressure wound therapy (NPWT) dressing (aka "the VAC") as a bolster. (See Figure 3) When an NPWT is used the graft is covered with a thin layer of bacitracin ointment, an adaptic dressing cut to the shape of the wound, the NPWT sponge also cut to the shape of the wound, secured to the surrounding skin, covered with an adhesive dressing and hooked up to the negative pressure device set at 75 mm Hg instead of the usual 100–125 mm Hg for open wounds. One unpublished study indicates that when the NPWT is used as a bolster it hastens the take of the skin graft allowing the dressing to be taken down in three days instead of the usual five days for standard bolster techniques. The factors attributed to its efficacy were total immobilization of the graft, elimination of fluid collections, and decreased bacterial contamination.

After the bolster is taken down the graft is covered with a thin layer of bacitracin, adaptic dressing, and dry dressing, changed twice a day for an additional week. Alternatively, grafts on extremities may be wrapped with an Unna's boot which is left intact for one week. Limb elevation must be continued during this time. After one week, dressings are removed and no further dressings are necessary as long as the skin graft had good take. Moisturizing cream is applied four times daily and as needed to help keep the graft skin moist and supple.

Grafts placed upon the lower extremity present a special problem. The capillary buds which bridge the interface between the graft bed and the graft are not only very delicate, they are also bridging a space with little or no support from surrounding connective tissue. If these capillaries are subjected to hydrostatic pressure from the weight of the vascular column of a standing patient, they are apt to rupture. This will lead to hemorrhage beneath the graft. Patients with split thickness skin grafts placed on the lower portion of the lower extremity have been found to have a much higher success rate if the extremity is kept elevated and the patient kept at complete bed rest for one week following application of a split thickness skin graft. This results in much better takes than if the patient was allowed to ambulate, even with the best of compression dressings.

Open grafts

Some surgeons find that grafts cared for in an open fashion have a higher success rate than those treated with occlusive dressings. In the open technique, the graft is placed upon the wound bed and left exposed. Success using this technique requires a very cooperative patient who will protect the graft. This may require restraining the extremity with the graft. It also requires nursing staff skilled in the observation and care of such grafts. The grafts must be "rolled out" with Q-tips moistened with saline as needed. In the first few hours post-op this will be needed very frequently, sometimes almost constantly. As the graft adheres, the necessity of rolling out a graft will become less frequent. If a pocket of blood, serum, or pus develops under the graft, the graft must be immediately incised with a pair of fine iris scissors, and the fluid collection rolled out and expressed. This requires a large expenditure of nursing time. Some patients are able and eager to manage the care of the graft after careful instruction. Advantages to this technique are numerous. Nursing staff become skilled in observing the signs of a successful graft. They will take pride in their part of the success of the graft. Patients in whom the nursing staff becomes highly involved do receive better care, and observation of a healing graft gives the surgeon a chance to educate staff on the process of wound healing in general. This is an ideal situation in which to teach the nuances of skin color changes.

When dealing with a difficult wound that has a less than optimal recipient bed for the graft, the open technique will give the skin graft a much better chance to succeed. Finally, if the open technique is routinely used, health care staff quickly become skilled in evaluating grafts which are not doing well and will institute corrective therapy promptly. If proper therapy is instituted at the appropriate time, failing grafts may be saved. HBO2 is frequently helpful.

Wound site infection can lead to the failure of the graft in one of two ways. A mixed infection may cause a graft to simply "melt" away in place. If pus forms underneath the graft the pus acts as a physical barrier between the graft and the recipient bed. We have already discussed the importance of "rolling out" pus from underneath a graft.

Two unpublished studies concerning the use of prophylactic antibiotics were performed at military hospitals. In both studies, wounds were assessed the morning of grafting by experienced surgeons. These surgeons identified wounds that were clean with a healthy recipient bed free from infection. Half were given penicillin as a prophylactic; the others were given a placebo. The studies were blinded. All other care was identical. Failure rates for grafts not treated with prophylactic antibiotics were double those treated. Most of the graft failures were due to an infection with mixed organisms that included *streptococcus*. By preventing the growth of the *streptococcus* species, the mixed infection was prevented. Only one week of treatment was given.

Occasionally, a graft may appear to have failed post-operatively, but the bed will have an abundance of hypertrophic capillaries. The wound will appear to be healthier than before the graft was placed, but the capillaries will be clearly exuberant. Before assuming that the graft has failed, it is appropriate to apply pressure to these wounds to reduce the exuberant capillaries. On rare occasions, the physician will find that "plugs" of the graft have established themselves deep within the capillary bed. With control of the hypertrophic granulations the plugs will spread, leading to rapid healing of the wound.

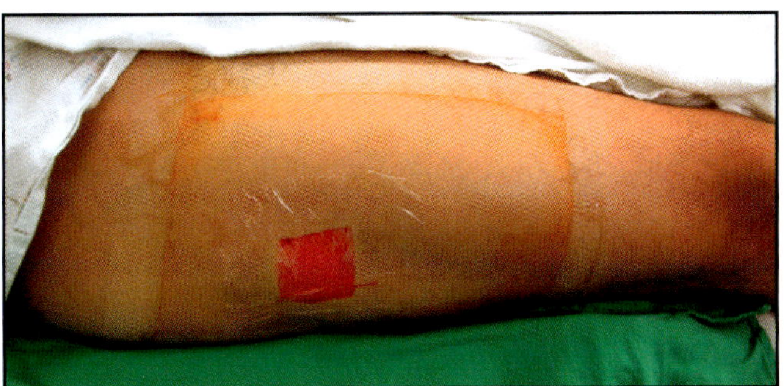

Figure 13. A split thickness skin graft donor site with a transparent dressing.

Donor Sites

Post-operative treatment of donor sites for split thickness grafts are as varied as there are surgeons. The two concerns for the donor site are postop pain, and the risk of infection. Exposure to air will usually obviate the risk of infection, but is very painful. Coverage with an opsite or tegaderm dressing will provide patient comfort.

These dressings are left in place and allowed to fall off on their own after a few weeks. Any significant drainage under-neath the dressings can be aspirated as needed. Any signs of infection must be treated very promptly and aggressively.

Donor sites for full thickness skin grafts are usually closed primarily. Post-operative care for donor sites for flaps that are covered by skin grafts are treated the same way as the previously described post-operative care for skin grafts in general.

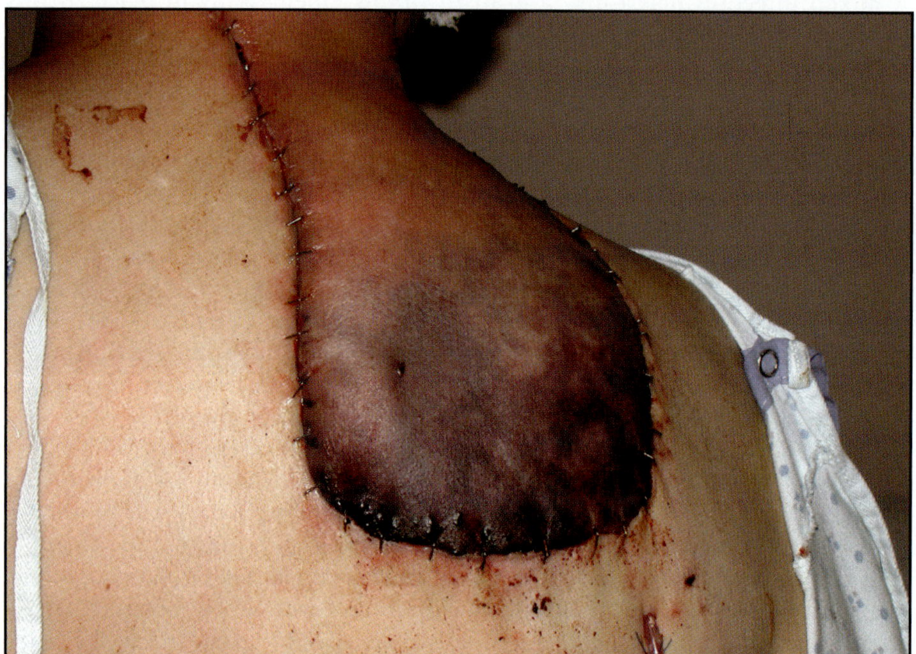

Figure 14. A flap showing advanced demarcation.

Flaps

Because flaps carry their own blood supply, they will heal in wounds that have poor or no blood supply. In fact, a flap placed in a poorly vascularized area will often provide blood supply to the tissue surrounding the flap. In this situation one will frequently find that within the relatively ischemic recipient site there exists a halo of well-vascularized skin a centimeter wide surrounding the flap.

Because flaps take their vascular supply with them and are usually large blocks of tissue, their survival depends upon maintaining blood flow through the vascular pedicle. Failure of circulation will almost always lead to failure of the flap. All health care workers caring for flaps must develop skill in assessing the color of flaps in the postoperative period. Any change in the color of a flap must be immediately reported and the cause found. If a correctable problem exists, it must be urgently remedied.

On rare occasions one will see a flap which looks good immediately postoperatively, and then several hours later develops a line of color demarcation across one portion. If the distal flap is cyanotic, the problem is probably due to obstruction of the venous return from the flap; if the flap is white, the problem is arterial. If either is left uncorrected, the distal portion of the flap will demarcate and die. The wound care specialist must immediately notify the operating surgeon of the problem. While waiting for the operating surgeon to arrive, the wound care specialist may remove a few sutures at the site of the line of demarcation. Sometimes the removal of a few sutures will allow the tissue to expand and restore circulation. Suture release may also reveal a large blood clot under the flap compressing the circulation. Evacuation of the clot will restore the circulation and preserve the flap. If the vascular pedicle has been kinked, the entire flap may have to be replaced in the donor area in order to restore the circulation. Replacing the flap in the donor area requires a return to the operating room. If an improvement in the color of the entire flap is noted, then nothing more may need to be done. However, the flap should still be monitored very carefully. More likely, the color will improve in a portion of the flap, but a line of demarcation will be established distal to the original line. This indicates the need for the removal of additional sutures until the entire flap has a healthy color. These are matters that must be dealt with promptly. They cannot be left until the morning. By that time the flap will have been lost.

If removal of the original sutures reveals a hematoma under the flap, the hematoma must be evacuated. Total removal of the hematoma will probably require a return to the operating room, but partial evacuation of the clot may be accomplished in the clinic area by forcing the hematoma out by rolling the area toward the suture line opening using a roll of gauze or a rolled up towel. This will be painful to the patient, since significant force is required. However, the pressure that the hematoma places on the vascular pedicle must be relieved. Even if the hematoma is evacuated, the patient may still need to return to the operating room so that the bleeding point which produced the hematoma can be identified and controlled.

If the flap is pale, the problem is probably due to the obstruction of the arterial supply to the flap. This pale color will be followed in a matter of hours by a cyanotic color. The operating surgeon must be notified immediately. Occasionally a kink in the arterial supply can be straightened out by returning the flap to the donor area. Search for a correctable problem should be attempted, but usually none will be found. The wound care specialist then faces the decision as to whether or not hyperbaric oxygen treatments should be initiated in an attempt to rescue the flap.

Hyperbaric oxygen will usually provide enough oxygen to enable the flap to survive as long as the treatments are continued. Once the treatments are stopped, the flap must have reestablished enough circulation to nourish itself, or it will demarcate and fail. If the flap was used to fill a void in otherwise healthy tissue, the flap will establish vascular connections to the surrounding tissue over a few days, during which HBO2 should be sufficient to nourish the flap. The treating hyperbaric facility will note that the flap will initially require multiple treatments each day. After a few days, the interval between treatments will gradually lengthen until further treatments become unnecessary. If, however, the flap was designed to bring healthy vascularized tissue to an area of ischemia, then the flap will be unable to form vascular connections from the surrounding tissue and will fail. In this situation, hyperbaric treatments may keep the flap alive, but the flap will ultimately die whenever the treatments are stopped. It is better to not start treatments unless ultimate success is likely.

SUMMARY OF GENERAL PRINCIPLES

The wound care specialist who is asked to care for a wound which is not doing well post-operatively must evaluate the situation in two ways. First, determine what is wrong with the healing process. Second, determine what it was that the surgeon was trying to accomplish with his initial procedure. Was the goal simple coverage, was it providing revascularity to the area, or was it improving aesthetics? The interaction of these two determinations will often lead to dramatically different courses of action in situations which seem superficially similar. Failing to understand in a global way the goals of reconstruction may lead to success for the wound care specialist, but failure for the patient. Finally, but perhaps most importantly, if the current care is not resulting in an improvement in the wound, then one's management strategy needs to be reassessed.

REFERENCES

These references to classical publications are listed for the wound care specialist who desires to understand the principles and knowledge which addresses thoughful wound management, and how it developed.

1. Gillies Sir H, Millard DR, Jr.: The Principles and Art of Plastic Surgery, Boston: Little Brown and Company, 1957.
    This two-volume work pictorially describes the techniques developed prior to the development of microvascular procedures. Although most of the cases would be handled differently today, the principles remain vital.

2. Peacock EE, Van Winkle W. Surgery and Biology of Wound Repair, Philadelphia: W.W. Saunders Company 1970.
    This scholarly work remains the classic description of the wound healing process at the cellular and subcellular level.

3. Grabb WC; Smith JW, Aston SJ. Plastic Surgery, A Concise Clinical Guide: Boston: Little Brown and Company 1991
    The medical student who reads this book will gain a basic understanding of plastic surgery. A general surgery resident can also read the book, and will find information he did not discover the first time he read it. Similarly, the plastic surgery resident, and the practicing plastic surgeon will all find it beneficial to reread. The wound care specialist will find much valuable information here.

4. McGregor IA.: Fundamental Techniques of Plastic Surgery, Edinburgh: Churchill Livingston 1995.
    As the title suggests, this book describes very clearly the fundamental techniques and reasons for the technique.

5. Janis JE, Attinger CE. Editors: Current Concepts in Wound Healing: Supplement to Plast. & Reconst. Surg. Vol 117 # 75, June 2006.
    The current state of knowledge is presented here.

REVIEW QUESTIONS

1.) The goal of the wound care specialist is to:
    a. Debride wounds as skillfully as possible so as to facilitate wound healing
    b. Handle wounds using sterile technique so as to prevent infection and cross contamination
    c. Obtain a healed wound in the shortest possible time, and at the least possible expense
    d. Try and heal the wound so the scar crosses Relaxed Skin Tension Lines.
    e. Always be sure that the latest and best available dressing and techniques are used in caring for wounds.

2.) The most important skill the wound care technician must develop is:
    a. Skill in debriding wounds
    b. Knowledge of the benefits and disadvantages of the many different types of wound dressings.
    c. Certification as a Hyperbaric Technologist
    d. Knowledge of the way and the rate at which wounds normally heal, and what they look like as they heal normally.
    e. Skill in using the ICD codebooks so as to assure proper payment is made for treatments.

3.) Split thickness skin grafts
    a. Do not contract, usually match the color of surrounding skin, and are more durable the thinner they are
    b. Usually contract, do not match the color of surrounding skin, and are less durable the thinner they are.
    c. Do not contract, do not match the color of surrounding skin, and are less durable the thinner they are.

4.) A flap instead of a split thickness skin graft must be used when:
    a. The recipient bed has poor blood supply
    b. A tendon crosses the recipient bed
    c. The wound is in a weight bearing area
    d. All of the above
    e. None of the above

5.) Heterografts or Xenografts:
    a. Will provide permanent coverage for a wound
    b. Should be thought of as biological dressings
    c. Will "take" even when not carefully immobilized.
    d. Have no role in the care of an infected wound
    e. Will not help predict the success of a subsequent autograft

6. A flap which has been placed in an area of radiation damaged skin turns white:
    a. Immediate HBO2 therapy must be started.
    b. A hematoma must be evacuated from beneath the flap
    c. The flap must be returned to the donor area in the clinical area while waiting for the operating surgeon
    d. All of the above
    e. None of the above

Answers: 1c, 2d, 3b, 4d, 5b, 6e

CHAPTER 11

MANAGEMENT OF THE PROBLEM POST-OPERATIVE WOUND

CHAPTER ELEVEN OVERVIEW

NOTES

MANAGEMENT OF THE PROBLEM POST-OPERATIVE WOUND

John S. Steinberg, Todd A. Derksen

OVERVIEW OF WOUND HEALING PROCESS

Skin is the largest of the human organs. While skin certainly has a significant role as a sensory organ, the principle responsibility is as a physical barrier for protection against environmental dangers. These potential threats include microorganisms such as bacteria, viruses and fungi, each of which can have the potential to create an opportunistic infection. Additionally, environmental dangers from temperature regulation, ultraviolet radiation, and dehydration can be causative factors in wound development. The presence of a physical skin defect is often the trigger in complicated wounds. These defects can include those which are created surgically.

In the most general of terms, skin consists of two principle layers: the epidermis and dermis. The process of wound healing depends upon the

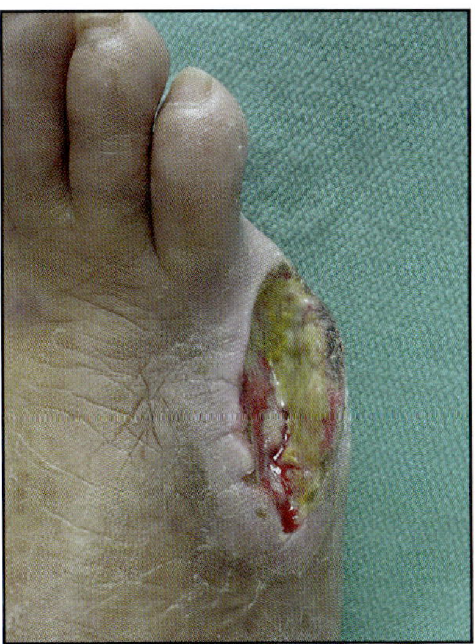

Figure 1. Failing wound site following toe amputation.

epidermis resurfacing the wound in order to re-establish a protective barrier. Prior to this occurring, the dermis must generate or posses appropriate structure and integrity to adequately protect the underlying surface.

WOUND CLASSIFICATION

Clinically validated wound classifications provide a common language to describe wounds and they also allow the healthcare team to understand the associated risks with each wound so as to guide treatment planning. For example, the appropriate classification and stratification of a heavily contaminated puncture wound confirms the higher risk for infection and can help guide the delivery of significantly more aggressive treatment. Classification systems also help us better understand and quantify risks of surgical wound sites based on the level of contamination identified.

The overall wound healing process depends greatly on the location, severity, and size of a given wound. The amount of tissue loss can directly correlate to the complexity of the expected healing course (1). Wounds with significant tissue loss often require healing via secondary intention and therefore result in significant scarring and poor predictability / organization. In contrast, the clean surgical wound heals by primary intention because this type of wound generally presents with minimal tissue loss and good approximation of skin edges is easily achieved. These wound types are also created under aseptic conditions and thus the possibility of infection is minimized. As dictated by good surgical technique, the surgeon should generally take care to follow natural tissue planes and then re-approximate and repair these planes to minimize postoperative hematoma, edema and inflammation as well as allowing the wound to heal through direct tissue approximation.

Following the initial process of hemostasis, there are three stages of wound healing: inflammatory, proliferative, and maturation. The inflammatory phase begins at the time of initial insult to the skin and deep tissues. This generally lasts throughout the first three days of wound healing. During these first moments of the wound, the process of hemostasis will progress to involve constriction of blood vessels, platelet aggregation, clot formation, fibrin mesh development, and will ultimately stop the bleeding vessel wall and begin the repair process (2). The damaged soft tissues release histamine which progressively dilates local capillaries and recruits inflammatory cells to the site of the wound. This process will typically result in the cardinal signs of inflammation which are localized edema, erythema, calor, dolor, and loss of function. Neutrophils in the wound site begin to ingest bacteria and cleanse small debris. Monocytes transform into macrophages as they react to chemotactic agents and extravasate from the blood vessels near the injured site. These cells also ingest bacteria, cleanse the wound, recruit other macrophages, stimulate formation of fibroblasts and release growth hormones for wound repair (3). The fibroblasts produce collagen which aids in the strength and integrity of wound in the form of scar tissue.

The proliferative phase starts from day 3 post-op and lasts for approximately 24 days. During this phase, the tensile strength of the surgically repaired wound edges increases as collagen continues to form. The amount of scar tissue formed during this period is directly dependent of the amount of local stress at the site. This is a particular challenge when performing surgery on the extremities which

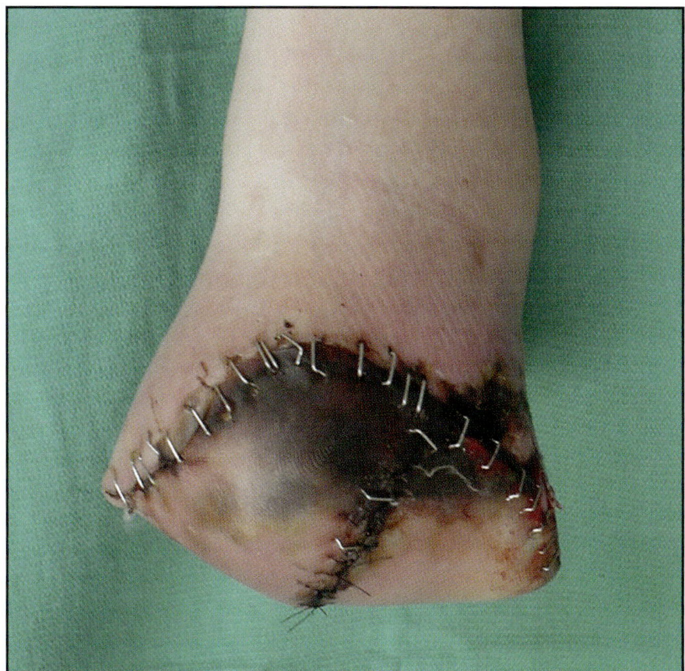

Figure 2. Ischemic limb with gangrenous tissue flaps necessitating more proximal amputation.

undergo a significant amount of motion and possibly even weight-bearing when compared to other areas of the body. Finally, in the maturation phase, the surgical wound will continue to strengthen and remodel for several months up to over a year. For details on the phases of acute wound healing see the Chin et al. chapter entitled "Biochemistry of Wound Healing in Wound Care."

FACTORS THAT AFFECT WOUND HEALING

Healing any wound, including a surgical wound can be influenced by a multitude of factors including environmental, physical, and metabolic. Other factors may include but are not limited to age, obesity, vascular disease, malnutrition, dehydration, anemia, smoking, edema, systemic disease, or drugs. Malnutrition, dehydration, and anemia can significantly increase the risk for surgical wound infection and other complications (4). Malnutrition is diagnosed by inadequate systemic and local supply of protein, vitamin C, zinc, and copper. These elements are required by fibroblasts for the synthesis of collagen. Zinc is also noted to play an important role in wound epithelialization. A decrease in serum albumin and transferrin is attributed to protein-calorie malnutrition. If a deficiency is suspected for any of these, simple lab tests may be performed with some values even having a predictive value for wound healing capacity. For example a serum albumin of less than 3.5 g/dl or a total lymphocyte count of less than 1500 both have a negative predictive value for healing a surgical wound site. Wound healing in the elderly population is altered by several factors: a less than optimal circulation/perfusion for wound healing is often encountered and even in the minimally invasive surgical wound created under controlled circumstances, the collagen is less pliable and the scar is less elastic in elderly patients. Smoking has repeatedly been associated with numerous post operative complications. These include delayed surgical healing both in soft tissue and bone, increased risk for infection, and increased risk of dehiscence. In fact, the effect of smoking a single cigarette on the peripheral vasculature is a decrease in the digital blood flow by 35–42% that persists up to 50 minutes. Therefore a pack per day smoker essentially has decreased blood flow to the surgical site for the entire time that they are awake. This effect is attributed to the nicotine and has been recorded with the transcutaneous nicotine patch as well. However, the effects of smoking are not limited to the vasoconstrictive properties of nicotine. Cigarette smoking also increases platelet adhesiveness thereby increasing the risk of arterial microvascular thrombolic occlusion and DVT. Carbon monoxide and hydrogen cyanide (both byproducts of cigarette smoking) decrease oxygen transport and cellular metabolism further reducing the body's capacity to repair a wound. In addition, excessive physical pressure in the post-operative wound caused by localized edema can hinder wound healing. Special caution should be followed in the immune-compromised patient, such as in the rheumatoid patient, or those who have a history of chronic steroid therapy. Chronic corticosteroid therapy depletes the body of it's vitamin A stores. Vitamin A plays a significant role in stimulating epithelialization and collagen deposition in fibroblasts. In an effort to reverse this impaired healing ability, it is critical that patients on chronic steroid therapy take oral and topical vitamin A supplements to reverse the impaired healing process (5). Additionally, patients on long term corticosteroid therapy have impaired bone healing and have a five–fold increased risk for fracture. Hypoxia decreases the body's resistance to infection, impairs fibroblast division, and collagen production (6). Therefore patients with vascular disease are more prone to wound complications. A resultant wound complication from vascular compromise can present as necrotic tissue and excessive drainage which will ultimately increase the risk of a wound infection. Proper pre-operative vascular screening is important for patients who are at risk for PVD. Screening exams may include ankle/brachial index (ABI) and transcutaneous oxygen partial pressure ($P_{tc}O_2$, or $TcpO_2$). Each of these tests has values that correlate with a negative outcome predictive value. Values for the ABI that predict a negative outcome follow a U shaped curve. Values of greater than 1.3, or less than 0.5 are indicative of lower extremity ischemia and probable failure to heal a wound. However, patients who have diabetes need a value of greater than 0.45 to have the same chance of healing as someone without diabetes. $TcpO_2$ values of greater than 40 mm Hg indicate a likelihood that the surgical site will heal.

Hyperglycemia in the postoperative period is also directly correlative to complications. A single glucose above 200 within the first 24 hours post-operatively has been found to increase the likelihood of surgical site infection fourfold after non-cardiac surgery (7). This phenomenon is most often cited in patients who are known to be diabetic, but it has also been identified as a concern in non-diabetics as well. It is very important to monitor glucose closely and to correct hyperglycemia in all populations to prevent infection or dehiscence.

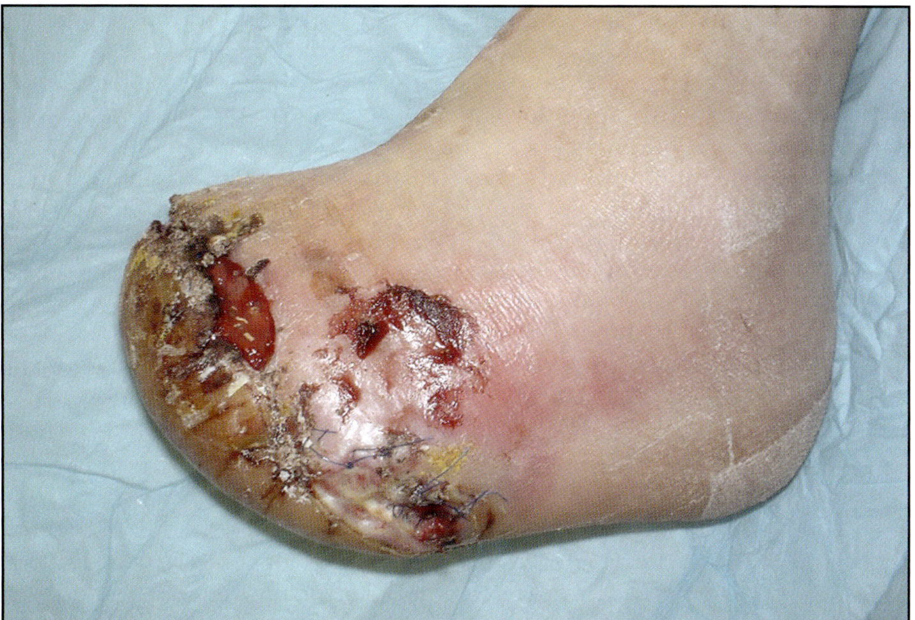

Figure 3. Infected wound following closure of a midfoot amputation.

PURPOSE OF DRESSING

Application of a dressing to a post operative wound serves to protect the underlying surface from bacterial contamination and trauma. In addition to providing an environment for optimal wound healing, a dressing will secondarily aid in hemostasis, absorption of drainage, and splintage of the surgical site. Dressing choices for elective surgical procedures are vary by type of wound, part of the body, and personal preference. Most surgeons apply non-adherent dressing such as Adaptic™, Xeroform®, Telfa®, or petroleum gauze. Others utilize an iodine gauze or simple dry sterile gauze dressing as the primary layer. Secondary dressings often add to the bulk or absorptive quality of the dressing and usually extend far beyond the surgical margins. Extremity surgical procedures often utilize a form of immobilization post operatively to reduce motion and to reduce edema. Splinting is often used following a bony procedure to provide the best possible protection of the surgical site. Edema is controlled by elevation of the effected part above heart level, compressive dressing, and cold therapy to the surgical site post operatively.

SUTURE AND DRAINAGE CARE

Common surgical wound closure techniques include adhesive strips, sutures, staples, or skin glue. Varieties of suturing techniques have been utilized to close surgical wounds depending on the nature and condition of the wound. Sutures are divided into several categories which include absorbable vs. non-absorbable, synthetic vs. natural, and braided vs. monofilament. The actual suture materials which are commonly used include nylon, polyester, stainless steel, cotton, silk, polyethylene, gut, and polyglycolic acid sutures. Wounds are often closed in layers with the deep layer closure using absorbable suture i.e., polyglactin (Vicryl) suture. The early stage of suture degradation via hydrolysis can trigger local inflammation in response to a foreign body reaction. This reaction can be to the suture or other absorbable surgical implants that may lead to the formation of a sterile abscess or even act as a nidus for an infection. There is a significant difference noted in the degree to which different suture materials cause reactivity. For example, stainless steel and polypropylene sutures are minimally reactive, while silk and natural gut suture materials cause significant local reactivity and can be associated with wound complications. The presence of one silk suture can alter the intrinsic immune resistance and lower the number of bacteria necessary to cause infection. The study by Edlich et al. (9) indicates that the usage of tape to close wounds shows a greatest degree of resistance to infection, followed by stapled wounds, and finally closure by sutures. Sutures are usually removed when wounds are clinically healed at 10–14 days post-operatively. The most important concept in suture removal is to cut one end of the suture as close to the skin surface as possible and then pull the long end of the suture away from the skin/incision site. The goal is to minimize the chance of iatrogenic inoculation of the contaminated suture into the subcutaneous structures. The type of suture material, the diameter and the quality of suture, and the tightness with which each suture was tied across the wound are all noted risk factors for infection. Another option for skin closure is topical skin adhesive or skin glue also called liquid suture. This skin glue forms a thin film over the surgical site and actually provides an antimicrobial barrier while maintaining closure. The film will fall off after 14–20 days alleviating the need for suture removal. Skin glue does not change the need for deep closure sutures and is not appropriate when there is tension at the surgical site.

Generally, post-operative wounds can be cleansed with a variety of antiseptic solutions throughout the healing process without concern for disruption the healing process. Chlohexidine (Hibiclens) and povidone-iodine (Betadine) are the most commonly used antiseptic solutions. A solution of povidone-iodine in 1:1000 dilution is effective against *Staphylococcus aureus* without being cytotoxic to tissue cells of the wound. It is common to observe some degree of erythema, edema, and sometimes calor in the normal post operative wound. This most often is a sign of local inflammation versus an actual early sign of infection. The presence of post operative infection is usually accompanied by constitutional signs and symptoms: nausea, chills, fever, vomiting, and increasing pain not relieved with appropriate analgesic medication.

In surgical procedures involving deep spaces or in which hemostasis may be a concern, a drain is often placed into the wound site post-operatively. The purpose of a drain is to prevent formation of hematoma, seroma, and other excessive drainage that may interfere with wound healing. The presence of a hematoma in a closed wound creates an environment which is at a heightened risk for infection and other wound complications. Oxygenation to a hematoma is limited and phagocytosis is often retarded. Drains can be either closed or open to the outside environment. Closed suction drains (i.e., Hemovac®, Jackson-Pratt) provide the most reliable source for negative pressure without exposing the wound depths to the outside environment. It is important to record the exact output of wound drainage on each shift.

Most drains are removed or replaced after 24–48 hours or when the total input is less than 10 mL in a 24-hour period. A drain left in place greater than 72 hours can place added infection risk on the site. If the wound site remains open post operatively, the surgeon may elect to utilize negative pressure wound therapy (Wound VAC®, KCI, San Antonio, Texas; or Blue Sky Versatile 1™ Wound Vaccum System, Blue Sky Medical, Carlsbad, California). This system uses a vacuum to create a closed circuit suction system via a porous sponge, surgical tubing, and a clear film dressing. This system is used to promote granulation and remove excess exudate in chronic and acute wounds.

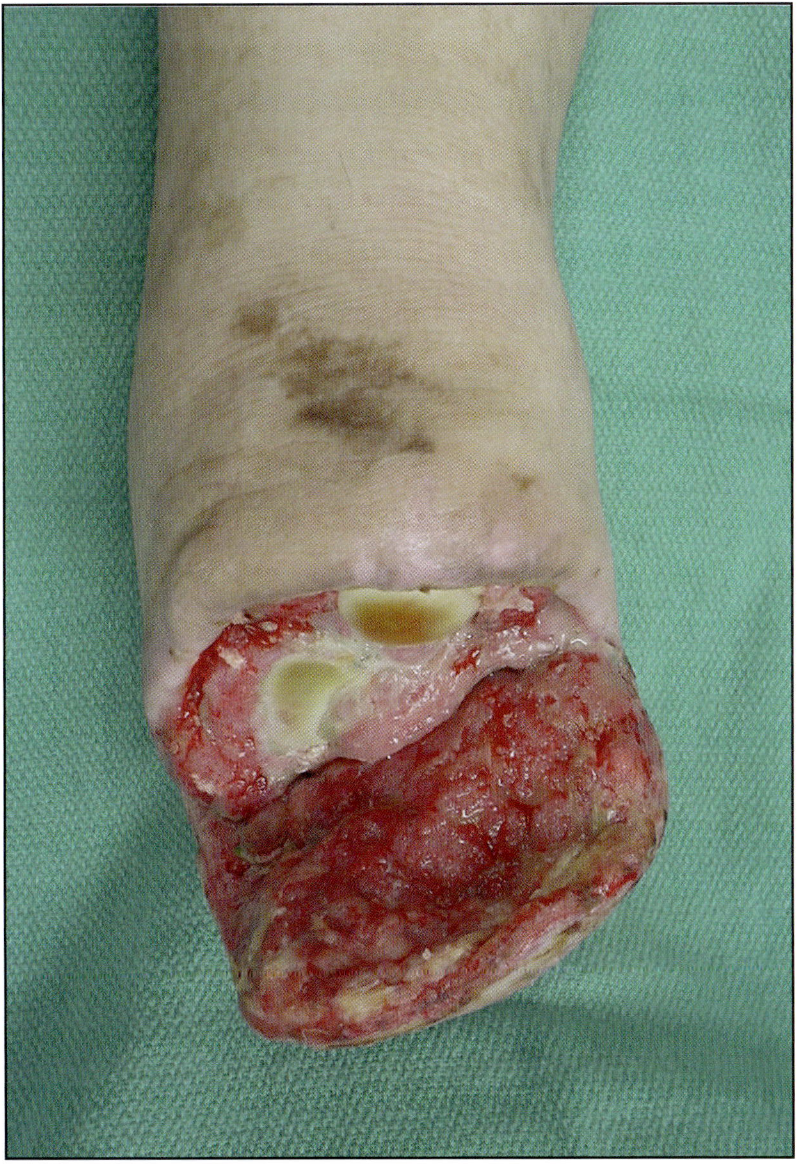

Figure 4. Problem wound site following Choparts Amputation with fibrous soft tissue base and desiccated bone and cartilage.

HEAT AND COLD THERAPY

Therapeutic application of heat or cold therapy at a surgical site can elicit local and systemic responses. External heat application will generally stimulate blood flow to the area via vasodilation and is appropriate after the inflammatory stage of healing is over. Heat application to a diabetic wound must be monitored closely to prevent iatrogenic burns to the insensate extremities of these patients. Cold therapy will induce vasoconstriction at the wound site and will reduce local inflammatory responses. Cold application can be used as an effective local anesthetic and can also serve to reduce cell metabolism and increase blood viscosity. Cold therapy is contraindicated in ischemic wounds or in patients with peripheral vascular disease.

POST-OPERATIVE WOUND INFECTION

Despite the advances in sterile technique and instrumentation, up to 84% of surgically "prepped" feet culture positive for bacteria just prior to skin incision. It is no surprise that infection of post-operative wounds in elective surgery occurs consistently in 1–2% of all cases. Post-operative infections generally make themselves evident on post-op day 3 or later. Body temperature fluctuation and increased white blood cell count with shifts to the left (presence of band cells) are reliable indicators of post-operative infection. Caution is needed when evaluating clinical indicators of infection in various patient groups, as emphasized in a study by Lavery et al. at the University of Texas Health Science Center in San Antonio which found that diabetic infections can occur *without* elevation of white blood cells and oral temperature. Diabetic patients will notice an abrupt elevation in their glucose levels prior to developing other systemic signs of infection. In the initial assessment of post-operative wounds, one should assess for drainage, fluctuance, erythema, temperature or odor. Fluctuance of a surgical wound often indicates hematoma, seroma, or perhaps an abscess. In addition, the presence of pain which is out of expected proportions can be a significant warning sign that infection is present. If any or all of these warning signs are present during the post operative period, the surgeon must decide on a course of action. Generally a few sutures/staples can be removed to allow drainage of the wound site and irrigation/exploration of the site. If significant infection is suspected, then a return to the operating room will most likely be necessary to open and explore/debride the site as needed. Inspection and culture of the wound exudate can also provide valuable information on infection. Staphylococcal infections possess odorless golden pus, where as Streptococcal infection generally shows serous to serosanguineous drainage with possible non-blanching erythema/petichiae and red streaking (lymphangitis) (10). Infected wounds require immediate action from the health care team. Quick gram stain obtained from the wound site allows early empiric antibiotic therapy and the choice of antibiotic will be adjusted accordingly with the result of deep tissue or bone cultures. The infected post operative wound should undergo formal incision and drainage with possible debridement of all necrotic tissue, foreign debris, hematoma, and dead space. These wounds are normally left open for management and will eventually be considered for closure when the clinical signs of infection have resolved. It has been proposed that if wound demonstrates three negative cultures then it is deemed ready for closure. In general, this is clinically challenging because all open wounds have a high predilection for sub-clinical bacterial contamination which would continually yield positive cultures despite the fact that no infection is present. Robson et al. found that wounds with delayed closure that contain 10^5 or less bacteria per gram of tissue progressed to uncomplicated wound healing whereas none of the wounds with greater than 10^5 bacteria per gram of tissue healed successfully (11). Quantitative cultures can assist in making this detailed wound assessment, but due to limited availability of this test, the provider is often faced with making this decision based mostly on clinical appearance of the wound site.

Regarding antibiotic therapy, it is important to remember that the most effective time to prescribe prophylactic antibiotics is 30–60 minutes before the surgical incision is made. Numerous studies have confirmed that pre-operative antibiotics have a better chance of preventing a surgical wound infection than does a post-operative prescription.

WOUND DEHISCENCE, HYPERTROPHIC SCARS, AND KELOIDS

Wound dehiscence is another common post operative complication. It involves gaping along the incision site and the skin is therefore no longer coapted. A wound dehiscence can be superficial and involve only the top skin layers, or it can be extensive and involve all deep layers of the wound closure. Post-operative wound dehiscence can be caused by infection, poor surgical placement of the incision, body's reaction to sutures, edema, hematoma, seroma, poor tissue perfusion, or intra operative tissue trauma. Some patients are at increased risk for post-operative dehiscence. These include patients with poorly controlled diabetes, other chronic diseases, poor skin integrity, rheumatoid patients on chronic steroid therapy, and geriatric patients. Initial treatment of wound dehiscence involves exploration and evaluation of the site. Once this has been assessed, one may want to consider debridement and culture. Once the site is deemed stable, the wound can be re-approximated with adhesive strips and compressive dressing to control edema and to reduce skin tension.

Patients with superficial wound dehiscence or macerated/exudative incisions can be treated aggressively using topical dressings. Cadexomer iodine (Iodosorb gel or Iodoflex, Smith & Nephew) cleanses the wound by absorbing fluid, pus, exudates, bacteria, enzymes and cellular residue. It also has a time-released antimicrobial that has been shown to effectively treat MRSA and other resistant bacteria. It is contraindicated in patients with iodine allergy or those with thyroid conditions. Absorptive dressings that contain silver ions can also be used over macerated or dehisced incisions. These dressings come as alginates, hydrofibers, foams, composites and packing strips. In addition to controlling the local exudates, these dressings also reduce bacterial load as a result of the antimicrobial properties from silver which is also active against MRSA and other resistant bacteria (12).

Wound dehiscence can be caused by hypertrophic tissue and keloid formation, especially in patients with a history of such a wound disorder. Hypertrophic scar is defined as raised, erythematous, pruritic lesions that remain confined within the original scar (13). Keloids have similar presentation as hypertrophic scars but generally extend beyond the border of the original scar. Wound contracture is part of the normal healing process in which the edges of wound are drawn toward center in attempts to spread wound closure. Scar contracture results from extra-cellular matrix degradation, contraction, and cross-linking during the remodeling phase that leads to an undesirable cosmetic result and rigid deformity. Keloid and hypertrophic scars are often treated with injections to reduce of break apart the collagen bulk or silicone padding to decrease the shear forces and pressure on the site.

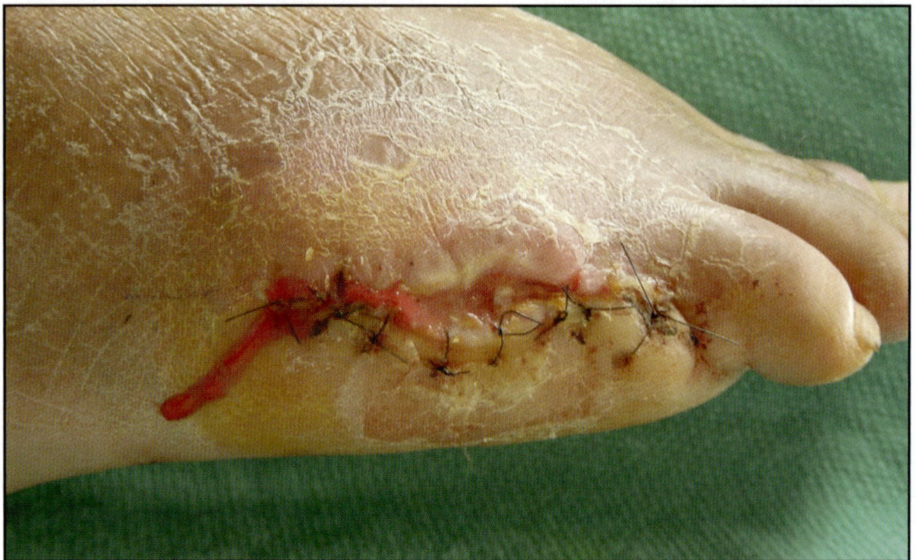

Figure 5. Dehiscent incision necessitating suture removal and debridement. Note the fibrous tissue and edema contributing to the wound.

CONCLUSION

In order to properly treat the post operative wound complication, one must first understand the nature and origin of the wound. A comprehensive evaluation of the patient's medical and surgical history is necessary in order to differentiate uncomplicated wounds from those that will require a high level of attention. Nothing can be taken for granted or assumed when evaluating these patients and their wounds. Generally, with proper supportive care, the majority of post operative wounds will heal uneventfully and rapidly. However, in those patients with complicating systemic illness or extenuating local wound concerns, a post operative wound can rapidly become a limb or life threatening entity. Providers should always be mindful that sometimes the most important tool to combat a post-operative wound is a proper *pre-operative* assessment of local and systemic wound risk factors.

REFERENCES

1. Cole S. Clients with wounds. In Potter PA, Perry AG (ed). *Fundamentals of Nursing concepts, Process & Practice* St Louis: Mosby-Year Book Inc, 1993; 1652-1693.

2. Wilczynski RJ. Wound dehiscence, hypertrophic scars, and keloids. *Clinics in Podiatric Medicine and Surgery* 1991; 8:359-365.

3. Stadelmann WK, Digenis AG, Tobin GR. Physiology and healing dynamics of chronic cutaneous wounds. *Am J Surgery* 1998; 176: 26s-38s.

4. Albritton JS. Complication of wound repair. *Clinics in Podiatric Medicine and Surgery* 1991; 8:773-785.

5. Arnold M, Barbul A. Nutrition and wound healing. *Plastic and Reconstructive Surgery*, June 2006; 117(7S): 42S-58S.

6. Davis JC. The use of adjuvant hyperbaric oxygen in treatment of the diabetic foot. *Clinic in Podiatric Medicine and Surgery* 1987; 4: 429-437.

7. Barie PS, Eachempati SR. Surgical site infections. *Surg Clin North Am* 2005; 85(6):1115–1135.

8. Jeter KF, Tintle TE. Wound dressings of the nineties: indications and contraindications. *Clinic in Podiatric Medicine and Surgery* 1991; 8: 799-815.

9. Edlich RF, Becker DG, Thacker JG,et al. scientific basic for selecting staple and tape skin closures. *Clinic in Plastic Surgery* 1990; 17: 571-581.

10. Joseph WS. Clinical and laboratory diagnosis of lower extremity infection. *J Am Pod Med Assoc* 1989; 79:505-510.

11. Robson MC, Stenberg BD, Heggers JP. Wound healing alterations caused by infection. *Clinics in Plastic Surgery* 1990; 17: 451-465.

12. Hess CT. Clinical Guide: *Wound Care 5th ed*. Lippincott, Williams and Wilkins, Philadelphia, PA. 2005.

13. Su CW, Alizadeh K, Boddie A, et al. The problem scar. *Clinics in Plastic Surgery* 1998; 25: 451-465.

14. Ostrander RV, Brage ME, Botte MJ. Bacterial skin contamination after surgical preparation in foot and ankle surgery. *Clinical Orthopedics and Related Research* 2003; 1(406): 246-252.

15. Pinzur MS, Sage R, Stuck R, et al. Transcutaneous oxygen as a predictor of wound healing in amputations of the foot and ankle. *Foot Ankle* 1992; 13(5): 271-272.

16. Stuck RM, Sage R, Pinzur M, et al. Amputations in the diabetic foot. *Clinics in Podiatric Medicine and Surgery* 1995; 12(1): 141-155.

17. Sivestro A, Diehm N, Savolainen H, et al. Falsely high ankle-brackial index predicts major amputation in critical limb ischemia. *Vascular Medicine* 2006; 11(2): 69-74.

REVIEW QUESTIONS

1.) The proliferative phase of wound healing lasts for approximately:
   a. 1 week
   b. 24 days
   c. 2 months
   d. 1 year

2.) The decreased digital blood flow from a single cigarette can persist up to:
   a. 10 minutes
   b. 25 minutes
   c. 40 minutes
   d. 50 minutes

3.) Chronic corticosteroid therapy depletes the body of:
   a. Vitamin A
   b. Copper
   c. PDGF
   d. Fibroblasts

4.) $P_{tc}O_2$ or $TcpO_2$ values of greater than _______ mm Hg indicate a likelihood that the surgical site will heal:
   a. 5
   b. 10
   c. 20
   d. 40

5.) The most effective time to administer prophylactic antibiotics is:
   a. 30-60 minutes before the surgical incision
   b. 30 minutes after surgical incision
   c. Continuous for three days following surgery
   d. 24 hours post surgery

Answers: 1b, 2d, 3a, 4d, 5a

CHAPTER 12

ARTERIAL INSUFFICIENCY ULCERS

CHAPTER TWELVE OVERVIEW

ARTERIAL INSUFFICIENCY ULCERS

Mellick T. Sykes, Ronald L. Blumoff

INTRODUCTION
Arterial Insufficiency Ulcers

Arterial insufficiency ulcers represent a late manifestation of peripheral arterial disease (PAD), a syndrome of chronic limb symptoms caused by progressive stenosis of the arteries (and consequent decreased blood flow) to the legs. Other historical terms for this syndrome include chronic limb ischemia, lower extremity occlusive disease (LEOD), lower extremity arterial disease (LEAD), or peripheral vascular disease (PVD).

Although atherosclerosis is by far the most common etiology, PAD may be caused by thromboangiitis obliterans (Buerger's Disease), inflammatory arteritis, radiation arteritis, adventitial cystic disease, popliteal aneurysm, or popliteal entrapment syndrome.

Ulceration of the feet may be caused by PAD alone; however, coexisting PAD may exacerbate ulcers with another etiology. Patients with refractory venous or neurogenic ulcers should be evaluated for occult arterial compromise.

Arterial insufficiency ulcers usually result from minor tissue trauma in the setting of decreased blood flow. Successful treatment focuses on meticulous wound care, avoidance of further trauma, and restoration of adequate blood flow.

PATHOPHYSIOLOGY
Blood Flow and Its Determinants

Blood vessels carry oxygen, nutrients, and immunologic factors to tissues. On a cellular level, these factors sustain tissue and combat infection. Toxic local waste products, greatly increased in areas of infection or wounding, are eliminated by blood flow. Regardless of other factors, an ulcer without adequate blood flow heals poorly.

What physical factors affect blood flow? Flow in an ideal laminar tube is described by Poiseuille's equation, which states that flow within a vessel is proportional to the driving pressure gradient, the fourth power of the radius, and is inversely proportional to the length of the tube:

$$\text{Flow} = \pi P R^4 / 8\eta L$$
$$\text{where}$$
$$P = \text{driving pressure; } R = \text{radius of the vessel;}$$
$$\eta = \text{viscosity; } L = \text{length of the vessel.}$$

Poiseuille's equation explains the profound effect of atherosclerosis on blood flow: a stenosis that decreases the vessel radius by one-half causes a sixteen-fold decrease in maximum blood flow. Energy losses caused by turbulence within and distal to a stenosis also result in diminished flow.

Atherosclerosis and Blood Flow

Atherosclerosis (AS) reduces flow by several mechanisms: 1) AS plaque narrows the vessel radius which diminishes distal flow exponentially; 2) irregular AS plaque produces turbulent flow which further lessens the energy and flow to distal tissue, and 3) the intimal "cap" over the plaque may ulcerate or dissect, releasing atheroembolic plaque or thrombus to occlude distal vessels.

Absolute and Relative Ischemia

Ischemia occurs when local tissue demands exceed the supply of blood flow.

$$\text{Ischemia} = \text{Demand} > \text{Supply}$$

Ischemia may be caused by increased demand, decreased supply, or both. PAD causes a drop in the absolute blood flow to a limb (absolute ischemia), which may or may not cause clinical symptoms depending on the tissue metabolic demands.

Exercise, infection, and trauma are high-metabolic processes which greatly increase the demand for blood flow. If this is unavailable due to PAD, exercise ends prematurely in claudication, infection spreads, wounds fail to heal, and tissue dies. The concept of relative ischemia refers to a discrepancy between the amount of blood available and the amount of blood needed to carry on cellular function. Relative ischemia arises when supply becomes inadequate, demand increases, or both.

Trauma and Ischemia

Arterial insufficiency ulcers commonly begin with minor or repetitive tissue injury, often initially unrecognized. In the setting of PAD, a seemingly trivial injury becomes a nonhealing ulcer or a portal for infection. It is this combination of poor arterial blood flow and tissue trauma that creates the arterial insufficiency ulcer. The wound, ulcer, or infection are secondary phenomena.

CLASSIFICATION

Fontaine's simple description of the classic stages of chronic limb ischemia is useful in understanding the progression of PAD. Rutherford's more recent scheme is complex and cumbersome for the practitioner, but facilitates accurate comparison of treatment groups (Table 1). Although these categories depict progressively severe symptoms, patients with PAD do not necessarily pass through all stages. Most Stage II claudicants never progress to critical limb ischemia, for example, and many diabetics present with Stage IV gangrene as the first manifestation of arterial occlusive disease.

Asymptomatic

PAD progresses insidiously. The initial asymptomatic phase (Fontaine Stage I) involves gradual narrowing of the major limb vessels accompanied by

TABLE 1. FONTAINE AND RUTHERFORD CLASSIFICATIONS OF CHRONIC LIMB ISCHEMIA

FONTAINE		RUTHERFORD				
Stage	Description	Grade	Category	Clinical Features	Objective Criteria	
I	Asymptomatic	0	0	Asymptomatic– no hemodynamically significant occlusive disease	Normal treadmill or reactive hyperemia test	
II	Intermittent Claudication	I	1	Mild claudication	Completes treadmill exercise*; AP after exercise > 50 mm Hg but at least 20 mm Hg lower than resting value	
			2	Moderative claudication		
			3	Severe claudication	Cannot complete treadmill exercise and AP after exercise < 50 mm Hg	
III	Ischemic rest pain	II	4	Ischemic rest pain	Resting AP < 40 mmHg; flat or barely pulsatile ankle or metatarsal PVR; TP < 40 mm Hg	CHRONIC CRITICAL LIMB ISCHEMIS: CCLI
IV	Ulceration or gangrene or both	III	5	Minor tissue loss–nonhealing ulcer, focal gangrene with diffuse pedal ischemia	Resting AP < 60 mm Hg; flat or barely pulsatile ankle or metatarsal PVR; TP < 40 mm Hg	
			6	Major tissue loss–extending above TM level, functional foot no longer salvageable	Same as category 5	

*TP=Toe Pressure; AP=Ankle Pressure; PVR=Pulse Volume Recording; *=Five minutes at 2mph on 12% incline*

a variable degree of collateralization by branch vessels such as the internal iliac, profunda femoral, geniculate, tibial and muscular arteries. Presence and severity of symptoms depend on a variety of individual factors including activity level, expectations, coexisting risk factors, rate and extent of luminal obliteration, and degree of collateral development. The duration of the asymptomatic phase may be decades; inactive patients may never manifest intermittent claudication.

Intermittent Claudication (IC)

As stenoses increase, most patients complain of exercise-induced cramping, aching, or tiredness of the calf, thigh, or buttock. The pain is reproducible by the same walking distance daily. Inclined surfaces are particularly difficult. Pain is relieved with brief rest maintaining the standing position. This is the classic picture of intermittent claudication (IC–Fontaine Stage II).

Vascular claudication must be distinguished from other common causes of leg pain with activity, particularly arthritis and spinal stenosis which affect the same older population. Arthritis symptoms are variable, lacking the reproducibility of vascular IC. Lumbospinal compression is not relieved while standing, and both onset and relief are more variable.

Rest Pain

With continued compromise of the arterial supply, patients experience ischemic rest pain (Fontaine Stage III). Rest pain may begin in a nocturnal pattern when the combined effects of leg elevation and central redistribution of cardiac output combine to further deprive the foot of circulation. Ischemic rest pain is typically located in the metatarsal and instep area. Patients may resort to sleeping in a chair or with the foot hanging off the bed.

Tissue Loss: Ulceration and Gangrene

With progression of PAD, minor trauma or infection produce ulcers or gangrene (Fontaine Stage IV). This category includes neuroischemic plantar ulcers which do not heal. Inactivity and sensory neuropathy may mask claudication and rest pain, allowing gangrene to be the first manifestation of PAD.

Critical Limb Ischemia (CLI)

Thus PAD may progress from a prolonged asymptomatic period into a phase of non-critical ischemic symptoms of claudication or diminished mobility, and finally to an end stage of critical limb ischemia (CLI) in which, without treatment, loss of limb is imminent.

CLI is defined as a combination of desperate clinical presentation (rest pain, ulceration, or gangrene) plus objective evidence that the pain or tissue lesion is caused predominantly by arterial insufficiency.

CLI includes Fontaine's Stages III and IV, and Categories 4, 5, and 6 of Rutherford's scheme (see Table1).

EPIDEMIOLOGY

Good population data on PAD in its most general form is scarce. Several factors contribute: much vascular disease is asymptomatic; other medical conditions besides ischemia may affect ambulation and produce ulcers, and objective testing has only recently been standardized. Recent interest in PAD by national medical organizations has provided a broader audience with screening and treatment guidelines.

Peripheral Arterial Disease (PAD)

Estimates of persons with PAD in the US are around 10 million. For every person with symptomatic PAD, three others have asymptomatic stenoses discovered by ABI screening.

Depending on the population and method of screening, prevalence ranges from 3% to 22%, increasing dramatically in the later decades of life. At age 60 the prevalence is 3–6%, rising to 20% for persons over 70.

Risk factors for development of symptomatic PAD are listed in Table 2. In contrast to coronary artery disease, few patients develop PAD without identifiable risk factors.

TABLE 2. RISK FACTORS FOR PAD

Risk Factors	Smoking Diabetes & IGT Advancing Age Male HTN	Hyperlipidemia Fibrinogen Homocysteine Polycythemia Thrombocytosis
Protective Factors	Mild-moderate ethanol intake	Regular exercise

Critical Limb Ischemia (CLI)

Critical limb ischemia has an estimated incidence of 300-1000 per million per year. Risk factors for development and progression of CLI include increased age, smoking, and diabetes. By age 60, roughly 15-20% of the population has PAD, 5% has claudication, and just under 1% has critical limb ischemia.

EVALUATION

Differential Diagnosis

Ulcers caused by venous disease or neuropathy must be distinguished from arterial ulcers. Table 3 summarizes characteristic diagnostic features of each group. Etiologies may coexist with additive effects and require combined treatment. For example, plantar ulcers—the classic *mal perforans* neuropathic ulcer—often have underlying arterial insufficiency (See Figure 1).

TABLE 3. DIFFERENTIAL DIAGNOSIS OF FOOT AND ANKLE ULCERS

Type	Ischemic	Venous	Neuropathic
Location	Toes, interdigital, heel, lateral malleolus	Lower leg (gaiter), above medial malleolus	Plantar
Pain	Present, relieved with dependency	Mild, relieved with elevation	Absent
Appearance	Pale, irregular, dry, poor granulation	Beefy red granulation	Deep tract, punched out
Pulses	Poor/absent	Present, may be hidden by induration	Normal
Skin	Trophic changes: thin, shiny, dry. Thick nails.	Stasis changes: thick, indurated, pigmented	Normal; callus
Bleeding	Poor	Venous	Brisk
Edema	None–muscular atrophy	Present	None
Risk Factos	For atherosclerosis, especially: Smoking, diabetes, age.	Varicose veins, prior DVT	Diabetes, immobility
Key Treatment	Revascularization	Compression	Off loading
If treatment lags suspect:	Renal failure, infection, restenosis	Occult ischemia, inadequate compression	Occult ischemia, osteomyelitits

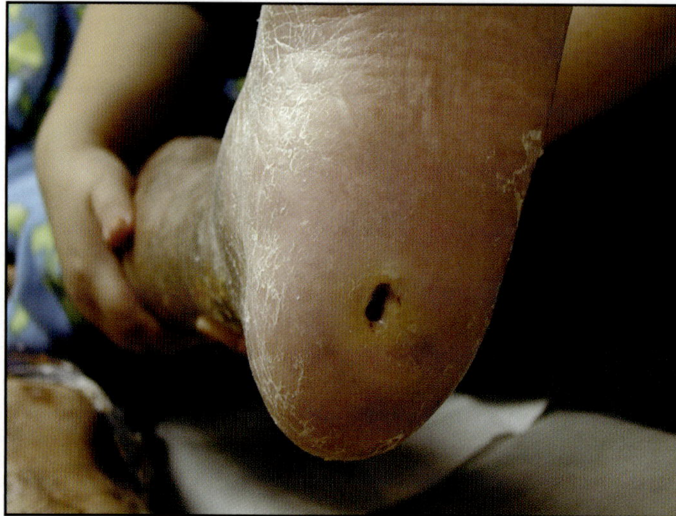

Figure 1. Plantar ulcer.

Symptoms

Symptoms of peripheral arterial disease depend on the severity and location of the arterial blockage; adequacy of collateral circulation; individual patient activity, expectations, and pain tolerance; and the influences of trauma and co-morbidities such as heart disease or diabetes.

Without neuropathy

In the presence of a foot ulcer, any exercise intolerance or foot pain suggests vascular insufficiency. A patient with vascular claudication or ischemic rest pain often blames arthritis or sciatica, delaying treatment.

Symptoms with neuropathy

Sensory neuropathy diminishes perception of pain. Diabetic neuropathy in particular predisposes a patient to foot trauma, and delays the recognition of such injury. The same neuropathy that permits foot trauma may also hide its progression into ulcer, infection, or gangrene. Resulting delay in treatment worsens chances for limb salvage.

Physical Examination

Because PAD patients generally have other medical issues which affect therapy and prognosis, physical examination should be thorough, then focused on the foot ulcer and the neurovascular status of the leg.

Pulses

The mainstay of evaluation of the arterial system remains the palpation of pulses in the lower extremity. Femoral, popliteal, and pedal (dorsalis pedis and posterior tibial) pulses should be palpated and characterized. Although many schemata exist, we prefer the simple scale of

    0 = absent
    1+ = palpable, but diminished
    2+ = normal

Together with critical inspection of the foot, a reliable diagnosis of CLI can usually be made on these bases alone.

Diminished or absent femoral pulses signify aortoiliac occlusive disease, often accompanied by a femoral bruit.

Popliteal pulses may be difficult to feel in muscular, obese, or edematous patients. Prominent or exaggerated popliteal pulses suggest aneurysm, which may cause ischemia by recurrent embolization. Use of two hands is needed to exert sufficient pressure for popliteal palpation (Figure 2).

Foot pulses deserve special attention. The dorsalis pedis pulse is the extension of the anterior tibial artery, and is felt superficially between the dorsal first and second metatarsal bones. A light touch is required, and the foot must be completely relaxed. Involuntary twitching of the extensor tendons may fool the inexperienced examiner into recording a dorsalis pedis pulse where none exists (Figure 3).

The posterior tibial pulse is felt posterior to the medial malleolus. A deeper vessel, it requires stronger pressure particularly if edema is present. Slight passive dorsiflexion of the foot often smoothes out the overlying flexor retinaculum (which buckles during plantar flexion), and discovers an elusive pulse (Figure 4A and B).

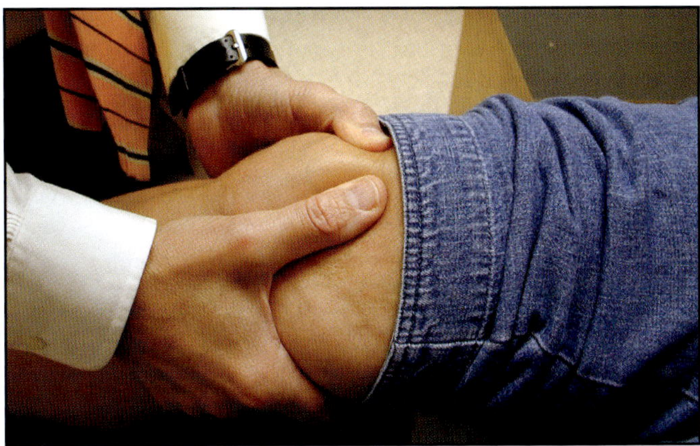

Figure 2. Popliteal pulse. Two hands and patience.

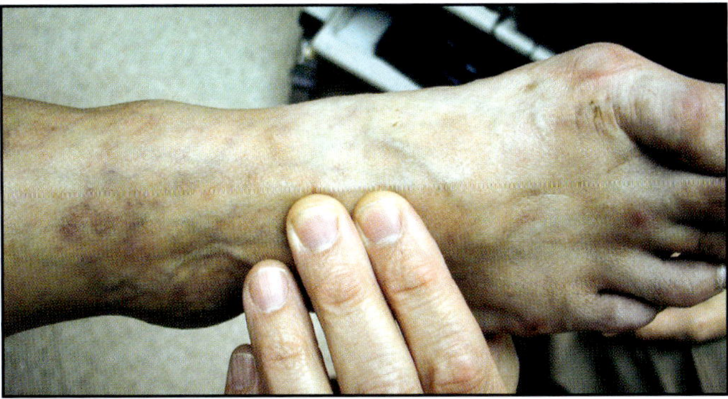

Figure 3. Dorsalis pedis pulse. Light touch.

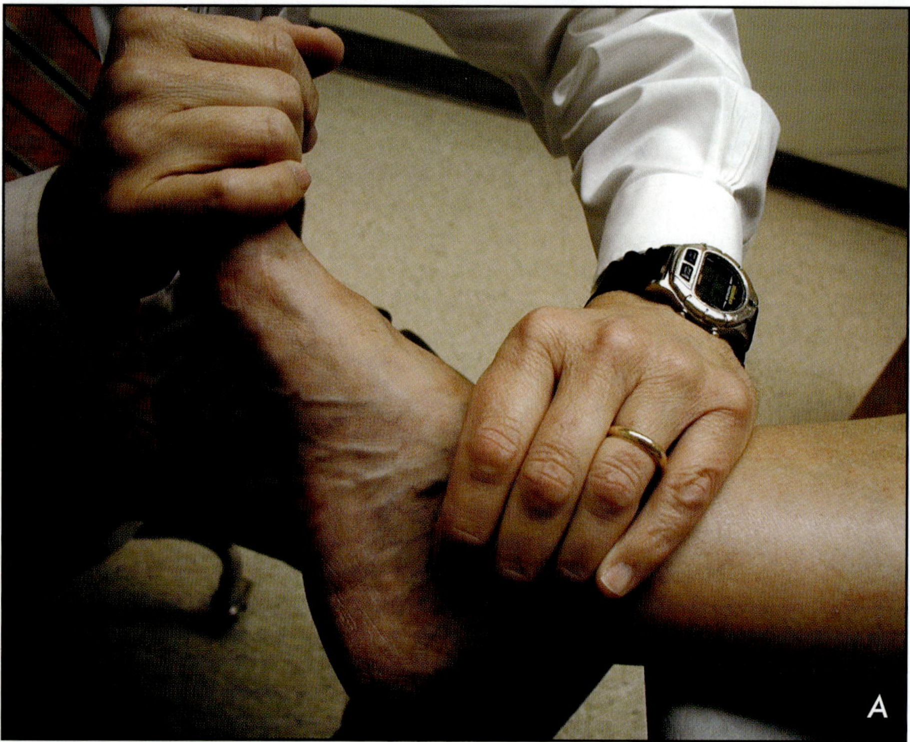

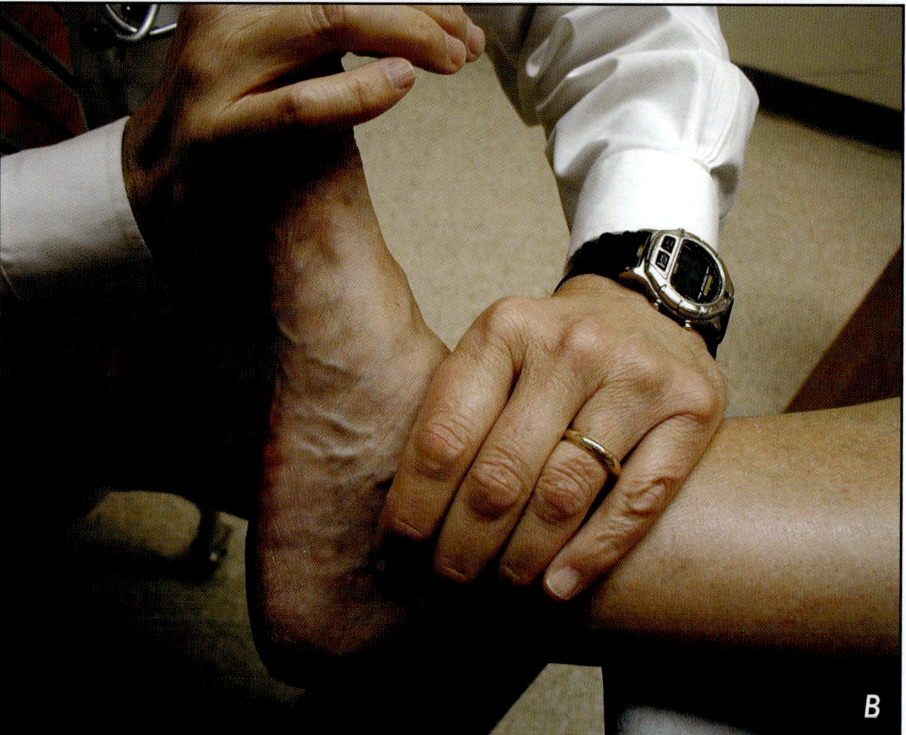

Figure 4. (A and B) Posterior tibial pulse palpation aided by gentle dorsiflexion of ankle.

Bedside Doppler exam

Particularly if a pulse cannot be palpated, a Doppler ultrasound probe should be used to elicit a signal over the artery. A normal arterial signal is triphasic, i.e., there are three components to the signal: 1) a sharp forward sound corresponding to systole, 2) a brief second sound of reversed flow, corresponding to elastic recoil from peripheral vessels, and 3) a period of forward diastolic flow corresponding to aortic valve closure.

As proximal stenoses progress the Doppler signal becomes biphasic, monophasic, or absent. Biphasic signals lack one of the aforementioned components, usually the period of reversal of flow or the forward diastolic flow. A monophasic signal exhibits a delayed upstroke, has a blunted peak, and no flow reversal or second component. Doppler signals are summarized in Figure 5.

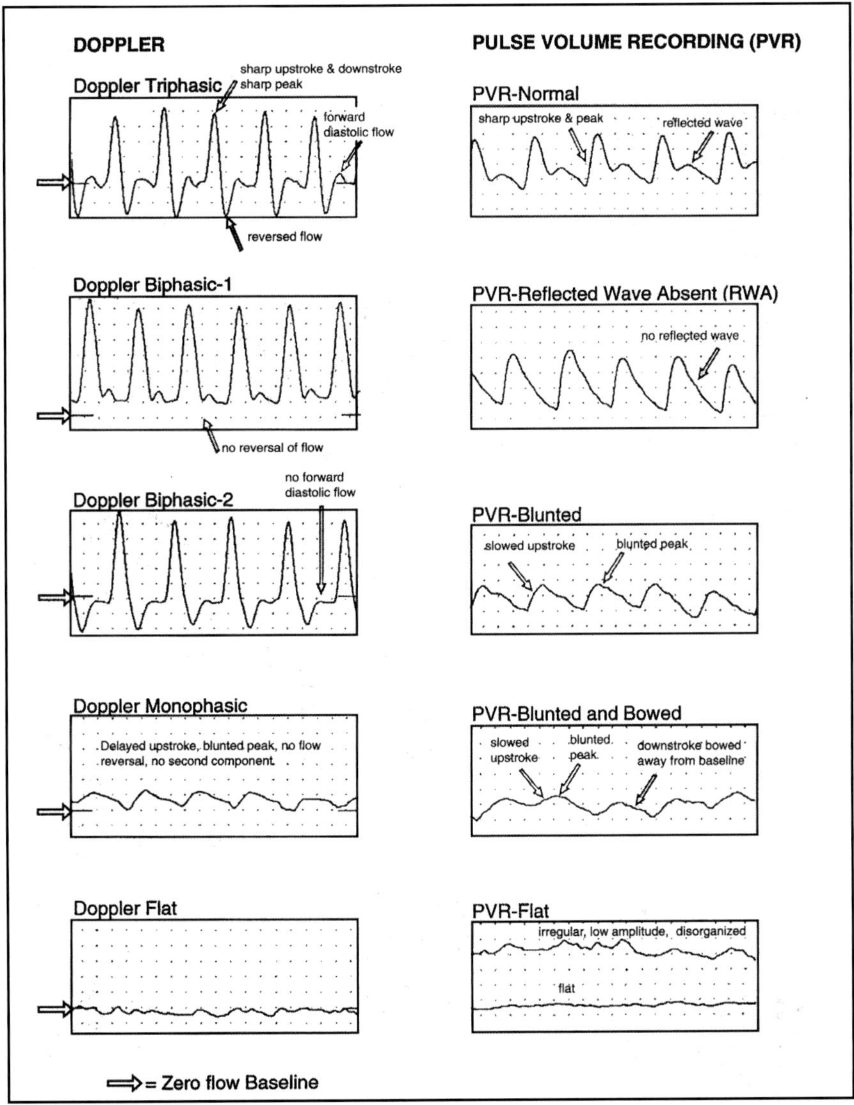

Figure 5. Doppler waveforms and pulse volume recordings. Information not dependent on vessel compression.

Visual inspection of the foot

The leg and foot should be inspected for other signs of arterial insufficiency. Trophic changes from chronic tissue malperfusion include: atrophy of skin and muscles, loss of distal pulp turgor, diminished lanugo hair, dependent rubor and elevation pallor, and nails which are hypertrophic from slow growth (Figure 6 A, B, C). The affected foot may be cooler than the other side. Signs of infection, such as cellulitis, plantar tenderness, or drainage should also be noted. Toes should be spread to find occult interdigital ulcers. The heel and plantar surface should be palpated for tenderness, suggesting deep infection.

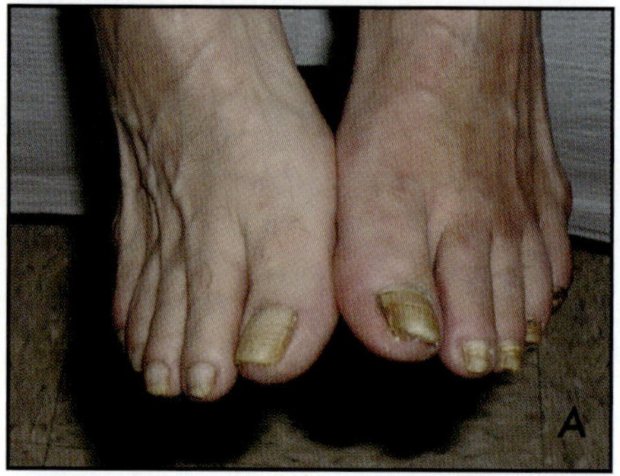
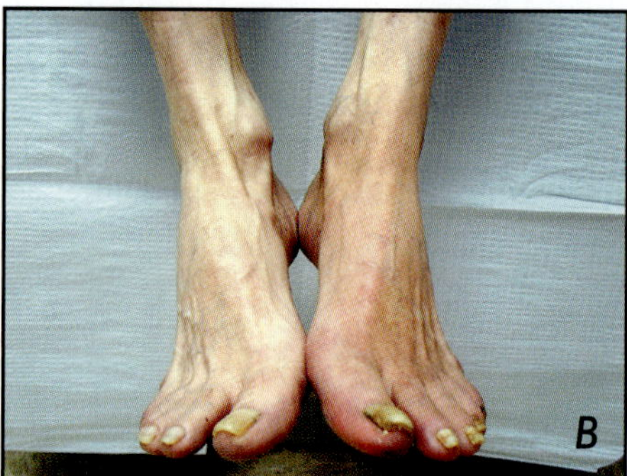
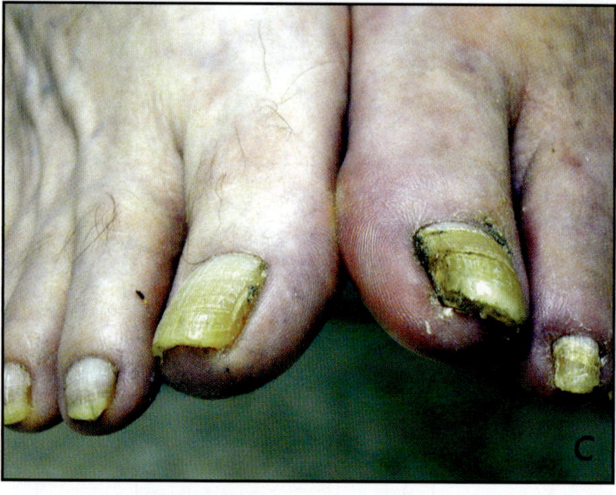

Figure 6 (A–C).
A. Trophic changes of PAD on left foot.
B. Dependent rubor of left foot.
C. Hypertrophic nails from slow growth.

Vascular Laboratory

Although the clinical diagnosis of PAD by pulse and foot examination is generally accurate, it is subjective and non-quantitative. Moreover, its accuracy is dependent on the experience and thoroughness of the clinician. The vascular laboratory enables an objective measurement of arterial circulation, localizes approximate levels of stenoses, and helps determine the role of revascularization for the individual patient.

Ankle-Brachial Index(ABI)

The standard test for PAD is the ankle-brachial pressure index (ABI or ABPI). This requires only a hand-held continuous wave Doppler and sphygmomanometer. It can be readily taught and is easy to perform (Figure 7).

The blood pressure in each of the patient's arms is taken and recorded. The higher systolic pressure will be used in the calculation. Next, the Doppler probe is positioned over the dorsalis pedis or posterior tibial pulse. A blood pressure cuff is placed around the patient's ankle and is insufflated to a pressure that causes the Doppler signal to disappear. The cuff is then slowly deflated. When the Doppler signal becomes audible again, the corresponding number on the sphygmomanometer dial is recorded. The ankle to brachial index is expressed as a ratio of the highest ankle pressure obtained divided by the higher systolic arm pressure. This process is repeated for the other leg.

A value over 0.95 is considered normal. Patients with claudication commonly have ABI's in the 0.6 to 0.9 range. An ABI of 0.5 or less categorizes individuals at risk for limb loss.

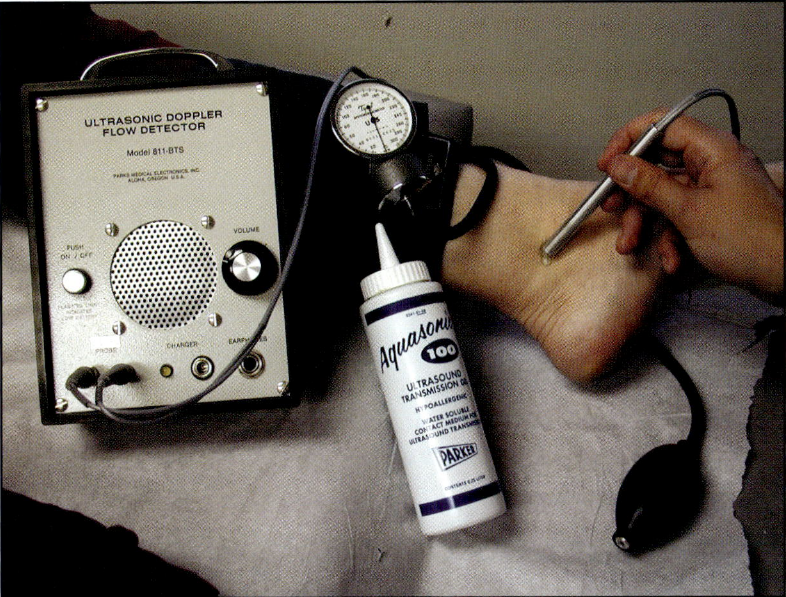

Figure 7. Simple Doppler equipment to measure ABI.

Limitations and pitfalls of the ABI: vessel calcification
The ABI test assumes that the occluding pressure in the cuff is resisted only by the intraluminal pressure of the artery, and therefore depends on readily compressible vessels to be accurate. Arteries which are stiff or calcified from diabetes or renal failure add unpredictable vessel wall resistance to the compressing cuff, and the cuff must be inflated well above the actual perfusion blood pressure to occlude the distal signal. As a result, the ankle pressure is erroneously overestimated and ischemia may not be recognized.

In this scenario, toe-brachial pressure index (TBI) may be useful: the toe vessels are almost always compressible. The vascular lab may also utilize tests that do not rely on compression of the blood vessels, such as plethysmography or Doppler wave form analysis to give a qualitative estimate of ischemia (Figure 5). Segmental pressures or waveform tracings allow an estimation of the level(s) of arterial stenoses present.

The vascular laboratory is a valuable resource and should be used liberally in the evaluation of foot pathology. Good vascular technicians generate reproducible results that accurately describe the presence or absence of arterial insufficiency, disease severity, and the level of involvement.

Other Non-Invasive Tests

Transcutaneous oxygen measurements offer information regarding cutaneous arterial flow, and are frequently used to guide amputation levels. They may be repeated after breathing 100% oxygen to determine possible benefit of hyperbaric oxygen therapy.

Duplex ultrasound may be used to quantify and localize PAD. It has not achieved in lower extremity testing the dominant role it has in evaluating cerebrovascular disease. Leg duplex testing is time consuming and technician dependent. Physiologic data produced is not as concise and reproducible as the ABI, and (15) is therefore less suited for follow-up comparison. Anatomic data produced is less precise than angiography, and therefore less useful for surgical planning. Advances in imaging, however, have increased its use.

Computed tomography (CT) and magnetic resonance (MR) angiography are improving with the computer technology on which they are based. Quality is uneven on older models, and study detail may be lacking compared with conventional angiography. However, they do not require arterial puncture, and play an increasingly valuable role in vascular imaging. For further details on noninvasive tests see Boccalandro's chapter entitled, "Chronic Critical Limb Ischemia and Limb Salvage."

Angiography

When revascularization is needed, angiography allows precise visualization of the vascular anatomy and pathology. Quality of arterial inflow, the location of arterial stenoses or obstructions, and the availability of outflow

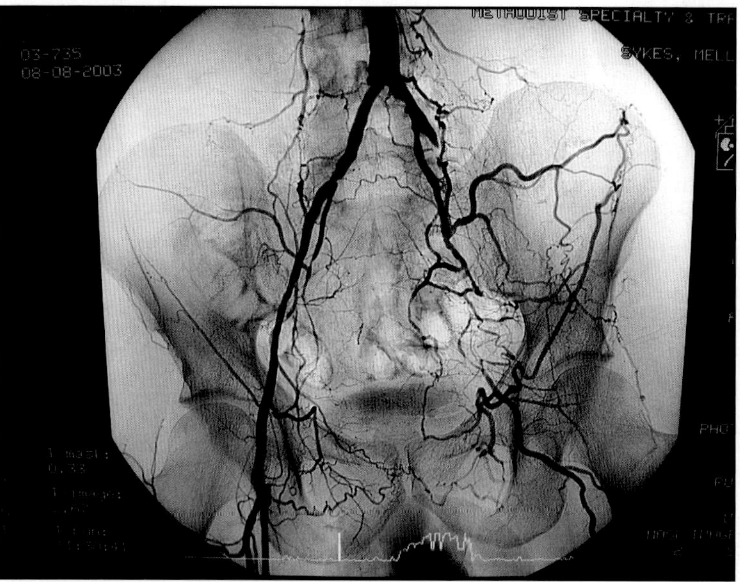

Figure 8. Left iliac artery occlusion.

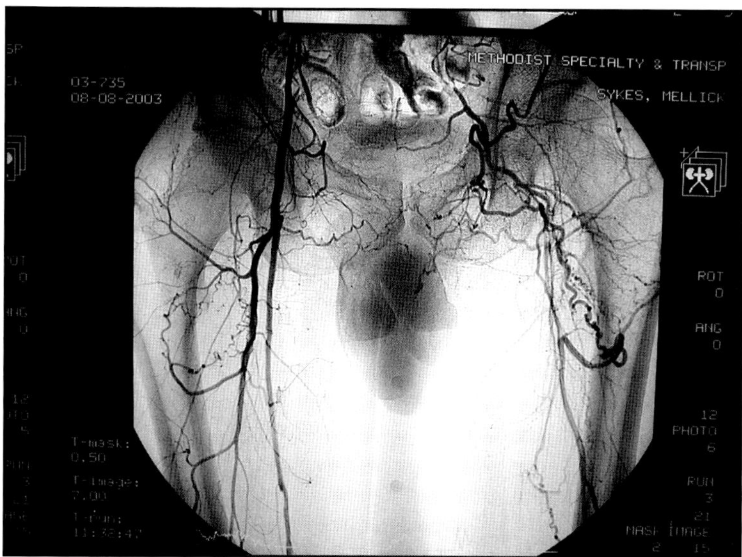

Figure 9. Left superficial femoral artery occlusion. Profunda femoral collateral.

targets allow planning of arterial reconstruction. A high quality diagnostic arteriogram remains the cornerstone of any revascularization procedure, open or endovascular (see Figures 8 and 9).

Risks of angiography are few but important to recognize, as many can be avoided with careful pre- and post-angio management. They include contrast-induced nephropathy, allergic reactions, and catheter vascular injury. Patients with renal insufficiency should be hydrated, and nephrotoxic drugs avoided; renal-protective agents such as acetylcysteine (Mucomyst), and sodium bicarbonate infusion should be considered. Steroid pretreatment regimens exist for patients with a history of contrast allergy. Widespread use of smaller catheter systems, non-ionic contrast agents, and digital subtraction imaging has significantly reduced the historic risk and discomfort of angiography.

TREATMENT
Urgency of Treatment

Critical limb ischemia heralds imminent limb loss, and should be approached aggressively. Simultaneous rapid evaluation of the wound and its arterial supply are carried out while optimizing risk factors that can be changed.

Three broad treatment options are available: 1) conservative, 2) revascularization (open or endovascular), or 3) amputation. These are not mutually exclusive, and often all occur in the same patient. Treatment must be individualized to the patient and to the local medical resources and talent.

Conservative Treatment

Usually, a non-healing ulcer is an absolute indication for intervention. However, revascularization—both endovascular and open—involves both peri-procedural risks, and longer term risk of graft, balloon, or stent failure.

Occasionally, therefore, it is reasonable to defer revascularization. In the presence of a small ischemic ulcer and modifiable risk factors a trial of medical therapy and intense wound care may be initiated. Close monitoring for failure is crucial in this setting.

Control of risk factors

Although risk factors for atherosclerosis take years to produce arterial narrowing, acute modification of risk factors appears to have a surprisingly beneficial affect on the healing of arterial insufficiency ulcers.

Smoking should stop, blood glucose levels should be controlled to a Hgb A1C less than seven, blood pressure should be less than 130/90, and hyperlipidemia treatment should reach an LDL < 100 mg%. Suspected hypercoagulable factors (elevated homocysteine, fibrinogen, hematocrit or platelet, etc) should be identified and treated.

Wound care

A number of wound treatment regimens may be used depending on the location and nature of the ulcer. These regimens are described elsewhere, but all follow the principles of regular debridement of devitalized tissue, control of infection, moist wound environment, protection from further trauma, and close follow-up. If ischemia is corrected, a number of wound care regimens may succeed; in the absence of revascularization, failure of healing is the rule regardless of wound care regimen.

Specific Presentations

Ulcers

Ischemic ulcers which are small, painless, and free of infection occasionally respond to maximum conservative care. If on close follow-up the lesion is healing, revascularization may be deferred until the next episode.

The metabolic requirements of intact skin are much lower than skin with a healing ulcer or infection. If a small ulcer can resolve without revascularization and the foot protected against similar trauma, the foot may stay healed for some time. Often years of productive ambulatory life are gained before revascularization is required. Vigilant follow-up, however, is necessary.

Infection

If cellulitis or drainage accompanies an ulcer, conservative care alone is less likely to succeed. Moreover there is greater danger of rapid deterioration of the foot. The thrombotic properties of many infections may spark a wildfire of sepsis, ischemia, and necrosis which threaten life as well as limb. Unless clear early improvement is noted, prompt correction of ischemia should be considered.

Deep infection requires urgent surgical drainage. Plantar space abscess may rapidly destroy a foot while producing remarkably little symptoms. Unexplained foot pain or plantar tenderness, erythema, or fullness suggests occult infection.

Rest pain

Despite the lack of overt tissue loss, the pain associated with this manifestation of CLI renders conservative care—largely narcotics and cessation of smoking—frustrating and futile for both physician and patient. Prompt angiography and revascularization are required.

If revascularization is unfeasible, amputation is necessary. Ischemic rest pain is so severe that relief and gratitude may be the dominant emotions after even major limb loss.

Wet gangrene

Tissue necrosis associated with infection requires emergent debridement and drainage, followed if possible by revascularization. Local metabolic requirements are high, and pulsatile flow to the foot is usually needed for limb salvage. Debridement must be aggressive, with deep cultures obtained to guide antibiotic therapy.

Dry gangrene

Dry tissue necrosis lacks an invasive nature, and does not produce sepsis unless it becomes secondarily infected. Revascularization should be performed first and allowed to mature before amputation. Often tissue which initially appears marginal will survive, permitting a lesser amputation (Figure 10 A, B, and C).

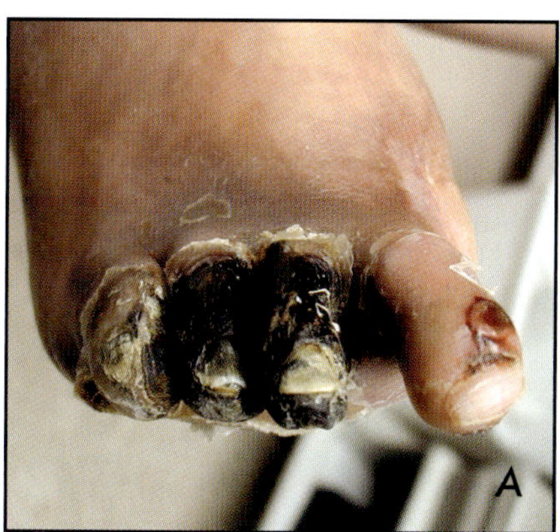

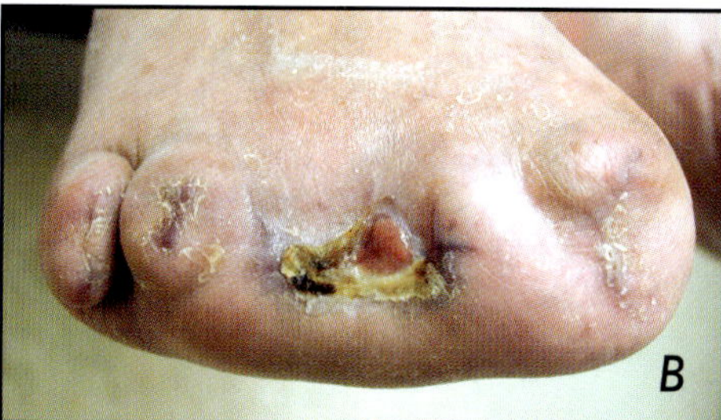

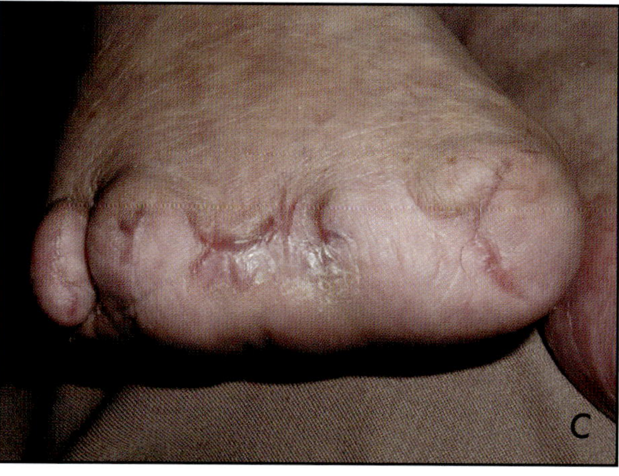

Figure 10 (A–C)).
A. Dry Gangrene. TMA or toe amputation after bypass?
B. Multiple toe amputations rather than TMA.
C. Healing toe amputations.

TABLE 4. DECISIONS FOR ANGIOGRAPHY

Angio Findings	Management
Normal vessels	Non-ischemic etiology
Straightforward bypass	Early revascularization
Difficult bypass	Maximum conservative care; revascularization if fails
"Heroic" bypass	Max conservative care; revascularization or amputation if fails.
No bypass possible	Conservative care; early amputation if fails.

Revascularization vs. Amputation

Not all patients with critical limb ischemia can be revascularized. Lack of autogenous conduit, unfit general health, and extensive necrosis beyond the midfoot may all preclude revascularization. Most patients, even those with significant co-morbidities, are able to successfully tolerate vascular procedures. The alternative of amputation is not an attractive one, carrying a similar anesthesia risk and greater disability. The most common impediment to limb salvage is lack of a suitable target vessel on angiography (Table 4).

Risks vs. Benefits

The surgeon must take into account the risks, discomfort, and costs of a proposed revascularization, weighing these against the expected benefit to be gained and the durability of the procedure. Heroic procedures with smaller chances of success have their place, but the clinician should strive to achieve a balance between therapeutic nihilism and exercises in futility.

Close follow-up and monitoring

Critical to the success of conservative treatment is a commitment to close follow-up by both patient and physician. If the ulcer worsens or healing lags, prompt revascularization is needed.

Modes of Revascularization

Two general techniques of improving blood supply exist: 1) **open** procedures including endarterectomy and bypass, 2) and **endovascular** procedures including balloon angioplasty, stenting, and thrombolysis. These techniques are not mutually exclusive and indeed complement each other.

Endovascular treatments are most successful for focal stenoses in larger vessels with good runoff. As atherosclerotic lesions become more diffuse, in smaller vessels, and with compromised runoff, the durability and flexibility of an open approach begin to outweigh its inherent risks and discomfort. The modern vascular surgeon with facility and experience in both techniques offers some objectivity regarding the best approach for an individual patient.

For more on revascularization techniques see the chapter by Boccalandro entitled "Chronic Critical Limb Ischemia and Limb Salvage."

Suprainguinal arterial disease

Aorto-bifemoral bypass (ABF) has a long record of durability for occlusive disease of the aorta and iliac arteries and is one of the success stories of the last century. Increasingly, however, endovascular angioplasty and stenting procedures have achieved comparable results with much less morbidity in the aorta and iliac arteries.

Infrainguinal arterial disease

Bypass utilizing autogenous vein is the preferred reconstruction for femoral, popliteal, or tibial occlusive disease. Flexibility of technique, freedom from infection, and superior patency make vein ideal. When autologous vein is unavailable, prosthetic conduits (PTFE, human umbilical vein, Dacron) offer reasonable short and medium-term patency rates to the popliteal artery. Tibial and pedal bypasses using prosthetic material have generally poor results despite numerous technical modifications and anticoagulation regimens.

Percutaneous angioplasty of SFA and popliteal lesions have had success in focal lesions with good runoff. Benefit is usually not long-term, but procedural risk to the patient is low, and often endovascular treatment lasts long enough to permit healing of the wound and conversion to a state of lesser metabolic demand. The long-term benefit of infrainguinal atherectomy and stent procedures remains uncertain at this writing.

Amputation

After successful revascularization, minor "clean-up" forefoot amputations are often necessary to achieve a functional result.

The below-knee amputation is so functional that effort should be made to preserve the knee joint if even rudimentary ambulation rehabilitation is considered. The difference in nursing care between a patient who can strap on a prosthesis to go to the bath or dining room, and one who must be carried into a wheelchair for such trips, is significant.

A non-ambulatory or markedly senile patient gains little by preserving the knee joint. Above-knee amputation in this setting is more likely to heal, avoids knee contractures, and lightens the patient who must be carried.

PROGNOSIS AND FOLLOW-UP

Prognosis

Of all claudicants, 3–22% will require revascularization or amputation in their lifetime. Over 80% remain stable and do not require intervention.

Of patients with CLI, about 20% will die in the first year, and 33% after two years; a diagnosis of rest pain, foot ulcer, or gangrene, therefore, carries a worse overall prognosis for survival than many cancers!

Follow-up

All revascularization procedures have the potential to fail with time, usually due to the build up of intimal hyperplasia at the sites of anastomosis, angioplasty, stenting, valve, clamp, or endarterectomy. Correction of such lesions before thrombosis of the reconstruction has significantly less morbidity, and exceedingly better results, than trying to salvage an acute thrombosis.

These facts suggest the wisdom of life-long follow-up by these patients. Regular clinical and vascular lab evaluations allow detection and correction of small problems at a treatable stage.

SUMMARY

Arterial insufficiency ulcers are common. Arterial insufficiency is a common factor in poorly healing ulcers with another primary etiology (see Figure 11).

The combination of chronic limb ischemia and minor foot trauma produces ulceration, gangrene, infection or rest pain. These end-stage manifestations of CLI portend limb loss unless treated.

Evaluation requires assessing the nature of the ulcer and its blood supply. Clinical history and physical exam can stratify risks of arterial insufficiency. Objective verification of ischemia is important and may be obtained by the vascular lab.

Treatment by risk factor modification and wound care may succeed in patients with simple small ulcerations. Most patients additionally require revascularization to prevent amputation.

Long-term follow-up of the ipsilateral reconstruction and contralateral extremity optimize results.

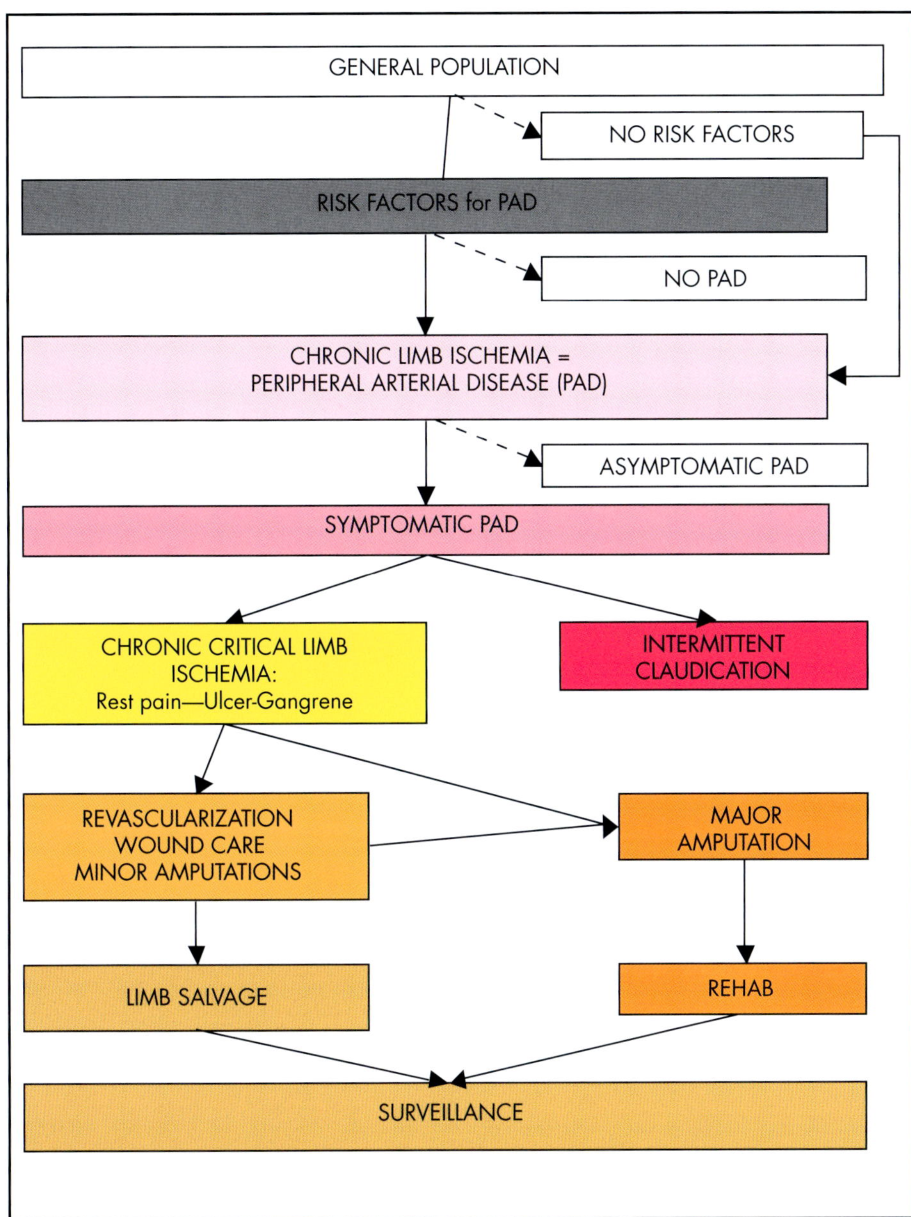

Figure 11. PAD algorithm.

REFERENCES

1. Management of Peripheral Arterial Disease (PAD); TransAtlantic Inter-Society Consensus (TASC). *Journal of Vascular Surgery* Jan 2000; 31(1). Part 2.

2. Criqui MH, Peripheral arterial disease: epidemiological aspects. *VascMed* 2001;6(3):3-7

3. Sykes MT, Godsey JB. Vascular evaluation of the problem diabetic foot, *Clinics in Podiatric Medicine and Surgery* 15(1), Jan 1998.

4. American Diabetes Association: *http://www.diabetes.org/main*

5. American Association for Vascular Surgery: *http://aavs.vascularweb.org/*

6. Transatlantic Inter-Society Consensus (TASC) on the Treatment of Peripheral Vascular Disease. *http://www.tasc-pad.org/*

7. Society of Interventional Radiology: *http://www.sirweb.org/*

8. American Heart Association: *http://www.americanheart.org/*

REVIEW QUESTIONS

1.) Atherosclerosis (AS) may reduce blood flow by :
   a. AS plaque narrows the vessel radius which diminishes distal flow exponentially
   b. Irregular AS plaque produces turbulent flow which further lessens the energy and flow to distal tissue
   c. The intimal "cap" over the plaque may ulcerate or dissect, releasing atheroembolic plaque or thrombus to occlude distal vessels
   d. All of the above

2.) Which of the following statements about ischemia is FALSE?
   a. Ischemia occurs when local tissue demands exceed the supply of blood flow
   b. Ischemia may be caused by increased demand
   c. Ischemia may be caused by decreased supply
   d. Peripheral arterial disease (PAD) causes a rise in the absolute blood flow to a limb

3.) Exercise, infection, and trauma are high-metabolic processes which greatly increase the demand for blood flow.
   a. True
   b. False

4.) Risk factors for development and progression of critical limb ischemia (CLI) include all of the following EXCEPT:
   a. Increased age
   b. Smoking
   c. Diabetes
   d. Edema

5.) When a Doppler ultrasound probe is used to elicit a signal over the artery, a normal arterial signal is
   a. Triphasic
   b. Biphasic
   c. Monophasic
   d. Absent

Answers: 1d, 2d, 3a, 4d, 5a

NOTES

CHAPTER 13

CHRONIC CRITICAL LIMB ISCHEMIA AND LIMB SALVAGE

CHAPTER THIRTEEN OVERVIEW

Chronic Critical Limb Ischemia and Limb Salvage

Fernando Boccalandro

DEFINITION OF CRITICAL LIMB ISCHEMIA AND LIMB SALVAGE

Peripheral vascular disease of the lower extremities comprises a clinical spectrum ranging from asymptomatic patients, to patients with chronic critical limb ischemia (CCLI) that might result in amputation and limb loss. Critical limb ischemia is a persistent and relentless problem that severely impairs functional status and quality of life, and is associated with increased cardiovascular mortality and morbidity. It can present acutely (i.e., distal embolization, external compression, acute thrombosis, etc.) or, in the majority of cases, as chronic critical limb ischemia, which will be the main focus of this chapter. Patients with CCLI are classified as having Fontaine Class III/IV or Rutherford Class 4, 5 or 6 peripheral vascular disease. Authors have proposed different definitions for CCLI, taking into account a variety of hemodynamic measurements in combination with clinical findings. Hemodynamic measurements are essential to confirm the diagnosis since some clinical manifestations can be caused by other non-vascular diseases. A practical and simple definition is the one proposed by the European Working Group on CCLI. This group defined CCLI as any of the following: the presence of ischemic rest pain requiring analgesia for more than two weeks; ulceration; or gangrene of the lower extremity with an ankle systolic blood pressure ≤50 mm Hg and/or toe systolic pressure ≤30 mm Hg (1). In general, patients with CCLI are defined as those patients in whom the natural course of the disease will lead to limb amputation within six months of the diagnosis. Limb salvage can be defined as any revascularization procedure (surgical or percutaneous) aimed at improving the blood flow with the purpose of preventing limb loss, and achieving pain resolution and complete wound healing.

PREVALENCE AND PROGNOSIS OF CRITICAL LIMB ISCHEMIA

The prevalence of peripheral vascular disease increases significantly with age, and can be estimated based on clinical symptoms, questionnaires and diagnostic vascular tests. As more sensitive vascular diagnostic tests became available for screening, the prevalence of this disease was found to be higher than expected based on clinical symptoms or epidemiological studies using vascular related questionnaires (2, 3). Using ankle brachial indexes and pulse wave recordings, it is estimated that among Americans 60 years and younger, the prevalence of peripheral vascular disease is 2.5%. This increases to 8.3% among those aged 60–69 years and to 18.8% in those 70 years and older, with a general male predominance (4). The mortality associated with peripheral vascular disease has remained stable over the past 50 years, whereas the mortality related to stroke and coronary artery disease has declined in the same period of time (5). Therefore, the mortality and morbidity associated with peripheral vascular disease is expected to grow significantly in the next decades due to the rapidly increasing elderly segment of the population. Currently, about 9.6% of all cardiovascular events are due to peripheral vascular disease, requiring 777,000 office visits and 63,000 hospitalizations, with 17,400 annual deaths attributed directly to this cause (4). The prognosis of patients with peripheral vascular disease is linked to its association with diabetes, advanced age, poor functional status, and advanced coronary and cerebrovascular atherosclerotic disease (6–8). It is very important for the wound care specialist to understand that the prognosis of patients with lower extremity vascular disease is determined by the extent of their associated coronary and cerebrovascular disease. Vascular disease is an "all over body" disease, so while peripheral vascular symptoms may bring the patient to the attention of a wound care specialist, their risk for cardiovascular and cardiac ischemic events exceeds the risk of limb loss. They have a 20–60% increase in the incidence of myocardial infarction, are two to six times more likely to die from a cardiac ischemic event (7, 9, 10), and are four to five times more likely to have a stroke or transient ischemic attack than those without lower extremity peripheral vascular disease (10). Smoking increases tenfold the risk for amputation and twofold the risk of death in these patients. Diabetes mellitus increases the risk of amputation sevenfold as compared to patients without diabetes (13). Among patients with peripheral vascular disease older than 50 years, it is estimated that only 1–2% will progress to CCLI, but this group of patients carry a poor prognosis. Patients suffering from CCLI have significant lifestyle limitations, increased healthcare expenditures, and significant loss of work and wages (14). Critical limb ischemia causes progressive worsening in their functional status and peak oxygen consumption that approximates the mortality of patients with chronic heart failure (1, 13). Only 50% of these patients are alive and with both lower extremities after one year; with a one-year mortality and amputation rate of 25% respectively (1, 14). Following a major amputation for CCLI, the one year survival rate is only 55% (15–17). Of these death, it is estimated that 70–80% are secondary to cardiovascular disease.

TABLE 1. DIFFERENTIAL DIAGNOSIS FOR CHRONIC CRITICAL LIMB ISCHEMIA

Atheroembolism
Aortic or popliteal aneurysms — Blue toe syndrome

Cardioembolism
Atrial fibrillation — Patent foramen ovale
Left ventricular thrombus — Endocarditis

Drugs induced
Ergotamine abuse — Cocaine abuse

Hematological diseases
Hyperhomocysteinemia — Leukemia
Antiphospholipid syndrome — Polycythemia
Sickle cell anemia — Thrombocytosis
Thalassemia

Insect bites
Brown recluse spider

Infectious diseases
Filariasis — Leprosy

Neurological causes
Radiculopathies — Spinal stenosis
Peripheral neuropathies

Systemic vasculitis
Polyarteritis nodosum — Thromboangitis obliterans
Wegner's disease — Essential cryoglobulinemia
Takayasu's disease — Giant cell arteridities

Chronic venous insufficiency

Sympathetic dystrophy

Vasospastic disorders
Raynaud's phenomenon/disease

Malignancy
Squamous cell carcinoma — Secondary metastases
Kaposi's sarcoma — Mycosis fungoides

Other causes
Gout — Pyoderma gangrenosum
Necrobiosis lipoidica — Vitamin B12 deficiency

PATHOPHYSIOLOGY OF CRITICAL LIMB ISCHEMIA

In the vast majority of cases, chronic CCLI is related to advanced atherosclerotic disease. Other diseases have to be kept in mind by the clinician, particularly in young patients, those with ulcers in atypical locations, or those with few or no risk factors for CCLI (Table 1). Chronic CCLI secondary to atherosclerosis develops when arterial stenosis reaches a critical point in which the blood flow supplied to the distal extremity is insufficient to provide the basal tissue oxygen demand. This occurs despite two compensatory mechanisms: post-stenotic arteriolar vasodilatation and development of collateral circulation (19). When the basal tissue oxygen demand cannot be met by the peripheral vascular system, ischemic injury occurs in the tissues leading to resting pain, tissue destruction, the appearance of ulceration, and gangrene. Patients are also threatened by severe microvascular dysfunction secondary to a local and systemic inflammatory response and a thrombotic milieu that worsens their poor capillary blood flow (19–21). Also reported in this group of patients are: impaired vasomotor response, vasospasm, increased platelet aggregation (19–22), impaired fibrinolysis (22), micro-thrombus formation, increased leukocyte activation and adhesion, increased capillary permeability with interstitial edema, and local activation of the immune system with increased levels of C-reactive protein in addition to other systemic inflammatory mediators (23–25). These changes seem to be accentuated in diabetics, which present with a combination of macro and micro angiopathy due to accelerated atherosclerosis, increased blood viscosity, thrombosis, and an enhanced inflammatory response (19, 22, 26); leading to a more distal and diffuse disease that might significantly limit the possibility of an effective revascularization. The presence of neuropathy in this later group also plays an important role in the pathogenesis of CCLI (27, 28). The lack of proper blood flow predisposes the ischemic tissues in diabetics to have extensive wounds with poor healing potential even after minor trauma (24). Diabetes mellitus predisposes the formation of early wet gangrene with polymicrobial infections that are difficult to treat due to the limited blood supply, predisposing them to the formation of deep wound infections and osteomyelitis (31).

CLINICAL MANIFESTATIONS OF CRITICAL LIMB ISCHEMIA

In evaluating patients with suspected CCLI, it is important to confirm the suspected clinical diagnosis, excluding the possibility of other diseases that might mimic vascular insufficiency, and to assess the severity of limb compromise in order to plan the best limb salvage strategy in a timely manner. The first step in patients with suspected limb ischemia should always be to rule out the presence of signs of acute critical limb ischemia since this represents a medical emergency requiring immediate revascularization (Figure 1). The signs of acute limb ischemia that require immediate attention and emergent revascularization can be remembered by the rule of the five "P's": Absence of Pulse, or the presence of resting Pain, Pallor, Paresthesia and Paralysis. Chronic CCLI is usually present in elderly patients with previous history of intermittent claudication, smokers, diabetics, or patients with a history of cerebrovascular or coronary artery disease. These patients present with one or all the four hallmarks of CLI: resting pain, non-healing ulcers, dry gangrene, and absence of palpable pulses.

Resting Pain

Patients with CCLI usually describe their pain as a throbbing pain, dull ache, or numbness that classically worsens when the patient elevates the leg, and thus, is worse in the evenings or nights. It is relieved by lowering the leg to a dependent position and, interestingly, in contrast to patients with intermittent claudication, the resting pain of CCLI can actually improve slightly with deambulation due to mild improvement in the arteriolar blood flow caused by the effects of gravity. In patient with diabetic neuropathy, resting pain secondary to vascular insufficiency might be difficult to differentiate clinically from neuropathic pain and frequently present together.

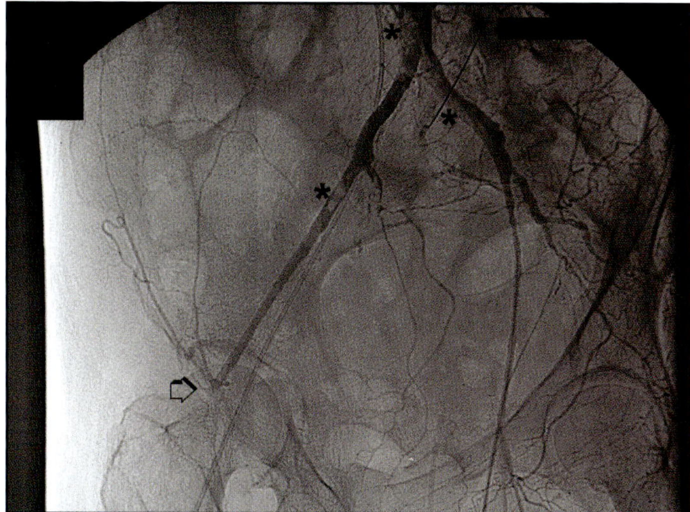

Figure 1. Patient presenting with acute critical limb ischemia. Angiography of a patient with severe peripheral vascular disease presenting with acute critical limb ischemia in the right lower extremity due to a total occlusion of the right common femoral artery (arrow) with extensive thrombus formation in the right external, common iliac arteries and aorta-iliac bifurcation (∗).

Non-Healing Ulcers

Ischemic ulcers usually appear in the distal areas of the extremities such as the tips of the toes, or at bony prominences. They are associated with severe pain and are generally dry, with irregular borders, are associated with a cold or cyanotic foot, and contain a base that can be pale, gray or black with gangrenous tissue (Figure 2). Diabetic patients with advanced sensory neuropathy may have advanced ulcers without significant pain or discomfort.

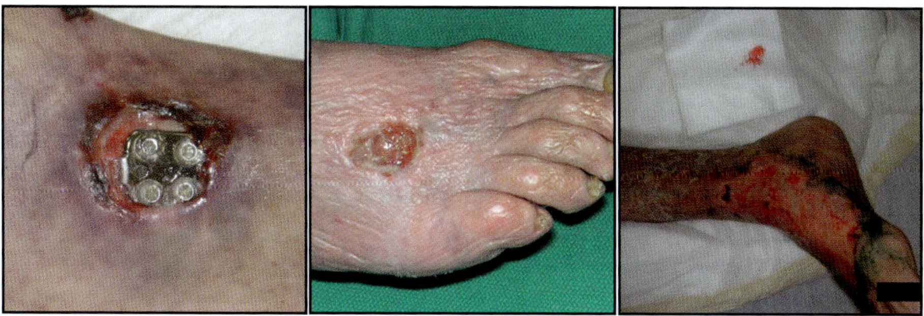

Figure 2. Nonhealing ulcer in patients with chronic critical limb ischemia.

Dry Gangrene

The presence of devitalized tissue is the end-stage clinical manifestation of CCLI. In the absence of neuropathy it usually appears as a very painful area of necrotic and dry tissue (Figure 3). If it becomes infected it can present with purulent and fetid drainage with signs of inflammation surrounding the necrotic area (wet gangrene).

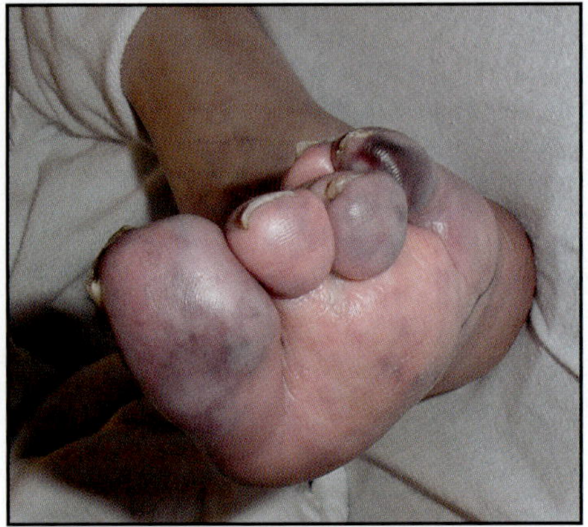

Figure 3. Gangrenous foot due to severe advanced chronic limb ischemia in a diabetic patient.

Absence of Palpable Pulses

Examination of distal pulses is important in patients in whom CCLI is suspected. Posterior tibial and dorsalis pedis pulses are almost always absent, except in selected patients with severe disease above the knee with an adequate collateral flow in whom distal pulses might be appreciated. Routinely, the physician should include examination of the popliteal and femoral pulses to localize, if possible, the area of vascular compromise. When distal pulses cannot be palpated, the use of a hand-held Doppler is strongly recommended to assess for distal blood flow.

Clinical Pearls

In patients with palpable pulses and suspected CCLI, the elevation/ dependency test is a simple and accurate bedside test: the limb is elevated for 60 seconds and then lowered (32). In the ischemic limb this process results in a purple, ruborous red color in the foot. Presence of faint pulses that disappear after a six-minute walk test are also very suggestive of severe peripheral vascular disease in patients with suspected CCLI and palpable pulses. The six-minute walk test can be done with no equipment in the outpatient setting and its results have a good correlation with a formal treadmill test. In an excellent review of the physical examination findings in patients with non-critical peripheral vascular disease, McGee et al. found that classic signs like abnormal resting coloration of the lower extremities, atrophic skin, lack of foot hair and abnormal capillary refill time were not associated with the presence or severity of peripheral vascular disease (32). In addition, a recent review reached similar conclusions regarding the limitations of clinical examination in non-critical peripheral vascular disease (33). For patients with CCLI it is likely that the aforementioned four clinical hallmarks have a better diagnostic accuracy since they represent a more advanced disease process when recognized in a more restricted segment of the population, and therefore with a higher pretest probability of advanced vascular disease. However, no data are available regarding the diagnostic accuracy of the classic clinical manifestations of end-stage peripheral vascular disease in the diagnosis of CCLI.

DIAGNOSTIC TESTS IN PATIENTS WITH SUSPECTED CRITICAL LIMB ISCHEMIA

Noninvasive vascular testing should be the next step after a thorough clinical history and physical examination. An ankle or toe systolic blood pressure and/or an ankle-brachial index (ABI) are two initial tests that can be easily performed at the bedside to confirm the clinical impression of CCLI. Other tests are needed to assess the severity and anatomic localization of the compromised vascular territories and to predict the likelihood of wound healing and limb salvage. In general, the diagnostic studies for CCLI can be classified into physiological studies, anatomic studies or studies that provide both physiological and anatomical information (Table 2). Physiological studies quantify the degree of vascular hypoperfusion in the affected extremity. Some physiologic studies serve also to estimate the likelihood of wound healing in patients with CCLI, and have become invaluable for decision making in wound care. Anatomical tests are based mainly in imaging diagnostic studies, and used primarily to evaluate the vascular anatomy.

TABLE 2. DIAGNOSTIC STUDIES FOR PATIENTS WITH CHRONIC CRITICAL LIMB ISCHEMIA

1) Physiological Studies
Quantify the degree of tissue hypoperfusion in the affected extremity;
May serve to estimate the likelihood of wound healing in patients with non-healing ischemic wounds
  Ankle systolic blood pressure
  Ankle-brachial index
  Toe systolic blood pressure
  Toe-brachial index
  Transcutaneous oximetry
  Laser Doppler imaging

2) Anatomical Studies
Serve to evaluate the vascular anatomy;
Used to plan limb salvage procedures
  Magnetic resonance arteriography (MRA)
  Computer tomographic angiography (CTA)
  Conventional angiography

3) Anatomical and Physiological Studies
Allows evaluation of the degree of tissue hypoperfusion;
Gives additionally anatomical information regarding the degree and localization of the underlying vascular compromise
  Segmental pressures
  Pulse volume recordings
  Arterial Duplex ultrasound with continuous-wave Doppler examination

PHYSIOLOGIC DIAGNOSTIC TESTS
Ankle Systolic Blood Pressure and Ankle Brachial Index (ABI)

The ABI is a well validated physiologic method in the diagnosis and management of patient with peripheral vascular disease. At the bedside, measurement of an ankle systolic blood pressure using a hand-held Doppler and an adequately sized blood pressure cuff is mandatory. The brachial blood pressure is compared to the dorsalis pedis or posterior tibialis. An ankle systolic blood pressure ≤50 mm Hg, in conjunction with the aforementioned physical findings, confirms the diagnosis of CCLI. The test is highly reproducible, simple, fast, readily available, cost-effective, portable and accurate with a reported sensitivity of 75–79% and a specificity of 97–100% for an ABI threshold of 0.90 for vascular stenosis greater than 50% (34). ABI values are often considered to be mildly to moderately diminished when they are between 0.41 and 0.90, and severely decreased when less than or equal to 0.40. The presence of an ABI below 0.4 identifies individuals who are at particularly high risk of subsequent development of CCLI and limb loss. Additionally, the ABI provides important survival prognostic information for patients with peripheral vascular disease (35, 36). and correlates well with disease progression (37). In patients with CCLI, the ABI is almost universally below 0.5. One important caveat of the ankle systolic pressure and ABI is the fact that diabetic patients or patients with chronic kidney disease with severe medial artery calcification and therefore advanced underlying peripheral vascular disease, might have falsely elevated distal pressures. This is due to a decrease in their vascular compliance with the presence of non-compressible pedal vessels resulting in ABI higher than 1.2 (35). This might confuse the physician with limited experience resulting in discordance between the clinical presentation of the extremity and the hemodynamic measurements obtained by Doppler. Therefore a patient with such ABI should undergo an alternate diagnostic method for further evaluation or a post-exercise ABI. If a variation of more than 12 mm Hg of interarm blood pressure is noted during the measurement of the upper extremity brachial blood pressures, the presence of upper extremity obstructive peripheral vascular disease should also be suspected and further investigated.

Toe Systolic Blood Pressure and Toe Brachial Index

A toe systolic blood pressure determination performed in the vascular laboratory not only confirms the diagnosis of CCLI (toe systolic pressure ≤ 30 mm Hg) and provides prognostic information, but also predicts the likelihood of wound healing. In patients with a toe systolic pressure <20 mm Hg the rates of spontaneous healing are estimated to be less than 30%, while in patients with a toe systolic pressure >30 mm Hg the spontaneous healing rates can be close to 90% (38–40). Toe systolic blood pressure may be a practical way to obtain a distal hemodynamic measure in patients with non-compressible pedal vessels since digital arteries are usually spared of severe calcification. Additionally a toe brachial index of 0.7 of less, confirms the diagnostic for peripheral vascular disease.

Transcutaneous Oximetry

Transcutaneous oximetry measures the transcutaneous oxygen pressure ($TcpO_2$) at the skin surface produced by heat-induced hyperemia. Transcutaneous oximetry serves as a practical functional test that evaluates the oxygen delivery to the ischemic tissues (41). It is used not only to evaluate the need for revascularization in patients with CCLI and non-healing ulcers ($TcpO_2$ <40 mm Hg), but also helps predicting the outcome of patients requiring an amputation and assisting in the selection of an adequate amputation level (42). Survival of skin grafts can be estimated by $TcpO_2$ (43), prognosis of wound healing can be anticipated with the use of hyperbaric therapy (44) and the effectiveness of percutaneous or surgical revascularization following limb salvage can be assessed by $TcpO_2$ (45). In one study of diabetic patients with non-healing ulcers, $TcpO_2$ monitoring showed that after successful revascularization it took 3–4 weeks for cutaneous oxygenation to improve, and reach optimal levels for wound healing (46). This might be important to take into account, since the patients may benefit from four weeks of delay from aggressive wound debridement or surgical procedures following revascularization to allow optimal tissue reperfusion.

Laser Doppler Perfusion

Laser Doppler perfusion imaging is being used to assess tissue perfusion in CCLI (47). Although laser Doppler imaging is a relatively new area of investigation, already there have been a substantial number of wound-related studies using this technique for CCLI (48). Laser Doppler perfusion imaging appears to be an excellent technique for assessing perfusion in lower limb ischemic wounds. From a practical point of view, it is quick, noninvasive, and involves no contact with the tissue at all, which is a great advantage for wound care, while providing a relative measure of blood flow. A wealth of data from single-point laser Doppler studies has proved the worth of this measure, and the advantages of imaging will hopefully enable researchers to continue further clinical studies to apply this technique soon in daily practice.

ANATOMIC DIAGNOSTIC TESTS
Magnetic Resonance Arteriography (MRA)

Magnetic resonance arteriography has recently become one of the preferred methods of evaluation of CCLI (Figures 4 and 5). It requires only a simple venipuncture of the arm and avoids the use of iodinated contrast while providing detailed anatomic information including grafts, infra-popliteal vessels, pedal and plantar arches. Assessment of the diagnostic accuracy of MRA depends on the technique used and the standard against which it is compared. Contemporary techniques employed include two-dimensional time of flight, 3D rendering imaging, contrast enhancement with gadolinium, digital subtraction, parallel imaging, cardiac gating, fluoro-triggering, sub-systolic thigh compression to eliminate venous contamination and stepping-table bolus chase three-dimensional MRA angiography (49, 50). A multicenter comparison study of MRA with intraoperative angiography found that both techniques had similar accuracy (51). Other studies have shown excellent correlation between MRA and conventional angiography (52). The use of MRA requires experienced technologists and radiologist, and is an expensive diagnostic modality. MRA gives information not only of stenotic areas, but also provides valuable anatomic information regarding the patency of the renal arteries as well as the distal aorta, iliac and common femoral arteries that are difficult to evaluate with duplex ultrasound. Some studies claim that MRA is superior to catheter angiography in detection of outflow vessels suitable for distal bypasses, and had been used in some centers as the sole imaging modality for surgical revascularization (53–55). Magnetic resonance angiography has several particular limitations. It tends to overestimate the degree of stenosis because of blood flow turbulence. Time-of-flight studies may overestimate occlusions owing to loss of signal from retrograde collateral flow. Metal clips and stents can cause artifacts that mimic vessel occlusions obscuring vascular flow. Patients with pacemakers and defibrillators and some

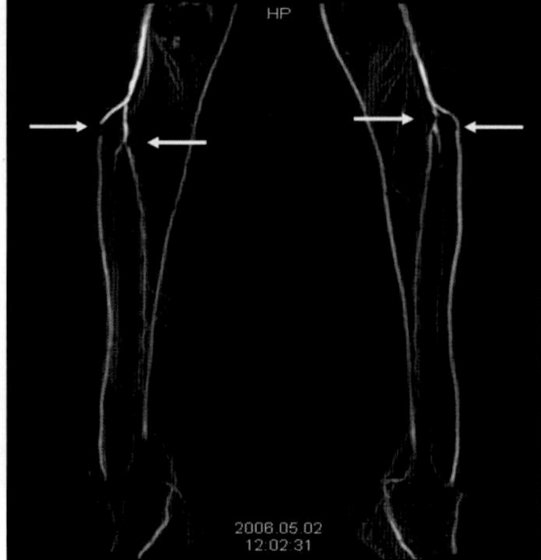

Figure 4 (above). Magnetic resonance angiography of the infra-popliteal vessels of a patient with critical limb ischemia. Note the presence of severe bilateral disease in both anterior tibial arteries and tibio-peroneal trunks.

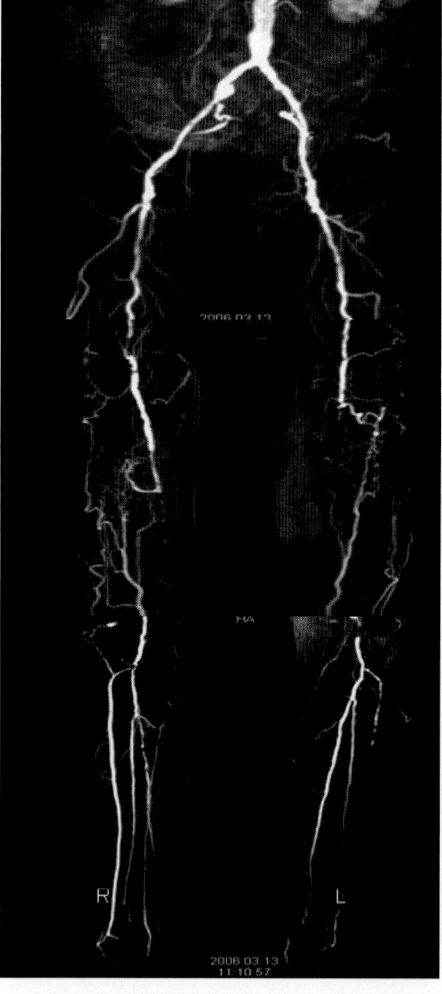

Figure 5. (right) Magnetic resonance angiography showing bilateral total superficial femoral artery occlusions in a patient with a nonhealing ulcer of the left lower extremity with distal run-offs filled by collateral flow. Note the poor distal run-offs in the left foot and evidence of multi-level peripheral vascular disease.

older generation cerebral aneurysm clips cannot be scanned safely. And although MRA with gadolinium had been considered generally non-nephrotoxic, on rare occasions had precipitated acute renal failure in patients with elevated creatinine levels. Since MRA has the advantages of not requiring arterial puncture and being unlikely to cause renal compromise, while still providing the same quality of information as traditional angiography, it is becoming the method of choice for anatomical assessment of the vasculature.

Computer Tomographic Angiography (CTA)

Computed tomographic angiography of the extremities has been increasingly used to diagnose the anatomic location and severity of stenosis of patients with peripheral vascular disease. In contrast to MRA, CT angiography requires intravenous injection of iodinated contrast, which opacifies the arteries. The final angiographic image is reconstructed from multiple cross-sectional images and then presented in projections similar to the appearance of conventional arteriography. The image can be rotated three-dimensionally in space to view any oblique projection with excellent resolution (Figure 6, 7). The latest generation of multidetector computed tomography scanners acquire up to 64 or more simultaneous images. The main advantages of this novel technology are the exceptionally short scan times, high spatial resolution, increased anatomic coverage, and capability to generate high-quality multiplanar reconstruction with three-dimensional renderings from raw data that can be reprocessed easily and quickly (56). The reported sensitivity and specificity of CTA for stenosis greater than 50% is approximately 86% and 90%; for 50–99% stenosis, sensitivity and specificity is 79% and 89%; and for occlusion, 85% and 98% when compared with conventional angiography (57). In general, above the knee CTA scores have slightly better concordance (86.1%) than below-knee readings (82.3%). Computed tomographic angiography has potential diagnostic advantages compared with conventional angiography. The three-dimensional images rendered by CTA, as in MRA, can be freely rotated in space, which permits better assessment of eccentric lesions. The use of intravenous injection of contrast during CTA fills all collateral vessels, and allows visualization of arteries distal to total occlusions that may be occult by catheter angiography. Additionally, tissues surrounding the opacified lumen of the artery can be evaluated such as aneurysms, vascular entrapment, masses, and cystic adventitial disease, which are not usually detected with conventional angiography. However, compared with conventional angiography it has less resolution. Venous opacification and dense calcification can obscure arterial filling and asymmetrical opacification of the legs may cause CTA to miss the arterial phase in some vessels during examination. Both CTA and conventional angiography require the use of ionizing radiation and iodinated contrast, which may limit its use in patients with renal dysfunction. Radiation doses in general can be less than those used in conventional angiography, but they are dependent on the computed tomography scanner and protocol used, and may vary considerably. Compared with MRA, CTA has potential advantages. Patients with pacemakers or defibrillators may be imaged safely with CTA. Metal clips, stents, and prostheses usually do not cause significant CTA artifacts. Computed tomographic angiography has higher resolution and can provide images of calcification in the vessel wall. Scan times are significantly faster with CTA

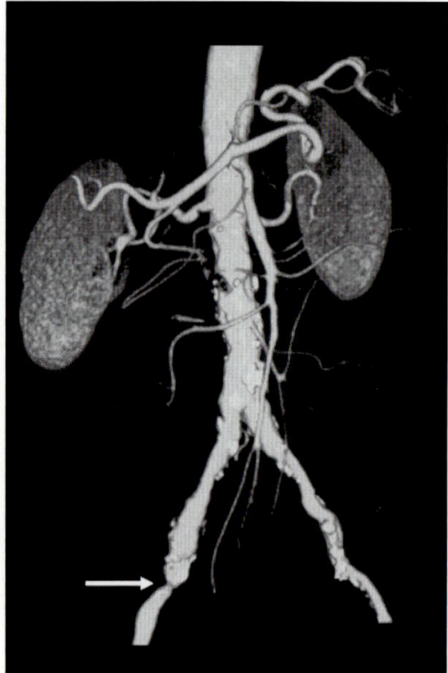

Figure 6. Computer tomographic angiography with three dimensional reconstruction of a patient with a non-healing ulcer due to a severe right iliac stenosis (arrow).

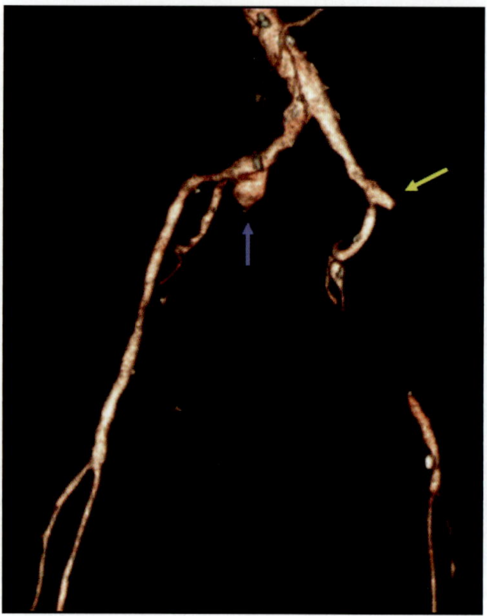

Figure 7. Computer tomographic angiography with three dimensional reconstruction of a patient with a non-healing ulcer due to a total left external iliac occlusion (green arrow). Additionally a right common iliac aneurysm was visualized (blue arrow).

than with MRA, and claustrophobia is usually not a problem for CTA. As with conventional angiography, it is recommended to obtain a creatinine level before this study can be performed.

Conventional Angiography

Although it represents an invasive test requiring the use of iodinated contrast, conventional contrast angiography with digital substraction is the historical "gold standard" for patients with CCLI. It allows a detailed evaluation of all the different parts of the vascular tree and, importantly, of the distal circulation and plantar arches. It can be performed from the retrograde approach using a femoral access or antegrade through the common femoral artery or the brachial/transradial approach (Figures 8–13). The use of digital substraction angiography that can eliminate the superimposing shadows of underlying tissues has enhanced the resolution of conventional angiography. Emphasis must always be placed in having an adequate visualization of the distal run-offs and plantar circulation, which becomes decisive in patients with CCLI when revascularization is considered. During conventional angiography, the "area of interest" is where the critically ischemic tissue is located, as well as the vasculature providing blood flow to this area. Imaging this area makes it possible to plan the best revascularization strategy aimed at improving blood flow specifically to the affected area. New digital angiographic systems provide better resolution with less radiation, and some newer systems allow enhanced three-dimensional evaluation with features

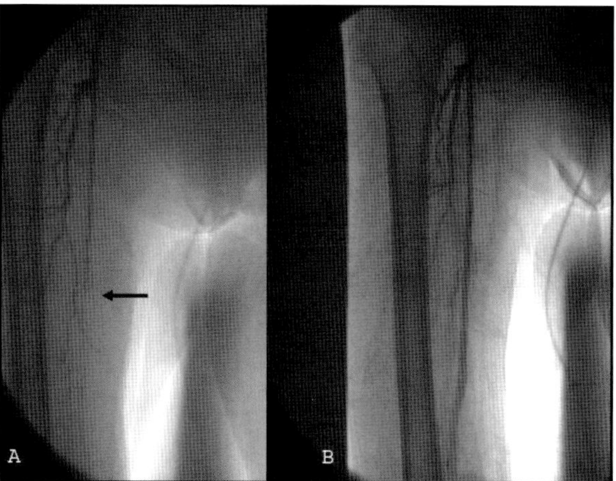

Figure 8. (A) Conventional angiography showing a long chronic total occlusion of the right superficial femoral artery (arrow) in a patient with chronic critical limb ischemia.
(B) Following percutaneous revascularization with laser assisted angioplasty and Nitinol stents implantation, with complete recanalization of the vessel.

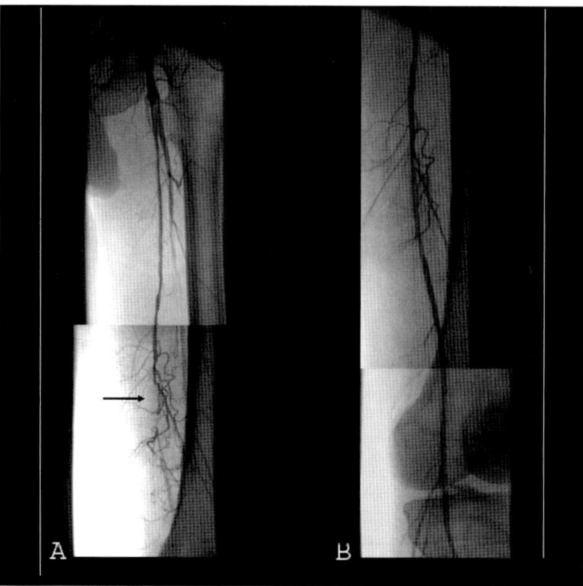

Figure 9. (A) Total occlusion of the left superficial femoral artery in a patient with critical limb ischemia (arrow).
(B) Following percutaneous revascularization using an atherectomy device with complete recanalization of the vessel.

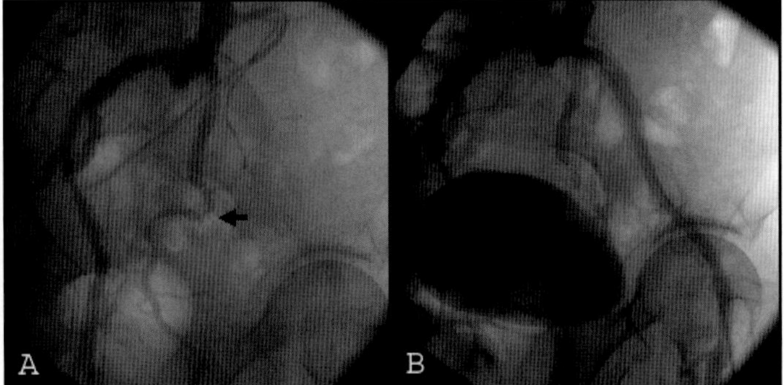

Figure 10. (A) A long chronic total occlusion of the left external iliac artery was found in this patient with non-healing ulcers of the left lower extremity.
(B) Following percutaneous revascularization with angioplasty and Nitinol stents implantation with complete recanalization of the vessel.

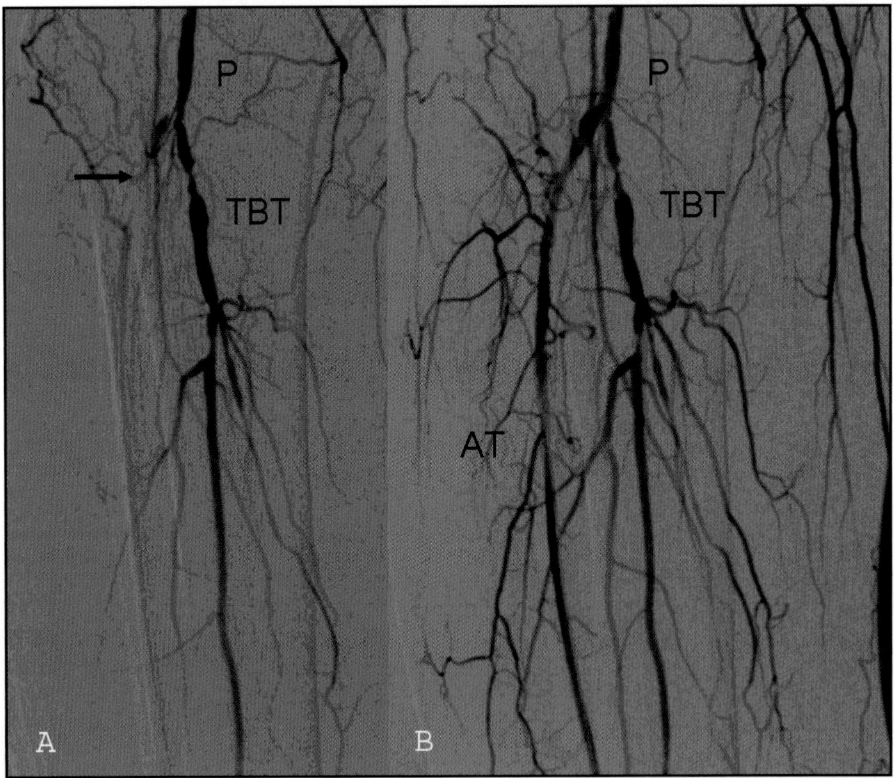

Figure 11. (A) Digital substraction angiography showing a total occlusion of the anterior tibial artery (arrow) in a patient with a gangrenous toe in the right lower extremity.
(B) Following percutaneous revascularization using an atherectomy device with complete reconstitution of this vessel. (AT: Anterior tibial artery, P: Popliteal artery, TBT: Tibio-peroneal trunk).

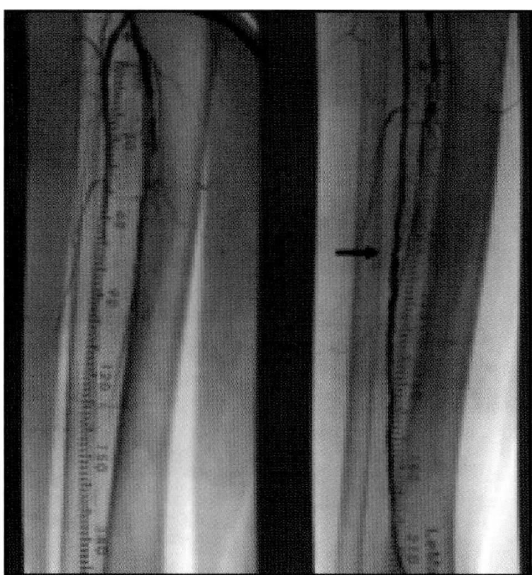

Figure 12. (A) Conventional angiography in a patient
with a non-healing ulcer showing no remaining vessels
below the knee.
(B) Complete percutaneous recanalization of the
anterior tibial artery following cryoplasty.

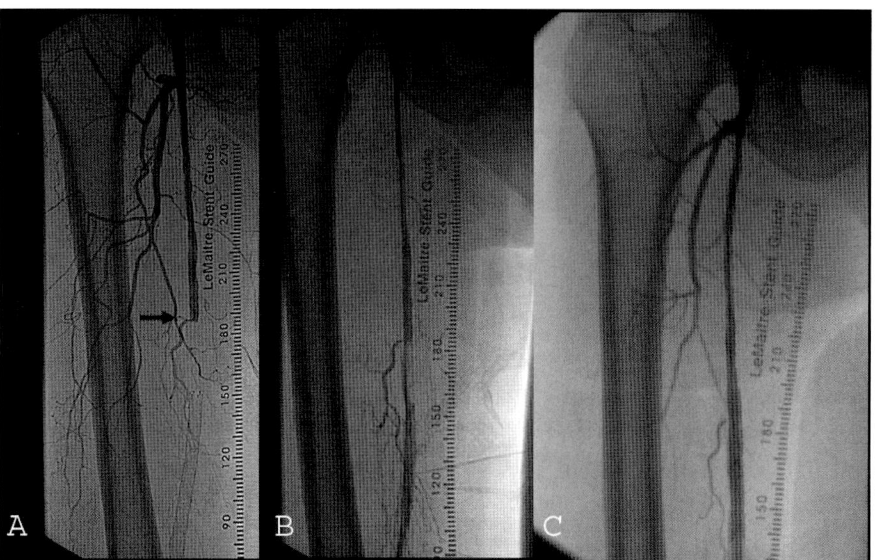

Figure 13. (A) Acute thrombotic occlusion of the superficial femoral artery (arrow) in a
patient with prior history of peripheral vascular disease and stent placement due to a
ruptured plaque proximal to the previously treated segment.
(B) After rheolytic thrombectomy with thrombolysis, using the pulse-spray technique,
showing the culprit ruptured plaque proximal to the stented segment.
(C) Final result after implanting a new stent over the atheromatous lesion.

such as, rotational angiography, three dimensional reconstructions, landmarking, and road-mapping modes that facilitate percutaneous interventions. Angiography is, at present, the only method for guiding percutaneous peripheral interventional procedures and therefore necessary for all percutaneous revascularization procedures.

ANATOMIC AND PHYSIOLOGIC DIAGNOSTIC TESTS
Segmental Pressures

Arterial pressures can be measured with plethysmographic cuffs placed sequentially along the extremity at different levels. Measurements are obtained at the upper and lower thigh, the upper calf, and the lower calf above the ankle. These systolic blood pressures obtained from the lower extremities can also be indexed relative to the brachial artery pressure, in a manner similar to the ABI. The use of segmental pressures is able to accurately determine the location and severity of individual arterial stenosis using a systolic pressure gradient of more than 20 mm Hg between adjacent segments. Using the distal ankle pressures, hemodynamic measurements can be obtained with the same validity as an ankle blood pressure. As with the ABI, segmental pressure measurements may be falsely elevated in patients with non-compressible vessels.

Pulse Volume Recordings

Arterial in the lower extremities derives a pulsatile flow from the cardiac cycle. This pulsatility leads to measurable volume changes with each cardiac cycle. Measurement of these cyclical volume changes can be documented by a pneumoplethysmograph or mercury-in-silastic strain gauges which provide qualitative or quantitative data regarding the limb perfusion in patients with peripheral vascular disease. Pulse volume recordings are used in a segmental fashion along the extremity from the thigh to the ankle to assess the change in volumes between diastole and systole. Thus, any sequential decrease in pulsatility (upstroke and/or amplitude), identifies a flow limiting stenosis in the extremity. Pulse volume recordings help to localize the site of an anatomic stenosis. It can be predictive of disease severity, limb perfusion before and after revascularization procedures and can assess disease progression, the risk of CCLI and amputation (58, 59). Pulse volume recordings are also useful in individuals with non-compressible vessels in which ABIs and segmental pressures may be falsely elevated.

Continuous-Wave Doppler Ultrasound

Spectral continuous-wave Doppler ultrasound is used to obtain velocity waveforms and to measure systolic blood pressure at sequential segments of the upper or lower extremity. It is a traditional component of a noninvasive peripheral arterial evaluation and usually combined with arterial Duplex ultrasound examination. Analysis of the morphology of the Doppler waveform can add useful localizing information, in addition to quantitative measurements of severity. Use of this technique allows estimation of disease location and severity, serves to follow-up disease progression, and to assess the effectiveness of revascularization in patients with CCLI.

Arterial Duplex Ultrasound

In experienced vascular laboratories, arterial duplex ultrasound is an accurate method that allows the precise localization and severity of arterial stenoses and the site in need of revascularization. As mentioned above, is usually combined with continuous-wave Doppler ultrasound for hemodynamic assessment. Duplex ultrasound includes imaging in grayscale and/or color format, and provides essential anatomic and well validated physiologic data when combined with continuous-wave Doppler ultrasound. Most of the clinical information is derived from duplex studies using analysis of the velocity of blood flow. Quantitative criteria used to diagnose stenoses are based on peak systolic velocity and peak systolic velocity ratios within or beyond the stenosis compared with the adjacent upstream vascular segments, the presence or absence of turbulence, and preservation of pulsatility. The sensitivity and specificity of color guided duplex ultrasound have been reported in experienced centers to be higher than 90% (60). Some practical limitations exist in the identification of aorto-iliac disease, severe calcified vessels, sequential stenosis and lesions below the knee that might limit its use in selected patients. A complete Duplex scanning also requires prolonged examination times, and a technologist with expertise to perform the test. This diagnostic modality can be useful in the follow-up of patients after percutaneous or surgical revascularization. Currently it is recommended after 4–6 weeks, and at three, six, and every 12 months after vascular surgery to guide the long-term secondary patency of previously placed venous bypass grafts (61, 62). Although advocated by many clinicians, the utility or cost effectiveness of Duplex ultrasound for "surveillance" of synthetic grafts and patients revascularized percutaneously has not yet been prospectively validated.

Which Diagnostic Method to Use First?

The first step in a patient with suspected CCLI is to gather a complete history and detailed physical examination. As part of this initial evaluation, a physiologic test to demonstrate the degree of hypoperfusion, such as an ankle-brachial systolic blood pressure/toe blood pressure or skin perfusion pressure should be obtained. Further tests depend largely on the clinical presentation and local expertise. Generally, when resting pain or gangrene is present the need for revascularization or amputation is certain. Thus, another physiologic test is not needed and the patient should be evaluated with an anatomical test to assess the underlying vasculature and the feasibility of revascularization. Usually an MRA or CTA is preferred, although Duplex ultrasound in centers with experience may provide the necessary information. Based on these initial results, an individualized revascularization strategy is made with the goal to achieve the best results for limb salvage. If surgery or amputation is contemplated, MRA or CTA in experienced centers might suffice as the sole diagnostic pre-operative imaging test. When the information provided by non-invasive methods is not diagnostic, conventional contrast angiography with digital subtraction is indicated.

For wound healing purposes, the best approach is to start with a functional test that estimates the likelihood of wound healing (transcutaneous oximetry, laser Doppler perfusion or skin perfusion pressure) combined with the ankle systolic blood pressure/toe blood pressure or ABI. If these tests show a reasonable prognosis for wound healing, a trial of intensive wound care and medical therapy should be attempted first. If this fails to achieve wound healing, or if the patient develops coexisting severe life-style limiting intermittent claudication, resting pain, or gangrene, or if the functional tests are suggestive of a poor healing potential; then an anatomic test is recommended (i.e. MRA, CTA or duplex ultrasound) to plan a revascularization procedure.

THERAPEUTIC OPTIONS FOR CRITICAL LIMB ISCHEMIA

Patients with CCLI have end-stage peripheral vascular disease and their therapeutic options are narrowed to either revascularization for limb salvage or amputation (63). Therefore, the presence of CCLI is a clear indication to pursue an aggressive arterial revascularization strategy to prevent limb loss and its associated mortality and morbidity. However, although a successful revascularization represents the cornerstone in the initial treatment of these patients, a comprehensive multidisciplinary team approach is considered necessary between the primary care physician, the wound care specialist, the radiologist and the vascular specialist, to offer the best care to this complex group of patients.

The primary care physician should identify the signs and symptoms of CCLI as soon as they are suspected, and should refer the patient as early as possible to the wound care specialist or to the vascular specialist for further assessment, while starting an adequate medical therapy. The wound care specialist plays a pivotal role in the care of these patients, managing the local wound care before and after revascularization, assessing the potential and following the progress of wound healing, and making the decision with the vascular specialists regarding the best timing for revascularization. All the team members should focus on improving the patient's modifiable risk factors and optimizing the patient's medical therapy to limit further disease progression without overlooking the high incidence of concomitant cardiac and cerebrovascular disease in these patients. Intensive medical therapy is mandatory in hopes of improving their poor prognosis. The vascular specialist (interventional cardiologist/radiologist in conjunction with the vascular surgeon) must make the best decision regarding the preferred revascularization approach, based upon the disease segment to be treated, the inflow and outflow present, the underlying operative risk of the patient, and the expected prognosis.

Three forms of revascularization therapy are available for limb salvage: endovascular therapy, surgical revascularization, and thrombolysis. For revascularization procedures in general, two end-points are usually considered for comparison, in addition to rates of complications. The end points are: clinical benefit seen after the procedure (i.e. limb salvage, survival, improvement in intermittent claudication, distance walked, quality of life, etc.) and the durability of the procedure (rates of documented patency). Due to the severe nature of their disease and the dismal overall prognosis associated with limb loss, limb salvage is the primary end-point in patients with CCLI. Rates of documented patency, although accounted for, are considerably less important than the clinical end-point of limb salvage (complete healing, resolution of pain and salvage of the limb). For all revascularization methods applied for

CCLI, the rates of limb salvage are superior to the long term angiographic patency rates following any given procedure.

Percutaneous Revascularization (Endovascular Therapy)

Historically, patients presenting with CCLI underwent arterial bypass surgery or amputation. In the past decade, endovascular therapy has revolutionized the treatment of patients with vascular disease, in particular in the group of patients with CCLI who have multiple medical problems, advanced age and a high surgical risk. Endovascular therapy is playing a leading role in providing effective revascularization and limb salvage while limiting the operative risk and post-operative recovery compared with vascular surgery.

Endovascular strategies for management of patients with CCLI have evolved considerably, in conjunction with the dramatic advances in endovascular technology and techniques. Thus, percutaneous strategies are increasingly being used to treat CCLI even in complex arterial lesions, such as lengthy occlusions of the iliac, femoral, and tibial arteries (Figures 8–13). Percutaneous endovascular technologies include numerous endovascular devices which are designed to treat peripheral arterial occlusive disease, such as percutaneous balloon angioplasty, bare metal stent placement, covered stent placement, drug eluting stent placement, re-entry catheters, blunt dissection catheters, atherectomy catheters, laser angioplasty, cutting balloons, thermal angioplasty, mechanical thrombectomy, rotational atherectomy and local delivered fibrinolysis. Advances have been made in all these innovative technologies, particularly in lesion modification, atheroablation, and other ingenious approaches. Nevertheless, most of the clinical data regarding limb salvage is derived from balloon dilatation and stenting procedures.

Regardless of the technique used, the angiographic goal of any endovascular therapy is to provide the distal extremity with an adequate inflow. Ideally, this would mean pulsatile blood flow through a patent tibioperoneal vessel with reconstitution of the pedal arch, thus providing adequate reperfusion to the area in jeopardy. Outcomes of endovascular therapy depend on anatomic and clinical factors. The durability of patency after percutaneous revascularization is greatest for lesions in the common iliac artery and decreases with more distal interventions. Durability also decreases with increasing length of the stenosis or occlusion, and in multi-level and diffuse lesions which are commonly seen in patients with CCLI. As with surgical revascularization, outcomes of endovascular therapy are also dependent on the distal vessel run-off. Higher success rates are seen in patients with focal and short stenosis, in mild diffuse distal disease, in non-diabetics, non-smokers and in patients with reconstituted pedal arches after the procedure (64). "Technical success" is defined as the successful restoration of flow during the endovascular procedure, whereas "clinical success" refers to subsequent evidence of clinical response as defined above.

In a recent series of patients with iliac disease treated mainly with angioplasty and conditional stenting, the technical success rate was 99%, with an initial clinical success rate of 99% (Figure 10). Overall, the cumulative primary patency rates at one, three, and five years were 76%, 59%, and 49% with only 7% of patients undergoing primary stent placement. The cumulative assisted primary and secondary patency rates at seven years were 98% and 99%; and the limb salvage rate at seven years was 93% (65). Saha et al. reported a primary patency following iliac stenting for CCLI after three years of 86% (66). In a contemporary series of 32 diabetic patients with CCLI, and using angioplasty as a primary revascularization method, Jacqueminet et al. was able to complete the procedure successfully in 78% of patients with a wound healing rate of 70% and a limb salvage rate 90%. Successful limb salvage was significantly associated with a higher post-procedure transcutaneous oxygen pressure and the presence of at least one patent pedal vessel by univariate analysis (67). Haider et al. reported the following outcomes on 180 patients two years after femoral-popliteal angioplasty: a primary cumulative patency rate of 75%, limb salvage rate of 90%, and survival rates of 88%. The 30 day mortality was 2.7%, and the complication rate was 8.3%. At two years, there was a restenosis rate (>50%) of 68% and 65% for the femoropopliteal and infrapopliteal angioplasty groups. Seven patients required repeat angioplasty of the same site, 30 underwent subsequent bypass, and 16 of 43 occluded limbs were amputated. A total of 153 comparative control patients underwent 162 bypass procedures during the same period. Primary cumulative patency, limb salvage, and survival for femoropopliteal bypass (n = 80) at two years were 69%, 87%, and 76%, respectively, and for infrapopliteal bypass were 53%, 57%, and 64% (n=82). The 30-day mortality for bypass was 5.2%, with a complication rate of 35%, and 31 limbs were amputated. Although there were relatively high restenosis rates for angioplasty patients, these data suggest that angioplasty, when used preferentially in anatomically suitable patients, provides very similar limb salvage rates with a lower morbidity and mortality when compared to surgical revascularization (68).

A recent randomized study suggested that for superficial femoral artery lesions, primary implantation of self-expanding Nitinol stents might be superior to percutaneous angioplasty alone, although the number of patients with CCLI in this study was small (69). Among stents, Nitinol self expandable stents appear to be superior compared with stainless steel stents in the femoropopliteal vessels, with a higher primary patency rate (Figure 8) (70, 71). For infrapopliteal disease, the use of coronary techniques are now widely accepted. These have demonstrated high rates of limb salvage despite having generally poor durability (Figures 11 and 12), emphasizing the difference between clinical outcome, mechanical function (72) and long term patency. Faglia et al. reported on a group of 191 patients with CCLI in whom 41% required infrapopliteal angioplasty and 51% multi-level angioplasty. A limb salvage rate of 94% with a significant improvement in both ABI and transcutaneous oximetry post-procedure (71, 73). Feiring et al. showed that successful below the knee stent-supported angioplasty for CCLI improves ankle brachial indexes, healed limited-amputations and ulcerations, relieved rest pain, and improved ambulation in up to 96% of patients (74). These success rates were comparable to tibial bypass procedures. In a preliminary study, the implantation of infra-popliteal drug eluting coronary balloon expandable stents showed a limb salvage rate of 94% (75). Clinical success with a percutaneous approach may be expected to be superior to angiographic patency because once wound healing has occurred, if restenosis or occlusion occur, collateral may then be sufficient to preserve tissue integrity provided there is no further injury. Compared to surgery, this revascularization modality carries a lower morbidity and mortality, requires a shorter hospital stay and does not preclude surgery. If permitted by the underlying anatomy, it is ideal for patients who are high-risk surgical candidates. In a report on ten years of experience treating multilevel disease, Kudo and colleagues demonstrated that an endovascular approach is feasible, safe, and effective for the treatment of CCLI (76). Despite low primary patency rates, high limb salvage rates (89%) were attributed to high assisted primary and secondary patency rates (76), highlighting the importance of close follow-up in these patients. In a group of patients with CCLI who were not suitable candidates for surgical revascularization, percutaneous techniques achieved a rate of limb salvage of 83% (77). Besides angioplasty and stenting, various techniques and technologies also have been shown to be useful as a stand-alone or adjunctive therapy. These include the use of atherectomy devices (78, 79) (Figures 9 and 11), cryoplasty (80, 81) (Figure 12), sub-intimal angioplasty (82–85), covered stents (73, 86), and laser assisted angioplasty (87–89) (Figure 8).

Today it is indisputable that endovascular therapy has a main role in the revascularization of patients with CCLI. Percutaneous revascularization has lower long-term patency rates than the rates of limb salvage. Therefore, close surveillance is warranted to maintain an adequate level of assisted secondary patency.

Surgical Revascularization

Currently there are different surgical techniques that allow long-lasting lower extremity revascularization for patients suffering from CCLI. New technologies are being developed to improve patency rates and to offer alternatives to traditional bypass surgery. The surgical options and results are dependent on the anatomical area being revascularized (aortoiliac, femoral or below the knee), the type of conduit used (venous versus prosthetic or composite grafts) and the quality of the graft inflow and outflow available. In different surgical series with unselected patients, limb salvage has been reported to be between 65–95% (71, 73, 90–93). Better success is attained when the lesion treated is higher in the vascular tree, with best outcomes in aortoiliac disease and worst outcomes when disease is present below the knee (94, 95). Satiani et al., reported a primary patency rate of 80% and limb salvage rate of 74% at five years following aortoiliac bypass in 77 patients with CCLI (92). In 112 patients undergoing infrainguinal bypass surgery for limb salvage, five years after operation, the assisted primary graft patency and limb salvage rates were 77% and 87% respectively (96). Hughes et al. reported their experience with distal arterial bypasses to the plantar and lateral tarsal arteries for ischemic limb salvage in 90 patients. Seventy-one grafts (72%) had inflow from the popliteal artery, 25 grafts had inflow from a femoral artery or a higher graft (26%), and two grafts had inflow from a tibial artery (2%). Conduits used were the greater saphenous vein in 67 patients (69%), upper extremity vein in 20 patients (20%), composite vein in ten patients (10%), and a polytetrafluoroethylene conduit in one patient (1%). There were 77 bypasses (79%) to plantar artery branches, and 21 bypasses (21%) to the lateral tarsal artery. Primary patency, secondary patency and limb salvage were 50%, 69%, and 63%, respectively, at five years. Greater saphenous vein grafts performed better than all other conduits, with a secondary patency rate of 82% versus 47% at one year (95). Nearly all studies that have compared autologous veins with prosthetic conduits for arterial reconstruction of the lower extremity have shown the superior patency of venous grafts (97). Prosthetic grafts are successfully used for aortoiliac disease with patency at five years close to 90% (92). However, the use of venous grafts have significantly improved patency rate compared with prosthetic grafts when anastomosed at the infrainguinal level (68% vs. 38% at five year) or below the knee (50% vs. 12% at five year); and therefore should be the preferred conduit for these anatomic sites if available (95, 98–100). When the greater saphenous vein is unavailable, alternate autologous veins are preferable to other graft materials especially for bypasses attached to the infrapopliteal arteries (99). Autologous veins can be used *in situ* or used in reverse fashion. In a study comparing both techniques, the *in situ* vein graft group had an overall limb salvage rate of 92% with an 88% cumulative patency rate at 4 to 18 months. The reversed autogenous vein graft group had a limb salvage rate of 86% with a 79% patency, supporting the use of *in situ* vein bypass grafting for limb salvage in this population (90). Unfortunately, many of patients with CCLI had no available autologous vein to harvest and their only choice is to place a prosthethic graft. Despite a low rate of long-term patency, prosthethic grafts achieve a high rate of limb salvage in patients with CCLI and are an acceptable alternative in patients with critical ischemia if autologous vein is not available (91, 94, 100). In 83 consecutive femorotibial bypass procedures in 70 patients with CCLI, thin-walled, ringed 6-mm polytetrafluoroethylene was used in patients in whom no autologous vein was available (100). After five years, 33 patients had died, mainly of cardiovascular causes. Primary patency was 64% after six weeks and 18% after five years. Secondary patency was 74% after six weeks and 22% after five years. Despite this poor durability, the limb salvage rate was 62% after five years. Newer surgical techniques such as distal interposition of vein patches and cuffs and arteriovenous fistulas aimed to improve the patency of prosthetic grafts are encouraging for limb salvage (98, 98, 101, 102). Also recently, remote endarterectomy has been used with good results in a small series of patients with CCLI (103). Besides the quality of the runoffs and the severity of the vascular disease, graft failure is not uncommon in patients undergoing limb salvage due to spontaneous thrombus formation, disease progression and graft or anastomotic neointimal hyperplasia. To limit disease progression, aggressive medical therapy should be instituted to try to control the risk factors and improve lipids, glucose, smoking and blood pressure control. Use of pharmacologic therapy to prevent graft failure remains uncertain, except for the use of antiplatelet agents. (i.e., aspirin and clopidrogel) In some cases of prosthetic grafts going to the femoropopliteal area or below, the use of warfarin (Coumadin) is also advocated by some vascular specialists. It is important not to overlook the surgical risk in patients with CCLI considering the strong correlation between peripheral vascular disease, coronary and cerebrovascular disease in this population. Therefore, a complete preoperative evaluation is mandatory before proceeding with vascular surgery to assure the best outcome in this high-risk population.

Thrombolysis

Systemic or direct thrombolysis by an infusion catheter directed into the occlusive zone or used with thrombectomy catheters (Possis device, Trellis device, etc.), is another therapeutic modality for patients with CCLI (Figure 13). Its role in acute limb ischemia is well established (104). This form of revascularization has been used both as a primary treatment and as an adjuvant therapy for patients undergoing endovascular therapy or surgical revascularization. Three studies have been completed comparing thrombolytic therapy to surgical revascularization for ischemic limbs using plasminogen activator and urokinase (TOPAS, STILE and the Rochester trial) as initial therapy (105). Thrombolysis reduces the need for any subsequent surgical procedure in approximately 40% to 60% of patients. However, recurrent ischemia is frequent, and the subsequent need for surgical revascularization is common for any native artery occlusion or chronic bypass graft occlusion. In patients with acute bypass graft occlusions, the incidence of recurrent ischemia is less and limb salvage at one year is enhanced when treated initially by thrombolysis. A possible survival benefit after thrombolysis was suggested in the Rochester trial and in the STILE trial for diabetics with femoral-popliteal occlusions. Major bleeding complications are seen in 1–2% of patients undergoing thrombolysis (104, 106). Based on a review of the current evidence regarding the infusion techniques for peripheral arterial thrombolysis published by the Cochrane Collaborators Database (107), it is recommended to reserve thrombolysis for patients with acute limb threatening ischemia, due to the high risk of bleeding or death associated with thrombolysis. Greater benefit is seen when the thrombolytic agent is delivered into the thrombus. Systemic intravenous thrombolysis is less effective compared with intra-arterial thrombolysis, and is associated with an increase in bleeding complications. High dose techniques, or adjunctive agents such as platelet glycoprotein IIb/IIIa inhibitors, may speed up thrombolysis, but these are not accompanied by lower amputation rates or a decreased need for adjunctive lysis of the thrombus with a high dose of the thrombolytic agent (107). No randomized study has been done comparing endovascular therapy versus thrombolysis or endovascular therapy plus thrombolysis versus surgical revascularization. Thrombolysis in CCLI plays an important role in occluded grafts and native vessels with large thrombus burden to facilitate endovascular or surgical therapy. However, it is not the preferred approach for localized or small thrombus since the use of catheter based techniques for thrombectomy have successfully managed this with a lower risk.

What revascularization method to use?

The decision of which revascularization method to use must always be individualized for each patient, taking into account the operative risk, risk factors, prognosis, vascular anatomy and the area to revascularize. Additionally, the local expertise of the center caring for the patient needs to be considered. Patients with CCLI are typically elderly with multiple co-morbidities and limited life expectancy. Therefore, in the majority of cases, a procedure which is minimally invasive with a reduced morbidity and mortality but lesser long-term patency, may be more appropriate than a more invasive, costly procedure with a better long-term patency. The recently published BASIL study is the only available randomized study comparing bypass surgery with percutaneous revascularization for CCLI (108). This multicenter study randomized 452 patients who presented to 27 hospitals in England with CCLI due to infrainguinal disease, to receive a surgery-first (n = 228) or an angioplasty-first (n = 224) strategy. The primary endpoint was amputation free survival after 5.5 years. At the end of follow-up, 55% patients were alive without amputation, 8% alive with amputation, 8% dead after amputation, and 29% dead without amputation, with no difference between both groups regarding amputation-free survival. There was no difference in health-related quality of life between the two strategies, but the hospital costs associated with the surgical strategy were about one third higher than those with an angioplasty based strategy. Therefore, the authors conclude that in patients presenting with severe limb ischemia due to infrainguinal disease and who are suitable for surgery or angioplasty, a bypass-surgery-first and a balloon-angioplasty-first strategy are associated with broadly similar outcomes, but in the short-term, surgery is more expensive than angioplasty. With the current techniques, most patients with CCLI can benefit from revascularization. Initially, the percutaneous approach is preferred by many centers in order to avoid a surgical procedure in a group of patients that are considered at high operative risk. However, the best treatment to achieve the highest rates of limb salvage and long-lasting revascularization can not be generalized; and in the best interest of the patient, needs to be individualized based on their underlying risk factors, comorbidities, severity of peripheral vascular disease, and anatomic characteristics.

Spinal Cord Stimulation

Spinal cord stimulation has been introduced as a treatment option for patients with CCLI. In a recent meta-analysis including 444 patients (61, 62, 109), this modality showed 11% (95% CI: 0.02–0.20) lower amputation rates after 12 months of follow-up compared to those treated with optimum medical therapy. In addition, patients receiving spinal cord stimulation required fewer analgesics and showed a significant clinical improvement. Transcutaneous oximetry measurements were found to be useful in selecting the most respondent patients (those with $TcpO_2$ values between ten and 30 mmHg), which had a rate of limb salvage as high as 83% with this therapy.

In a systematic review based on the Cochrane Peripheral Vascular Diseases Group (61, 62, 110), the authors conclude that limb salvage after 12 months was significantly higher in the spinal cord stimulation group (RR 0.71, 95% CI: 0.56 to 0.90) compared to medical therapy alone. Significant pain relief occurred in both treatment groups, but was more prominent in the spinal cord stimulation group, in which the patients required significantly less analgesics. Overall, no significantly different effect on ulcer healing was observed between the two treatments. Complications of this therapy consisted of implantation problems (9%; 95% CI: 4–15%) and changes in stimulation requiring reintervention, (15%; 95% CI: 10–20%). Infections of the lead or pulse generator pocket occurred less frequently (3%; 95% CI: 0–6%). The overall risk of complications of additional spinal cord stimulation group treatment was 17%, (95% CI: 12–22%), indicating a number needed to harm of six. A cost comparison was made in only one study, reporting average overall costs at two years, of \$46,700 in the spinal cord stimulation group and \$36,600 in the conservative group. Therefore, currently there is some limited evidence to favor spinal cord stimulation over standard conservative treatment to improve limb salvage. The benefits of spinal cord stimulation against the possible harm of relatively mild complications, the availability of this therapy and costs must be considered.

Amputation

All efforts of revascularization and wound healing are directed towards limb salvage in CCLI. An aggressive stand to preserve the jeopardized extremity is justified in patients with CCLI because patients undergoing a major limb amputation have generally a dismal prognosis with a 30-day mortality of approximately 10% (111), 30% at one-year, and close to 50% at only two-years (112–114). Moreover, amputees due to CCLI have a poor quality of life and functional outcome with higher post-operative complications (115), lower independence (111), high incidence of depressive symptoms (116), significant progression to a higher level of limb loss and high usage of health services utilization reaching up to 4.3 billion dollars yearly for Medicare beneficiaries nationwide (114). In general, patients with diabetes and renal disease have the worst outcomes developing CCLI at earlier ages. Despite the dismal scenario for patients suffering from CCLI who are not candidates for revascularization, amputation is an important treatment option. It effectively controls systemic life-threatening infections originating from the affected limb, cures untreatable resting pain, and might accelerate and improve the rehabilitation, independence and mobility of patients who have no revascularization options. The healing of minor (interphalangeal or transmetatarsal) amputations may be facilitated by pre-operative revascularization. This is an ideal approach to limb salvage (113). If this is not possible, a major amputation will be required. Ideally a below the knee amputation should be then considered, and if not possible, an above the knee amputation may be necessary. It is difficult to predict the potential for ambulation after an amputation because the morbidity associated with delayed wound healing and the challenges involved in rehabilitation (111). In determining the level of amputation, it is necessary to consider the potential for effective rehabilitation versus the likelihood of post-operative complications. More distal amputations have a better rehabilitation potential, but also have a higher risk of incomplete healing, necessitating further stump revisions, possible subsequent amputations, and delayed rehabilitation if the ischemic limb has inadequate perfusion. Therefore, before the level of amputation is chosen it is essential to consider the following factors besides the overall cardiopulmonary condition of the patient: Non-invasive or invasive assessment of the arterial perfusion in the affected limb to guarantee effective healing (usually a calf pressure > 70 mm Hg, ankle or toe pressure > 30 mm Hg, or a transcutaneous oximetry value > 40 mm Hg), adequate knowledge of the underlying vascular anatomy of the limb, the presence or absence of infection (i.e., cellulitis, osteomyelitis, etc), adequate glucose control in diabetics, appropriate nutrition, and attention to any additional mechanical features that might compromise wound healing after the amputation (i.e., gait abnormalities, trauma of the stump, inadequate prosthesis fittings, infection, neuropathy, combined venous and arterial insufficiency, etc). In patients undergoing an amputation, adequate evaluation of the contra-lateral limb is also compulsory, since peripheral arterial disease is most of the time symmetrical with subsequent contra-lateral amputations seen in 23% of patients (117). Therefore, it is important to have a thorough evaluation of the vascular supply and overall clinical status of the contra-lateral limb before proceeding with surgery. Although amputation is considered the end of effort of revascularization, it should not be considered the end of medical therapy of these patients. Amputees require intensive medical therapy and a comprehensive wound care and rehabilitation program. Aggressive medical therapy is essential to facilitate wound healing and to improve the overall prognosis of these patients. Therefore, intensive risk factor modification and medical therapy is mandatory during and after amputation to optimize the outcomes of these patients with end-stage vascular disease.

Medical Therapy for Patients with Critical Limb Ischemia

As a consequence of coexisting coronary and cerebrovascular disease, there is an increased risk of myocardial infarction, stroke, and cardiovascular death in patients with lower extremity peripheral vascular disease. Patients with CCLI show a high incidence of comorbidities in vascular diseases and high prevalence of modifiable risk factors for atherosclerotic vascular disease. Despite this, the use of evidence-based medical therapy in this group of patients is notoriously suboptimal (61, 62, 118). Therefore, it is fundamental for the team members to expand the focus of therapy well beyond local wound care and revascularization. To provide the best overall prognosis of this high-risk population, the team must apply an aggressive medical therapy and risk factor modification program.

All patients should be counseled to stop using tobacco products, maintain an adequate weight (body mass index <25 Kg/m^2), and to follow a heart healthy diet. Blood pressure should be treated towards a goal of less than 140/90 mmHg (130/85 mm Hg for diabetics and patients with chronic kidney disease), diabetes mellitus to a goal of Hemoglobin A1c of less than 7%, LDL-cholesterol should be lowered to less than 100 mg/dl (and if possible to less than 70 mg/dl) and non-HDL cholesterol should be less than 130 mg/dl for patients with triglycerides levels above 200 mg/dl (119). Treatment with a hydroxymethyl glutaryl coenzyme-A reductase inhibitor (statin therapy) is strongly recommended to achieve the mentioned lipid goals to any patient with a LDL-cholesterol above 100 mg/dl. Therapy with a fibric acid derivative (also known as fibrates) can be useful for patients with low HDL-cholesterol, normal LDL cholesterol, and elevated triglycerides or a non-HDL cholesterol above target. Based on the results of the HOPE trial (120), it is recommended that Angiotensin Converting Enzyme (ACE) inhibitors be considered as treatment for patients with asymptomatic or symptomatic lower extremity peripheral vascular disease to reduce the risk of adverse cardiovascular events regardless of the blood pressure. Beta-blockers reduce the risk of myocardial infarction and death in patients with coronary atherosclerosis (121). A meta-analysis of 11 placebo-controlled studies in patients with intermittent claudication found that beta-adrenergic blockers did not adversely affect walking capacity and therefore can be used safely in patients with CCLI with documented coronary artery disease or hypertension (122). Aspirin, in daily doses of 75–325 mg, is recommended as an effective antiplatelet therapy to reduce the risk of myocardial infarction, stroke, or vascular death in all patients. Clopidogrel (75 mg per day) is recommended as an effective alternative antiplatelet therapy to aspirin to reduce the risk of MI, stroke, or vascular death in

TABLE 3. MEDICAL THERAPY FOR PATIENTS WITH CHRONIC CRITICAL LIMB ISCHEMIA

1) Arterial Hypertension Management:
Goal for blood pressure:
< 140/90 mm Hg for all patients
< 130/85 mm Hg for diabetes mellitus and patients with chronic kidney disease

2) Diabetic Management:
Goal for Hb A1c:
< 7%

3) Lipid Management:
Goal for LDL-cholesterol:
< 100 mg/dl and strongly consider a goal of < 70 mg/dl

Goal for non-HDL cholesterol for patients with triglycerides > 200 mg/dl:
< 130 mg/dl

Consider use of hydroxymethyl glutaryl coenzyme-A reductase inhibitors (statin therapy) in all patients with lipid concentrations above goals.

4) Medical Therapy:
a) Aspirin 81–325 mg daily if no contraindications for all patients.

b) Clopidrogel 75 mg daily can be an effective alternate to aspirin therapy.

c) Angiotensin Converting Enzyme (ACE) inhibitors should be considered for all patients if no contraindications.

d) Beta-adrenergic blockers can be used safely in patients with chronic critical limb ischemia and should be prescribed to all patients with known coronary *atherosclerosis.*

e) Oral anticoagulation therapy with warfarin (Coumadin) is not generally indicated to reduce the risk of adverse cardiovascular ischemic events in individuals with atherosclerotic lower extremity disease, but might be considered in selected patients following bypass surgery.

f) Cilostazol has no defined role in patients with CCLI. However, a therapeutic trial of cilostazol should be considered in all patients with lifestyle-limiting claudication in the absence of left ventricular dysfunction.

g) Pentoxyfiline has no role in patients with CCLI.

individuals with atherosclerotic lower extremity vascular disease, and may be superior to aspirin in this setting (123). Oral anticoagulation therapy with warfarin (Coumadin) is not generally indicated to reduce the risk of adverse cardiovascular ischemic events in individuals with atherosclerotic lower extremity disease, although it may have a role in selected patients undergoing bypass surgery. Cilostazol has no defined role in patients with CCLI, however a therapeutic trial of cilostazol should be considered in all patients with lifestyle-limiting claudication in the absence of left ventricular dysfunction. Pentoxyfiline has no role in patients with CCLI. Table 3 is a summary of medical therapy considerations for patients with critical limb ischemia.

FOLLOW-UP FOR THE PATIENT AFTER LIMB SALVAGE

In patients who undergo limb-salvage, a multidisciplinary team approach between the vascular specialist, primary care physician, and the wound care specialist is necessary to achieve the best long-term results, prevent further recurrences of CCLI, and improve the patient's overall cardiovascular outcome. All patients should receive intensive medical therapy as described. A periodic vascular examination including records with ankle-brachial indexes, and preferably complete Duplex ultrasound is recommended during follow-up visits to assure adequate distal limb perfusion and vascular patency. If the patient underwent surgical revascularization with a venous graft, attention to the whole length of the graft, peak velocities with translesional velocity ratios, and inflow and outflow examination of the conduit needs to be noted by Duplex imaging. This group of patients have a high incidence of thrombus formation, graft failure and restenotic lesions (61, 62). Currently Duplex imaging is recommended after four to six weeks, and three, six, and every 12 months after vascular surgery with venous grafts to guide their long-term secondary patency. After percutaneous and surgical revascularization utilizing prosthetic conduits, a similar strategy is advocated by many vascular experts using periodical duplex ultrasound examinations or other non-invasive tests to detect early problems. The importance of this regular surveillance program needs to be underscored, since its goal is to attempt an early treatment of any problematic areas (generally using the endovascular approach) before the distal flow gets further compromised, preventing any symptoms or manifestation of recurrent CCLI. Whether this intensive mode of follow-up leads to a better long-term outcome than regular clinical follow-up is intuitive, but still needs to be proven by randomized clinical studies for patients undergoing prosthetic grafts placement and endovascular revascularization. There are no current data available regarding follow up of patients post-revascularization with new imaging technology such as CTA and MRA, but the cost of these new modalities and the potential radiation exposure for CTA, may be important drawbacks for its widespread use in daily practice compared with follow-up with Duplex ultrasound imaging.

FUTURE TREATMENT OPTIONS FOR LIMB SALVAGE

Many efforts are devoted to try to improve the revascularization outcomes in patients suffering from CCLI. New bare-metal stents are being developed to avoid stent fatigue and fracture. New alloys and designs improve their durability, specifically for infrainguinal interventions. Covered stents are now being used for lower extremity interventions hoping to decrease the incidence of restenosis with encouraging initial results (73). One area of intense research is the prevention of restenosis in the peripheral vasculature, in which the use of drug eluting stents may hold a bright future, despite the negative results reported in their first clinical trial (124). Intravascular ultrasound guided atherectomy devices and mini-atherectomy devices to target the smallest vessels are currently under development as an attempt to avoid flow limiting dissections and barotrauma in the infragenicular vasculature. Novel pharmacological approaches are also being studied to enhance vascular growth and collateral vessels formation, such as local endovascular delivery of growth factors, gene therapy, and cell transplantation for end-stage peripheral arterial disease. Hypoxia inducible factor-1alpha, fibroblast growth factor-4, Del-1 and hepatocyte growth factor have entered clinical trials. Stem-cell therapy or factors mobilizing bone marrow progenitor cells and endothelial progenitor cells have provided evidence for a new avenue for therapeutic angiogenesis and also hold a bright future in this area (125). Clinical tests are underway on new surgical techniques including the use of robotic surgery, new endoscopic techniques, and innovative graft materials intended to prevent graft thrombosis and to improve graft patency (102, 126, 127).

MANAGEMENT ALGORITHM FOR LIMB SALVAGE

As a guide for the clinician, we provide this simplified algorithm to help in the management of patients with CCLI (Figure 14).

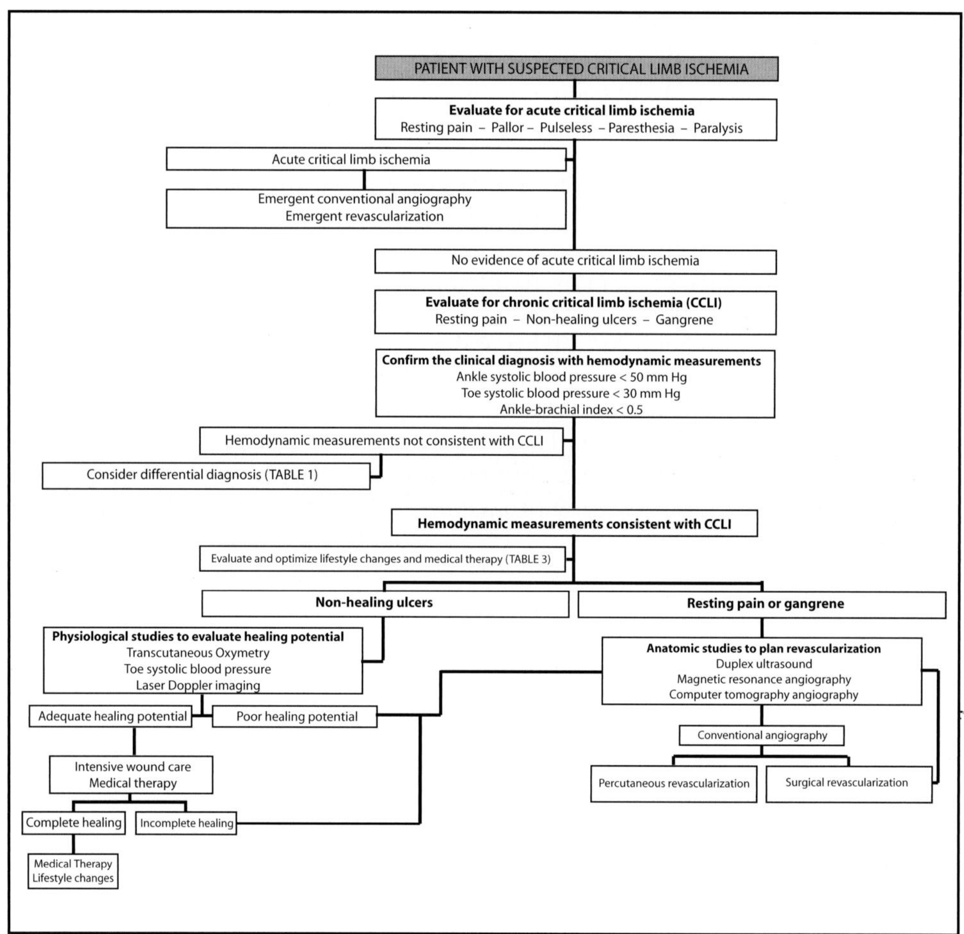

Figure 14. Management algorithm for patients with critical limb ischemia.

REFERENCE

1. Second European Consensus Document on chronic critical leg ischemia *Circulation* 1991; 84(4 Suppl):IV1-26.

2. Goessens BM, Visseren FL, Algra A, et al. Screening for asymptomatic cardiovascular disease with noninvasive imaging in patients at high-risk and low-risk according to the European Guidelines on Cardiovascular Disease Prevention: the SMART study. *J Vasc Surg* 2006; 43(3):525-532.

3. Criqui MH, Fronek A, Barrett-Connor E, et al. The prevalence of peripheral arterial disease in a defined population. *Circulation* 1985; 71(3):510-515.

4. Kannel WB. The demographics of claudication and the aging of the American population. *Vasc Med* 1996; 1(1):60-64.

5. Murabito JM, Evans JC, D'Agostino RB, Sr., et al. Temporal trends in the incidence of intermittent claudication from 1950 to 1999. *Am J Epidemiol* 2005; 162(5):430-437.

6. Criqui MH. Peripheral arterial disease and subsequent cardiovascular mortality. A strong and consistent association. *Circulation* 1990; 82(6):2246-2247.

7. Criqui MH, Langer RD, Fronek A, et al. Mortality over a period of 10 years in patients with peripheral arterial disease. *N Engl J Med* 1992; 326(6):381-386.

8. Criqui MH. Peripheral arterial disease-epidemiological aspects. *Vasc Med* 2001; 6(3 Suppl):3-7.

9. Newman AB, Sutton-Tyrrell K, Vogt MT, et al. Morbidity and mortality in hypertensive adults with a low ankle/arm blood pressure index. *JAMA* 1993; 270(4):487-489.

10. Zheng ZJ, Sharrett AR, Chambless LE, et al. Associations of ankle-brachial index with clinical coronary heart disease, stroke and preclinical carotid and popliteal *atherosclerosis*: the *Atherosclerosis* Risk in Communities (ARIC) Study. *Atherosclerosis* 1997; 131(1):115-125.

11. Dormandy JA, Murray GD. The fate of the claudicant--a prospective study of 1969 claudicants. *Eur J Vasc Surg* 1991; 5(2):131-133.

12. Valentine RJ, Grayburn PA, Eichhorn EJ, et al. Coronary artery disease is highly prevalent among patients with premature peripheral vascular disease. *J Vasc Surg* 1994; 19(4):668-674.

13. Dormandy JA, Rutherford RB. Management of peripheral arterial disease (PAD). TASC Working Group. TransAtlantic Inter-Society Concensus (TASC). *J Vasc Surg* 2000; 31(1 Pt 2):S1-S296.

14. Weitz JI, Byrne J, Clagett GP, et al. Diagnosis and treatment of chronic arterial insufficiency of the lower extremities: a critical review. *Circulation* 1996; 94(11):3026-3049.

15. Ebskov B, Ebskov L. Major lower limb amputation in diabetic patients: development during 1982 to 1993. *Diabetologia* 1996; 39(12):1607-1610.

16. Ebskov B. Relative mortality and long term survival for the non-diabetic lower limb amputee with vascular insufficiency. *Prosthet Orthot Int* 1999; 23(3):209-216.

17. Kazmers A, Perkins AJ, Jacobs LA. Major lower extremity amputation in Veterans Affairs medical centers. *Ann Vasc Surg* 2000; 14(3):216-222.

18. Criqui MH, Langer RD, Fronek A, et al. Coronary disease and stroke in patients with large-vessel peripheral arterial disease. *Drugs* 1991; 42 Suppl 5:16-21.

19. Coats P, Wadsworth R. Marriage of resistance and conduit arteries breeds critical limb ischemia. *Am J Physiol Heart Circ Physiol* 2005; 288(3):H1044-H1050.

20. Erren M, Reinecke H, Junker R, et al. Systemic inflammatory parameters in patients with atherosclerosis of the coronary and peripheral arteries. *Arterioscler Thromb Vasc Biol* 1999; 19(10):2355-2363.

21. Robless PA, Okonko D, Lintott P, et al. Increased platelet aggregation and activation in peripheral arterial disease. *Eur J Vasc Endovasc Surg* 2003; 25(1):16-22.

22. Koksal C, Ercan M, Bozkurt AK. Hemorrheological variables in critical limb ischemia. *Int Angiol* 2002; 21(4):355-359.

23. Barani J, Nilsson JA, Mattiasson I, et al. Inflammatory mediators are associated with 1-year mortality in critical limb ischemia. *J Vasc Surg* 2005; 42(1):75-80.

24. Ngo BT, Hayes KD, DiMiao DJ, et al. Manifestations of cutaneous diabetic microangiopathy. *Am J Clin Dermatol* 2005; 6(4):225-237.

25. Tzoulaki I, Murray GD, Lee AJ, et al. C-reactive protein, interleukin-6, and soluble adhesion molecules as predictors of progressive peripheral *atherosclerosis* in the general population: Edinburgh Artery Study. *Circulation* 2005; 112(7):976-983.

26. Greenman RL, Panasyuk S, Wang X, et al. Early changes in the skin microcirculation and muscle metabolism of the diabetic foot. *Lancet* 2005; 366(9498):1711-1717.

27. Wu S, Armstrong DG. Risk assessment of the diabetic foot and wound. *Int Wound J* 2005; 2(1):17-24.

28. van Schie CH. A review of the biomechanics of the diabetic foot. *Int J Low Extrem Wounds* 2005; 4(3):160-170.

29. Singh N, Armstrong DG, Lipsky BA. Preventing foot ulcers in patients with diabetes. *JAMA* 2005; 293(2):217-228.

30. D'Ambrogi E, Giacomozzi C, Macellari V, et al. Abnormal foot function in diabetic patients: the altered onset of Windlass mechanism. *Diabet Med* 2005; 22(12):1713-1719.

31. Lipsky BA, Berendt AR, Deery HG, et al. Diagnosis and treatment of diabetic foot infections. *Plast Reconstr Surg* 2006; 117(7 Suppl):212S-238S.

32. McGee SR, Boyko EJ. Physical examination and chronic lower-extremity ischemia: a critical review. *Arch Intern Med* 1998; 158(12):1357-1364.

33. Khan NA, Rahim SA, Anand SS, et al. Does the clinical examination predict lower extremity peripheral arterial disease? *JAMA* 2006; 295(5):536-546.

34. Lijmer JG, Hunink MG, van den Dungen JJ, et al. ROC analysis of noninvasive tests for peripheral arterial disease. *Ultrasound Med Biol* 1996; 22(4):391-398.

35. Almahameed A. Peripheral arterial disease: recognition and medical management. *Cleve Clin J Med* 2006; 73(7):621-4

36. Leng GC, Fowkes FG, Lee AJ, et al. Use of ankle brachial pressure index to predict cardiovascular events and death: a cohort study. *BMJ* 1996; 313(7070):1440-1444.

37. McLafferty RB, Moneta GL, Taylor LM, Jr., et al. Ability of ankle-brachial index to detect lower-extremity atherosclerotic disease progression. *Arch Surg* 1997; 132(8):836-840.

38. de Graaff JC, Ubbink DT, Legemate DA, et al. Evaluation of toe pressure and transcutaneous oxygen measurements in management of chronic critical leg ischemia: a diagnostic randomized clinical trial. *J Vasc Surg* 2003; 38(3):528-534.

39. Vitti MJ, Robinson DV, Hauer-Jensen M, et al. Wound healing in forefoot amputations: the predictive value of toe pressure. *Ann Vasc Surg* 1994; 8(1):99-106.

40. Varatharajan N, Pillay S, Hitos K, et al. Implications of low great toe pressures in clinical practice. *ANZ J Surg* 2006; 76(4):218-221.

41. Sheffield PJ. Measuring tissue oxygen tension: a review. *Undersea Hyperb Med* 1998; 25(3):179-188.

42. Poredos P, Rakovec S, Guzic-Salobir B. Determination of amputation level in ischaemic limbs using $tcpO_2$ measurement. *Vasa* 2005; 34(2):108-112.

43. Tejerina C, Reig A, Codina J, et al. Application of transcutaneous PO2 determinations for the postoperative monitoring of skin grafts. *Burns* 1992; 18(1):49-50.

44. Fife CE, Buyukcakir C, Otto GH, et al. The predictive value of transcutaneous oxygen tension measurement in diabetic lower extremity ulcers treated with hyperbaric oxygen therapy: a retrospective analysis of 1,144 patients. *Wound Repair Regen* 2002; 10(4):198-207.

45. Hanna GP, Fujise K, Kjellgren O, et al. Infrapopliteal transcatheter interventions for limb salvage in diabetic patients: importance of aggressive interventional approach and role of transcutaneous oximetry. *J Am Coll Cardiol* 1997; 30(3):664-669.

46. Caselli A, Latini V, Lapenna A, et al. Transcutaneous oxygen tension monitoring after successful revascularization in diabetic patients with ischaemic foot ulcers. *Diabet Med* 2005; 22(4):460-465.

47. Cobb J, Claremont D. Noninvasive measurement techniques for monitoring of microvascular function in the diabetic foot. *Int J Low Extrem Wounds* 2002; 1(3):161-169.

48. Khan F, Newton DJ. Laser Doppler imaging in the investigation of lower limb wounds. *Int J Low Extrem Wounds* 2003; 2(2):74-86.

49. Pereles FS, Collins JD, Carr JC, et al. Accuracy of stepping-table lower extremity MR angiography with dual-level bolus timing and separate calf acquisition: hybrid peripheral MR angiography. *Radiology* 2006; 240(1):283-290.

50. Ersoy H, Zhang H, Prince MR. Peripheral MR angiography. *J Cardiovasc Magn Reson* 2006; 8(3):517-528.

51. Baum RA, Rutter CM, Sunshine JH, et al. Multicenter trial to evaluate vascular magnetic resonance angiography of the lower extremity. American College of Radiology Rapid Technology Assessment Group. *JAMA* 1995; 274(11):875-880.

52. Huegli RW, Aschwanden M, Bongartz G, et al. Intraarterial MR angiography and DSA in patients with peripheral arterial occlusive disease: prospective comparison. *Radiology* 2006; 239(3):901-908.

53. Kreitner KF, Kalden P, Neufang A, et al. Diabetes and peripheral arterial occlusive disease: prospective comparison of contrast-enhanced three-dimensional MR angiography with conventional digital subtraction angiography. *AJR Am J Roentgenol* 2000; 174(1):171-179.

54. Carpenter JP, Owen RS, Baum RA, et al. Magnetic resonance angiography of peripheral runoff vessels. *J Vasc Surg* 1992; 16(6):807-813.

55. Owen RS, Carpenter JP, Baum RA, et al. Magnetic resonance imaging of angiographically occult runoff vessels in peripheral arterial occlusive disease. *N Engl J Med* 1992; 326(24):1577-1581.

56. Hiatt MD, Fleischmann D, Hellinger JC, et al. Angiographic imaging of the lower extremities with multidetector CT. *Radiol Clin North Am* 2005; 43(6):1119-27, ix.

57. Bui TD, Gelfand D, Whipple S, et al. Comparison of CT and catheter arteriography for evaluation of peripheral arterial disease. *Vasc Endovascular Surg* 2005; 39(6):481-490.

58. Gale SS, Scissons RP, Salles-Cunha SX, et al. Lower extremity arterial evaluation: are segmental arterial blood pressures worthwhile? *J Vasc Surg* 1998; 27(5):831-838.

59. Kaufman JL, Fitzgerald KM, Shah DM, et al. The fate of extremities with flat lower calf pulse volume recordings. *J Cardiovasc Surg* (Torino) 1989; 30(2):216-219.

60. de Vries SO, Hunink MG, Polak JF. Summary receiver operating characteristic curves as a technique for meta-analysis of the diagnostic performance of duplex ultrasonography in peripheral arterial disease. *Acad Radiol* 1996; 3(4):361-369.

61. Mattos MA, van Bemmelen PS, Hodgson KJ, et al. Does correction of stenoses identified with color duplex scanning improve infrainguinal graft patency? *J Vasc Surg* 1993; 17(1):54-64.

62. Laborde AL, Synn AY, Worsey MJ, et al. A prospective comparison of ankle/brachial indices and color duplex imaging in surveillance of the in situ saphenous vein bypass. *J Cardiovasc Surg* (Torino) 1992; 33(4):420-425.

63. Marston WA, Davies SW, Armstrong B, et al. Natural history of limbs with arterial insufficiency and chronic ulceration treated without revascularization. *J Vasc Surg* 2006; 44(1):108-114.

64. Surowiec SM, Davies MG, Eberly SW, et al. Percutaneous angioplasty and stenting of the superficial femoral artery. *J Vasc Surg* 2005; 41(2):269-278.

65. Kudo T, Chandra FA, Ahn SS. Long-term outcomes and predictors of iliac angioplasty with selective stenting. *J Vasc Surg* 2005; 42(3):466-475.

66. Saha S, Gibson M, Torrie EP, et al. Stenting for localised arterial stenoses in the aorto-iliac segment. *Eur J Vasc Endovasc Surg* 2001; 22(1):37-40.

67. Jacqueminet S, Hartemann-Heurtier A, Izzillo R, et al. Percutaneous transluminal angioplasty in severe diabetic foot ischemia: outcomes and prognostic factors. *Diabetes Metab* 2005; 31(4 Pt 1):370-375.

68. Haider SN, Kavanagh EG, Forlee M, et al. Two-year outcome with preferential use of infrainguinal angioplasty for critical ischemia. *J Vasc Surg* 2006; 43(3):504-512.

69. Schillinger M, Sabeti S, Loewe C, et al. Balloon angioplasty versus implantation of nitinol stents in the superficial femoral artery. *N Engl J Med* 2006; 354(18):1879-1888.

70. Sabeti S, Schillinger M, Amighi J, et al. Primary patency of femoropopliteal arteries treated with nitinol versus stainless steel self-expanding stents: propensity score-adjusted analysis. *Radiology* 2004; 232(2):516-521.

71. Faglia E, Mantero M, Caminiti M, et al. Extensive use of peripheral angioplasty, particularly infrapopliteal, in the treatment of ischaemic diabetic foot ulcers: clinical results of a multicenter study of 221 consecutive diabetic subjects. *J Intern Med* 2002; 252(3):225-232.

72. Das T. Optimal therapeutic approaches to femoropopliteal artery intervention. *Catheter Cardiovasc Interv* 2004; 63(1):21-30.

73. Saxon RR, Coffman JM, Gooding JM, et al. Long-term results of ePTFE stent-graft versus angioplasty in the femoropopliteal artery: single center experience from a prospective, randomized trial. *J Vasc Interv Radiol* 2003; 14(3):303-311.

74. Feiring AJ, Wesolowski AA, Lade S. Primary stent-supported angioplasty for treatment of below-knee critical limb ischemia and severe claudication: early and one-year outcomes. *J Am Coll Cardiol* 2004; 44(12):2307-2314.

75. Bosiers M, Deloose K, Verbist J, et al. Percutaneous transluminal angioplasty for treatment of "below-the-knee" critical limb ischemia: early outcomes following the use of sirolimus-eluting stents. *J Cardiovasc Surg* (Torino) 2006; 47(2):171-176.

76. Kudo T, Chandra FA, Ahn SS. The effectiveness of percutaneous transluminal angioplasty for the treatment of critical limb ischemia: a 10-year experience. *J Vasc Surg* 2005; 41(3):423-435.

77. Tefera G, Hoch J, Turnipseed WD. Limb-salvage angioplasty in vascular surgery practice. *J Vasc Surg* 2005; 41(6):988-993.

78. Zeller T, Rastan A, Schwarzwalder U, et al. Midterm results after atherectomy-assisted angioplasty of below-knee arteries with use of the Silverhawk device. *J Vasc Interv Radiol* 2004; 15(12):1391-1397.

79. Kandzari DE, Kiesz RS, Allie D, et al. Procedural and clinical outcomes with catheter-based plaque excision in critical limb ischemia. *J Endovasc Ther* 2006; 13(1):12-22.

80. Fava M, Loyola S, Polydorou A, et al. Cryoplasty for femoropopliteal arterial disease: late angiographic results of initial human experience. *J Vasc Interv Radiol* 2004; 15(11):1239-1243.

81. Joye JD. The clinical application of cryoplasty for infrainguinal peripheral arterial disease. *Tech Vasc Interv Radiol* 2005; 8(4):160-164.

82. Aarts F, Blankensteijn JD, Van der Vliet JA, et al. Subintimal angioplasty of supra- and infrageniculate arteries. *Ann Vasc Surg* 2006.

83. Spinosa DJ, Leung DA, Matsumoto AH, et al. Percutaneous intentional extraluminal recanalization in patients with chronic critical limb ischemia. *Radiology* 2004; 232(2):499-507.

84. Yilmaz S, Sindel T, Yegin A, et al. Subintimal angioplasty of long superficial femoral artery occlusions. *J Vasc Interv Radiol* 2003; 14(8):997-1010.

85. Treiman GS, Treiman R, Whiting J. Results of percutaneous subintimal angioplasty using routine stenting. *J Vasc Surg* 2006; 43(3):513-519.

86. Wiesinger B, Beregi JP, Oliva VL, et al. PTFE-covered self-expanding Nitinol stents for the treatment of severe iliac and femoral artery stenoses and occlusions: final results from a prospective study. *J Endovasc Ther* 2005; 12(2):240-246.

87. Laird JR, Zeller T, Gray BH, et al. Limb salvage following laser-assisted angioplasty for critical limb ischemia: results of the LACI multicenter trial. *J Endovasc Ther* 2006; 13(1):1-11.

88. Biamino G. The excimer laser: science fiction fantasy or practical tool? *J Endovasc Ther* 2004; 11 Suppl 2:II207-II222.

89. Boccalandro F, Muench A, Sdringola S, et al. Wireless laser-assisted angioplasty of the superficial femoral artery in patients with critical limb ischemia who have failed conventional percutaneous revascularization. *Catheter Cardiovasc Interv* 2004; 63(1):7-12.

90. Hurley JJ, Auer AI, Binnington HB, et al. Comparison of initial limb salvage in 98 consecutive patients with either reversed autogenous or *in situ* vein bypass graft procedures. *Am J Surg* 1985; 150(6):777-781.

91. Kalra M, Gloviczki P, Bower TC, et al. Limb salvage after successful pedal bypass grafting is associated with improved long-term survival. *J Vasc Surg* 2001; 33(1):6-16.

92. Satiani B, Liapis CD, Evans WE. Aortofemoral bypass for severe limb ischemia. Long-term survival and limb salvage. *Am J Surg* 1981; 141(2):252-256.

93. Chang BB, Paty PS, Shah DM, et al. Results of infrainguinal bypass for limb salvage in patients with end-stage renal disease. *Surgery* 1990; 108(4):742-746.

94. Connors JP, Walsh DB, Nelson PR, et al. Pedal branch artery bypass: a viable limb salvage option. *J Vasc Surg* 2000; 32(6):1071-1079.

95. Hughes K, Domenig CM, Hamdan AD, et al. Bypass to plantar and tarsal arteries: an acceptable approach to limb salvage. *J Vasc Surg* 2004; 40(6):1149-1157.

96. Nicoloff AD, Taylor LM, Jr., McLafferty RB, et al. Patient recovery after infrainguinal bypass grafting for limb salvage. *J Vasc Surg* 1998; 27(2):256-263.

97. Hobson RW, O'Donnell JA, Jamil Z, et al. Below-knee bypass for limb salvage. Comparison of autogenous saphenous vein, polytetrafluoroethylene, and composite dacron-autogenous vein grafts. *Arch Surg* 1980; 115(7):833-837.

98. Lauterbach SR, Torres GA, Andros G, et al. Infragenicular polytetrafluoroethylene bypass with distal vein cuffs for limb salvage: a contemporary series. *Arch Surg* 2005; 140(5):487-493.

99. Albers M, Romiti M, Brochado-Neto FC, et al. Meta-analysis of alternate autologous vein bypass grafts to infrapopliteal arteries. *J Vasc Surg* 2005; 42(3):449-455.

100. Klinkert P, van Dijk PJ, Breslau PJ. Polytetrafluoroethylene femorotibial bypass grafting: 5-year patency and limb salvage. *Ann Vasc Surg* 2003; 17(5):486-491.

101. Aracil-Sanus E, Mendieta-Azcona C, Cuesta-Gimeno C, et al. Infragenicular bypass graft for limb salvage using polytetrafluoroethylene and distal vein cuff as the first alternative in patients without ipsilateral greater saphenous vein. *Ann Vasc Surg* 2005; 19(3):379-385.

102. Ducasse E, Chevalier J, Chevier E, et al. Patency and limb salvage after distal prosthetic bypass associated with vein cuff and arteriovenous fistula. *Eur J Vasc Endovasc Surg* 2004; 27(4):417-422.

103. Martin JD, Hupp JA, Peeler MO, et al. Remote endarterectomy: lessons learned after more than 100 cases. *J Vasc Surg* 2006; 43(2):320-326.

104. Allie DE, Hebert CJ, Lirtzman MD, et al. Continuous tenecteplase infusion combined with peri/postprocedural platelet glycoprotein IIb/IIIa inhibition in peripheral arterial thrombolysis: initial safety and feasibility experience. *J Endovasc Ther* 2004; 11(4):427-435.

105. Weaver FA, Toms C. The practical implications of recent trials comparing thrombolytic therapy with surgery for lower extremity ischemia. *Semin Vasc Surg* 1997; 10(1):49-54.

106. Giannini D, Balbarini A. Thrombolytic therapy in peripheral arterial disease. *Curr Drug Targets Cardiovasc Haematol Disord* 2004; 4(3):249-258.

107. Kessel DO, Berridge DC, Robertson I. Infusion techniques for peripheral arterial thrombolysis. *Cochrane Database Syst Rev* 2004;(1):CD000985.

REVIEW QUESTIONS

1.) The three cardinal clinical manifestations of chronic critical limb ischemia include:
   a. Resting pain, non-healing ulcers and dependent cyanosis.
   b. Cyanosis, wet gangrene and paresthesias.
   c. Gangrene, non-healing ulcers and resting pain.
   d. Severe intermittent claudication, dry gangrene and non-healing ulcers.

2.) In a patient with suspected chronic critical limb ischemia, the following results will confirm the diagnosis:
   a. An ankle blood pressure of 20 mm Hg and an ankle-brachial index (ABI) of 0.2.
   b. Toe blood pressure of 60 mm Hg and transcutaneous oximetry value of 70 mmHg.
   c. Absence of palpable pulses and an ABI of 0.6.
   d. Transcutaneous oximetry of 70 mm Hg and a toe blood pressure of 60 mm Hg.

3.) Medical care of a diabetic patient with an ischemic non-healing ulcer should include:
   a. Use of ACE inhibitors, a target HbA1c less than 8% and a blood pressure goal of 140/90 mm Hg.
   b. An LDL-cholesterol less than 100 mg/dl, a blood pressure less than 130/80 mm Hg and the use of pentoxyfiline.
   c. An HbA1c less than 7%, an LDL-cholesterol less than 100 mg/dl and antiplatelet therapy.
   d. Use of beta-blockers, ACE inhibitors and aspirin.

4.) In a patient with critical limb ischemia and renal insufficiency with suspected severe calcific peripheral vascular disease and no palpable left femoral pulse in need of revascularization, the preferred diagnostic test is:
   a. Conventional angiography.
   b. Duplex ultrasound imaging.
   c. Magnetic resonance angiography.
   d. Computer tomographic angiography.

5.) In an 85-year-old smoker male reporting resting foot pain with an ABI of 1.4 the management should include:
   a. Analgesics and antibiotics.
   b. A full Duplex ultrasound of the lower extremities or transcutaneous oximetry.
   c. Analgesics for foot pain. No further work-up needed since the ABI is normal, this patient has arthritis.
   d. Smoking cessation, Beta-blockers and aspirin.

Answers: 1c, 2a, 3c, 4c, 5b

CHAPTER **14**

VENOUS DISEASE

CHAPTER FOURTEEN OVERVIEW

NOTES

VENOUS DISEASE

Patrick N. Kimbrell, Valerie Larson-Lohr

INTRODUCTION

Chronic venous insufficiency (CVI) is related to over 70% of the lower extremity ulcers treated in the United States today (1) with an estimated 500,000 to 1 million people afflicted with venous disease in the United States. These numbers are sure to increase as the population continues to age.

Despite this high prevalence, venous ulcers remain a multidisciplinary problem. This clinical challenge has lead to increasing interest over the last decade in finding effective treatments for CVI and related venous ulcer disease.

Recent history has been dominated by a lack of trained clinical specialists in the community, leading to long periods of ineffective and sometimes inappropriate treatment. During this period, data on patient healing and recurrence rates for both physician and nursing based management programs are generally dismal (2).

Once thought to be an easily treatable disease, clinicians have begun to realize that appropriate venous management remains a continuing challenge despite recent publications of useful management guidelines. Although CVI and venous ulceration risk increases with age it is not exclusively a disease of the elderly. Over 40 percent of patients report the occurrence of their first venous ulcer prior to age 50 and 13 percent before age 30 (3).

Of those ulcers that heal, recurrence rates are reported as high as 72 percent at one year.

The importance of improving clinical treatment and outcomes becomes even more paramount when coupled with data concerning treatment costs. In the United States alone, estimated annual healthcare expenditures for venous disease is between $1.9–2.5 billion per year with each case costing approximately $40,000 (4). These estimates do not account for an additional loss of over two million workdays annually and the significant negative impact on the quality of life of those patients suffering from venous disease. It is clear the morbidity associated with venous disease is substantial. This chapter is written with the goal of educating the medical practitioner on the etiology, patho-physiology, evaluation, and current effective treatment of patients suffering from venous stasis and associated venous ulcer disease of the lower extremities.

VENOUS ANATOMY AND PHYSIOLOGY

The veins of the leg are divided into the superficial and deep systems based on their position relative to the fascia. The deep veins that form the popiteal and femoral veins lie within the fascia and are responsible for the venous return from the leg in a cephalad direction back towards the heart. The superficial veins consist of the long saphenous vein, which runs along the medial side of the leg, the short saphenous vein running at the back of the calf from foot to knee and numerous superficial tributaries. These vessels lie outside the fascia and are responsible for the venous return from the skin and subcutaneous fat. Communicating veins called perforators join the two systems. The deep and superficial veins are equipped with one-way bicuspid valves that normally prevent retrograde flow. The perforators also contain bicuspid valves that allow blood flow in a single direction, from the superficial system to the deep system.

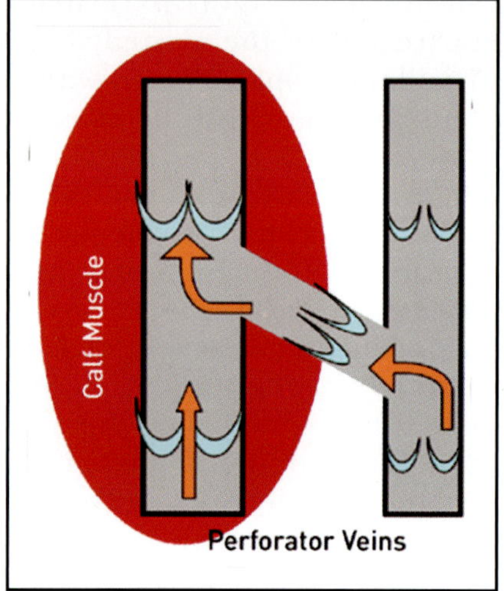

Figure 1. Venous flow from superficial veins to deep veins.

In the healthy venous leg system, standing venous pressure is high at approximately 80 mm Hg. In the supine position, venous pressure is low at approximately 10 mm Hg. During high-pressure states, the venous valves open and blood flows is unidirectional. During low-pressure states, venous valves close. Thus, venous valves direct blood flow only in the presence of a pressure differential. During walking, the foot is dorsal flexed; the calf muscle compresses the deep veins producing internal pressure up to 250 mm Hg, emptying the deep veins of blood in a cephalad direction, back to the heart. When the foot is plantar flexed the pressure in the deep veins drops causing to fill with blood through the open perforators (1, 5). The cycle repeats with each step or muscle contraction, maintaining appropriate venous blood flow back to the heart.

PATHOLOGY OF VENOUS INSUFFICIENCY

Damage or disease to the venous leg system often results in a progressive disruption of the normal venous blood flow. If valves in the superficial veins are affected venous return from the skin will be impaired. This will result in backflow into the superficial system and engorgement of the superficial veins forming varicosities. If the perforator valves are impaired, the action of the calf muscle pump will cause blood to flow in a retrograde fashion to the superficial veins contributing to varicosities. When the valves of the deep veins are affected, continued pressure produced by the calf muscle pump on the perforator valves might cause them to become incompetent. No matter the cause, depending on the degree of valve damage, obstruction or muscle pump dysfunction, the normal drop in venous pressure with ambulation or leg exercise does not occur. The pressure may drop minimally or stay the same as during ambulation. This situation has been called venous hypertension or venous insufficiency (Figure 2). Persistently high hydrostatic pressures in the superficial venous system extend the thin walled veins and capillaries. This eventually over comes the tissue osmotic gradient in the dermal capillaries leading to leakage of fluid and plasma contents into the surrounding tissue, (Figure 3) resulting in leg edema (venous stasis).

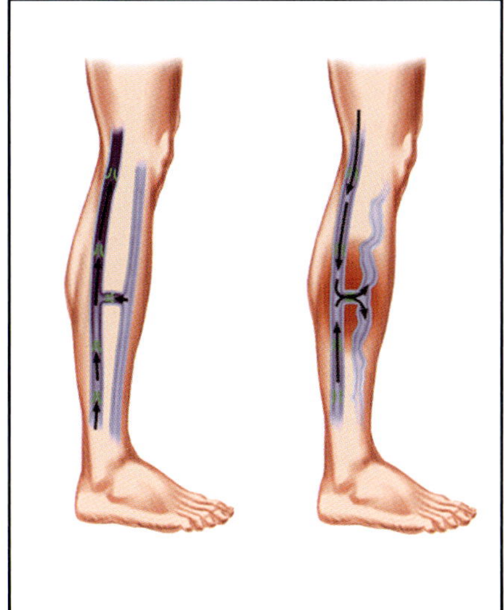

Figure 2. Venous blood flow, normal versus venous insufficiency.

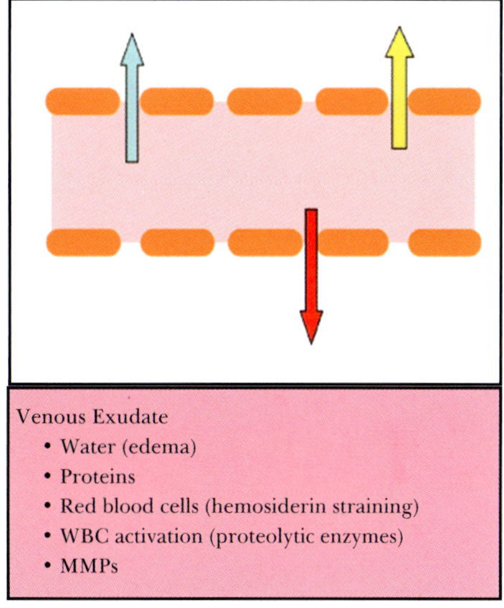

Figure 3. Leaking venous capillaries.

CLINICAL FEATURES OF VENOUS INSUFFICIENCY

The most obvious clinical feature of CVI is the edematous leg(s). Patients describe this type of edema as insidious in onset, initially in involving the feet and ankles, worse after activity and resolving after bed rest or extremity elevation. Over time (years), if the venous disease remains untreated, the persistent high venous pressures lead to progressive valvular damage and incompetence. The edema worsens and begins to involve the entire leg, most often below the knee with a heavy, aching discomfort that improves with bed rest or elevation but does not fully resolve. Varicosities are frequently present due to engorgement of the superficial venous system. As edema worsens it can become a barrier to tissue oxygenation by increasing the diffusion distance between capillaries and cells. The resulting relative tissue hypoxia has a negative impact on tissue integrity, normal wound repair and wound closure.

Hyperpigmentation can form in the ankle area and extend to the anterior shin in chronic venous stasis patients (Figure 4). The hyperpigmentation, also termed hemosiderin staining, is due to extravasated blood into the tissue with the process of edema formation as well as bleeding from ruptured venules. As these tissue bound blood cells lyse, hemosiderin (iron containing pigment) and melanin are deposited resulting in progressive hyperpigmentation and contributing to chronic inflammation and therefore fibrosis of the involved skin.

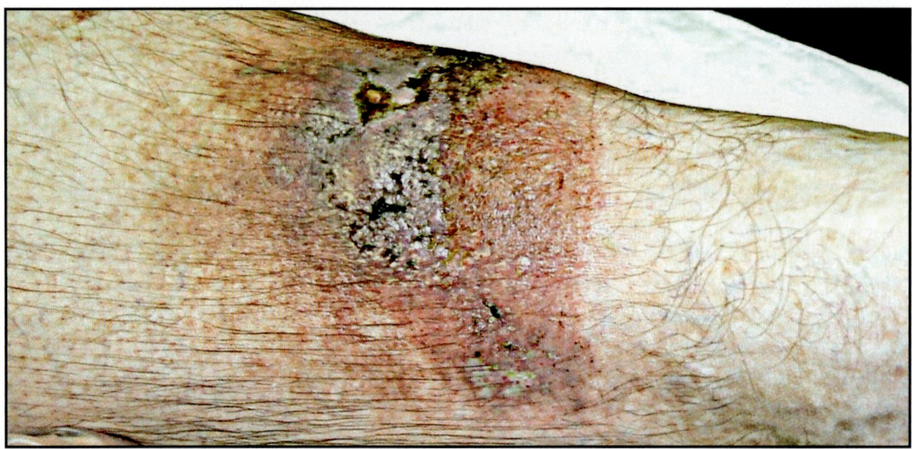

Figure 4. Hyperpigmentation or hemosiderin staining.

The surrounding dermal and subcutaneous tissue of the ankle and calf can become quite indurated and fibrotic, with a waxy feel and eczematous appearance that has been termed lipodermatosclerosis (Figure 5). Also, venous ulcers frequently develop in the lipodermatosclerotic skin; scarring may be seen signifying prior ulceration and will be discussed later. The classic inverted

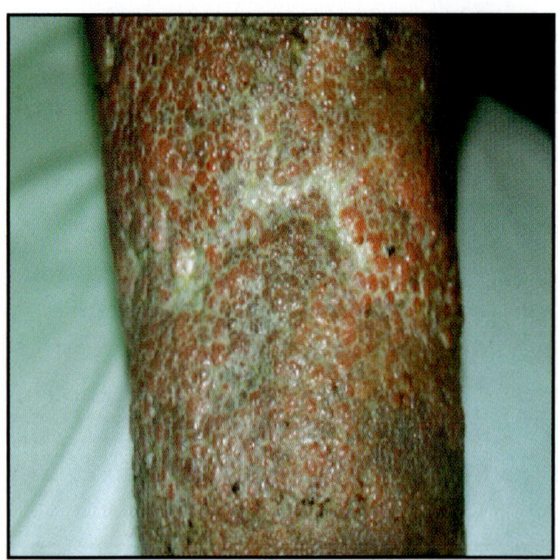

Figure 5. Limpodermatosclerosis.

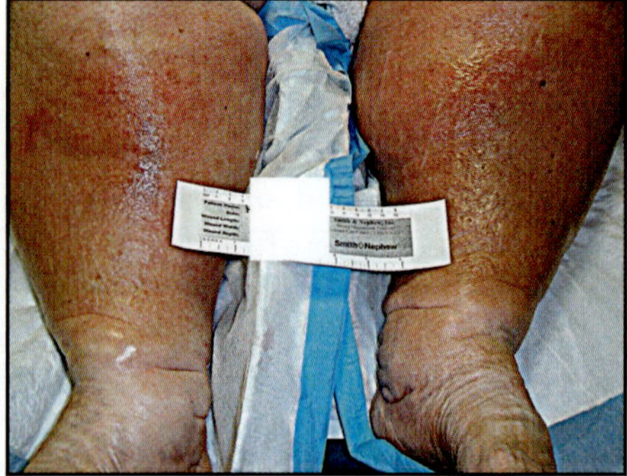

Figure 6. Inverted bottle shape of CVI due to ankle fibrosis with mild dermatits.

bottle appearance of the leg (Figure 6) found in many chronic venous stasis patients is associated with fibrosis of the distal calf and ankle of patient with lipodermatosclerosis. Fibrosis is believed to result from chronic inflammation stemming from the cumulative deposits of plasma protein in the tissue and persistent edema which stimulate fibroblasts to deposit collagen inappropriately in the affected skin.

Dermatitis is a frequent finding in the moderate to severely edematous leg and usually involves the anterior shin or ankle. It is often bilateral, causing inflammation, pruritus and warmth of the involved skin. (Figure 7). The etiology is unclear but may be due to a loss of the skin's ability to respond appropriately to allergens and often develops after the use of topical preparations that may not have caused a skin reaction before the presence of venous edema. This is supported by our observations that this dermatitis

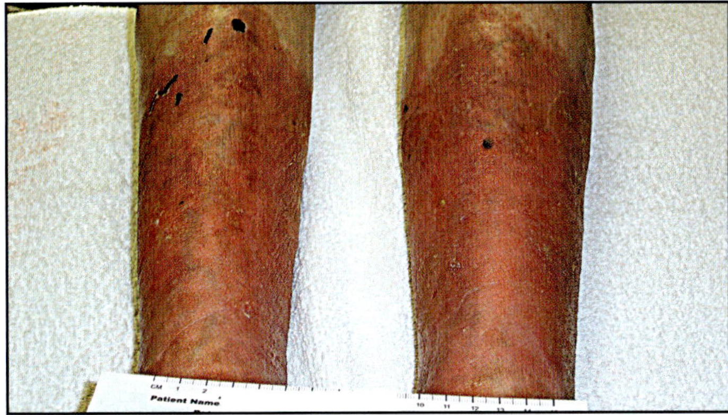

Figure 7. Bilateral venous dermatitis.

almost always resolves as the patient's edema is controlled. Stasis dermatitis is frequently mistaken for cellulitis by the inexperienced clinician.

A small group of severely edematous patients with stasis dermatitis exhibit a weeping and sometimes blistering of the skin (Figure 8). An amber colored, slightly viscous fluid exudes from the friable area of erythematous tissue or from the skin pores. These transudates are the same protein rich plasma that constitutes the tissue edema.

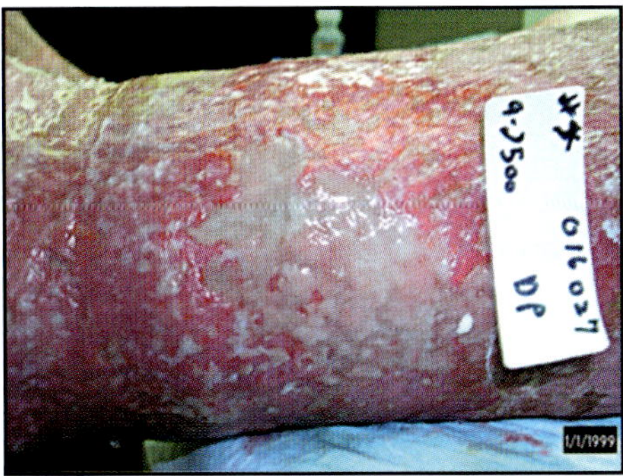

Figure 8. Weeping venous dermatitis.

Long standing venous edema places an increased demand on the lymphatic system of the legs and over time may result in the formation of secondary lymphedema. This will be discussed by Fife in the chapter entitled, "Lymphedema: An Epidemic Hidden in Plain View."

VENOUS ULCERS

One of the major complications of unrecognized, untreated or poorly treated venous stasis disease is the occurrence of venous ulcers (Figure 9). Venous ulcers constitute the largest group of ulcer patients found in developed countries with studies showing venous ulcers to account for as much as 76 percent of all ulcers seen in a community (3). Sixty-one percent of venous stasis patients report their first ulcer before age 65, an ulcer duration of more than one year was reported by 54 percent of patients with the vast majority (72 percent) reporting recurrent ulcerations (6).

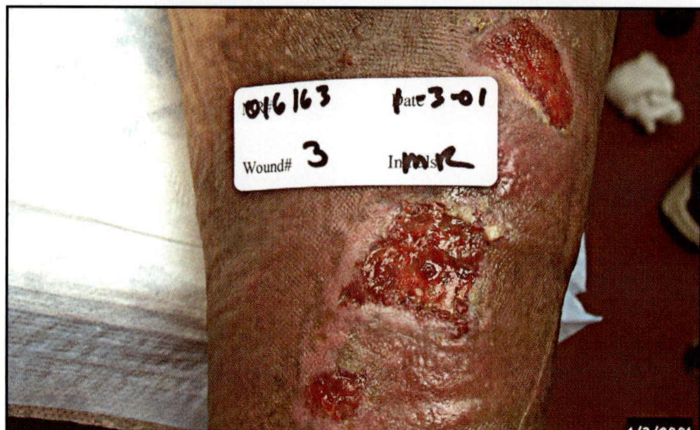

Figure 9. Venous ulcers.

Pathology

While the mechanisms causing venous hypertension and therefore venous edema, are generally understood, the pathology leading from venous hypertension to breakdown, delayed healing and recurrence of ulceration is still under investigation. Three main theories have been proposed to explain the pathology. A number of researchers have found the presence of fibrin deposits in both pre-lipodermatosclerotic tissue and peri-ulcer tissue (7,8). The role of fibrin in the pathology can be viewed two different ways. There is support for the finding of fibrinogen polymerizing to fibrin and forming cuffs around the capillaries (9, 10). It is hypothesized that the fibrin cuffs act as a barrier to oxygen and nutrients and ultimately contribute to cellular death. Other researchers have proposed that the fibrinopeptides released during fibrin formation stimulate replication and migration of fibroblasts and monocytes. This causes the development of fibrotic tissue and along with the deposition of fibrin may make the tissue more sensitive to ulceration (11). Some researchers have questioned whether the fibrin cuffs are the primary cause of tissue ischemia (12).

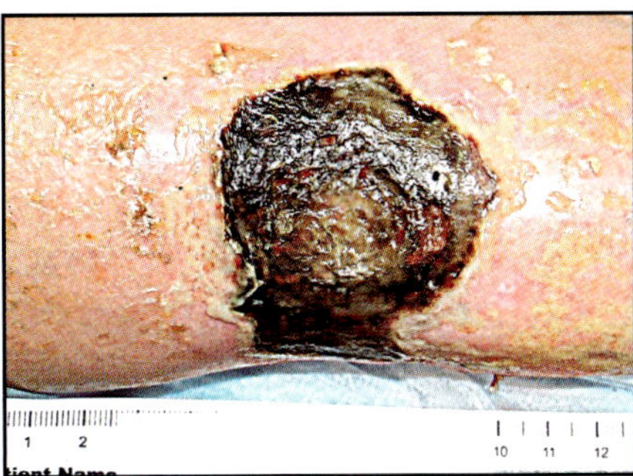

Figure 10. Arterial ulcer.

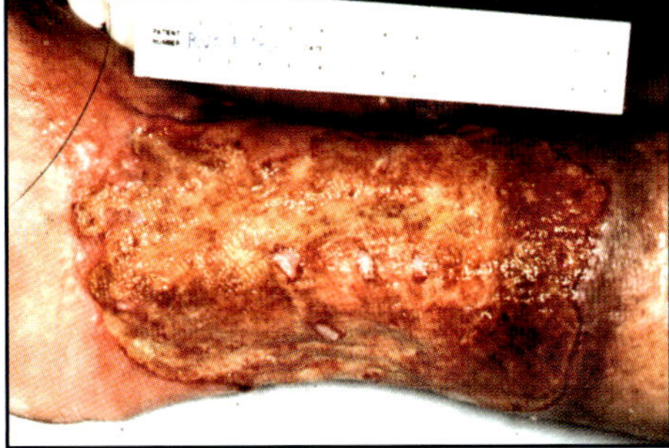

Figure 11. Fibrinous slough in venous ulcer bed.

Researchers such as Coleridge-Smith et al. (13) believe it is the venous hypertension that damages the endothelial cell causing white cell adherence and release of inflammatory mediators. The release of mediators creates changes in the capillaries and vasculature, which increases their permeability, leaking plasma and other components into the tissues.

The "trap" hypothesis by Falanga and Eaglstein (11) proposes that the increased permeability of capillaries and leakage of macromolecules into the tissue produce an environment where growth factors and matrix material are bound. When these components are bound, they are unavailable for use in repair and regeneration of tissue.

It is most likely that the pathology leading to risk for venous ulcer formation is multi-factorial, involving to various degrees, persistence of edema, chronic inflammation, hemosiderin deposition and tissue fibrosis. These factors together may contribute to an oxygen diffusion deficit and a retarded or disordered tissue healing response.

These hypotheses on the pathophysiology of venous ulceration continue to be tested and may one day lead to alternative therapeutic approaches for treatment.

Clinical Features Of Venous Ulcers

Although venous ulcer formation may be a spontaneous event, in our experience, the most common instigating factor is trauma to the ankle or calf region of a patient suffering from venous edema, particularly in patients with extensive lipodermatosclerosis. These traumatic wounds often fail to progress through an orderly healing process and instead begin to deteriorate until the level of severity is sufficient to prompt the patient to seek medical help.

Venous ulcers are found below the knee, vary in size, and although most are found above the medial malleolus (61 percent), lateral, tibial, and calf ulcers are common. Venous foot ulcers are rare. Venous ulcers generally have an irregular but well defined border as compared to arterial or vasculitic ulcers, which are usually round or punched out (Figure 10). The wound edges of venous ulcers are usually flat and nearly flush with the wound bed or, in chronic states, may have a steep elevation from the wound bed. The wound edges are usually not undermined. The wound bed usually displays friable, congested, purple appearing granulation tissue and can sometimes contain scattered epithelial islands. The patient frequently

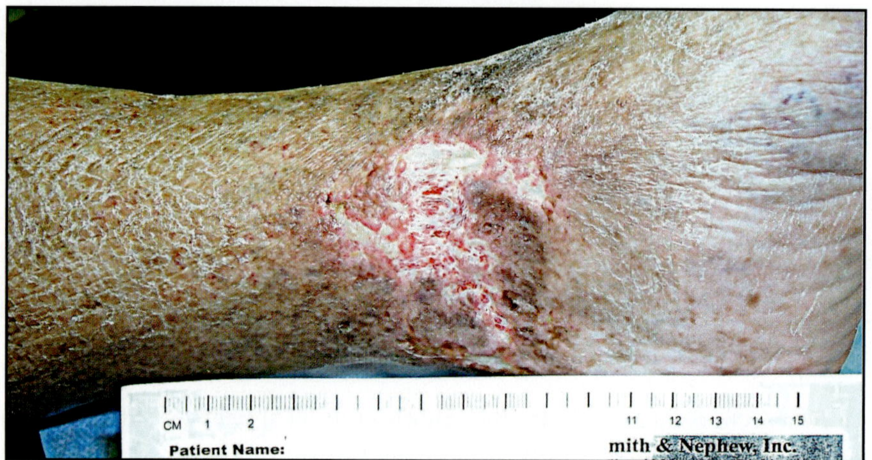

Figure 12. Atrophe blanche.

reports an odor and copious amber or yellow tinged, slightly viscous drainage from the ulcer, which may dry to form a fibrinous slough (Figure 11) within the wound bed. Pruritus of the surrounding skin is often reported.

Skin surrounding venous ulcer is usually indurated, eczematous, inflamed and hyperpigmented, especially if the ulcer is within an area of lipodermatosclerosis. When lipodermatosclerosis is not present, ulcers may be found in an area of white atrophic skin, atrophic blanche is a type of vasculopathy sometimes associated with venous insufficiency (Figure 12). Black eschar, necrosis, tendon, or bone exposure is rarely ever seen with pure venous ulcers and, if found, should lead the examiner to investigate the diagnosis of an arterial or vasculitic component.

Pain, when present, is usually relieved by elevation of the extremity and is more often associated with ulcer debridement or dressing changes. It has been our observation that exquisitely painful venous ulcers are often associated with a concomitant arterial or vasculitic component, infection or are in areas that involve the periosteum of underlying bone.

OTHER DIAGNOSTIC CONSIDERATIONS

The diagnosis of venous stasis, CVI, and venous ulceration is most often a clinical determination and for the experienced clinician is usually a straightforward diagnosis made from information obtained from a careful history and physical exam.

A description of the history of the disease process leading to problematic edema and/or ulceration is very important. As previously stated, the initial onset of symptoms is most often described as an insidious onset of edema which worsens over time (years), eventually involving the entire leg(s) below the knees with a heavy aching discomfort that improves with bed rest or elevation but does not fully resolve. Stasis skin changes appear and finally slow healing or non-healing ulcers may form. A history of recurrent ulceration is also important to note, since this tends to favor a venous etiology, especially if the recurrence is at the same site.

Past medical history may reveal risk factors associated with the formation of venous insufficiency, foremost being a history of deep venous thrombosis (DVT), which has been associated with 37 percent of venous ulcer patients (6). Other risk factors include leg trauma, surgical history involving the knee, calf or thigh, employment involving long hours standing, morbid obesity, pregnancy, advanced age, CHF, immobility or paralysis, and congenital vein wall weakness.

The physical exam focuses on the vascular status of the lower extremities, presence and extent of edema, appearance of any ulcerations and the skin immediately adjacent to any ulcers. When evaluating a possible venous ulcer, most important in the differential diagnosis is the exclusion of arterial insufficiency as a primary cause of the ulcer or a contributing factor. The clinician should be aware that CVI and arterial insufficiency co-exist in about 20 percent of elderly patients with venous ulcers (1). In contrast to venous ulcers, arterial ulcers tend to be painful, punched out, containing black eschar and often involve deep tissues, tendon, and even bone.

The ankle-brachial index (ABI) is a helpful, easily performed and reproducible non-invasive test for indirectly determining the presence, absence, or degree of arterial disease in the lower extremities. An ABI is determined by dividing ankle systolic pressures by the highest resting brachial systolic pressure (Figure 13). The resulting values have a range of indications. An ABI of 0.9–1.1 generally correlates with normal arterial perfusion. An ABI of 0.7–0.9 correlates with adequate perfusion. ABIs of 0.5–0.7 generally correlates with clinically significant arterial occlusive disease. An ABI of < 0.5 correlates with severe arterial occlusive disease and would benefit from a vascular consult. ABI's in diabetics with calcified vessels can be misleading, demonstrated by ABIs of > 1.1, the values can be misleading or inaccurate. Further vascular evaluation may be indicated to determine the extent of arterial occlusion in this group of patients.

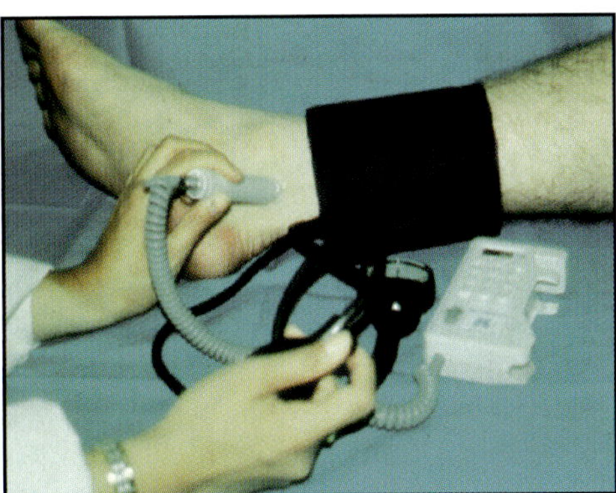

Figure 13. ABI being performed.

Biopsy can be useful in diagnosis, especially when evaluating the atypical appearing ulcer. Basal cell carcinomas are known to arise from chronic ulcers and can appear as exuberant granulation tissue that tends to roll over onto the wound edge. Biopsies from sites within the ulcer bed generally do not deteriorate and usually heal up to the level of the original bed. In contrast, biopsies of non-ulcerated skin in an area of venous stasis changes may have difficulty healing (1). In our experience with ulcers that are suspect for infection, tissue biopsy from the edge of the ulcer bed, sent for culture are more accurate in identifying the invasive organisms. Swab cultures have a greater tendency to sample skin flora and organisms that colonize chronic wounds.

Occasionally a more definitive diagnostic test may be helpful in verifying venous insufficiency when the history and physical is not compelling. Today, the definitive test for CVI is duplex venous scanning (14,15). This ultrasound test scans the deep and superficial veins during function to detect and quantify venous reflux. Duplex scanning has replaced the previous standard, venogram study. Duplex scanning is non-invasive, provides accurate data and is usually less expensive.

MEDICAL TREATMENT

When considering the treatment of venous insufficiency and venous ulcers it is important to remember that the underlying pathophysiology leading to clinically significant problems has to do with the failure of the muscle pump, followed by venous hypertension, leg edema and finally ulceration. If this muscle pump defect is appropriately augmented, 86 percent of all venous ulcers will heal (16).

Compression Therapy

Compression therapy is the application of external pressure to the lower extremities in such a way as to promote the return of blood from the peripheral veins to the central circulation, therefore counteracting venous hypertension. Other benefits of compression therapy include: stimulation of fibrinolysis, increased local oxygenation and the return of an environment that is favorable for wound healing (14). Ideally, external compression of 30–40 mm Hg is needed to ensure adequate venous return from the lower extremities (17). This pressure must be applied in a gradient fashion so that compression delivered to the ankle is higher than that delivered to the knee. Compression bandages should be the first line of treatment for CVI and CVI with ulceration. Gradient compression stockings should only be used for maintenance therapy after compression dressings have controlled the clinically significant pathology of edema and venous ulcer are healed or nearly healed.

During the treatment phase either short-stretch or long-stretch compression therapy can be used. Short-stretch dressings assist the calf muscle pump by compressing lower extremities by resisting changes in force during walking. Because of the mechanism of resisting change in force, the short-stretch dressing will have low resting and high working pressures. This means that the patient has to be ambulatory for the ideal edema control effect of this inelastic dressing.

One of the oldest and often most familiar compression dressing is the Unna's boot (Figure 14). This is a medicated bandage that can be impregnated with zinc oxide, calamine, glycerin, sorbitol, or magnesium silicate depending on the manufacturer. To be applied correctly, the Unna's boot must be wrapped in a gradient fashion with 50 percent overlap. This dressing will stiffen as it dries which will cause a resistance in force when the calf muscle presses against it during ambulation. In order to ensure adequate pressures are maintained between dressing changes, an ace wrap or coban (3M Health Care, St. Paul, MN) should be applied over the Unna's boot in a

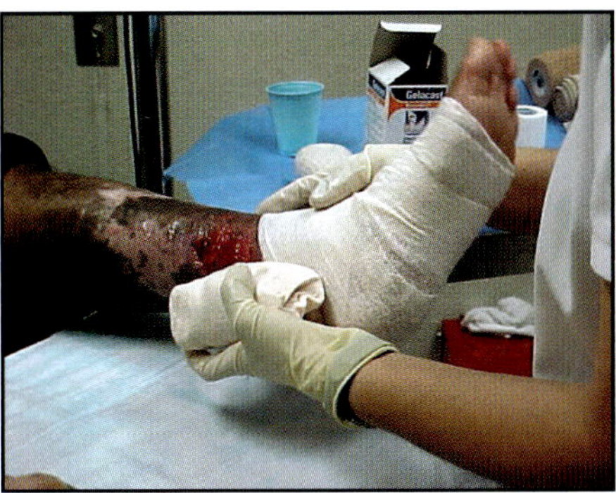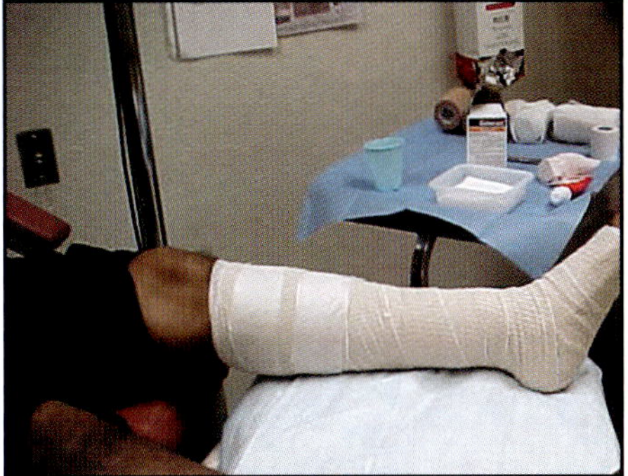

Figure 14. Unna boot's placement with four-inch ACE wrap covering.

spiral fashion with 50 percent overlap. The Unna's boot can be left in place for up to seven days between changes.

The long-stretch dressings are extensible bandage(s) that increase in length when force is applied and returns to original length after the force is removed. These dressings are able to supplement the calf muscle pump both with and without patient ambulation.

In a multi-layered, long-stretch dressing, the pressure developed beneath any bandage is governed by the tension in the fabric, the radius of the curvature of the limb and the number of layers applied. Applying a bandage with a 50 percent overlap produces two layers of fabric, which generates a pressure twice that produced by a single layer. The sub-bandage pressure may be calculated using a simple formula derived from the Laplace equation:

$$P = (TN \times 4630)/CW$$

Where:

P = pressure in mm Hg

T = bandage tension (in kgf)

N = number of layers applied

C = circumference of the limb (in cm)

W = bandage width (in cm)

The sub-bandage pressure is therefore directly proportional to bandage tension but inversely proportional to the radius of the curvature of the limb to which it is applied. This means that a bandage applied with constant tension to a limb of normal proportions will automatically produce gradient compression with the highest pressure at the ankle and will gradually reduce pressure up the leg as the circumference increases.

A common multi-layered long-stretch bandage is Profore® (Smith & Nephew, Largo, FL). This dressing has four distinct layers (Figure 15). The first layer is an absorbent padding bandage that is wrapped in a spiral fashion with 50 percent over lap from just below the toes to the knee. This layer cushions and redistributes pressure away from boney prominences. The second layer is a light conforming bandage also wrapped in a spiral fashion with 50 percent overlap. It provides added absorbency, elasticity plus smoothes out the first layer. Bandages three and four are the compression layers. Layer three is wrapped in a figure-eight technique with 50 percent

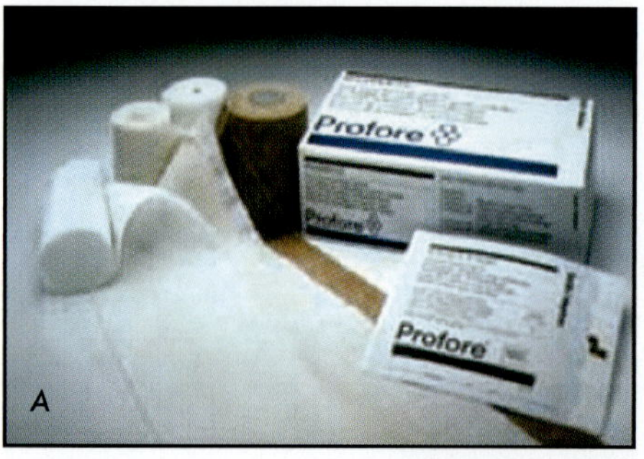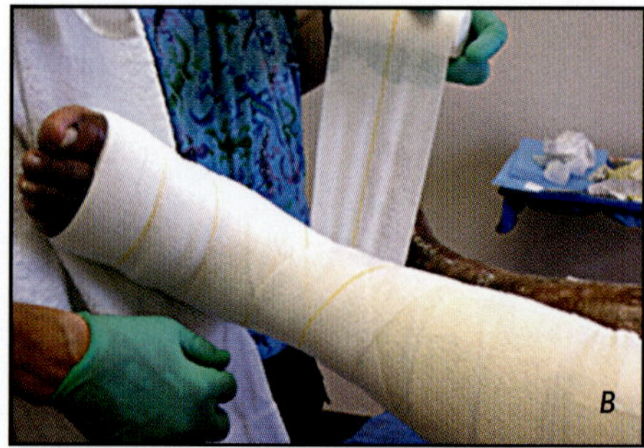

Figure 15 (A–B). Profore® four-layer compression dressing.

overlap and 50 percent stretch. By wrapping in this manner, 17 mm Hg compression is applied. The fourth layer is cohesive layer that is wrapped in spiral fashion with 50 percent overlap and 50 percent stretch. This layer will provide an additional 20 mm Hg pressure. Total pressure for all four layers at the ankle is 40 mm Hg (17). The degree of pressure can be altered by the amount of stretch applied in layers three and four. This multilayered dressing can be left in place for up to seven days.

In 2006, 3M introduced the *Coban 2 Layered Compression System®* using new technology which allows for two layers to produce the equivalent pressure as the four-layered Profore® (Smith & Nephew, Largo, FL). The inner layer is a lamination of polyurethane foam that when the second layer is applied over it, the inner layer adheres to the skin and prevents slippage of the dressing. It does this without damaging the skin (Figure 16).

The *Coban 2 Layered Compression System®* in a pilot study demonstrated increase in patient comfort, decreased sleep interference, decrease in mobility interference and little effect on the selection of pants or shoes while wearing the compression dressing. These factors lead to increased compliance by the patient (33).

Applications of compression dressings are not without complications. Only trained and experienced clinicians should apply the dressings. If the dressing is applied too tightly, tissue necrosis over bony prominences can occur. If arterial disease is present and the compression dressing is wrapped too tightly or the incorrect type of compression dressing is applied, microvascular occlusion may occur, that can result in increased leg pain and tissue necrosis. A bandage that is too loose can result in the bandage slipping, loosing compression, bunching at the ankle and causing friction or rub wounds on the leg.

Prior to making the decision to use either the short-stretch or long-stretch compression the degree of arterial disease needs to be considered. An ankle-brachial index (ABI) should be obtained before applying compression. In our experience, patients who have an ABI of 0.8 and above will generally do well with a four-layer long-stretch dressing or *Coban 2 Layered Compression System®*. Profore Lite® (Smith and Nephew, Largo, FL), which is a three-layer long-stretch dressing, has been used successfully in those patients with ABIs between 0.6–0.8. This particular dressing, when appropriately applied, produces 23–24 mm Hg pressure at the ankle. Short-stretch dressings have been used successfully in patients with ABIs as low as 0.5. Ankle pressures

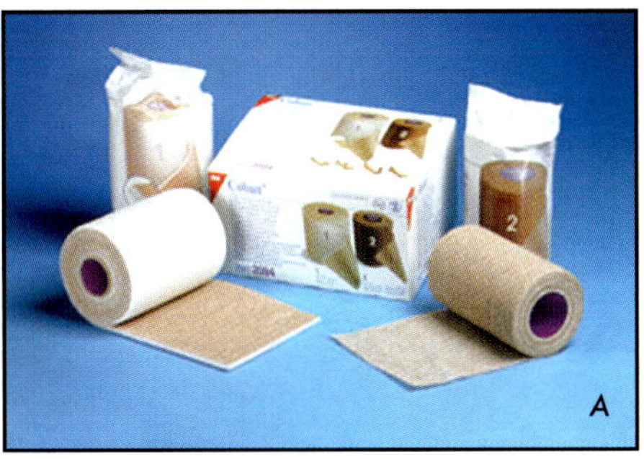 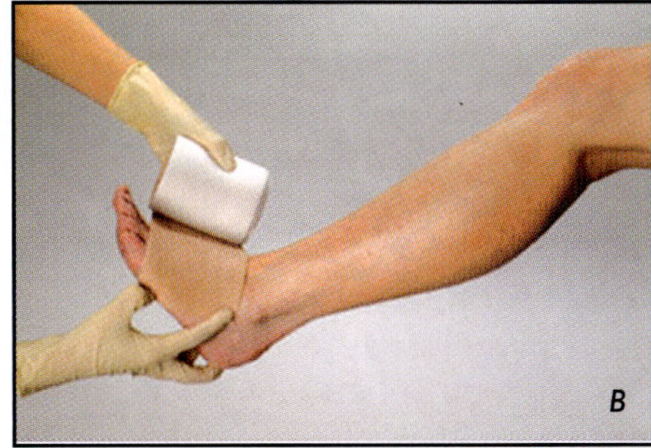

Figure 16 (A–B). Coban 2 Layered Compression System.

with short-stretch dressings have a wide variability in pressure, ranging from 18-55 mm Hg. This is dependant upon application technique, product and secondary wrap (18). Care needs to be taken not to compromise the arterial flow through the extremity and only clinicians experience in application of compression dressings should do the wrapping of the extremity.

Leg circumference measurements should be obtained before the initial wrapping and then with each dressing change. Measurements should be taken at the instep, ankle, and the thickest part of the calf. This will provide an objective method in determining edema reduction during subsequent visits.

A review was performed by Cullum et al. (19) utilizing the Cochrane Database. The objective of this review was to examine effectiveness of compression bandaging in the management of venous ulcers. A total of 22 randomized controlled trials were reviewed. Nine trials addressed multilayered systems compared with non-elastic compression or single layered short-stretch dressings. It was found that the multilayered dressings were more effective in healing than the inelastic or short-stretch dressings. In three trials that looked at the difference in four-layered versus other high pressure, long-stretch dressings, there was no difference. The reviewer's conclusion was that 1) Compression increases ulcer healing rates compared with no compression; 2) Multilayered systems are more effective than single layered systems; 3) There is no significant difference between the different types of multilayered dressings and 4) High compression is more effective than low compression in ulcer resolution.

Sequential compression pumps are also used to treat CVI, venous ulcers, and lymphedema (20). This mechanical device consists of a leg sleeve with inflatable chambers at the ankle, calf, and thigh connected to a pump that can be programmed to deliver sequential and gradient pressure in a cyclic manner. While pumps are expensive, they can be useful in recalcitrant cases that fail other compression modalities.

Lifetime Maintenance Compression

After edema is well controlled and ulcers healed, the patient moves into the maintenance phase of therapy. External gradient pressure must be maintained to sustain the benefits achieved through treatment by continuing to augment the calf muscle pump. This goal can be achieved by fitting the patient into an appropriate prescription gradient compression stocking. These stockings are available in four classes based on the external pressure maintained at the ankle.

Class	Ankle Pressure
I	20–30 mm Hg
II	30–40 mm Hg
III	40–50 mm Hg
IV	≥ 60 mm Hg

For stockings to be effective in maintaining control they must deliver an ankle pressure between 20–50 mm Hg. There are several manufacturers of stockings which offer ready-made sizes, knee or thigh length. However, they must be measured to fit, accounting for differences in leg and foot size in order to afford patient comfort and provide appropriate therapeutic gradient compression. An experienced stocking fitter should be used as part of the treatment team during this stage of therapy in order to obtain the best results. In our experience, coordinating the removal of the final compression wrap with placement of an appropriate gradient stocking affords the best fit and encourages patient compliance since they witness the importance the clinician places in maintaining edema control at all times.

We are aware of practitioners who have instigated appropriate and successful CVI treatment with gradient compression wraps only to allow the patient to leave their last clinic visit without maintenance gradient stockings on their legs. Many of these patients will return to a state of uncontrolled venous edema in less than 48 hours without continued gradient compression.

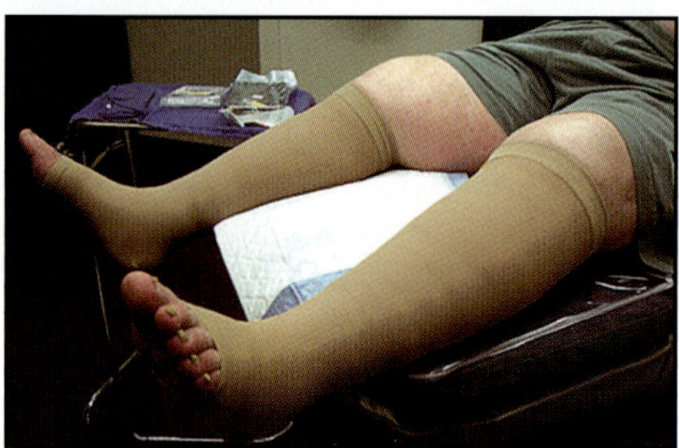

Figure 17. Patient wearing gradient compression stockings.

In selecting the appropriate compression stocking class, our experience has shown the majority of patients will benefit and maintain control of their venous disease when placed in a measured to fit 30–40 mm Hg stocking (Figure 17). Very active and working patients may need a 40–50 mm Hg stocking to maintain control since they spend a majority of the day upright and ambulatory. A few patients will be unable to tolerate 30–40 mm Hg stocking either due to concomitant moderate arterial disease or severe frailty leading to a difficulty in donning these stockings. These patients can be placed on a trial of 20–30 mm Hg stockings. Over the counter stockings (< 20 mm Hg) do not produce enough gradient compression to control clinically significant venous insufficiency and are best used to treat mild or early edema in individuals who are trying to prevent venous stasis from occurring.

Compression stockings must not be confused with elastic stockings used for DVT prophylactic such as TED hose. TED hose is a brand name of anti-embolism (blood clot) stockings. These DVT prophylactic stockings deliver moderate compression ($\cong 18$ mm Hg) but are not designed and are inadequate for the maintenance of CVI. This can also be said about Ace wraps that are unable to deliver gradient compression.

Wound Management

Compression therapy has become the corner stone for treatment of CVI and venous edema. There is less agreement on what topical therapies should be applied to assist ulcer healing. In our experience, once venous edema is controlled venous ulcers begin to respond to the same therapies advocated for treating the problem wound. These therapies include: infection control, improving arterial perfusion, debridement of non-viable tissue, controlling edema, inflammation and exudate, avoiding pressure and trauma, and moist wound care. Although discussed elsewhere in this book, two areas are worth elaborating on further in the context of venous ulcer care, infection, and dermatitis.

During the initial evaluation, the treating clinician is often faced with the complexity of distinguishing cellulitis from dermatitis in an erythematous and edematous leg. This task becomes easier as the clinician gains experience. The infected venous ulcer will usually be unilateral, exquisitely tender, with a noticeable increase in drainage. The ulcer bed will become increasingly friable, deteriorate and enlarge. The patient usually has systemic symptoms of fever and malaise.

This contrasts with venous dermatitis, which is often bilateral, with a slight increase in pain or puritis and frequently associated with an acute increase in the severity of their leg edema or concomitant use of topical agents to the affected skin. The ulcer bed usually remains stable or may slowly deteriorate in episodes of severe dermatitis. The patient will frequently report prior episodes of the same erythema without systemic symptoms and an unimpressive response to antibiotics, but improvement with decreased activity, leg elevation and rest.

The infected ulcer should have tissue cultures and appropriate antibiotics started immediately before continued therapy can prove effective. With the infection resolving, compression and wound care can continue.

Stasis dermatitis will respond well to the edema control of compression therapy usually resolving completely. We have also seen improved resolution of dermatitis by adding a topical steroid preparation such as clocortolone pivalate (Cloderm 0.1%) to the involved skin under compression during the initial and sometimes second compression wrap(s). Other clinicians advocate the use of a short course of systemic steroids tapered slowly over six weeks, always coupled with edema control (1).

Drug Therapy

Drug therapy specific for the treatment of CVI is an area of active investigation. The following brief reviews will summarize selected research covering the adjunctive use of systemic medications touted to improve venous ulcer healing.

In a study of 20 patients that were randomized to either aspirin and compression or placebo and compression, 38 percent of the patients who received aspirin closed at four months while the patients who received the placebo report no wound closures at four months (21). It is concerning that the overall healing rate in this study is so low, especially with no closed ulcers in the placebo group.

Several research groups have investigated the efficacy of Daflon for use in CVI. Daflon is a venotropic drug, which increases venous tone, improves lymphatic drainage, and protects microcirculation. In one double-blind, randomized controlled trial involving 200 patients, the patients that received Dalfon 500mg, two tablets daily, for two months demonstrated a significant reduction in ankle circumference (22). Blume et al. confirmed these findings in a second study (23). The mechanism of action of Daflon in edema control is thought to be the drug's ability to inhibit inflammatory reactions and to decrease capillary permeability. Another study with Daflon was undertaken to look at venous ulcer healing (24). This was a double-blind, randomized, controlled multi-center trial of 105 patients. Both groups were similar in characteristics, had ulcers that had not shown any healing in three months and the patients agreed to wear elastic compression therapy. In the patients who had ulcers $\leq$ 10 cm, improved healing rates were demonstrated at two months in those patients who received Daflon. In patients who had ulcers > 10 cm, no ulcers were reported healed.

To date, pentoxifylline appears to be the most promising of the systemic agents to be used as an adjunct in the treatment of CVI. A recent 12-month double-blind placebo controlled trial involving 85 patients demonstrated significant improvement in the healing rate in those patients receiving pentoxifylline 400 mg three times per day (25). It was also noted that a decrease in reflux and an increase in pO_2 was greater in the pentoxifylline group (p = < 0.05). In a study by Falanga, which was multi-center, randomized, placebo-controlled, and involved 131 patients, improved healing was demonstrated with pentoxifylline. Patients were divided into 3 groups, placebo, 400 mg pentoxifylline three times daily or 800 mg pentoxifylline three times daily. All patients were in compression dressings (26). The patients who received 800 mg pentoxifylline (three times daily) healed faster than the patients who received the placebo (p = 0.043). More than 50 percent of both groups of patients receiving pentoxifylline were ulcer free at week 12 compared to 50 percent of the placebo group at week 16.

SURGICAL INTERVENTION

A variety of surgical interventions have been tried in the management of venous ulceration and venous hypertension with limited reported success. Surgical studies have reported that fewer than five percent of patients with venous hypertension are likely to benefit from surgery (27). This section will give an overview of current surgical venous interventions.

Surgical interventions for chronic venous insufficiency are based on the abnormal physiological disturbance diagnosed in patients with this clinical disorder. After a careful physical examination, extensive ultrasound evaluation including provocative testing is frequently necessary to specifically

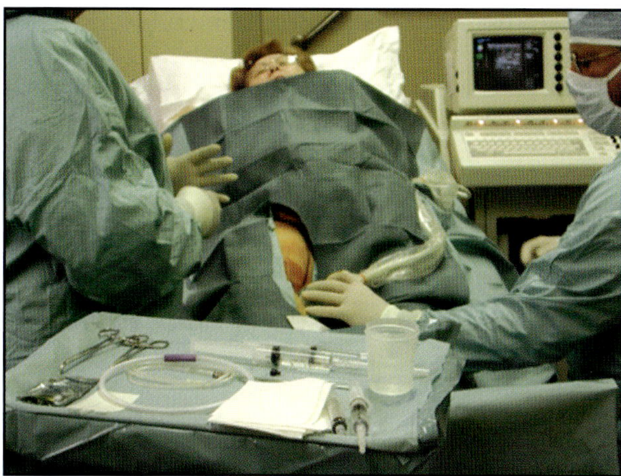

Figure 18. Venous surgery.

delineate the venous physiologic abnormality. From a hemodynamic point of view, the clinical picture of chronic venous insufficiency is either caused by obstruction, reflux or a combination of the two; surgical therapy can then be directed in an attempt to correct the demonstrated hemodyamic defect (Figure 18).

Superficial venous reflux has traditionally been treated by greater or lesser saphenous vein extirpation combined with excision of associated varicosities. Despite the presence of concomitant deep venous or perforator incompetence, a beneficial physiological response in the deep and perforating systems is frequently noted with removal of the superficial venous system alone. Clinical improvement in both deep and perforator reflux and early ulcer healing has also been observed (34, 35). However, open techniques have progressively higher long term recurrence rates, approaching 50%. Recently endovascular, catheter based technologies have been available as percutaneous alternatives to saphenous vein stripping. These outpatient procedures are performed alone or in combination with microphlebectomy

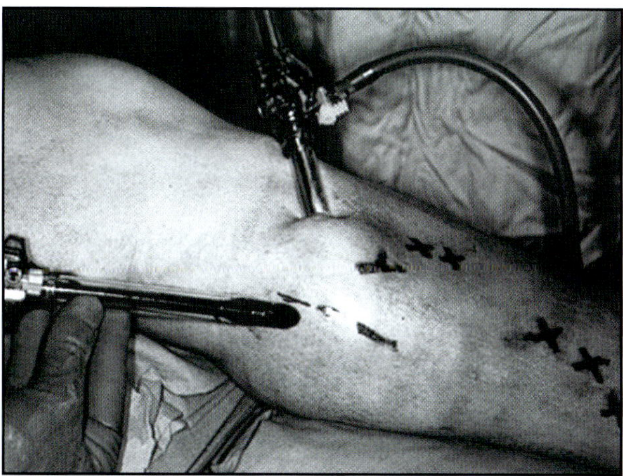

Figure 19. Subfacial Endoscopic Perforator Vein Surgery (SEPs).

or sclerotherapy. Radiofrequency ablation or endovenous laser therapy is applied under ultrasonic guidance to obliterate the greater saphenous vein. Success rates equal or exceed traditional open surgical techniques. Significant complications such as venous thrombosis, pulmonary emboli or wound infection are rare (36, 37).

Treatment of perforator vein incompetence by SEPS (subfacial endoscopic perforator vein surgery) is usually relegated to those patients who recur after superficial venous surgery or those with perforator reflux in the absence of superficial reflux (Figure 19). This procedure has a lower complication rate than the older Linton procedure but selection of patients and long term results still need to be determined (30, 31).

Venous valvuloplasty and autogenous venous valve transplantation are employed in those patients with deep venous insufficiency who fail aggressive medical management. Venous valve transplants have been used in research trials with limited success for brief periods of 6 months or less and are recommended only in patients with few remaining therapeutic options (32). Cryopreserved valve transplantation continues to be plagued with high failure rates with a few notable exceptions (39, 40).

Deep venous obstruction with or without associated reflux has traditionally been treated medically. Obstruction of the inferior vena cava, iliac veins (May-Thurner Syndrome), or the deep veins of the lower extremities may be the predominant abnormality in up to one third of post thrombotic limbs (41). Enthusiasm for venous thrombectomy with or without bypass, though infrequently performed, has been dampened by high thrombosis rates. Recent advances in endovenous dilation and stenting, either in combination with thrombolytic therapy or alone, have been shown to improve both the venous hemodynamics and clinical picture of those patients with a significant obstructive venous component.

Skin grafting has had the greatest appeal of surgical interventions but with variable long-term success. Recurrence is high if used as the sole therapy for venous ulcer closure, but has an excellent success rate when used on recalcitrant ulcers when edema has been controlled preoperatively and patients are placed in maintenance compression post-operatively (28, 29).

Clinical and research efforts persist to further define the role of surgical treatment for chronic venous insufficiency.

CONCLUSION

As the trend evolves in industrialized nations towards an increasingly older population, we can expect a increasing prevalence of venous disease, with venous ulcers continuing to account for as much as 70 percent of lower extremity wounds. The challenge for health care is to find ways to treat this population in an effective and cost efficient manner.

Today, compression therapy must be viewed as the mainstay of treatment, and has been shown to effectively heal 86 percent of all venous ulcers. Unfortunately many practitioners continue to unsuccessfully manage these ulcers with topical care only, neglecting to control the underlying venous hypertension and CVI. Appropriate topical therapy must be an adjunct to compression therapy if we are to succeed. Even today, patients usually receive treatment only after their edema is very severe or when an ulcer appears. The key to effective treatment and cost containment may be in recognizing the early signs and symptoms of venous hypertension. Therapy implemented early for edema control and maintenance, before venous ulcers appear, can greatly reduce the costs associated with managing problem wounds while significantly improving quality of life for millions of people.

ACKOWLEDGEMENTS

Special thank you to Ronald L. Blumoff, M.D., F.A.C.S. for his input and advice on the surgical intervention section of this chapter.

REFERENCES

1. Falanga V. Venous ulceration. *J Dermatol Surg Oncol* 1993 Aug; 19(8):764-71.

2. Lorimer KR, Harrison MB, Graham ID, et al. Assessing venous ulcer population characteristics and practices in a home care community. *OWM* 2003 May; 19(5):32-43.

3. Callam MJ, Harper DR, Dale JJ, et al. Chronic ulcer of the leg:clinical history. *Br Med J* 1986; 294:1389-91.

4. Simon D, McCollum C. Approaches to venous leg ulcer care within the community: compression, pinch skin grafts and simple venous surgery. *OWM* 1996; 42(2):34-40.

5. Goldman MP, Fronek A. Anatomy and pathophysiology of varicose veins. *J Dermatol Surg Oncol* 1989; 15:138-145.

6. Nelzen, Berguist D, Lindhagen A. Venous and non-venous leg ulcers:clinical history and appearance in a population study. *Br J Surg* 1994; 81:182-187.

7. Claudy AL, Mirshahi M, Soria C, et al. Detection of undegraded fibrin and tumor necrosis factor-alpha in venous leg ulcers. *J AM Acad Dermotl* 1991; 25:623-7.

8. Stacey MC, Burnand KG, Pattison M, et al. Changes in the apparently normal limb in unilateral venous ulceration. *Br J Surg* 1987; 74:936-9.

9. Browse NL, Burnand KG. The cause of venous ulceration. *Lancet* 1982; 2;243-5.

10. Burnand KJ, Clemenson G, Whimster I, et al. The effect of sustained venous hypertension on the skin capillaries of the canine hind limb. *Br J Surg.* 1982;69: 41-44.

11. Falanga V, Eaglestein WH. The trap hypothesis of venous ulceration. *Lancet* 1993;341:1006-8.

12. Dormandy JA. Pathophysiology of venous leg ulceration-an update. *Angiology* 1997; 48:71-5.

13. Coleridge-Smith PD, Thomas P, Scurr J, Dormandh JA. Causes of venous ulceration: a new hypothesis? *Br Med J* 1988; 296:1726-7.

14. Reichardt LE. Venous ulceration: Compression as the mainstay of therapy. *JWOCN* 1999; 26(1):39-47.

15. Sandeman D, Shearman CP. Clinical aspects of lower limb ulceration. In:Mani J, Falanga V, Shearman CP, Sendeman D. (eds) *Chronic Wound Healing* London, WB Saunders, 1999; 4-25.

16. Cordts PR, Hanrahan LM, Rodriguez AA, et al. A prospective, randomized trial of Unna's boot versus Duoderm CGF hydroactive dressing plus compression in the mangement of venous leg ulcers. *J Vasc Surg* 1992; 15:480-6.

17. Moffatt CJ, O'Hare L. Venous leg ulcerations: treatment with high compression bandaging. *Ostomy/Wound Management* 1995; 41:16-25.

18. Moore Z. Compression bandaging: are practitioners achieving the ideal sub-bandage pressures? *J Wound Care* 2002; 11(7):265-8.

19. Cochrane Database Rev. 2001; (2): cd000265.

20. Cahall E, Spence Rk. Practical nursing measures for vascular compromise in the lower leg. *Ostomy/Wound Manage* 1995; 41:16-32.

21. Layton AM, Ibbotson SH, Davies JA, et al. Randomized trial of oral aspirin for chronic venous leg ulcers. *Lancet* 1994; 8916:164-5.

22. Laurent R, Gilly R, Frilleux C. Clinical evaluation of a venotropic drug in man. *Int Angiol* 1988; 7(suppl 2):39-43.

23. Blume J, Langenbahn H, De Champvallins M. Quantification of edema using the volumeter technique: therapeutic application of Daflon 500 mg in CVI. *Phlebology* 1992; 7 (suppl 2):37-40.

24. Guilhour JJ, Dereure O, Marezin L, et al. Efficacy of Daflon 500 mg in venous leg ulcer healing: a double blind, randomized, controlled versus placebo trial in 107 patients. *Angiology* 1997 J; 48(1):77-85.

25. DeSanctis MT, Belcaro G, Cesarone MR, et al. Treatment of venous ulcers with pentoxifylline: a 12-month, double-blind, placebo controlled trial. Microcirculation and Healing. *Angiology.* 2002; Jan-Feb; 53 Suppl 1:s49-51.

26. Falanga, V. Care of venous leg ulcers. *Ostomy/Wound Management* 1999; 45(suppl1a):33s-43s.

27. Arnold, TE, Stanely JC, Fellows EP, et al. Prospective, multicenter study of managing lower extremity venous ulcers. *Ann Vasc Surg* 1994; 8356

28. Turczynski R, Tarpila E. Treatment of leg ulcers with split skin grafts: early and late results. *Scand J Plast Reconstruc Surg Hand Surg* 1999 Sep; 33(3):301-5.

29. Kirsner RK, Falanga V. Techiques of split-thickness skin grafting for lower extremity ulcerations. *J Dermatol Surg Oncol* 1993; 19:779-783.

30. Kalra M, Gloviezki P. Subfascial endoscopic perforator vein surgery: who benefits? *Semin Vasc Surg.* 2002 Mar; 15(1):39-49.

31. Kalra M, Glovieczki P. Surgical treatment of venous ulcers: role of subfascial endoscopic perforator vein ligation. *Surg Clin North AM.* 2003 Jun; 83(3):671-705.

32. Dalsing MC, Raju S, Wakefield TW, et al. A multicenter, phase I evaluation of cryopreserved venous valve allografts for the treatment of chronic deep venous insufficiency. *J Vasc Surg.* 1999 Nov; 30(5): 854-64.-62.

33. Schnobrich E, Solfest S, Bernatchez S, et al. 7-Day in-use assessment of a unique, innovative compression system. 3M Medical Division.

34. Blomgren L B, Johansson G, Dahlberg-Akerman A, et al. Changes in superficial and perforating vein reflux after varicose vein surgery. *J Vasc Surg* 2005;42:315-320.

35. Mendes R, Marston W, Farber M, et al. Treatment of superficial and perforator incompetence without deep venous insufficiency; Is routine perforator ligation necessary? *J Vas Surg* 2003;38:891-5.

36. Van Rij A, Jiang P, Solomon C, et al. Recurrence after varicose vein surgery: A prospective long term clinical study with duplex ultrasound scanning and air plethysmography *J Vasc Surg* 2003;38:935-43.

37. Goldman M. Regarding "Deep vein thrombosis after radiofrequency ablation of greater saphenous vein: A word of caution" *J of Vasc Surg* 2005;41:737.

38. Mozes G, Kalra M, Swenson, L, et al. Extension of saphenous thrombus into the femoral vein: A potential complication of new endovenous ablation techniques. *J Vasc Surg* 2005;41:130-5

39. Neglen P, Raju S. Venous reflux repair with cryopreserved vein valves. *J Vasc Surg* 2003;38:1139-1140.

40. Garcia-Rinaldi R, Revuelta J, Martinez M, et al. Implantation of cryopreserved pulmonary allograft monocusp match to treat nonthrombotic femoral vein incompetency. *Tex Heart Inst J* 2002;29:92-9.

41. Neglen P, Thrasher T, Raju S. Venous outflow obstruction: An underestimated contributor to chronic venous disease *J Vasc Surg* 2003;38:879-85

REVIEW QUESTIONS

1.) Chronic venous insufficiency edema is due to:
   a. Long term increase in salt consumption
   b. Uncontrolled diabetes and hypertension
   c. Venous valve incompetence and loss of leg muscle pump
   d. Pulmonary congestion and cardiac failure

2.) The mainstay of treatment for CVI is:
   a. Daily diuretic therapy
   b. Strict bedrest
   c. Salt reduction and blood pressure control
   d. Gradient compression wraps

3.) Venous ulcer will heal with:
   a. Topical wound care only
   b. Only if surgery is performed
   c. By leaving wounds open to air
   d. Comprehensive wound care after the venous edema is controlled

4.) Which answer is true about CVI and arterial insufficiency?
   a. Venous and arterial insufficiency co-exist in about 20% of CVI patients
   b. An ABI is a useful screening test to perform as part of the initial evaluation of all CVI patients
   c. Arterial ulcers usually have necrotic eschar while venous ulcers usually have purple granulation tissue
   d. All of the above

5.) Once venous edema is treated, maintenance therapy consists of:
   a. Daily use of fitted gradient compression stockings to maintain edema control
   b. Daily diuretic use to maintain edema control
   c. Edema is resolved and unlikely to return
   d. Fitted gradient compression stockings only if patient notices severe edema of legs

Answers: 1c, 2d, 3d, 4d, 5a.

CHAPTER 15

LYMPHEDEMA: AN EPIDEMIC HIDDEN IN PLAIN SIGHT

CHAPTER FIFTEEN OVERVIEW

NOTES

Lymphedema, an Epidemic Hidden in Plain Sight

Caroline E. Fife

INTRODUCTION

Lymphedema is a little-understood disease afflicting the lymphatic system, most commonly of the extremities, but occasionally involving the trunk, head, or genital area, and which can complicate the healing of wounds or skin conditions. Patients who have lymphedema must have this pathological condition addressed first since the chronic skin conditions caused by the disease do not respond to treatments purely targeted at the skin. Regardless of etiology, the results of the damaged, obstructed, or dysfunctional lymphatic system in the affected limb(s) cause massive swelling, sometimes of elephantine proportions.

A recent UK study reported a crude prevalence of 1.33 individuals per 1000, with an associated increase in age (5.4 per 1000 in those aged >65 years), and a gender bias toward women (2.15 per 1000 for women versus 0.47 per 1000 for men) (1). Because of the explosive increase in morbid obesity in the USA and continuing high levels of breast cancer, both factors affecting secondary lymphedema, it is certain that the incidence of lymphedema will rise, and perhaps increasingly affect younger patients.

Despite these attention-getting numbers, lymphedema represents an "orphan" disease, primarily because the lymphatic system does not neatly fall into any medical specialty, and consequently few physicians are well versed in its pathophysiology or treatment.

ANATOMY OF THE LYMPHATIC SYSTEM

While the body's rich capillary network retains blood cells, the porosity of its vessels permits leakage of fluid into the interstitial "third" space to bathe cells and remove cellular waste. Nonresorbed fluid is normally collected via the extensive network of the lymphatic system for its long journey proximal to the thoracic duct where it is returned to the circulatory system. Besides removal of this fluid, the lymphatic system also entrains macromolecules and pathogens that might be potentially harmful to the body. Extremities contain both superficial and deep lymphatic channels, which facilitate lymph flow from superficial to and from distal to deep proximal.

Based on the Starling principle governing fluid movement across the walls of exchange vessels (2, 3), it was thought that a relatively small amount of capillary ultrafiltrate was returned to the circulation via the lymphatics, with the bulk of the ultrafiltrate being reabsorbed by venules. However, recent evidence suggests that this is a gross underestimation. In part this is due to a revision of the Starling parameters, particularly the interstitial forces and interstitial oncotic pressure (4–6), but also the discovery that lymph nodes can concentrate lymph (4). Although 2–4 L of postnodal lymph are returned to the circulation every day, at least 8 L of efferent lymph and perhaps more are produced on a daily basis (3, 4) Lymph also carries and returns to the general circulation approximately 240 g of protein per day (7). Without this protein carriage, the resultant edema and loss of protein to the body would have serious pathological consequences within 24 hours. In Figure 1, note the dilated superficial lymphatics that are attempting to return fluid to the heart, easily visible in a patient with congestive heart failure.

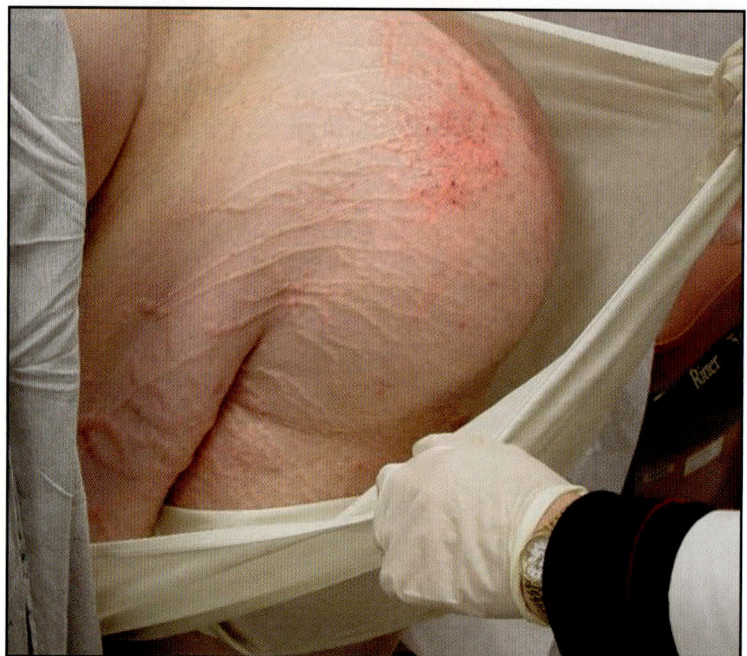

Figure 1. Dilated superficial lymphatics in a patient with congestive heart failure. The overhanging pannus is to the left of the image, and the buttocks to right.

Under the dermis, the superficial lymphatic plexus comprises lymphatics with a diameter of 10–60 µm composed of a single layer of endothelial cells, which rest on a discontinuous basement membrane (8). This membrane is composed of type IV collagen that is attached to the surrounding connective tissue by anchoring filaments. Stretching of the filaments allows the interendothelial clefts between cells to expand, permitting interstitial fluid and macromolecules to enter the lumen of the lymphatics (8). See Figure 2.

The superficial lymphatics are connected to the deeper lymphatics of the dermis via precollectors, the collecting ducts. Unlike the superficial lymphatics, the collecting ducts possess a thin layer of smooth muscle surrounding the endothelial cells, as well as unicuspid and bicuspid valves spaced at 6-20 mm intervals to prevent lymph backflow. These lymphangions possess contractile properties similar to small venules, and generate 5–7 action potentials per minute, causing 1–30 pulsations per minute. The end result is that the lymph is propelled unidirectionally in a peristaltic fashion. See Figure 1. In addition, proximal flow of the lymph to the deeper lymphatic channels and nodes is aided by arterial pulsation, muscle contraction, and skin distention. Venous insufficiency, peripheral arterial disease, and diseases causing muscle paralysis instigate lymphostasis and swelling, which is why certain skin-focused therapeutic interventions, such as kinesiotaping, can decrease the resultant edema. Interestingly, research suggests that in primary lymphedema a considerable volume of lymph is removed by high-resistance, small-diameter lymphatics, resulting in microvascular hypertension (9). In addition, under such conditions, contractions of the few preserved large proximal lymphatic collectors are enhanced.

The level of fluid in the interstitial spaces is carefully regulated to avoid dehydration (too little fluid) or edema (too much fluid). Normally, the transport capacity of the lymphatic system far exceeds the loads typically placed upon it, but when this functional reserve is unavailable, the result is lymphedema. The shortfall in reserve can be the effect of mechanical insufficiency (contractility failure or valve incompetence) or a massive increase in lymph volume due to congestive heart failure, increased venous pressure, capillary injury, or hypoproteinemia from chronic renal insufficiency or malignant ascites (2). Regardless of the etiology, a buildup of protein-rich fluid in the superficial tissues occurs, sometimes known as "localized high-protein edema."

LYMPHEDEMA PATHOPHYSIOLOGY

Lymphedema is diagnosed as primary or secondary on the basis of its etiology: if the defect is in the lymph-conducting pathways it is primary; if the cause is due to extralymphatic factors, it is secondary (10). The causes of primary lymphedema are poorly understood, but typically involve inadequate development or function of the lymphatics, often the outcome of lymph vessel hypoplasia, aplasia, or dysplasia.

Primary lymphedema is diagnosed during three general age categories. Congenital lymphedema, which represents about 10–15% of primary patients, is present at birth, and can affect any anatomical area. A family history of such disorders suggests Milroy's disease, which affects the lower extremities,

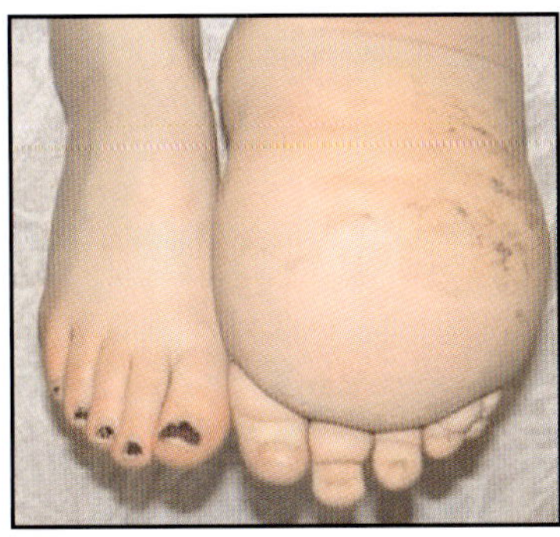

Figure 2. Severe changes to the foot of a patient with KTW Syndrome. Note the small port wine stain on the left foot.

although rarer genetic syndromes do occur, and the lymphedema can be associated with hemangiomas, lymphangiomas, port wine stains, and Klippel-Trenaunay-Weber (KTW) syndrome (telangectasias, excessive long bone growth). Figure 2 shows severe lymphedema of the foot in a 12-year-old patient with KTW syndrome.

While a few of the missense mutations responsible for congenital lymphedema belong to the vascular endothelial cell growth factor genes, and mutations of the homeobox gene (master control gene), Prox1 are probably involved, the identity of most still remain to be discovered (11). Lymphedema "Praecox" is by far the most common secondary lymphedema (75%) presenting at an average age of 17, with three-quarters of the patients being female. Familial factors might be responsible, including Meige's disease (similar to Milroy's disease). Finally, Lymphedema "Tarda" has a typical onset after age 35 with a slightly higher incidence than congenital lymphedema. The estimated total incidence of primary lymphedema in the USA is one in 6,000, which means approximately 50,000 individuals in the current population need treatment (12). Primary lymphedema is usually asymmetrical in presentation, although on close inspection the paired "normal" element in half of the cases manifests some degree of lymphedema.

Secondary lymphedema is the most common type of lymphedema, and worldwide, filariasis is the most common cause. Obstruction of the lymphatic system by filarial organisms is estimated to affect 15 million individuals (13). In developed countries, significant causes of secondary lymphedema include surgery, radiation therapy, malignancy, infection, and trauma. For women, following breast cancer surgery, the incidence of secondary lymphedema

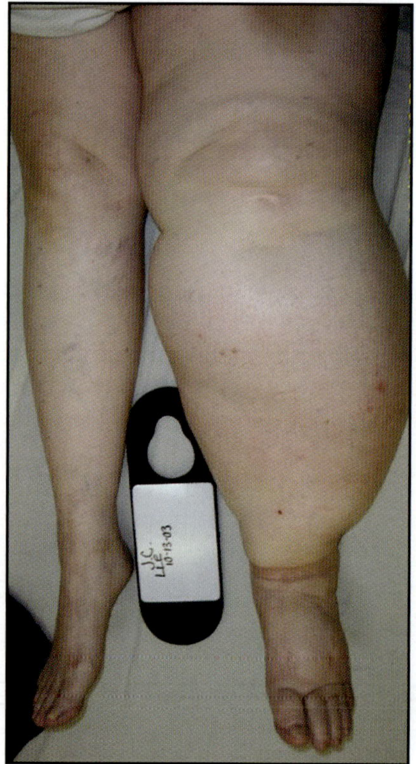

Figure 3. Secondary lymphedema of the left leg after treatment for uterine cancer, which included pelvic radiation.

varies from 6–63% (14–16), and for men recovering from prostate cancer treatment, up to 70% can develop symptoms (17), depending on the range of lymphatic exploration and the nature of the surgery. In many cases, the lymphedema can take anywhere from three months to five years to appear as shown in an Australian study of the incidence of lymphedema following treatment for gynecological cancer (18), and can be triggered by minor episodes of trauma, and such activities as heavy lifting or even air travel. Figure 3 shows lymphedema of the left leg in a woman after treatment with radiotherapy and surgery for uterine cancer.

It must be stressed that the development of secondary lymphedema is not really the end result of a simple lymphatic obstruction mechanism, as had been thought previously. For example, in secondary lymphedema resulting from breast cancer treatment, the forearm can be swollen, but not the hand. In this particular scenario, Modi et al. (19) elegantly demonstrated that although the edema is epifacial—ie, outside the fascia bordering the arm musculature, mainly in the subcutis—it is not the epifascial lymph drainage rate constant that is responsible for the severity of the swelling, but rather the subfacial lymph drainage rate constant. In other words, the rate at which lymph drains from the subfascia correlated with the degree of limb swelling. The implication is that the pathology of the disease involves the deeper lymphatic system, as well as the dermal lymphatics.

Variations in lymphatic transport capacity might also be partially controlled by genetics, which will affect to what degree breast cancer survivors subsequently develop lymphedema. As Ferrell has put it, "Whether one develops lymphedema secondary to cancer or trauma, or one was born with a severely impaired system that leads to primary lymphedema, there is increasing evidence that the same set of genes is involved in lymphedema. As we learn more about the genetic aspects of lymphedema, I would not be surprised to find that the dividing line between what we historically believe to be primary and secondary lymphedema will become quite blurred (20)."

CLINICAL FEATURES ASSOCIATED WITH LYMPHEDEMA

Inflammation of the skin, subcutaneous tissue, lymph nodes, and the lymphatic system is a basic feature of lymphedema, which can lead to chronic pain, functional impairment, and recurrent cellulitis in patients with primary or secondary lymphedema. Indeed, the stages of untreated lymphedema severity are attributable to the inflammatory processes associated with lymphostasis (21). In many cases the diagnosis of lymphedema starts with the

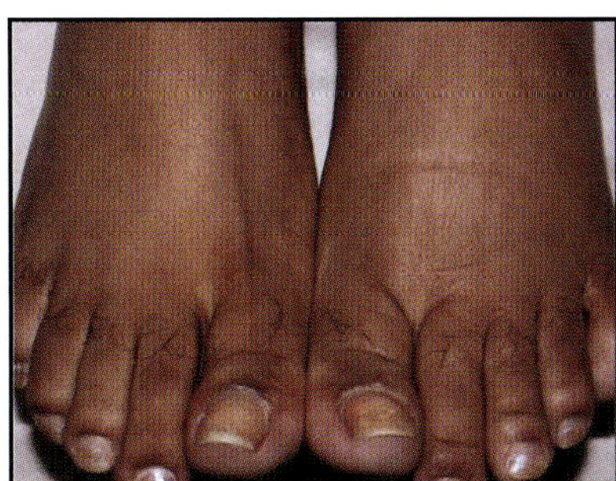

Figure 4. Subtle foot changes in a patient who has a positive "Stemmer's Sign" on the left foot. Note the impression left from her sandal.

appearance of "Stemmer's Sign," the inability to pinch a fold of skin at the base of the second toe due to thickening (2). While the changes to the foot are pronounced in Figure 2, they are very subtle in Figure 4. On careful inspection, the indentation from the patient's sandal on the left foot is apparent. She also has a positive Stemmer's Sign.

Progressive infiltration of neutrophils, macrophages, and fibroblasts caused by the accumulation of protein in the third space leads to deposition of collagen, and further destruction of intact lymphatics through fibrosis of their delicate structures. These processes are often observed through the appearance of dermal changes that include dry or flaky skin, hyperkeratosis, skin creases, fibromas, lymphangiomas, and papillomas, as seen in Figure 5. Eventually, significant limb distortion can occur, as seen in Figure 6. Extreme lymphedema manifests itself as elephantiasis, an extremely apt term.

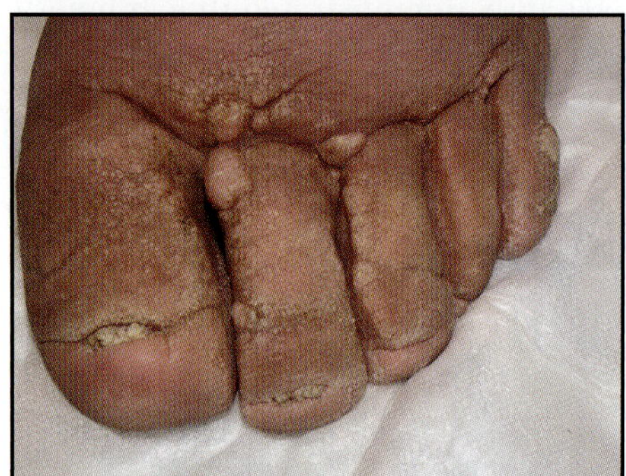

Figure 5. Fibromas of foot.

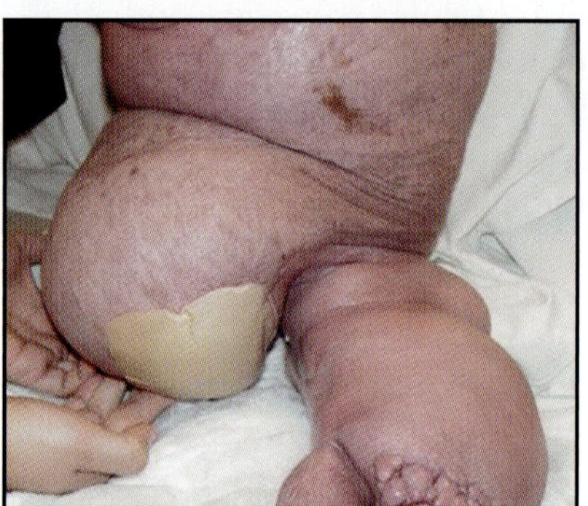

Figure 6. Note the limb distortion and the papillomas of the foot just visible.

Most clinicians utilize the 3-stage classification for a lymphedematous limb developed by the International Society of Lymphology as a consensus document (22), shown in Table 1. Within each stage, the severity of an affected limb can be assessed based on the increase in limb volume: minimal (<20%); moderate (20–40%); severe (>40%). In essence, Stage I represents a reversible condition, while Stage II introduces fibrotic conditions and places the patient at risk for infection, and Stage III involves elephantiasis with concurrent papillomas, significant hypertrophy of the underlying affected tissues, substantial limb distortion, the appearance of a "wooden" skin texture, and often lymphorrhea (weeping of lymph through the skin), and skin breakdown. There has been also increasing discussion on the use of a Stage 0, which would represent a latent or subclinical condition in which lymph transport impairment is evident, but no swelling is apparent.

Massive localized lymphedema (MLL) is a syndrome seen in morbidly obese patients. It is characterized by the appearance of a benign overgrowth of lymphoproliferative tissue, comprising fibrotic and edematous fibroadipose tissue (23), and because of its large size and similarity to a sarcoma, has often been termed as a pseudosarcoma (24), as seen in Figure 7. Although termed rare, in our practice, we have not found this to be uncommon in morbidly obese patients, defined as being at least 100 lb over one's ideal weight or having a body mass index of 40 or higher. In general, such patients only seek

TABLE 1. CLASSIFICATION OF LYMPHEDEMATOUS LIMBS BY STAGE ACCORDING TO THE INTERNATIONAL SOCIETY FOR LYMPHOLOGY

Stage	Symptoms
I	Early accumulation of fluid relatively high in protein Pitting possible Subsides with limb elevation
II	Pitting manifest Tissue fibrosis apparent in later stage II and pitting might not be visible Limb elevation alone rarely reduces swelling
III	Lymphostatic elephantiasis Trophic skin changes, such as acanthosis, fat deposits, and warty overgrowths Pitting absent

treatment when the expanding tissue mass becomes of sufficient size as to interfere with their daily activities, or when excoriation or wound breakdown occurs. The patient in Figure 7 is immobile, because the mass on her left thigh makes ambulation difficult. Note that she has evidence of venous insufficiency with a wound visible on the left lower leg, as well as hemosiderin deposits.

Treatment of MLL is difficult. Bandaging these enlargements, most commonly found on the lower extremities, is difficult, since they are rather spherical and thus not easily amenable to compression techniques. Morbidly obese patients cannot bandage themselves. The masses are a collection of fat, engorged lymphatics and inflammatory tissue, and thus will decrease somewhat but not resolve with compression. Surgical removal is the only way to eradicate them, and most third-party payors consider this a cosmetic procedure, even though in some cases, the enlargements limit ambulation. Furthermore, we have seen these masses return if patients fail to control their weight. Massive localized lymphedema is directly related to the disease of morbid obesity and cannot be treated unless that overarching issue is addressed.

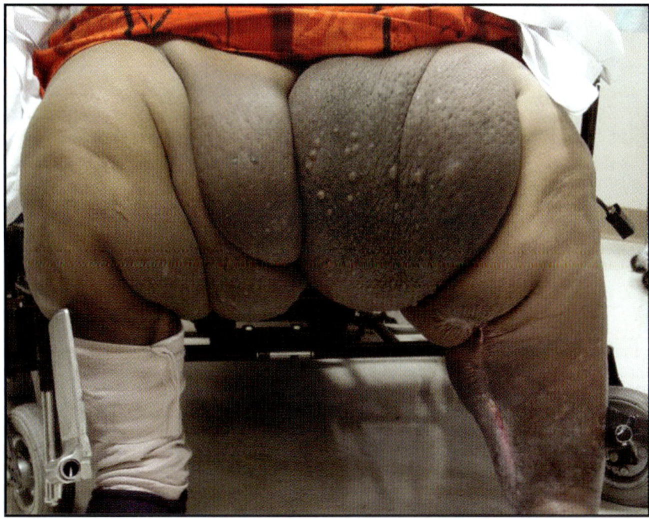

Figure 7. Massive localized lymphedema in an obese patient with venous stasis.

Lipedema is a syndrome often mistaken for lymphedema (25). It is a genetically mediated disease that involves the pathological accumulation of fat on the lower body and is most commonly seen in women. Initially, there are features that differentiate lipedema from lymphedema. The most significant distinction is that in lipedema, the feet are spared, with leg enlargement initially affecting the ankle and lower leg in a "pantaloon" distribution (Figure 8), whereas, in (primary) lymphedema, the feet are commonly the first area affected. Furthermore, in lipedema, both legs are symmetrically affected. In later life, the fatty depositions can occlude the lymphatic system, which can lead to secondary lymphedema. Thus, in advanced states, a syndrome of lipolymphedema can develop as shown in Figure 9. This morbidly obese patient began with lipedema and developed secondary lymphedema. Note that her feet are now affected. Table 2 shows the primary distinguishing features of lipedema and lymphedema that assist in differential diagnosis.

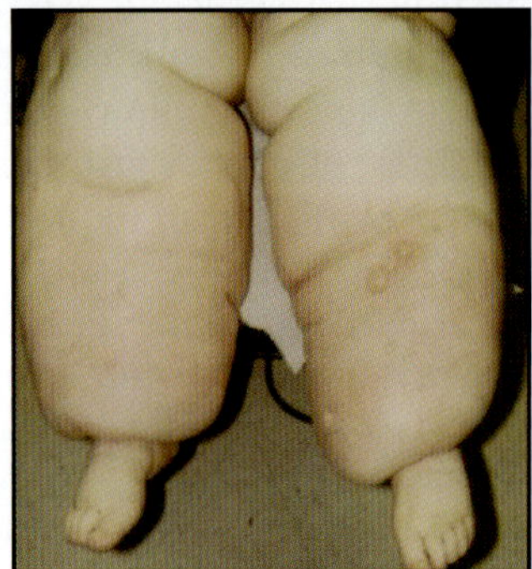

Figure 8. Lipedema with pantaloon distribution.

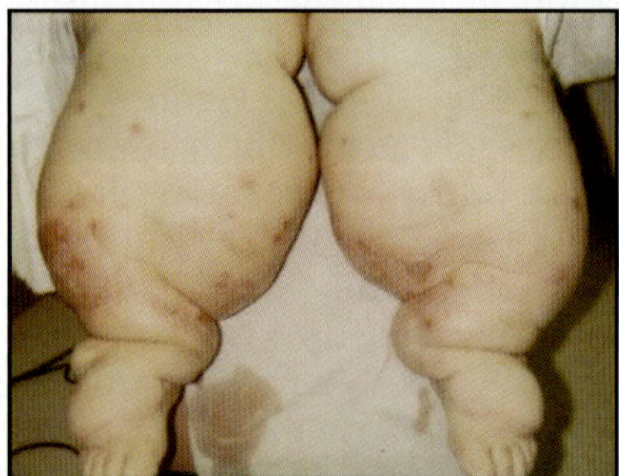

Figure 9. Morbidly obese patient with lipedema and now secondary lymphedema. Note the collection of massive localized lymphedema and the "peu d'orange" changes to the left medial thigh due to fluid accumulation.

TABLE 2. FEATURES ASSOCIATED WITH LIPEDEMA AND LYMPHEDEMA THAT ASSIST IN DIFFERENTIAL DIAGNOSIS

Features Associated with Lipedema	Features Associated with Lymphedema
Feet normally spared until secondary lymphedema occurs	Feet normally the first area to be affected
Legs bilaterally affected	Legs unilaterally affected, although a small amount of swelling might be observed with the other leg
"Pantaloons" common	"Pantaloons" rare
Upper torso and arms unaffected	Arms and other areas of the upper torso can be affected
Areas affected are tender to touch	Areas affected are not usually tender to touch, except in Stage III

Women with lipedema are often described as having upper and lower bodies that "do not match," which gives rise to small breasts but dramatically enlarged hips and thighs that do not respond to dietary modifications. An increase in weight results in the preferential deposition of fat below the waist, but weight loss tends to occur in the upper body, making the enlarged legs very diet resistant. Besides the aching dysthesia and facile leg bruising that accompanies the disease, sometimes referred to as "painful fat syndrome," the disfigurement and absolute need to control weight to prevent further fat deposition is a demoralizing issue for these women. Liposuction can result in cosmetic improvement, although there is controversy regarding whether this procedure can be safely performed below the knee, and whether it can further damage lymphatics. Furthermore, it is considered cosmetic and thus not covered by payors, despite the pathological basis of lipedema.

Several other clinical conditions can be confused with lymphedema, including myxedema due to hyperthroidism or hypothyroidism, and chronic venous insufficiency or venous occlusion. A number of pathological states are responsible for the venous edema that results from increased capillary pressure and filtration, leading to an excess of protein-poor interstitial fluid. These include pulmonary hypertension, congestive heart failure, renal disease, liver disease, malnutrition and malabsorption syndromes, anemia, and some sepsis conditions. In addition, a surprising number of drugs can cause leg edema, such as calcium channel blockers, beta blockers, nonsteroidal anti-inflammatories, steroids, hormones (estrogen/progesterone) (26), as well as insulin, cyclophosporine, growth hormone, amantadine, and immuno-therapeutics, including the interleukins. Careful assessment of the presenting edema is necessary to determine its etiology before initiating treatment (25).

THE BIOCHEMICAL FACTORS UNDERLYING LYMPHEDEMA

Although the development of fibrotic modules and limb distortion are sequiturs of the undesirable skin and subcutaneous tissue changes that reflect imbalances in growth factors, proteases, and cytokines present in the interstitial spaces (27), we are only just beginning to understand the biochemical factors involved. Edema should increase the barrier to oxygen diffusion, and thus serious regional oxygen deficiency followed by reperfusion periods ought to occur in lymphedematous tissue (28). Tissue fibrosis should also lower oxygen levels. However, Nemeth et al. (29) found that edema did not account for the low transcutaneous oxygen pressures ($TcpO_2$) found in ulcerated edematous limbs, and moreover $TcpO_2$ measurements in the edematous arms of women who had unilateral mastectomy showed no difference compared to their control (unaffected) arms (30). Further, while therapy both improved the levels of edema and fibrosis, the $TcpO_2$ levels remained the same. These results suggest that we have an incomplete understanding of oxygen levels in lymphedematous tissue. For example, how does the oxygen level of lymphedematous tissue vary over time? Is there a threshold edema level that is required for oxygen levels to fall? Clearly, further research will be needed to explain how edema and tissue oxygen levels are related.

If oxygen levels in lymphedematous tissue are low, hyperbaric oxygen (HBO2) treatment ought to have a positive effect. Hyperbaric oxygen therapy has been investigated as a treatment for lymphedema in women after breast cancer and radiotherapy, but the effect was modest (31, 32). What is intriguing is that in one trial (31), VEGF-C levels had begun to rise. Unlike VEGF (vascular endothelial growth factor), the expression of VEGF-C does not appear to be regulated by hypoxia (33), but rises in response to proinflammatory cytokines, which indicates a role in inflammatory responses (34).

Inflammation and Oxidative Stress

Earlier, it was indicated that inflammation is a universal characteristic of lymphedema. Studies in humans have shown that cytokine levels are raised in lymphedema, most likely due to infiltrating immune cells, but the inflammation is local, rather than systemic (35). For example, in one report of patients with peripheral leg edema it was shown that gene expression for CD14, CD44, IFNγR, TNF-α, TNFR1 and other cytokines was upregulated (36). In contrast, studies of genetically engineered Chy mice, which are used as models for Milroy's disease, indicate that inflammation does not have a major role in lymphedema in the early stages (3–4 months) (37). However, the finding of lowered levels of IL-4 suggests a reduced immunological defense ability, which might be responsible for an increase in the proinflammatory IL-2 and IL-6 cytokines that are observed at a later stage of the disease (11–13 months). Earlier work linked inflammatory changes to the level of protein in the interstices (38, 39), but it is also clear from more recent investigations that this is far from a simple relationship (35).

Perhaps one of the most fascinating findings has been that chronic lymphedema leads to increased oxidative stress. By measuring oxidative biomarkers such as reduced and oxidized glutathione, and the lipid peroxidation products malondialdehyde (MDA) and 4-hydroxynonenal (HNE) in the blood of lymphedema patients, healthy control subjects, and patients who had undergone cancer treatment but had not developed lymphedema, Siems et al. demonstrated that MDA levels were threefold higher in the serum of lymphedema patients, who also had reduced levels of GSH and higher levels of oxidized GSH compared to the other two groups (28). Further, after manual lymph drainage, both plasma MDA and HNE levels increased. These are important results, because enhanced formation of reactive oxygen species and peroxidized lipids is detrimental to tissue. Similar findings were also found for lipidema (40).

Another interesting aspect is that VEGFR-3, which is a primary modulator of lymphatic endothelial proliferation and survival (41), might also protect against oxidative damage in endothelial cells (42). Since some primary forms of lymphedema are a result of VEGFR-3 gene mutations, this might also explain why patients with this hereditary form of the disease can be more susceptible to oxidative stress. The source of oxidative stress in lymphedema is postulated to be periods of regional hypoxia/re-oxygenation, coupled with the finding that interstitial fluid is much more vulnerable to oxidation than plasma (43).

There are still many missing pieces to the biochemical puzzle of lymphedema. In particular, we do not have a full understanding of the sequence of events in the development of secondary lymphedema, and why certain patients who are at risk for the disease, do not in fact develop it. In the long-term, more research in this area is likely to prove fruitful because of better definition for those at risk and novel therapies.

WOUNDS AND SKIN CHANGES

Skin breakdown and chronic wounds can occur with lymphedema, although in some patients it can be hard to ascertain whether they were the cause or effect of lymphedema. Maceration, cellulitis, and inflammation are part of the clinical picture of lymphedema, as exemplified in Figure 10. In general, wounds should be handled in the normal way, controlling bioburden, debriding nonviable tissue as necessary, and managing drainage, although the latter can be challenging underneath compression bandages. While commercial bandaging products are excellent, newborn diapers can be extremely useful in assisting with copious drainage. Just as in venous insufficiency, wounds will usually heal once the edema is controlled, but the challenges to edema control in the patient with lymphedema are legion. In patients with morbid obesity, issues such as limited mobility, management of skin folds, massive localized lymphedema, the limited financial resources, which can occur if patients are unable to be gainfully employed, and sometimes an attitude of helplessness, all contribute to a difficult clinical picture. However, what is perhaps most important to understand is that wounds are not likely to heal if edema is not controlled. Edema management is a core principle for wound management regardless of whether the patient has venous insufficiency, or lymphedema, or both.

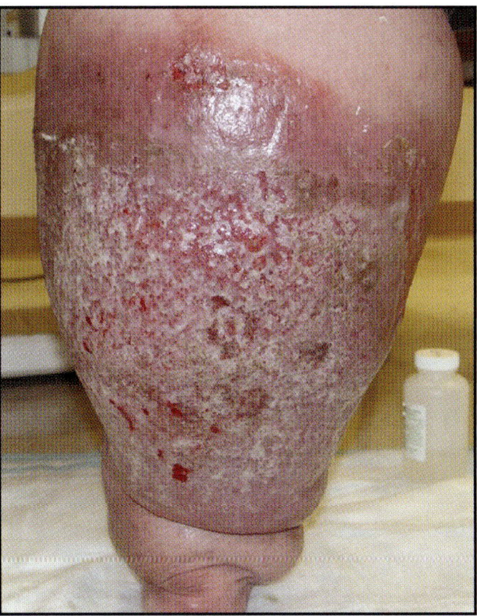

Figure 10. Obese patient with secondary lymphedema and cellulitis.

Skin changes are inevitable with lymphedematous conditions because macrophages acquire adipose tissue, thus causing deposits of subcutaneous fat in the affected extremities that cannot be removed by the body. In addition, fibrosis occurs in mid-stage lymphedema, which can be irreversible. The integration of compression into the wound management plan is a substantial challenge. Dressings must be chosen on the basis of their ability to remain for the duration of time until the next bandaging session, how well they will perform under sustained compression (i.e., will they rub, irritate, or leave marks in the skin), and whether they have sufficient absorptive properties, odor control, comfort, and a host of other practical considerations, including cost.

INITIAL TREATMENT OF LYMPHEDEMA

Although clinicians who treat venous disease are familiar with the concept of compression bandaging, the treatment of lymphedema requires a much more aggressive and extensive regimen that goes beyond simple compression treatment. A coordinated program of manual lymph drainage (MLD), compression bandaging, and skin care, often referred to as complete decongestive therapy (CDT) (44), is required to reduce the volume of the affected extremities to a near normal level. In addition, both the patient and any caregiver(s) must receive training to care for the condition. The initial phase of intensive treatment typically lasts four weeks, with the patient being seen 2–5 days a week. When serial measurements of the affected extremity or extremities reflect a size approaching that of the unaffected extremity, or demonstrate that the affected extremity appears to have reached its minimal volume, patients move to the second (maintenance) phase of treatment, which is long term and managed through the use of garments and other devices (45).

Diagnostic Testing

Lymphoscintigraphy is now considered to be the safest and most accepted method of diagnostic testing for lymphedema. Although the reliability of the test varies, lymphoscintigraphy has been used to differentiate between primary and secondary lymphedema (8, 46) and can be used to monitor the results of MLD (46, 47). Typically, technetium (Tc^{99}) in an unfiltered sulfur colloid is injected intradermally near a digit (finger or toe) on the affected limb. The flow of this substance is then traced with a gamma camera and a computer is used to create images of the lymph flow and calculate the speed of uptake. Magnetic resonance imaging is also increasingly being used to image the lymphatics.

Manual Lymph Drainage

In essence, MLD seeks to promote the functioning of lymphatics in transporting lymph from areas where it is less efficient. Historically, the method had its origins in the manual pumping techniques developed by Still, Vodder, and Miller several decades ago (48). Today, the procedure involves a specific sequence of manual strokes of a particular intensity, direction, and duration by trained therapists, beginning at the lymphatics of the neck, to facilitate movement of lymph to the thoracic duct, continuing with treatment of unaffected areas and finally affected areas (49, 50). When combined with compression bandaging, MLD assists in improving edema and the pain associated with it, although the results of randomized controlled trials show that the effect is only small to moderate (51, 52) However, MLD has been demonstrated to be more effective than mechanical pumping over time in reducing the volume of edematous extremities (53). Manual lymph drainage therapy can also utilize sticks, rollers or other cylindrical, flexible, and malleable material to improve its efficacy, but these procedures must be used with care to prevent trauma and subsequent infection (54).

MLD should be provided only by trained therapists. In the USA, there are a variety of certifying agencies with varying criteria for certification. The basic requirements suggested by the Lymphology Association of North America (LANA) (available at: *http://www.lymphnet.org/pdfDocs/nlntraining.pdf*) include:

- A specialized training involving 135 hours of CDT coursework from one lymphedema training program
- Coursework to consist of 1/3 theoretical instruction and 2/3 practical lab work teaching methods directly aimed at the treatment of lymphedema
- Proof of satisfactory completion of 12 credit hours of college-level human anatomy, physiology, and/or pathology from an accredited college or university
- A current unrestricted licensure in a related medical field.

Third party coverage policy pertaining to MLD is confusing at best. Thanks to grass roots movements by breast cancer survivor groups, MLD is covered by Medicare and most health care organizations for lymphedema resulting from cancer treatment. However, Medicare regards MLD as a means to train patients or caregivers to provide therapy rather than utilizing it as a treatment to reduce edema. Consequently, there is a "lifetime" limit on the number of sessions that can be provided for a lymphedema episode. Other health care organizations categorize MLD as a "physical therapy modality," and can exclude coverage on this basis.

In addition to limits on the number of "lifetime MLD visits," Medicare does not recognize massage therapists (MTs) as "licensed professionals" and thus MLD therapy cannot be billed to Medicare beneficiaries if provided by MTs, even if they are LANA certified. However, any physical therapist (PT) or occupational therapist (OT) is permitted to bill Medicare for the provision of MLD, even if these individuals have not received MLD training. It is estimated that in the U.S.A., at least half of the individuals certified to provide MLD therapy are massage therapists. Thus, the Medicare ruling that precludes massage therapists from being reimbursed for MLD services has resulted in the closure of many lymphedema treatment centers. This has caused in a crisis of access for Medicare beneficiaries with lymphedema.

Compression Bandaging

The type of bandage employed in CDT is different from the "long stretch" bandage, examples of which include ace wraps or cohesive bandages. Mostly made of cotton, washable and reusable, CDT bandages have little elasticity when maximal tension is applied. The effect is that tension is not applied to tissues at rest, but rather that the bandage constitutes a protective shell against which muscles contract when active, thus increasing the efficiency of the pump (high working pressure, low resting pressure) (55). The bandaging technique is key: bony prominences and underlying skin are protected by layers of foam and viscose-cotton or polyester padding under the bandages (56), which must be applied using a distal to proximal gradient (57), and worn 24 hours a day in the initial stages. Unlike compression bandaging for venous disease, which typically does not extend beyond the knee in the lower extremity, the multilayer bandaging for lymphedema often extends to the groin, and to the axillae for arm bandages (58). In addition, "bags" composed of foam chips applied underneath the bandages can be used to disperse fibrotic areas (56). Toes and fingers are almost always bandaged (see Figure 11). Slippage of bandages is common in the first several days and so frequent adjustments are necessary.

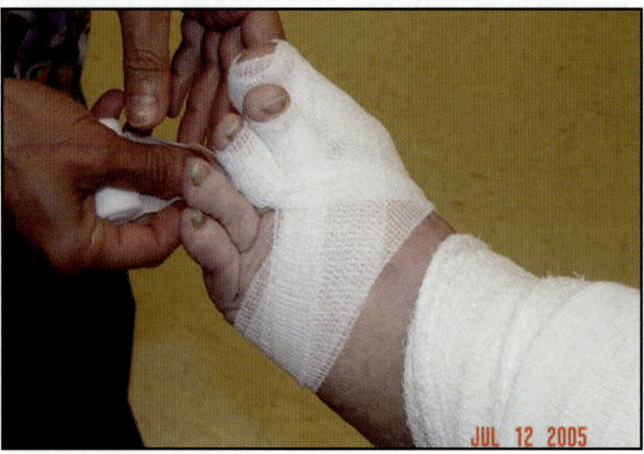

Figure 11. Toe bandaging.

MLD bandaging can be an integral part of wound care, and Figure 12A–C show the healing progression of a patient with an almost circumferential venous stasis ulcer who also had secondary lymphedema with foot swelling. Standard venous bandaging for over a year had effected no improvement in his wound. However, he responded to intensive MLD therapy in conjunction with skin grafting. Compression bandaging was performed over the skin graft to enhance the "take" of the graft and complete healing was achieved (Figure 12C).

Moffatt et al. suggest that the intensity of treatment in the initial phase and bandaging pressure be modified according to the type of patient presenting (59). For patients who do not have arterial occlusive disease and are not obese or elderly, they suggest a daily treatment with relatively high compression (>45 mm Hg); for patients who are obese or elderly with no arterial disease problems, the treatment frequency is reduced to three times weekly with the same compression. Even with low-stretch bandages, Compression therapy must be provided with care to frail patients who might have an element of arterial disease. Only very experienced caregivers, preferably physicians with expertise in lymphology should be managing these patients. Moffatt and colleagues recommend the "standard" intensive therapy frequency and a compression of 35–40 mm Hg for patients who have venous disease (59). In addition, toe bandaging is crucial. Probably the most important item for

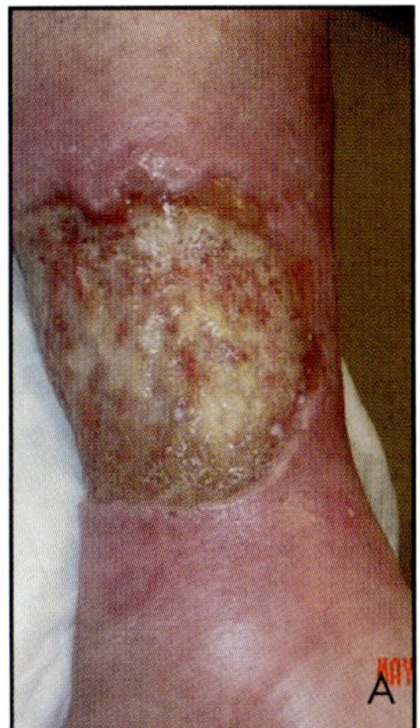
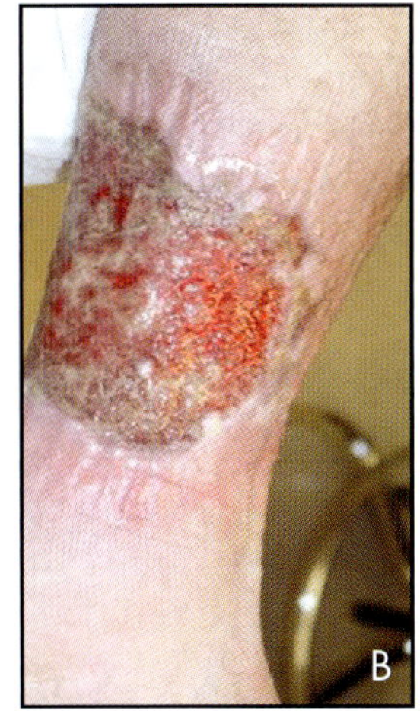
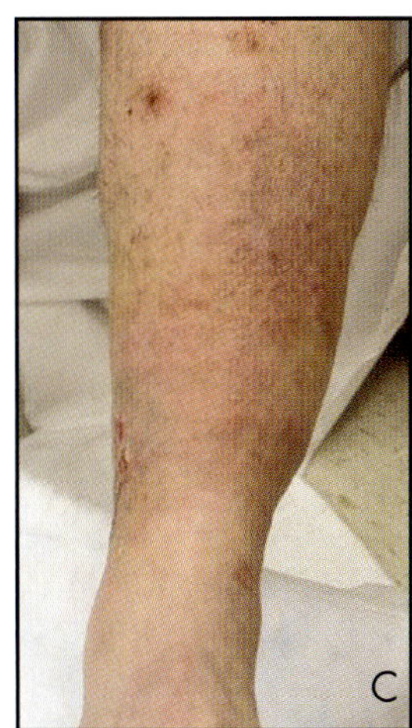

Figure 12 A-C. (A) Initial wound. (B) Granulating wound. (C) Healed wound.

patients and caregivers to learn is religious compliance with bandaging; many trials have often noted incompliance after a period of time either in the initial or maintenance phase of treatment (60, 61).

Foldi et al. (62) have outlined the science behind compression bandaging and suggest the following mechanisms at work:

- A reduction in capillary filtration
- A shift of fluid into non-compressed parts of the body
- An increase in lymphatic reabsorption and stimulation of lymphatic transport
- An improvement in the venous pump in patients with veno-lymphatic dysfunction
- A breakdown of fibrosclerotic tissue.

The strongest evidence to date for these mechanisms points to stimulation of lymph transport. For example, several studies have followed the effects of compression bandaging using dispersion of fluorescent dye (63), dynamic measurement of lymph parameters (64), and lymphoscintigraphy (65, 66). Foldi et al. (62) also suggest that the development of fibrosis is a result of upregulation in lymphedematous tissue, which can be reversed after compression bandaging, MLD, skin care, and remedial exercises (36).

Exercise

Since the intent behind compression bandaging is to raise the efficiency of local muscle pumping action, exercise must also be a component of CDT. As many patients have limited range of motion with the affected limb, this also improves the rehabilitation process. The exercises are designed to induce rhythmical, serial contractions in the affected areas of the limbs while the patients are wearing compression bandages. Again, compliance is important to maintain minimal edema and prevent reoccurrence, as over time some patients think that exercises can be discontinued when their condition improves.

Skin Care

For secondary lymphedema due to filariasis, the focus is on hygiene and skin care to prevent secondary infections (13), but the reduction of dermal colonization by bacteria and fungi is also an important goal for all lymphedema patients. This is accomplished by addressing chafing, dryness, cracking and other problems commonly encountered because of the lymphedema, or associated bandaging regimens. Use of nondrying soaps on a daily basis to remove skin debris and bacteria followed by drying, especially between the toes, and application of moisturizers to the skin will prevent skin cracking and cellulitis. For patients with advanced lymphedema who demonstrate fissured, keratinified skin, lactic acid products can assist with desquamation, and Olivamine™-containing formulations are useful in reducing superficial inflammation. In addition, the avoidance of cuts, pin pricks, hangnails, insect bites, contact allergens or irritants, pet scratches and burns to the affected extremity, as well as heat, especially saunas and hot tubs, will help prevent skin problems (67).

Bandages themselves can create further skin issues. Bandages can rub and irritate, and obese patients might have fungal or yeast infections of the skin that worsen under bandages. In addition, moisture from perspiration under hot bandages can cause maceration, and redundant skin folds must be carefully padded or they can break down. One of the most fascinating new products is a silver-impregnated, moisture-wicking fabric that can be placed into skin folds underneath bandages (InterDryAg Textile with Silver Complex, by Coloplast of Atlanta, GA) (68). It might also be necessary to work closely with a dermatologist to manage these challenging skin issues.

MAINTENANCE PHASE TREATMENT

Although exercise and skin care are important facets of long-term, maintenance treatment, and some patients might need compression bandaging, the use of compression garments, augmented by other devices to assist in MLD, are the mainstays of maintenance programs designed to minimize edema.

Compression Garments

Anti-embolism or "TED" hose do not constitute compression garments for any patient, including patients with venous disease. Even prescription compression garments at pressures of 20–30 mm Hg are usually insufficient for the management of lower extremity lymphedema (although they might be appropriate for venous stasis patients). On the other hand, garments with 20–30 mm Hg compression can be very satisfactory for mild upper extremity lymphedema. In some circumstances, garments with pressures as high as 40–50 mm Hg might be needed. However, such high compression can only be used in patients without arterial insufficiency and moreover can be difficult to don.

Patients who cannot be fitted with "off the shelf" garments can benefit from custom garments, but these are expensive. Garments can be manufactured for any area of the body, including the chest and face. Many lymphedema patients require custom garments for the hand, such as gloves, open finger "gauntlets," or even foot "gloves," which allow each toe to be placed in compression. However, some patients are unable to utilize compression garments due to irregularly shaped extremities or problems with donning or removal due to obesity or arthritis. Compression garments are not worn at night on any area of the body. Even with faithful use, compression garments do not always completely control swelling, and in such instances, patients might need to resort to bandaging at nighttime (69).

Compression garments must usually be replaced twice a year and this can present a significant financial burden for patients. Medicare covers garments only for patients with venous stasis ulcers and patients must have an open ulcer at the time that the garment is purchased for Medicare coverage policies to apply. Thus, if a wound continues to be closed, subsequent garments will not be covered by Medicare. Medicare does not cover custom fitted garments at all. Most private insurers will cover garments if physicians write a letter of medical necessity.

In cases in which compression garments cannot be used due to daily living activity limitations, semi-rigid devices, such as the Circaid™, Legassist™ or Farrow wrap (Figure 13), can help. While requiring special consideration for footware, these products include interlocking Velcro™ straps that assist the muscle pump, are easy to apply, and are surprisingly well accepted by patients who cannot utilize other garments. Velcro strap devices are not covered by Medicare for any reason (including stasis ulcerations), but represent a cost-effective way to manage edema. For patients who cannot afford garments or Velcro devices, their only option might be long-term use of short-stretch bandages. However, Medicare will not cover these supplies if no wounds are present, so patients will also have to purchase their own bandages (although there are some discount suppliers), and patients have to have a caregiver willing and able to apply bandages correctly. These limitations to long-term edema management options result in a "revolving door" problem with most lymphedema patients whose only access to supplies is via the outpatient clinic.

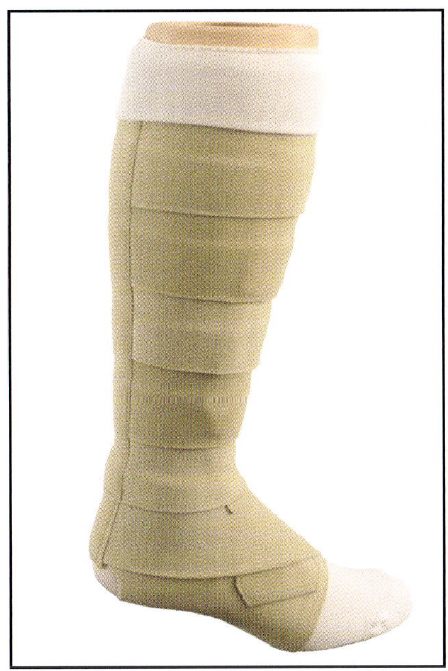

Figure 13. Farrow wrap

Pneumatic Pumps and Other Devices

In the last 10–15 years, a variety of other devices designed to mitigate edema have come on the market. The use of mechanical pumps is still controversial, and contraindicated in active deep vein thrombosis or active infection of the affected limb (67). Two randomized trials have been carried out to evaluate the use of intermittent pneumatic compression versus no treatment (70), and decongestive lymphatic therapy (71). Both involved lymphedema developing from breast cancer treatment. In the former trial, although substantial reduction in edema occurred with pump use compared to controls, the results failed to achieve statistical significance (70); in the latter trial, the results of volume reduction between the control case and the pump augmentation case were significant (71). With increasing evidence that pumps can make a significant difference in the reduction of edema as an adjunct treatment, there is probably a place for them in patients with intractable lymphedema and/or pelvic lymphedema (72). Early versions of these pumps might have been associated with increased genital swelling, but newer, multichambered, gradient, sequential pumps, which have pelvic attachments that might reduce genital swelling, are probably more efficient than older model pumps (73, 74), because they "produce a linear pressure wave from distal to proximal portions of the limb."

Other static devices designed to improve lymphatic return include the Reid Sleeve™ and the JOVI Pak™. While the Reid Sleeve™ is a dense foam product, the JOVI Pak™ is a quilted device that is custom fitted, and contains sewn channels intended to enhance lymphatic return. A "leotard"-like compression garment is worn over the device. Another process that can be used is termed kinesiotaping, which involves utilizing a specialized cotton tape applied to edematous areas. The idea behind this product is that body movement stretches the tape and lifts the skin, stimulating the superficial lymphatics. Although this technique has not been rigorously tested in lymphedema, it might be beneficial for those areas of the body that are hard to bandage, including the abdomen, genitalia, or face. Employment of any kind of kinesiotaping can be a useful addition if daily use of compression garments, self-MLD, and nightly bandaging have failed to control swelling.

Pharmaceuticals

At one time, both diuretics and benzopyrones were often prescribed for lymphedema. However, diuretics have been shown to be detrimental, causing hypotension, dehydration, and electrolyte imbalance through an associated, increased interstitial oncotic pressure that causes a rapid reoccurrence of edema (67, 75). Coumarin, a benzopyrone, was thought to enhance lymphangion contractility, and macrophage-induced proteolysis (76, 77), but a large (140 women) randomized, placebo-controlled trial failed to show any benefit (78), and it is not recommended now.

REVIEW OF KEY CLINICAL POINTS

Table 3 shows some key points to be determined when evaluating a patient with possible lymphedema in order to determine the etiology and optimal treatment. In general, the examination process should be directed at

TABLE 3. KEY POINTS TO BE DETERMINED IN PATIENTS PRESENTING WITH LYMPHEDEMA

Consideration	Key Points To Be Determined	Tests/Measurements
Edema	Time of onset (gradual, sudden, precipitating event)? Course? Familial involvement?	Volume measurement(s)
Prior edematous episodes	Has the patient had prior lymphedema episodes? If so, what treatment was provided, when, and how effective was it? What tests were given and what diagnoses were made?	
Affected limbs	Which extremities are affected? Severity of edema? Infection present?	Range of motion; strength; sensation, girth; photographic measurements; fungal/bacteriological identification
Unaffected extremities	Are the unaffected extremities truly unaffected?	Comparison to affected limbs (girth, etc.)
Patient History	Medications taken? History of surgeries? Previous treatments?	
Cancer	Has the patient had cancer treatment in the last five years? If so, what kind, and when was it given (radiation field data; surgical node dissection data)?	
General Health	Are daily living activites affected? What is the level of pain?	Body weight; BMI
Travel	Has the patient recently visited a filariasis-endemic area?	Filarial antibody testing
Sleep patterns	Where does the patient usually sleep? Does the patient sleep in chairs? Is immobility a factor? Does the patient suffer from sleep apnea?	
Skin	What is the condition of the skin?	Inspect visually for color, scarring, infection signs, papillomas, edma distribution; check for thickening, fibrosis, pitting, nodules, palpable nodes, and tenderness; Stemmer's Sign; check condition of nails
Wounds/Ulcers	Are wounds or ulcers present? if so, what kind, how many, and what stage if appropriate?	Measure size, depth; determine wound bed characteristics and drainage; document location (Photographs)
Comorbidites	What other significant comorbidities are present? Are major organ diseases present?	CTs, MRIs, other tests as necessary
Type of lymphedema	If the diagnosis is lymphedema, is it primary or secondary?	Nuclear scintigraphy; MRI

determining whether the edema is due to other pathological conditions or lymphedema. If lymphedema is present, it is also important to ascertain whether this is a new onset, or if other lymphedematous episodes have occurred.

Once a diagnosis of lymphedema is established, it is important that the clinician work with the patient to delineate realistic goals. For example, with an elderly patient, an incremental improvement might be all that is needed to improve the quality of life. For a young patient who is focused on the acquisition of visually normal extremities, more aggressive treatments might be warranted. Patients who are morbidly obese and do not control their weight during treatment are not likely to respond well to therapy.

TREATMENT FAILURE

There is no cure for lymphedema and some patients do not respond well to treatment. Further, the success of the treatment will depend on the patient's adherence to the care plan. For cancer survivors who have already experienced many psychological and physical traumas, discovering they have lymphedema can be a bitter blow. Similarly, for young lymphedema patients, the likelihood that they will require compression garments and/or bandaging for the rest of their lives can be a difficult issue.

Although there is no evidence to suggest that CDT exacerbates active cancer, textbooks often suggest a prohibition of CDT until cancer is treated out of fear that CDT will cause metastasis via the lymphatic system. It seems unlikely that CDT can cause metastasis beyond that which can naturally occur due to the mechanical activity of the lymphatic system. A logical approach would be not to perform CDT until cancer treatment has been initiated. However, once a patient has been diagnosed with metastatic disease and is under treatment for their cancer, there is no reason not to initiate CDT, as many cancer patients find uncontrolled edema the most distressing part of their advanced metastatic disease. Lymphedema therapy can also be part of a palliative care plan that greatly improves quality of life. Nevertheless, for cancer survivors presenting with recurrent lymphedema, it is crucial to determine whether the cancer has reoccurred before initiating CDT.

Proper training for patients and their caregivers is essential for long-term management. Improper bandaging or self-inflicted injury arising from poor technique is one major reason for CDT failure. Dementia, paralysis, morbid obesity, heart, liver, or renal failure, and other comorbidities often make patients unsuitable for CDT, or unable to fully participate in such a program, and thought should be given in such cases before deciding upon the best course of treatment. Finally, there is no substitute to daily compression for most lymphedema cases, and clinicians will frequently have to deal with patients who think that medication or the use of pumps will be sufficient to manage their condition without ongoing compression. In this regard, the clinician is both an educator and counselor, providing emotional support and encouragement, emphasizing the fact that early, consistent control is the key to preventing long-term disfigurement, limb distortion, and recurrent cellulitis.

Support groups might be helpful to the patient, and organizations, such as the National Lymphedema Network (*http://www.lymphnet.org*), can provide opportunities for the patient to network with other individuals who have lymphedema, as well as providing geographically useful information related to certified caregivers and therapists.

CONCLUSION

There is hope in the future that newer treatments currently being piloted will translate into simpler, more efficacious treatments. Principally these are gene therapies for primary lymphedema, and use of VEGF factors in secondary lymphedema (79). While these advanced treatments are based on a better biochemical understanding of the disease, there are still many obstacles to overcome, and they will be expensive. This is a problem for an orphan disease with few advocates in mainstream medicine, and for which most treatments are already not covered by Medicare or other insurance.

ACKNOWLEDGEMENT

We are grateful to Marissa J. Carter who has provided invaluable assistance getting the references for this chapter.

REFERENCES

1. Moffatt CJ, Franks PJ, Doherty DC, et al. Lymphoedema: an underestimated health problem. *Q J Med* 2003;96:731–738.

2. Williams A. An overview of non-cancer related chronic oedema—a UK perspective. Worldwide Wounds, 2003. Available at: *http://www.worldwidewounds.com/2003/april/Williams/Chronic-Oedema.html*. Accessed December 7, 2006.

3. Levick JR. Capillary filtration-absorption balance reconsidered in light of dynamic extravascular factors. *Exp Physiol* 1991;76:825-857.

4. Kirkman E, Sawdon M. Capillary dynamics and interstitial fluid lymphatic system. *Anaesth Intensive Care Med* (2004);5:38-42.

5. Michel CC. Fluid exchange in the microcirculation. *J Physiol* (Lond) 2004;557:701-702.

6. Levick JR. Revision of the Starling principle: new views of tissue fluid balance. *J Physiol* (Lond) 2004;557:704.

7. Levick JR. Changing perspectives on microvascular fluid exchange. In: Jordan D, Marshall J, eds. *Cardiovascular Regulation* London: Portland Press; 1999:127-152.

8. Szuba A, Shin WS, Strauss HW, et al. The third circulation: radionuclide lymphoscinctigraphy in the evaluation of lymphedema. *J Nucl Med* 2003;44:43-57.

9. Wen S, Dorffler-Melly J, Herrig I, et al. Fluctuation of skin lymphatic capillary pressure in controls and in patients with primary lymphedema. *Int J Microcirc Clin Exp* 1994;14:139-143.

10. Mortimer PS. ABC of arterial and venous disease. Swollen lower limb—2: lymphoedema. *BMJ* 2000;320:1527-1529.

11. Detmar M, Hirakawa S. The formation of lymphatic vessels and its importance in the setting of malignancy. *J Exp Med* 2002;196:713–718.

12. Swirsky J, Sakett Nannery D. Coping with lymphedema. Garden City Park, NY: Avery Publishing group; 1998:12.

13. Seim AR, Dreyer G, Addiss DG. Controlling morbidity and interrupting transmission: twin pillars of lymphatic filariasis elimination. *Rev Soc Bras Med Trop* 1999;32:325-328.

14. Mortimer PS, Bates DO, Brassington HD, et al. The prevalence of arm oedema following treatment for breast cancer. *Q J Med* 1996;89:377-80.

15. Querci della Rovere G, Ahmad I, Singh P, et al. An audit of the incidence of arm lymphoedema after prophylactic level I/II axillary dissection without division of the pectoralis minor muscle. *Ann R Coll Surg Engl* 2003;85:158-161.

16. Petrek JA, Heelan MC. Incidence of breast carcinoma-related lymphedema. *Cancer* 1998;83(12 Suppl American):2776-2781.

17. MD Anderson Cancer Center. Lymphedema. News in Cancer 2003. Available at: *http://www.mdanderson.org/departments/andersonnet/display.cfm?id=cdbf14a0-d2d6-4c0a-937d517e4ba3bb37&method=displayfull*. Accessed December 19, 2006.

18. Ryan M, Stainton MC, Slaytor EK, et al. Aetiology and prevalence of lower limb lymphoedema following treatment for gynaecological cancer. *Aust N Z J Obstet Gynaecol* 2003;43:148-151.

19. Modi S, Stanton AWB, Mellor RH, et al. Regional distribution of epifascial swelling and epifascial lymph drainage rate constants in breast cancer-related lymphedema. *Lymphat Res Biol* 2005;3:3–15.

20. Lymphatic research Foundation. Lymphedema genomics field exploding. *Lymphatic Res Matters* 2001;2:3.

21. Casley-Smith J. Alterations of untreated lymphedema and its grades over time. *Lymphol* 1995;28:174-85.

22. International Society of Lymphology. The diagnosis and treatment of peripheral lymphedema. *Lymphol* 2003;36:84-91.

23. Goshtasby P, Dawson J, Agarwal N. Pseudosarcoma: massive localized lymphedema of the morbidly obese. *Obes Surg* 2006;16:88-93.

24. Farshid G, Weiss S. Massive localized lymphedema in the morbidly obese: a histologically distinct reactive lesion simulating liposarcoma. *Am J Surg Pathol* 1998;22:1277-1283.

25. Rudkin GH, Miller TA. Lipedema: a clinical entity distinct from lymphedema. *Plast Reconstr Surg* 1994:841-7; discussion 848-849.

26. Ely JW, Osheroff JA, Chambliss ML, et al. Approach to leg edema of unclear etiology. *J Am Board Fam Med* 2006;19:148-160.

27. MacLaren JA. Skin changes in lymphoedema: pathophysiology and management options. *Int J Palliat Nurs* 2001 Aug;7(8):381-8.

28. Siems WG, Brenek R, Beier A, et al. Oxidative stress in chronic lymphedema. *Q J Med* 2002;95:803-809.

29. Nemeth AJ, Falanga V, Alstadt SP, et al. Ulcerated edematous limbs: effect of edema removal on transcutaneous oxygen measurements. *J Am Acad Dermatol* 1989;20:191-197.

30. Mayrovitz HN, Sims N, Brown-Cross D, et al. Transcutaneous oxygen tension in arms of women with unilateral postmastectomy lymphedema. *Lymphology* 2005;38:81-86.

31. Teas J, Cunningham JE, Cone L, et al. Can hyperbaric oxygen therapy reduce breast cancer treatment-related lymphedema? A pilot study. *J Women's Health* (Larchmt). 2004;13:1008-1018.

32. Gothard L, Stanton A, MacLaren J, et al. Non-randomised phase II trial of hyperbaric oxygen therapy in patients with chronic arm lymphoedema and tissue fibrosis after radiotherapy for early breast cancer. *Radiother Oncol* 2004;70:217-224.

33. Enholm B, Paavonen K, Ristimaki A, et al. Comparison of VEGF, VEGF-B, VEGF-C and Ang-1 mRNA regulation by serum, growth factors, oncoproteins and hypoxia. *Oncogene* 1997;14:2475-2483.

34. Ristimaki A, Narko K, Enholm B, et al. Proinflammatory cytokines regulate expression of the lymphatic endothelial mitogen vascular endothelial growth factor-C. *J Biol Chem* 1998;273:8413-8418.

35. Olszewski WL. Pathophysiological aspects of lymphedema of human limbs: 1. lymph protein composition.

36. Földi E, Sauerwald A, Hennig B. Effect of complex decongestive physiotherapy on gene expression for the inflammatory response in peripheral lymphedema. *Lymphology* 2000;33:19-23.

37. Karlsen TV, Larkkainen MJ, Alitalo K, et al. Transcapillary fluid balance consequences of missing initial lymphatics studied in a mouse model of primary lymphedema. *J Physiol* 2006;574(Pt 2):583-596.

38. Knight KFR, Collopy PA, McCann JJ, et al. Protein metabolism and fibrosis in experimental canine obstructive lymphedema. *J Lab Clin Med* 1987;110:558–66.

39. Gaffney RM, Casley-Smith JR. Excess plasma proteins as a cause of chronic inflammation and lymphedema: biochemical estimations. *J Pathol* 1981;133:229-242.

40. Siems W, Grune T, Voss P, et al. Anti-fibrosclerotic effects of shock wave therapy in lipedema and cellulite. *Biofactors* 2005;24:275-282.

41. Jussila L, Alitalo K. Vascular growth factors and lymphangiogenesis. *Physiol rev* 2002;82:673-700.

42. Wang JF, Zhang X, Groopman JE. Activation of vascular endothelial growth factor receptor-3 and its downstream signaling promote cell survival under oxidative stress. *J Biol Chem* 2004;279:27088-27097.

43. Kurtel H, Granger DN, Tso P, et al. Vulnerability of intestinal interstitial fluid to oxidant stress. *Am J Physiol* 1992;263:G573–578.

44. Foldi E. The treatment of lymphedema. *Cancer* 1998;83(12 Suppl American):2833-2835.

45. Ko DS, Lerner R, Klose G, et al. Effective treatment of lymphedema of the extremities. Arch Surg 1998;133:452-7.

46. Yuan Z, Chen L, Luo Q, et al. The role of radionuclide lymphoscintigraphy in extremity lymphedema. *Annals Nucl Med* 2006;20:341-344.

47. Ferrandez JC, Laroche JP, Serin D, et al. Lymphoscintigraphic aspects of the effects of manual lymphatic drainage. *J Mal Vasc* 1996;21:283-9.

48. Chikly BJ. Manual techniques addressing the lymphatic system: origins and development. *J Am Osteopath Assoc* 2005;105:457-464.

49. Fiaschi E, Francesconi G, Fiumicelli S, et al. Manual lymphatic drainage for chronic post-mastectomy lymphedema treatment. *Panminerva Med* 1998;40:48-50.

50. Korosec BJ. Manual lymphatic drainage therapy. *Home Health Care Manage Practice* 2004;16:499-511.

51. McNeely ML, Magee DJ, Lees AW, et al. The addition of manual lymph drainage to compression therapy for breast cancer related lymphedema: a randomized controlled trial. *Breast Cancer Res Treat* 2004;86:95-106.

52. Johansson K, Albertsson M, Ingvar C, et al. Effects of compression bandaging with or without manual lymph drainage treatment in patients with postoperative arm lymphedema. *Lymphology* 1999;32:103-10.

53. Johansson D, Lie E, Ekdahl C, et al. A randomized study comparing manual lymph drainage with sequential pneumatic compression for treatment of postoperative arm lymphedema. *Lymphology* 1998;31:56-64.

54. de Godoy JM, Batigalia F, Godoy Mde F. Preliminary evaluation of a new, more simplified physiotherapy technique for lymphatic drainage. *Lymphology* 2002;35:91-93.

55. Leduc O, Peeters A, Bourgeois P. Bandages: scintigraphic demonstration of its efficacy on colloidal protein reabsorption during muscular activity. In: Progress in Lymphology XII. Exerpta medica, International Congress series 887. Nishi M, Uchino S, Yabuki S, eds. Amsterdam: Elsevier, 1990;421-3.

56. Williams AF, Keller M. Practical guidance on lymphoedema bandaging of the upper and lower limbs. In Euro Wound Manage Assoc Focus Document: lymphoedema bandaging in practice. London: MEP Ltd., 2005;10-14.

57. Lawrence D, Kakkar VV. Graduated, static, external compression of the lower limb. *Br J Surg* 1980;67:119-121.

58. Casley-Smith JR, Boris M, Weindorf S, et al. Treatment for lymphedema of the arm—the Casley-Smith method. *Cancer* 1998;83(12 Suppl American):2843-2860.

59. Moffatt CJ, Morgan P, Doherty D. The lymphoedema framework: a consensus on lymphoedema bandaging. In Euro Wound Manage Assoc Focus Document: lymphoedema bandaging in practice. London: MEP Ltd., 2005;5-9.

60. Vignes S, Porcher R, Arrault M, et al. Long-term management of breast cancer-related lymphedema after intensive decongestive physiotherapy. *Breast Cancer Res Treat* 2006 Jul 7; [Epub ahead of print].

61. Mondry TE, Riffenburgh RH, Johnstone PA. Prospective trial of complete decongestive therapy for upper extremity lymphedema after breast cancer therapy. *Cancer J* 2004;10:42-48; discussion 17-19.

62. Foldi E, Junger M, Partsch H. The science of lymphoedema bandaging. In Euro Wound Manage Assoc Focus Document: lymphoedema bandaging in practice. London: MEP Ltd., 2005;2-4.

63. Franzeck UK, Spiegel I, Fischer M et al. Combined physical therapy for lymphedema evaluated by fluorescence microlymphography and lymph capillary pressure measurements. *J Vasc Res* 1997;34:306-311.

64. Olszewski WG. Lymph pressure and flow in limbs. In: Olszewski WG (ed). Lymph Stasis: pathophysiology, diagnosis and treatment. Boca Raton, FL: CRC Press, 1991.

65. Casley-Smith JR. Changes in the microcirculation at the superficial and deeper levels in lymphoedema: the effects and results of massage, compression, exercise and benzopyrones on these levels during treatment. *Clin Hemorheol Microcirc* 2000;23:335-343.

66. Földi E, Földi M, Weissleder H. Conservative treatment of lymphoedema of the limbs. *Angiology* 1985;36:171-180.

67. Harris SR, Hugi MR, Olivotto IA, et al. For the Steering Committee for Clinical Practice Guidelines for the Care and Treatment of Breast Cancer. Clinical practice guidelines for the care and treatment of breast cancer: 11. Lymphedema. *CMAJ* 2001;164:191-199.

68. Ostomy Wound Management. Silver dressing manages moisture, odor, and inflammation in skin folds. *Ostomy Wound Manage* 2006;52:78.

69. Badger CM, Peacock JL, Mortimer PS. A randomized, controlled, parallel-group clinical trial comparing multiplayer bandaging followed by hosiery versus hosiery alone in the treatment of patients with lymphedema of the limb. *Cancer* 2000;88:2832-2837.

70. Dini D, Del Mastro L, Gozza A, et al. The role of pneumatic compression in the treatment of postmastectomy lymphedema. A randomized phase III study. *Ann Oncol* 1998;9:187-191.

71. Szuba A, Achalu R, Rockson SG. Decongestive lymphatic therapy for patients with breast carcinoma-associated lymphedema. A randomized, prospective study of a role for adjunctive intermittent pneumatic compression. *Cancer* 2002;95:2260-2267.

72. Miranda F Jr., Perez MC, Castiglioni ML, et al. Effect of sequential intermittent pneumatic compression on both leg lymphedema volume and on lymph transport as semi-quantitatively evaluated by lymphoscintigraphy. *Lymphology* 2001;34:135-41.

73. Zanolla R, Monzeglio C, Balzarini A, et al. Evaluation of the results of three different methods of postmastectomy lymphedema treatment. *J Surg Oncol* 1984;26:210-213.

74. Gan JL, Chang TS, Liu W. The circulatory pneumatic apparatus for lymphedema of the limb. *Eur J Plast Surg* 1994;17:169-172.

75. Farncombe M, Daniels G, Cross L. Lymphedema: the seemingly forgotten complication. *J Pain Symptom Manage* 1994;9:269-276.

76. Piller NB, Morgan RG, Casley-Smith JR. A double-blind, cross-over trial of O-(B-hydroxyethyl)-rutosides (benzopyrones) in the treatment of the arms and legs. *Br J Plast Surg* 1988;41:20-27.

77. Casley-Smith JR, Morgan RG, Piller NB. Treatment of lymphedema of the arms and legs with 5,6-benzo-pyrone. *N Engl J Med* 1993;329:1158-1163.

78. Loprinzi CL, Kugler JW, Sloan JA, et al. Lack of effect of coumarin in women with lymphedema after treatment for breast cancer. *N Engl J Med* 1999;340:346-350.

79. Karkkainen MJ, Saaristo A, Jussila L, et al. A model for gene therapy of human hereditary lymphedema. *Proc Nat Acad Sci* 2001;9812677-12682.

REVIEW QUESTIONS

1.) Lymphedema can occur when:
    a. The volume of lymph exceeds the transport capacity
    b. There is a mechanical obstruction in the system
    c. There is a congenital insufficiency of the function of the lymphatic system
    d. All of the above

2.) World wide, the most common cause of lymphedema is primary lymphedema
    a. True
    b. False

3.) The incidence of lymphedema after breast cancer may be related to the following:
    a. The stage of cancer
    b. The agressiveness/type of treatment (surgery, chemo, etc)
    c. The underlying lymphatic transport capacity, which varies from patient to patient
    d. Whether the patient maintains a normal post operative body weight
    e. All of the above

4). Lymphedema bandaging differs from venous stasis bandaging in:
    a. The use of only short stretch bandaging (no high stretch)
    b. The use of extensive padding underneath the bandages
    c. The inclusion of toe and/or finger bandaging
    d. Bandages which often extend to the groin or axillae
    e. All of the above

5. Reasons for failure of complete decongestive physiotherapy include:
    a. Metastatic cancer
    b. Failure to maintain a reasonable weight
    c. Failure of the patient to adhere to the treatment regimen
    d. Undiagnosed systemic disease such as renal or cardiac insufficiency
    e. All of the above

Answers: 1d, 2b, 3e, 4e, 5e

CHAPTER **16**

DIABETIC FOOT WOUNDS

CHAPTER SIXTEEN OVERVIEW

NOTES

DIABETIC FOOT WOUNDS

Khurram H. Khan, Todd A. Derksen, John S. Steinberg

INTRODUCTION

The primary goal in the treatment of diabetic foot ulcers is to attain closure as expeditiously as possible. Over 85% of all diabetic related lower extremity amputations are preceded by an ulceration. It is well noted that quick resolution of a foot ulcer combined with appropriate intervention to reduce the rate of recurrence can lower the risk of developing a secondary infection and can decrease the probability of lower extremity amputation in the patient with diabetes.

The multidisciplinary healthcare team approach for the treatment of diabetic foot ulcers is efficacious and has been proven to improve the outcome and long-term prognosis of these patients. The foot specialist and/or primary care provider is often the first professional contacted for evaluation and management of the diabetic foot ulcer (Figure 1 and 2) and therefore can serve as an effective "gate keeper" for the purpose of integrating the other specialties in the treatment of this pathology. This chapter incorporates the essential principles of diabetic wound care recommended by the American Diabetes Association (ADA), the Agency for Health Care Policy and Research, the Center for Disease Control (CDC), and the U.S. Department of Health and Human Services (HHS).

EPIDEMIOLOGY

Diabetes is the sixth leading cause of death in the United States. According to the CDC, from 1980 to 2005, the prevalence of diabetes more than doubled from 5.8 million to 14.7 million. About 800,000 new cases of diabetes are diagnosed in the United States each year. Approximately 20.8 million Americans, or 7% of the population, have diabetes and 6.2 million of those are undiagnosed due to the silent nature of most symptoms. One in every 400–600 children and adolescents have type 1 diabetes.

In 1991, the U.S. Department of Health and Human Services, Public Health Service published a report on Diabetes and Chronic Disabling Conditions. Healthy People 2000 listed the national health promotion and disease prevention objectives. One Healthy People 2000 goal was to reduce the incidence of diabetes to 2.5 cases per 1,000 people and reduce the prevalence to 25 cases per 1,000 people. These objectives were never met. Healthy People 2010 seeks to decrease lower extremity amputations

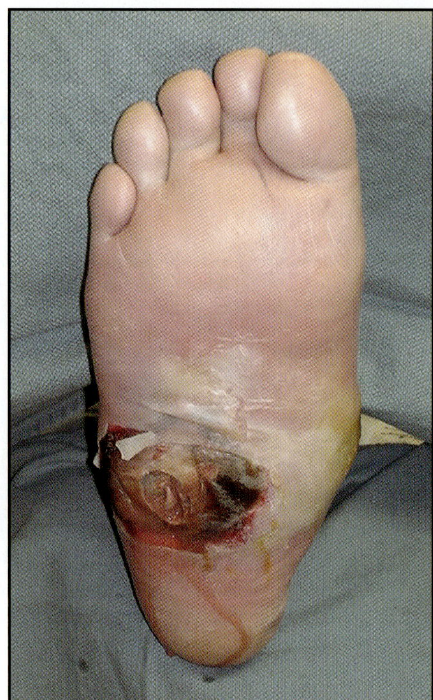

Figure 1. Infected Diabetic Foot Ulceration with involvement of soft tissues and bone.

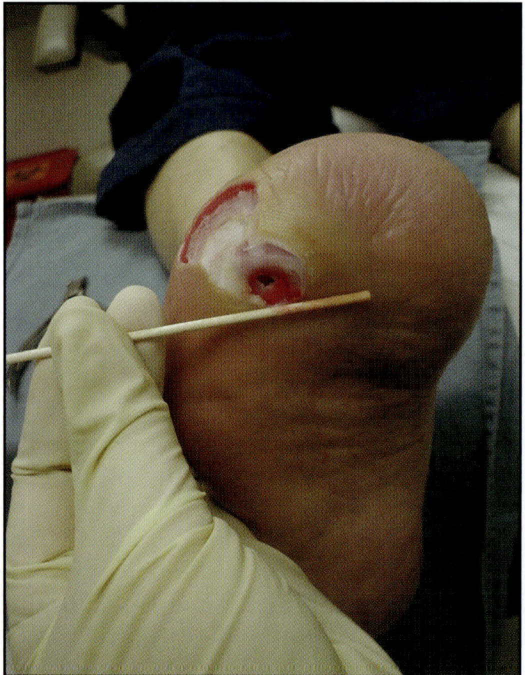

Figure 2. Patient with prior midfoot amputation now presents with new pressure ulceration and deep probing sinus.

secondary to diabetes and its complications to 11 per 1,000. These lower extremity complications in patients with diabetes significantly impact the overall wellbeing of the patient, and therefore have commanded much recent attention in the public health arena. An average of 54,000 diabetic foot amputations were performed each year between 1989 and 1992. In 1996 the number increased to over 86,000 amputations. Cost is one evident reason for this increased public health attention to lower extremity amputations in diabetics. The total direct and indirect dollars spent each year on lower extremity amputation was over 132 billion dollars in 2002, and the average cost of a transtibial amputation is between 40 and 60 thousand dollars. Yet in 2004 only 67.7% of diabetics reported receiving a foot examination within the last year and 65.8% reported examining their feet on a daily basis.

Etiology

The lifetime risk for foot ulceration in a person with diabetes is estimated at 15%. Most foot ulcerations are plantar lesions which result from neuropathy in the face of increased pressure. The pivotal events that cause skin breakdown, and ultimately foot ulceration, can be identified in three main categories:

1. Low pressure over prolonged exposure periods of time, i.e., pressure sores from bed rest. It takes ~ 2 lbs/in^2 to cause blanching of the skin. This amount of pressure over 15 minutes negatively affects microcirculation and tissue oxygenation. Common anatomic sites for these ulcers to present are the heel and the sacrum. These are also known as pressure ulcers, bed sores, or decubitus ulcerations.

2. High pressure over a short period of time, i.e., puncture wounds from a foreign object. Pressure >100 lbs/in^2 (70 N/ cm^2) will puncture the skin. This is seen most commonly on the plantar surfaces of the foot from puncture wounds due to a metallic or wooden object. These generally present as acute infections and can have a high risk for amputation due to the possible inoculation from a penetrating object.

3. Moderate pressure in a repetitive setting, i.e., neuropathic ulcers from weight bearing. This is the primary causative factor in plantar foot ulcer development in diabetics. Multiple studies have attempted to quantify this pressure but no clear pressure threshold has been demonstrated. However, peak plantar pressures analyzed with computerized gait analysis systems have demonstrated 70 N/cm^2 (100 psi) as a focal point. Repetitive pressures in excess of this have a high risk for neuropathic ulceration (sensitivity of 70.0% and specificity of 65.1%).

Risk Factors

The etiology of ulceration has been studied extensively. Most literature sources agree that there are three fundamental risk factors for foot ulceration. These risk factors, which have been demonstrated time and time again, include neuropathy, deformity/limited joint mobility, and pivotal trauma. Other factors which are less proven but still associated either directly or indirectly with ulcers include ischemia, male sex, and previous history of ulceration.

NEUROPATHY

Peripheral neuropathy is the most common type of neuropathy affecting persons with diabetes. It is a key factor in the development of diabetic foot ulcers. Neuropathy is generally considered to be a multifactorial disorder incorporating metabolic and vascular defects, which result in neuronal demyelination and atrophy. The effects of these mechanisms produce a combination of motor, autonomic and sensory deficits.

Motor deficit is exemplified by weakness of the anterior tibial compartment and pedal intrinsic muscular atrophy leading to digital instability and associated increased peak pressures around the resultant deformities. Autonomic neuropathy is associated with multiple foot complications including dry, fissured skin secondary to insufficient sweat gland activity. The fissured skin can lead to ulceration and infection if left untreated. Bounding pedal pulses and a pathologic increase in pedal perfusion can develop from decreased arteriolar tone and the resultant uncontrolled vasodilatation reactive to the autonomic dysfunction.

Sensory deficiency as a result of diabetic peripheral polyneuropathy is a commonly associated finding and has been identified as an important risk factor in the development of diabetic foot ulcers. The probability of developing these wounds increases dramatically when sensation is lost in the presence of faulty biomechanics and resultant deformity. These areas of bony prominence yield increased foot pressures and a heightened level of risk for skin and tissue breakdown.

One of the most dramatic and potentially devastating outcomes of peripheral sensory/autonomic neuropathy is the development of Charcot neuroarthropathy. Charcot is a disease process where multiple bones in the foot become demineralized and fracture concomitantly. These multiple fractures collapse and consolidate to form a malunion unless there is an intervention. This malunion then disrupts normal biomechanics and frequently results in plantar bony prominences of the foot. One of the most common deformities is the rocker bottom foot (Figures 3 and 4). The actual pathogenesis of Charcot is still unknown but the predisposing factors are peripheral neuropathy with increased peripheral blood flow. The resultant foot deformities from Charcot neuroarthropathy are especially worrisome since the foot is already insensate and now may have significant bony deformity which can further increase peak plantar pressures and the risk for ulceration.

Various diagnostic tests are employed when the clinician is assessing the level and degree of peripheral sensory neuropathy. Two of the more commonly used tests are the 5.07 Semmes-Weinstein Monofilament (SWMF) and the Vibration Perception Threshold exam (VPT). The Semmes-Weinstein device is a simple monofilament of nylon which delivers 10g of force when applied to the skin and is an easily reproduced exam. The Vibration Perception Threshold exam is commonly performed with a tuning fork, but is more accurately performed with a calibrated electrical device known as the Biothesiometer® or VPT Meter. A study in Diabetes Care, 2000 showed that clinical examination and a 5.07 SWMF test had 99% sensitivity in identifying patients at risk for foot ulcerations especially when the tests are used in conjunction with each other. These tests should be repeated twice yearly for progressively developing neuropathic conditions and for those persons at high risk for developing loss of protective sensation.

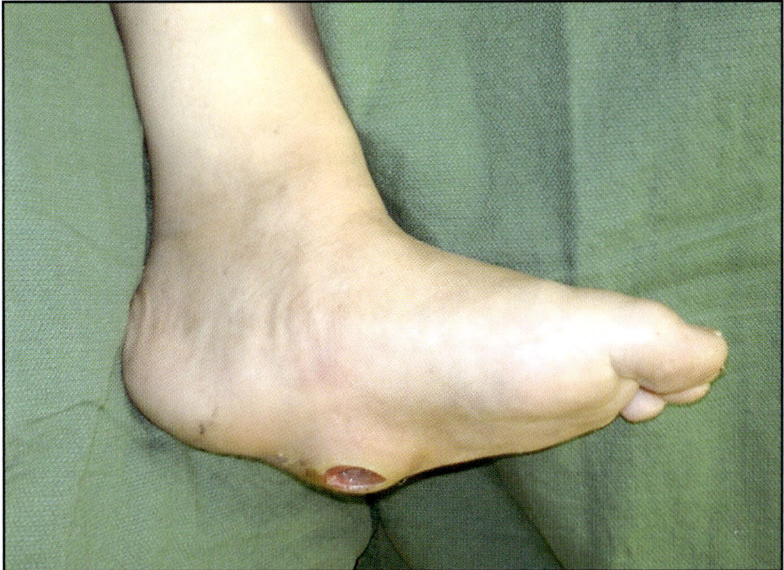

Figure 3. Severe Charcot Foot Deformity with plantar ulceration.

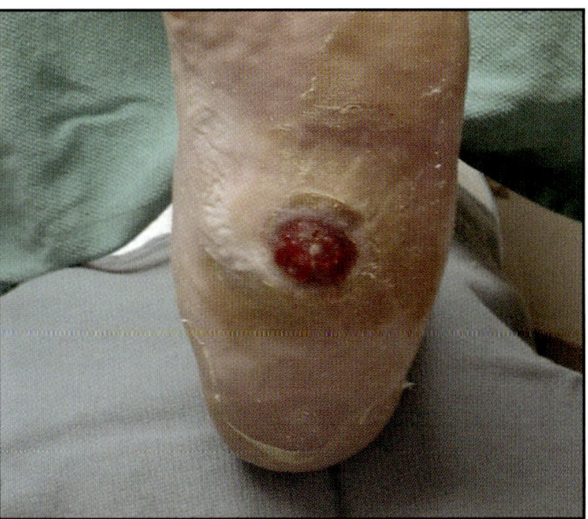

Figure 4. Typical Charcot Plantar Midfoot Ulceration due to rocker bottom foot type with increased pressures.

Rigid Deformity/Limited Joint Mobility/Pivotal Event

Recognizing biomechanically altered gait patterns and prescribing the appropriate off-loading is imperative if one is to attain healing of an ulcer and decrease the probability of developing a new one.

High compressive and frictional forces occur around areas of deformity. These deformities can include simple foot ailments such as bunions, hammertoes, and prominent metatarsals. Multiple techniques are available to off-load areas of increased peak pressure. The use of simple felt or plastizote insoles for redistribution of weight bearing forces is commonly prescribed in the treatment of an acute ulceration. Recently, some removable walking casts have been shown to be very effective and statistically as efficacious as the total contact cast. However, the total contact cast is still considered the gold standard for off loading since it is a custom molded device and applied on a weekly basis to allow for regular wound care to the site. Once healed, long-term management of the patient may incorporate use of custom molded orthoses and/or specialized supportive footwear to decrease the probability of redeveloping an ulcer.

VASCULAR DISEASE

The risk factors associated with development of peripheral atherosclerosis disease are similar to those associated with the development of coronary atherosclerosis.

Those are:
- Genetics
- Obesity
- Diabetes
- Smoking
- Dyslipidemia
- Hypertension
- Hypercoagulabilty
- Hyperhomocysteinemia

Non-invasive vascular studies are a helpful screening tool for peripheral vascular disease in the patient with diabetes. Angiograms and other invasive vascular studies are more conclusive and are generally warranted in patients who are likely to require a peripheral arterial bypass or an endovascular procedure. Coordinated care with an interventional radiologist, vascular surgeon, and / or cardiologist is an integral component of the team approach.

Persons with diabetes and lower extremity peripheral arterial disease have a very consistent pattern noted anatomically: Multisegmental occlusion distal to the trifurcation of the popliteal artery at the level just distal to the knee. Vascular reconstructive surgery of the impaired limb may be required prior to debridement and/or partial amputation foot surgery. Other options include endovascular surgeries (i.e., laser/plaque excision) for which long term yields are still widely debated but show significant promise. Vasodilator medications have not been found to promote wound healing in the ischemic foot. The newest research area is in gene therapy for reestablishing microcirculation, and is currently undergoing phase III trials in centers all over the world. These new non-surgical treatment modalities from pharmaceuticals to gene therapy may lead to a new field of vascular medicine which would specialize in the medical management of peripheral arterial disease.

The peripheral arterial disease (PAD) diagnosis carries a worse 5, 10, and 15 year prognosis than breast cancer or Hodgkin's disease. Fifty-five percent of those with PAD die from myocardial infarction.

In the New England Journal of Medicine in 1998, a study of 1300 non-diabetics and 1059 diabetics assessed long term outcome over the course of seven years. Patients with diabetes had a 20% incidence for myocardial infarction vs. 4% in non-diabetics. In patients with a previous history of myocardial infarction, there was a 45% incidence of repeat MI in persons with diabetes, vs. 20% incidence in persons without diabetes (14).

Classifications

Wound assessment calls for the use of a common language that can be easily interpreted from one practitioner to the next. Wounds can be described by: location, size (such as cross sectional measurements), depth and/or level of tissue involved, color and type of wound surface (i.e., red granulation tissue, fibrous or necrotic), exudate, odor, sinus track and/or tunneling. A description of the surrounding tissue should note such factors as cellulitis, edema, color (rubious, pallorous) and/or callus tissue.

Classifications were developed to bring these descriptions together to help simplify and help standardize charting so as to be reproducible from clinician to clinician.

Basis for classification, including:

- Staging
- Predicting outcome
- Identifying management strategy

One of the first and most often used classification systems is the Meggit/Wagner Classification 0–5, where:

0: Skin Intact
1: Superficial ulcer without penetrating to the deep layers
2: Deeper tissues involved and there is abscess
3: Deep involvement with osteomyelitis
4: Gangrene, localized
5: Gangrene, generalized

Basic structure of this classification is:
0–2: Graduation based on depth
3: Deep and infected
4–5: Gangrene (i.e., critical limb ischemia)

A problem with this type of wound classification system is that one can not combine different categories of pathology in order to accurately identify and define the multiple processes occurring concurrently. For example, an infected wound is easily classified according to the Meggit/Wagner System, but an infected/ischemic wound is difficult to properly assess and describe with this limited system.

The ADA consensus on ulcer classification was developed to help with communication between non-specialists in primary care and specialists. It is linked to an action plan and is loosely compatible with the Wagner System.

ADA Classification:

0: Intact

1: Superficial

2: Deep

3: Complicated (ischemia, infection, both)

A wound classification system for diabetic foot wounds was developed at the University of Texas (UT) Health Science Center at San Antonio, Texas. The UT Wound Classification System is based on depth of wound and state of wound (i.e., ischemic, infected) (see Table 1).

The UT Wound Classification System takes into account only the known risk factors (see Table 2) that ultimately influence the prognosis of a given wound site (depth, infection, and ischemia)

TABLE 1. UNIVERSITY OF TEXAS CLASSIFICATION SYSTEM FOR DIABETIC FOOT WOUND

Stage/Comorbidites: "Is the wound infected, ischemic, or both?"		Grade/Depth: "How deep is the wound?"			
		0	**I**	**II**	**III**
	A	Pre- or post-ulcerative lesion completely epithelialized	Superficial wound not involving tendon, capsule or bone	Wound penetrating to tendon or capsule	Wound penetrating to bone or joint
	B	Pre- or post-ulcerative lesion completely epithelialized with infection	Superficial wound not involving tendon, capsule or bone with infection	Wound penetrating to tendon or capsule with infection	Wound penetrating to bone or joint with infection
	C	Pre- or post-ulcerative lesion completely epithelialized with ischemia	Superficial wound not involving tendon, capsule or bone with ischemia	Wound penetrating to tendon or capsule with ischemia	Wound penetrating to bone or joint with ischemia
	D	Pre- or post-ulcerative lesion completely epithelialized with infection and ischemia	Superfical wound not involving tendon, capsule or bone with infection and ischemia	Wound penetrating to tendon or capsule with infection and ischemia	Wound penetrating to bone or joint with infection and ischemia

From: Armstrong DG, Lavery LA, Harkless LB. Diabetes Care 1998; 21: 855-859.
Also from Lavery LA, Armstrong DG, Harkless LB. J Foot Ankle Surg 1996; 35:528-531

TABLE 2. UNIVERSITY OF TEXAS RISK CLASSIFICATION SYSTEM FOR DIABETIC FOOT WOUNDS

Category 0: No Neuropathy	Category 1: Neuropathy, No Deformity	Category 2: Neurpathy, with Deformity	Category 3: History of Pathology
Patient diagnosed with DM Protective sensation intact Ankle-Brachial Index (ABI) > 0.80 and toe systolic pressure > 45 mm Hg Foot deformity may be present No history of ulceration	Protective sensation absent ABI > 0.80 and toe systolic pressure > 45 mm Hg No history of ulceration No history of neuroarthropathy No foot deformity	Protective sensation absent ABI > 0.80 and toe systolic pressure > 45 mm Hg No history of ulceration No history of neuroarthropathy Foot deformity present	Protective sensation absent ABI > 0.80 and toe systolic pressure > 45 mm Hg History of ulceration, amputation or neuroarthropathy Foot deformity present
Treatment	**Treatment**	**Treatment**	**Treatment**
Possible shoe accommodations Patient education Follow-up every 6–12 months	Possible shoe accommodations Patient education Quarterly visits every 3–4 months	Custom-molded, extra depth shoes Possible prophylactic surgery Patient education Follow-up every 2–3 months	Custom-molded, extra depth shoes Possible prophylactic surgery Patient education Follow-up every 1–2 months
Category 4A: Neuropathic Wound	**Category 4B: Acute Charcot's joint (Neuroarthropathy)**	**Category 5: Infected Diabetic Foot**	**Category 6: Ischemic Limb**
All UT stage A wounds Protective sensation absent ABI > 0.80 and toe systolic pressure > 45 mm Hg Foot deformity present No acute neuroarthropathy	Protective sensation absent ABI > 0.80 and toe systolic pressure > 45 mm Hg Non-infected neuropathic ulceration may be present Diabetic neuroarthropathy present	All UT stage B wounds Protective sensation may be present Infected wound Neuroarthropathy may be present	All UT stage C, D wounds Protective sensation may be present ABI < 0.80 or toe systolic pressure < 45 mm Hg or pedial transcutaneous oxygen tension < 40 mm Hg Ulceration may be present
Treatment	**Treatment**	**Treatment**	**Treatment**
Wound care regimen Pressure reduction program Possible surgical intervention Patient education Frequent follow-up visits	Wound care regimen if ulcer present Pressure reduction program Thermometric and radiographic monitoring Patient education Frequent follow-up visits	Debridement of infected, non-viable tissue and/or bone as indicated Possible hospitalization, antibiotic treatment regimen Medical management of diabetes	Vascular consultation, possible revascularization If infection present, treatment same as for Category 5

From: Armstrong DG, Lavery LA, Harkless LB. J Amer Pod Med Assn *1996; 86:311-316.*
Also from Lavery LA, Armstrong DG, Vela SF, et al. Arch Intern Med *1998; 158(2);157-162.*

NATURAL HISTORY
Treatment Options

The essential therapeutic objectives for the management of any plantar ulcer include:

- Establishing the level of vascular perfusion, and introducing measures to correct it as discussed above.
- Eradicating/protecting against infection via appropriate debridement
- Off-loading the areas of greatest pressure
- Maintaining a moist wound environment
- Maintaining metabolic control and nutritional status
- Frequently evaluating the response to directed treatment
- Patient education and compliance

Management of the diabetic foot ulcer should be initiated with a detailed and proper assessment of its etiology. This incorporates a careful medical history and physical examination with appropriate use of non-invasive studies. A complete examination involves assessing many factors, such as: the peripheral vascular status, neuropathy and sensory deficiency, limited joint mobility and signs that may suggest the presence of soft tissue infection or osteomyelitis, and secondary factors including serum glucose levels, glycosylated hemoglobin (HbA1c), CBC with differential, hepatic and renal profiles with electrolyte balance, nutritional status.

Some members of a team-approach include: podiatry, vascular surgery, plastic surgery, internal medicine, infectious disease, endocrinology, nephrology, cardiology, radiology, orthopedics, orthotist/prosthetist, nursing, and a certified diabetes educator with a nutritional background. Depending upon the degree of severity and the contributing factors, additional specialists may need to be consulted. Patient compliance and knowledge of their disease has been identified as a significant factor in the expected prognosis and the prevalence of both ulceration and limb loss.

DEBRIDEMENT

The removal of non-viable/necrotic and infected tissue is an integral component in the treatment of ulcerative wounds. The types of debridement available include: surgical, mechanical, autolytic, enzymatic and larval. Autolytic debridement occurs naturally in a moist wound environment when arterial perfusion and venous drainage are maintained. The best use of enzymatic debridement is generally as a follow up technique to surgical and mechanical debridement. This staged debridement method will serve to efficiently remove the gross, non-viable tissue by surgical and mechanical means, while leaving the maintenance and finishing debridement to the enzymatic component. Additionally, enzymatic debridement is employed when the patient is not a candidate for surgical or mechanical debridement methods. Mechanical debridement has been demonstrated to be of direct benefit to the wound site by ridding the site of non-viable/necrotic tissue, allowing cell activation through active bleeding, and through stimulation of the healing pathways. Wet-to-dry dressings were previously used as a common means of mechanically debriding the wound site but are generally non-specific and have therefore been mostly replaced with wet-to-moist dressings. Irrigation is another form of mechanical wound debridement and is commonly utilized at the time of surgery as well as during dressing changes. Flush irrigation under pressure (4–15 psi) appears to be more effective in reducing the bacterial count than low-pressure flush or scrubbing with a saline-soaked sponge. Additionally, pulse lavage systems can be efficacious in removing foreign debris. A 35 ml syringe with an 18-gauge needle or a 19-gauge angiocath delivers pressure at 8 psi and is an alternative measure for providing pressure irrigation when pulse lavage is not available in the operating room or not practical for daily dressing changes. Sharp surgical

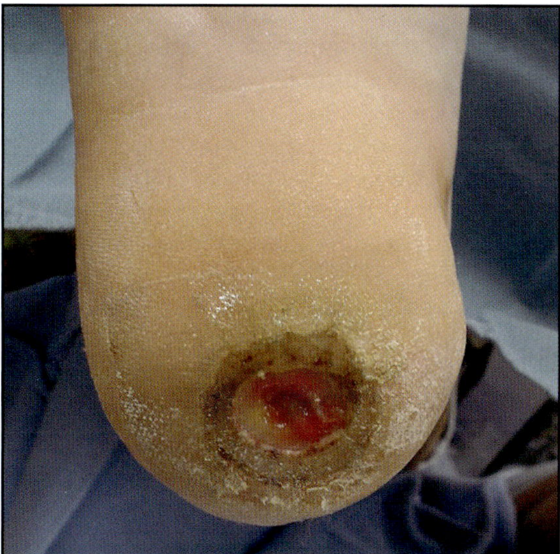

Figure 5. Plantar heel ulceration pre-debridement.

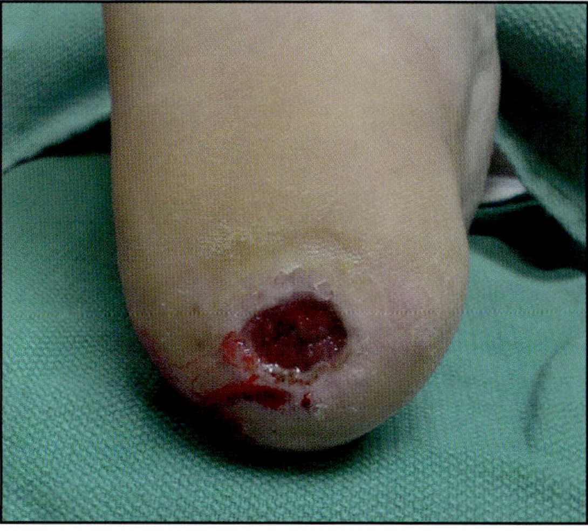

Figure 6. Plantar heel ulceration post-debridement.

debridement is primarily performed with basic hand instrumentation of blades, scissors, curettes, ronguers, and tissue nippers (Figures 5 and 6).

Regular wound debridements have been shown to be effective in stimulating healing of recalcitrant ulcers by converting a chronic wound environment into an acute wound environment. This technique serves to positively influence the nature of wound exudate and the bioactive environment. Hydrosurgery (Smith and Nephew Versajet®) is based in fluid jet technology and has been introduced for the use of selective surgical debridement of wounds. This technology has been recently approved by the FDA for use in burns. Its ability to excise and aspirate the unwanted tissue employs the Venturi effect. The device provides for the ability to select the strength of debridement and therefore facilitating the debridement of wounds in very thin tissue layers. This removes only what's necessary and leaves viable tissue behind for ultimate use in limb salvage.

Larval therapy is another modality available for wound debridement. While this modality has been around for greater than 70 years it has been largely ignored until just a few years ago. While there are no randomized, controlled studies to report on the efficacy of larval therapy for diabetic foot wounds, there are several studies showing that larval therapy is effective and efficient in decubitus ulcers and venous stasis ulcers. There are also numerous case series and retrospective studies offering some level of evidence in diabetic wounds. In one of the larger retrospective studies, Sherman concluded that among diabetic cohorts at a VA institution, maggot debridement was more effective and efficient then their conventional protocol in treating chronic wounds (74). The combination of evidence from larval therapy in all types of wounds suggests that this modality, while not necessarily a first choice, should no longer be a last choice. There are certainly some social hurdles to overcome before larval therapy can be accepted as mainstream therapy. For more details on debridement see the Emhoff and Ferro chapter entitled "Wound Debridement."

INFECTION

Infection needs to be treated both locally and systemically. Systemic interventions consist of oral or parenteral antibiotics and good glycemic control. Local intervention consists of surgical management and local wound care. Surgical management, consisting of drainage, decompression and debridement, is a key component in the management of infected wounds and includes the removal of all non-viable tissue including bone from the wound as well as the surrounding callus tissue. This aggressive form of wound debridement on a regular basis can expedite the rate at which a wound heals and has been shown in a recent study to increase the probability of attaining full secondary closure. As a surgical disease, osteomyelitis requires resection of bone and possibly associated joint structures or even partial amputation of the foot. With respect to the assessment of infection, it is indeed the overall clinical impression that is of primary importance; culture results are viewed as one aspect of the patient's total presentation.

Medical therapy should be guided, based on culture and sensitivity. For non-limb threatening infections, treatment should be aimed at Staph and Strep.

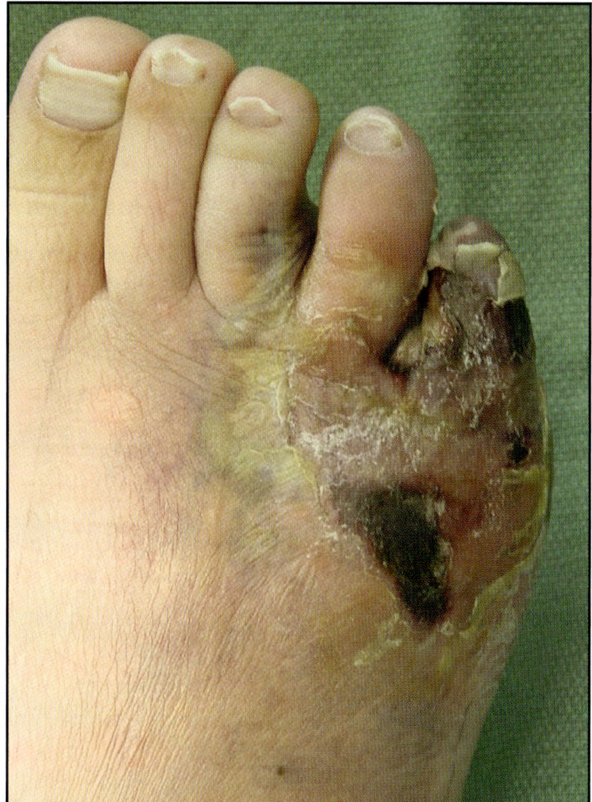

Figure 7. Interdigital ulceration with ischemia and infection.

Most diabetic foot infections are polymicrobial (Figure 7) and thus require broad-spectrum and/or mixed antibiotic coverage initiated empirically. The medications utilized are modified based primarily upon clinical response; culture results and, when needed, repeated cultures are also considered in the overall therapeutic management of the diabetic foot infection. For more information see the Le Frock chapter entitled "Post-Operative Surgical Site Infections (SSIs) and Non-Necrotizing Skin and Soft Tissue Infections."

WOUND CARE

Generally a moist wound environment has been shown to facilitate the healing process. Additionally, the bandage applied should provide protection from trauma and local contamination, allow gaseous exchange, thermally insulate the wound, absorb excess exudates and provide for removal without traumatizing the wound surface. The type of dressing used varies depending on the size and depth of the defect, its location on the foot and the quality of the wound surface. Wet to moist dressings are a common method of wound management that require frequent reassessment and dressing changes up to several times daily to balance the wound between maceration and desiccation. The solution used in the wet to moist dressing can be tailored to the wound. Normal saline may be used in clean wounds while dilute Dakin's solution or dilute acetic acid may be used to decrease the bacterial load in grossly infected wounds. Another wound characteristic important in the selection of the type of product to use varies between different degrees of absorbent dressings for exudative wounds versus those that encourage moisture for dry non-exudative defects.

Categories of wound dressings are discussed in detail by V. Larson Lohr and C.A. Fleck in their chapter entitled "Modern Wound Dressings—Principles, Form and Function," which includes the following:

1. Hydrocolloids, alginates, or foams: absorbent dressings for exudative wounds.
2. Films or hydrocolloids: occlusive or semi-occlusive dressings for dry non-exudative wounds
3. Hydrogels: add moisture to dry wounds and facilitate autolytic debridement.
4. Impregnated dressings: decrease drying, prevent dressing adherence and reduce bacterial content within the wound (i.e., Adaptic® or Xeroform®)
5. Topical medications such as antibiotics and antiseptics.
6. Silver impregnated dressing for superficially infected wounds with a high bioburden (surface bacterial load)
7. Negative pressure dressing removes exudates and promotes formation of granular tissue.

Chronic wounds are those in which healing has terminated or is not occurring in a timely fashion. The length of time a wound must exist without signs of appreciable healing until it is considered chronic is not well defined. Ulcers are in constant evolution and regular reassessment of an ulcer's response to a given treatment program is necessary to avoid continuing ineffective interventions and to prevent over utilization of healthcare resources. Once it has been established that a particular treatment is ineffective, a systematic evaluation of the basic etiological factors usually provides the information necessary to alter the plan of care and re-establish the healing process.

The primary goal in treating the chronic ulcer is to convert it to an acute wound that will then contain the active matrix needed for healing. The basic principles of treatment discussed for the acute ulcer apply here and include: providing the required arterial perfusion, off-loading pressure from the involved area, resolving any infective processes, surgically debriding necrotic tissue, and assessing patient compliance. Overall systemic management is imperative. Such factors as chronic hyperglycemia with serum levels of 180–200 or higher (HbA1c >9) can interfere with wound healing. Thus, reassessment requires analysis of all aspects of the patients care and, as mentioned previously, a multidisciplinary approach is most efficacious toward achieving that end.

When all of the above have been addressed and active signs of healing have not developed, then genetically engineered wound care products, such as endogenous or exogenous growth factors or bioengineered alterative tissues may be helpful to resolve the chronic wound. When used at the proper time in the proper wound, these agents have been shown to provide an optimal wound environment and encourage chemotaxis and mitogenesis of platelets, neutrophils, fibroblasts, monocytes, as well as other components that form the cellular basis for good wound healing.

There are numerous biologic agents available that may promote wound healing if they are used in the appropriate setting. Regranex®, a hydrogel with recombinant DNA platelet-derived growth factor, has been shown in clinical studies to be of benefit in some non-healing ulcers. The tissue engineered human dermal equivalent used in Dermagraft® has also shown promise in clinical trials for some non-healing wounds. Apligraf®, another living cell bioengineered alternative tissue product, is a construct that contains both dermal and epidermal cells in an attempt to more closely approximate the structure and biology of human skin. Integra is a bovine collagen based biologic product that is now being utilized to granulate over bone and other deep tissues. GraftJacket and other cadaver based products are also being used with some success. Negative pressure wound therapy has been shown to be very effective in closing deep wounds, and reducing the time to heal ulcers by removing excess exudates, decreasing bacterial load, promoting granulation tissue formation, maintaining a moist wound environment, and helping to draw wound edges together. It has been shown that wounds with $TcpO_2$ values less than 20 mm Hg have a 39x increased risk of non-healing. Systemic hyperbaric oxygen (HBO2) of 100% O_2 at 2–2.4 absolute atmospheres has been shown to produce O_2 partial pressures of 1200 mm Hg within arterial circulation. Although a critical $TcpO_2$ value to predict healing with HBO2 has not been established a periwound value of greater than 200 mm Hg while receiving HBO2 treatment is a strong indicator that the wound will heal. The increased partial pressure of O_2 increases the diffusion distance of O_2 into tissue from 60 microns to up to 250 microns. Several randomized, controlled trials have demonstrated the benefit of HBO2 in the management of diabetic foot ulcers (see the chapter by C.E. Fife entitled "Hyperbaric Oxygen Therapy Applications in Wound Care"). However, HBO2 is a modality reserved for those ulcers that have a $TcpO_2$ less than 40 mm Hg because tissues with values above 40 mm Hg should be able to heal without supplemental oxygen. Since most treatment options will only be effective if there are sufficient arterioles and capillaries present, HBO2 is used to generate them. HBO2 therapy has been shown to produce neovascularization, significantly reduce the risk of major amputation, and may improve the chance of healing. Current Medicare reimbursemant policy limits the use of HBO2 to diabetic foot ulcers of Wagner Grade III or higher.

While systemic HBO2 may be of benefit, another modality, topical oxygen applied only to the extremity has not been clearly shown to be effective in clinical trials. A variety of other modalities have also been advocated for the chronic wound such as electrical stimulation, end-diastolic compression boot, ultrasound, ESWT and others. Efficacy for many of these has not been clearly demonstrated and studies regarding their use are still pending.

OFF-LOADING

The study of pedorthics is concerned with the design, manufacture, modification and fit of shoes and foot orthoses to alleviate problems caused by disease, congenital condition, overuse or injury. Pedorthic devices can help reduce shear, shock, and transfer from sensitive or painful areas. Proper treatment can correct or support flexible deformities while serving to accommodate fixed deformities through control of motion and joint function.

Many modifications can be made to shoes which enable treatment of symptoms. Some of these modifications can be made to the sole and flare of the shoe such as in the treatment of Charcot deformity/ulceration with rocker soles.

Extended steel shank modifications can be used to accommodate for altered foot function following amputations of the forefoot. Cushion heel modifications can be used to absorb impact and reduce stress to the heel and ankle. These modifications can diminish the moment of force that bends the knee as well as reduce the demand for ankle plantarflexion.

Total contact orthoses are used to help relieve pressure and support/control joint motion. There are many materials that are available to help with the proper function of the orthoses including trilaminar material to make a device accommodative. Rigid material can be used to make an orthotic functional by physically modifying the contact surface of the plantar foot. There are many moldable and non-moldable coverings which can be used in combination.

Custom molded shoes can be used for those with a severe deformity that will not be accommodated in over-the-counter shoes or devices. People with amputations or unusual foot sizes may also benefit. Reducing pressure on the diabetic foot ulcer is a vital component of effective wound management. A small or superficial ulcer can benefit from the use of a healing sandal made from a surgical shoe containing an insole of felt or plastizote, which can then be apertured to properly off load ulcers. Plastizote can be custom molded to the foot or, depending on its density, can be used for its thermoplastic properties to dynamically mold around areas of increased pressure during ambulation. It should be noted however, that if the etiology of the ulceration involves ankle equinus, it will likely not respond to a shoe type device. Rather, these ulcerations require immobilization at the ankle (cast or removable cast walker boot) in order to remove the plantar pressures caused by tendo-achilles contracture. Total avoidance of weight bearing with the use of bed rest, crutch assisted ambulation, or wheel chair are the most effective methods to off-load the ulcerated foot, however patient compliance to these devices is generally low at best. The total contact cast has been accepted as the best overall method to reduce weight from a specific area of increased pressure and apply a more even distribution of weight bearing forces across the entire forefoot. Some studies have shown a Removable Cast Walker can be modified to function as a TCC coined "instant total contact cast." These modifications to a standard RCW to increase patient adherence to pressure off-loading may increase both the proportion of ulcers that heal and the rate of healing of diabetic neuropathic wounds.

Following healing of an ulcer, walking/running style footwear and extra-depth shoes can be accommodated with various orthoses for long-term management. In the presence of significant deformity, custom molded shoes can be used to accommodate deformity and decrease pressure on areas of prominence and thus decrease the possibility of recurrence of a diabetic ulcer. Molded ankle foot orthoses and similar devices (CROW) may support the otherwise unstable foot and ankle segments and thus decrease ulcerative risk. Reducing the possibility (or the degree) of obesity may be helpful in decreasing plantar pressures in the ulcer prone foot and should be part of the overall goals of a nutrition management program. More details are provided in the chapter by Bosker and LaFontaine entitled "Orthotics and Prosthetics in Wound Care."

SURGERY

The goal of curative and prophylactic diabetic foot surgery is to heal any existing ulcer and/or prevent the development of future ulcers. It is achieved by decreasing focal pressures through surgical reduction of associated bony prominence or soft tissue dysfunction while preserving pedal stability. Surgery is performed either in response to an ulcer history (prior or current) or as prophylactic surgery to decrease the probability of developing future ulcers. It is also indicated in cases of non-reversible ischemia resulting in amputation. Surgery includes incision and drainage of a deep abscess, debridement of necrotic tissue for the acute active infection, and ablative with partial or total foot amputation. Definitive surgery is applied with vascular analysis and intervention as needed. The literature supports the conclusion that diabetes is not a contraindication for prophylactic foot surgery and is especially worth considering for those patients who cannot be accommodated by footwear modifications and related orthoses. Pre-operative assessment of the vascular supply is the key to success and noninvasive tests should be performed to ensure adequate blood supply for healing.

Amputation is an unfortunate, but common sequela of ulceration and the level of amputation is determined by the area in which viable bone and soft tissue are noted. Additionally, the specific procedure selected takes into consideration the anticipated post-operative functional capacity of the patient. A variety of forefoot, midfoot, rearfoot, and leg amputations are available when other treatments fail.

Closure can be achieved through primary, secondary, or delayed primary means. Secondary wound healing is commonly utilized for patients when dealing with an infection that necessitates tissue resection to the extent that primary closure is not a viable option. Keeping the wound open allows for daily irrigation and wound packing may be required. Delayed primary closure may be used when a wound infection has resolved. Plastic surgical techniques utilizing skin grafts and flaps are other options that may be utilized to avoid secondary wound healing and accelerate ulcer resolution. Primary closure can be considered for non-infected wounds or those where there is confidence that the infection has been fully eradicated during the definitive surgery. All patients must be assessed on an individual basis for the selection of the surgical procedure and closure technique that best meets their needs. A recent study has shown that transmetatarsal amputation healing can be expected in a majority of diabetic patients after adequate revascularization, but cannot be predicted by angiographic findings. It was also shown that primary closure in a non-infected amputation had a better healing rate than when the TMA was left open (12% vs. 58% p<0.01)

There is also strong evidence that an Achilles tendon lengthening (TAL) should be considered/performed for forefoot ulcerations. Mueller (69) demonstrated in a randomized clinical study that patients treated with either a total contact cast (TCC) alone or with a TAL and a TCC healed their ulcerations at an equal rate. However, the patients that received the TAL were 4x less likely to reulcerate in the first seven months and 2.1x less likely at two years. While the long term financial or mortality effect has not been investigated, it stands to reason that if there is no longer an ulcer present, both of these important factors are reduced.

CONCLUSION

The literature consistently demonstrates that the treatment of diabetic foot ulcers is best accomplished by utilizing a multidisciplinary team approach. The primary care doctor is the key in coordinating the integration of the necessary specialists in the management of the ulcerated patient. It is of utmost importance to coordinate the efforts of everyone involved because each action has a cause and effect that must be balanced. For example, local debridement of necrotic/infected tissue will not heal in the presence of untreated systemic infection, ischemia, or poor blood glucose control. Any one of the prior mentioned interventions would be completely ineffective without the others. Members of the "team approach" may include physicians in any of the following specialties: family practice, internal medicine, endocrinology, infectious disease, neurology, radiology and imaging, vascular disease, podiatrists/orthopedics, orthotics and prosthetics, and others as necessary. Therefore, treatment of diabetic foot ulcers requires a thorough understanding of local and systemic factors involved in the development of open wounds and their healing mechanisms. Necrotic tissue must be removed and excised. Additionally, weight bearing forces and shear must be removed from the wound surface through effective off-loading. The ultimate goal of wound healing can only be attained with coordinated surgical and medical interventions which serve to create the proper environment for healing.

REFERENCES

1. Centers for Disease Control and Prevention. National diabetes fact sheet: general information and national estimates on diabetes in the United States, 2005. Atlanta, GA: *U.S. Department of Health and Human Services, Centers for Disease Control and Prevention* 2005.

2. Frykberg RG. Diabetic foot ulcers: current concepts, *J Foot Ankle Surg* 37:440-446, 1998.

3. Pham H, Armstrong DG Harvey C, et al. Screening techniques to identify people at high risk for diabetic foot ulceration: a prospective multicenter trial. *Diabetes Care* 2000 May;23(5):6006-11

4. National Institute of Diabetes and Digestive and Kidney Diseases. National Diabetes Statistics fact sheet: general information and national estimates on diabetes in the US, 2000. Bethesda, MD: US Dept. of Health and Human Services, National Institutes of Health, 2002.

5. Levin ME. Preventing amputation in patients with diabetes. *Diabetes Care* 1995;18:1383-94.

6. Reiber GE, Vileikyte L, Boyko EJ, et al. Casual pathways for incident lower-extremity ulcers in patients with diabetes from two settings. *Diabetes Care* 1999 Jan; 22(1):157-62.

7. Frykberg RG, Armstrong DG, Giurini J, et al. Diabetic foot disorders: a clinical practice guideline. American College of Foot and Ankle Surgeons. *J Foot Ankle Surg* 2000; 39(5 Suppl):S1-60. Review.

8. Armstrong DG, Lavery LA, Harkless LB. Validation of a diabetic wound classification system. The contribution of depth, infection, and ischemia to risk of amputation. *Diabetes Care* 1998 May;21(5):855-9.

9. Brand P, Yancey P. Pain: The Gift Nobody Wants. Harper Collins 1993.

10. Armstrong DG, Peters EJ, Athanasiou KA, et al. Is there a critical level of plantar foot pressure to identify patients at risk for neuropathic foot ulceration? *J Foot Ankle Surg* 1998 Jul Aug; 37(4):303-7.

11. Andrew JM, Boulton AI, Vinik JC, et al. Diabetic Neuropathies: A statement by the American Diabetes Association. *Diabetes Care* 2005 28:956-962

12. Carman TL. A primary care approach to the patient with claudication. *American Family Physician* February 15, 2000:61(4):1027-1034.

13. Brand FN, et al. Diabetes, intermittent claudication and risk of cardiovascular events. The Framingham study. *Diabetes* 38:504-509;1989.

14. Haffner SM, et al. Mortality from coronary artery disease in subjects with type 2 diabetes and in non-diabetic subjects with and without prior myocardial infarction. *N Eng J Med* 1998;339:229-234.

15. Hankey GJ, Norman PE, Eikelboom JW. Medical treatment of periperal aterial disease. *JAMA* 2006 Feb 1;295(5):547-53.

16. Lumsden AB, Rice TW. Medical management or peripheral arterial disease: a therapeutic algorithm. *Journal of Endovascular Therapy* 2006 Feb;13 Suppl 2:II19-29.

17. Frykberg RG, Team approach toward lower extremity amputation prevention in diabetes. *J Am Pod Med Assoc* 87:305-312, 1997.

18. Caputo GM, Cavanagh PR, Ulbrecht JS, et al. Assessment and management of foot disease with diabetes. *N Engl J Med* 331:854-860, 1994.

19. Rodeheaver GT, Pettry D, Thancker JG, et al. Wound cleansing by high pressure irrigation. *Surgery of Gynecology and Obstetrics* 1975 September;141(3):357-62.

20. Mosti G, Iabichella ML, Picerni P, et al. The debridement of hard to heal leg ulcers by means of a new device based on fluidjet technology. *International Wound Journal* 2005 December;2(4):307-314.

21. American Diabetes Association: Preventative Foot Care in Diabetes: Position statements and ADA statements. *Diabetes Care* 29:S75-S77, 2006.

22. Lansdown AB, William A, Chandler S, et al. Silver absorption and antibacterial efficacy of silver dressings. *Journal of Wound Care* 2005 April;14(4):155-160.

23. U.S. Department of Health and Human Services, Public Health Service: Diabetes and Chronic Disabling Conditions. Healthy People 2000: nation health promotion and disease prevention objectives. Washington, D.C.: Government Printing Office, 1991:442-474. (DHHS publ. no. PHS 91-50212).

24. Eaglstein WH, Falanga V. Chronic Wounds, Surg Clin N. A. 77:689-700, 1997.

25. Armstrong DG, Peters EGJ, Athanasiou KA, et al. Is there a critical level of plantar foot pressure to identify patients at risk for neuropathic foot ulceration? *J Foot Ankle Surg* 37:303 307, 1998.

26. Boulton AJ. Lowering the risk of neuropathy, foot ulcers, and amputations. *Diabet Med* 998;15 Suppl 4:S57-9.

27. Frykberg RG. The team approach in diabetic foot management. *Advances in Wound Care* 1998;11:71-7.

28. Diabetes Control and Complications Trial Research Group. DCCT protocol. Springfield, Virginia: U.S. Department of Commerce, National Technical Information Service, 1988 (publication no PB88-116462-AS).

29. Lazarus GS, Cooper DM, Knighton DR, et al. Definitions and guidelines for assessment of wounds and evaluation of healing. *Arch Derm* 130:489-493, 1994.

30. Toursarkissian B, Shireman PK, Harrison A, et al. Major lower extremity amputation: contemporary experience in a single Veterans Affairs institution. *Am Surg* 2002 Jul; 68(7):606-10.

31. Thomson FJ, Veves A, Ashe A, et al. A team approach to diabetic foot care - the Manchester experience. *The Foot* 2:75-82,1991.

32. Faglia E, Favales F, Aldeghi A, et al. Change in major amputation rate in a center dedicated to diabetic foot care during the 1980's: Prognostic Determinants for Major Amputation. *J Diabetes Complications* 1998. Mar-Apr;12(2):96-102.

33. Fernando DJS, Masson EA, Veves A, et al. Relationship of limited joint mobility to abnormal foot pressures and diabetic foot ulceration. *Diabetes Care* 14:8, 1991.

34. William D, Enoch S, Miller D, et al. Effect of sharp debridement using curette on recalcitrant nonhealing venous leg ulcers: a concurrently controlled, prospective cohort study. *Wound Repair Regen* 2005 Mar-Aprl;13(2):131-7.

35. Fauci AS, Braunwald E, Isselbacher KJ, et al, (eds). *Harrison's Principles of Internal Medicine,* 14th Edition. New York, NY: McGraw Hill , 1998.

36. Edmonds ME, Blundell MP, Morris ME, et al. Improved survival of the diabetic foot: the role of a specialized foot clinic. *Q J Med* 232:763, 1986.

37. Marazzi M, Stefani A, Chiaratti A, et al. Effect of enzymatic debridement with collagenase on acute and chronic hard-to-heal wounds. *J Wound Care* 2006 May;15(5):222-7.

38. Armstrong DG, Harkless LB. Outcomes of preventative care in a diabetic foot specialty clinic. *J Foot Ankle Surg* 37:460-466, 1998.

39. Wagner FW. The dysvascular foot: a system for diagnosis and treatment. *Foot Ankle* 2:64, 1981.

40. American Diabetes Association. Consensus Development Conference on Diabetic Foot Wound Care. *Diabetes Care* 22(8), August 1999. 1354-1360.

41. Armstrong DG, Lavery LA, Harkless LB. University of Texas Classification System for Diabetic Foot Wounds. *Diabetes Care* 1998 21:855-859.

42. Grayson ML. Diabetic foot infections: antimicrobial therapy. *Infect Dis Clin NA* 9:143-161, 1995.

43. Hamer ML, Robson MC, Krizek TJ, et al. Quantitative bacterial analysis of comparative wound irrigations. *Ann Surg* 181:819-822, 1975.

44. Gross A, Cutright DE, Bhaskar SN. Effectiveness of pulsating water jet lavage in treatment of contaminated crushed wounds. *Am J Surg* 124:373-377, 1972.

45. Armstrong DG, Lavery LA, Wu S, et al. Evaluation of removable and irremovable cast walkers in the healing of diabetic foot wounds: a randomized controlled trial. *Diabetes Care* 2005 Mar;28(3):551-4.

46. Steed DL, et al. [and Diabetic ulcer study group]. Clinical evaluation of recombinant human platelet derived growth factor for the treatment of lower extremity diabetic ulcers. *J Vasc Surg* 21:71-81, 1995.

47. McNeely MJ, Boyko E, Ahroni JH, et al. The independent contributions of diabetic neuropathy and vasculopathy in foot ulceration: how great are the risks? *Diabetes Care* 18:216-19, 1995.

48. Venturi ML, Attinger CE, Mesbahi AN, et al. Mechanisms and clinical applications of the vacuum-assisted closure (VAC) device: a review. *American Journal of Clinical Dermatology* 2005;6(3):185-194

49. Evans D, Land L. Topical negative pressure for treating chronic wounds. The Cochrane Database of Systemic Reviews 2001, issue1. Art No.: CD001898. DOI: 10.1002/14651858.CD001898

50. Kranke P, Bennett M, Roeckl-Wiedmann I, et al. Hyperbaric oxygen therapy for chronic wounds. The Cochrane Database Reviews 2004, Issue1.art.No.:CD004123.DOI:10.1002/14651858.CD004123.pub2.

51. Armstrong DG, Lavery LA. Negative pressure wound therapy after partial diabetic foot amputation: a multicentre, randomized controlled trial. *Lancet* 2005 Nov 12 Vol 366 issue 9498 pgs 1704-1710.

52. Veves A, Murray H, Young MJ, et al. The risk of ulceration in diabetic patients with high foot pressures: a prospective study. *Diabetologia* 35:660, 1992.

53. Young MJ, Breddy JL, Veves A, et al. The prediction of diabetic neuropathic foot ulceration using vibratory perception thresholds: a prospective study. *Diabetes Care* 17:557-560, 1994.

54. Guzman B, Fisher G, Palladino SJ, et al. Pressure removing strategies in neuropathic ulcer therapy. *Clin Pod Med Surg* 11:3390353, 1994.

55. Shaw JE, His WL, Ulbrecht JS, et al. Mechanism of plantar unloading in total contact casts: implications, designs, and clinical use. *Foot Ankle Int* 18:809 817.

56. Lavery LA, Vela SA, Lavery DC, et al. Reducing dynamic foot pressures in high risk diabetic subjects with foot ulcerations. *Diabetes Care* 19:818-821, 1996.

57. Janisse DJ. A scientific approach to insole design for the diabetic foot. *The Foot* 1993; 3:105-108.

58. Kozak GP, Campbell DR, Frykberg RG, et al. (eds). Management of diabetic foot problems. Philadelphia, PA: WB Saunders, 1995.

59. Steed DL. The role of growth factors in wound healing. *Surg Clin N.A.* 77:575-586, 1997.

60. Gentzkow GD, Iwasaki SD, Hershon KS, et al. Use of Dermagraft, a cultured human dermis, to treat diabetic foot ulcers. *Diabetes Care* 9:350-354, 1996.

61. Eaglstein WH, Falanga V. Tissue engineering and the development of Apligraf a human skin equivalent. *Supplement to Advances in Wound Care*, 11:1-7, 1998.

62. Reger SI, Hyodo A, Negami S, et al. Experimental wound healing with electrical stimulation. *Artif Organs* 1999 May;23(5):460-2.

63. Spencer S. Pressure relieving interventions for preventing and treating diabetic foot ulcers. The Cochrane Database of Systemic Reviews 2000, Issue 3. Art. No.: CD002302.doi: 10.1002/ 14651858.CD002302

64. Catanzariti AR, Blitch EL, Karlock LG. Elective foot and ankle surgery in the diabetic patient. *J Foot Ankle Surg* 34:23-41, 1995.

65. Armstrong DG, Lavery LA, Stern S, et al. Is prophylactic diabetic foot surgery dangerous? *J Foot Ankle Surg* 35:585-589, 1996.

66. Kozak GP, Campbell DR, Frykberg RG, et al, (eds). Management of Diabetic Foot Problems. Philadelphia, PA: WB Saunders, 1995.

67. Fleischli JG, Laughlin TJ. Electrical stimulation in wound healing. *J Foot Ankle Surg* 1997 Nov Dec; 36(6):457-61.

68. Toursarkissian B, Hagino RT, Khan K, et al. Healing of transmetatarsal amputation in diabetic patient: is angiography predictive? *Annals of Vascular Surgery* 2005 November;19(6):769-773.

69. Mueller MJ, Sinacore DR, Hastings MK, et al. Effect of Achilles tendon lengthening on neuropathic plantar ulcers: a randomized clinical trial. *JBJS Am* 85:1436-1445, 2003.

70. Lin SS, Lee TH Wapner KL. Plantar forefoot ulceration with equinus deformity of the ankle in diabetic patients: the effect of tendo-Achilles lengthening and total contact casting. *Orthopedics* 19(5):465-75, 1996.

71. Armstrong DG, Stacpoole-Shea S, Nguyen H, et al. Lengthening of the Achilles tendon in diabetic patients who are at high risk for ulceration of the foot. *JBJS Am* 81:535-538, 1999.

72. Armstrong DG, Nguyen HC. Improvement in healing with aggressive edema reduction after debridement of foot infection in persons with diabetes. *Arch Surg* 2000 Dec;135(12):1405-9.

73. Jude EB, Unsworth PF. Optimal treatment of infected diabetic foot ulcers. *Drugs Aging* 21(13):833-850, 2004

74. Sherman RA. Maggot therapy for treating diabetic foot ulcers unresponsive to conventional therapy. *Diabetes Care* 26(2): 446-451, 2003.

75. Barnes RC. Point Counterpoint: Hyperbaric oxygen is beneficial for diabetic foot wounds. *Clinics Infectious Diseases* 43:188-192, 2006.

REVIEW QUESTIONS

1.) Which of the following is NOT considered a fundamental or primary risk factor for the <u>development</u> of diabetic foot ulceration?
   a. Ischemia
   b. Neuropathy
   c. Deformity / Limited Joint Mobility
   d. Pivotal Trauma

2.) Approximately ____% of all diabetic related lower extremity amputations are preceded by an ulceration.
   a. 25
   b. 45
   c. 65
   d. 85

3.) Autonomic neuropathy commonly results in:
   a. Dry fissured skin
   b. Bunion deformity
   c. Ingrown toenails
   d. Ganglion Cysts

4.) The essential therapeutic objectives for the management of any plantar diabetic foot ulcer include all of the following EXCEPT:
   a. Off-loading the areas of greatest pressure
   b. Maintaining a moist wound environment
   c. Removal of all granulation tissue
   d. Patient education and compliance

5.) Which dressing would be best suited for a wound with high levels of surface bacterial contamination (bioburden)?
   a. Hydrogel
   b. Silver Impregnated
   c. Hydrocolloid
   d. Petroleum gauze

Answers: 1a, 2d, 3a, 4c, 5b

NOTES

Chapter **17**

PRESSURE ULCERS: TOWARDS A NEW UNDERSTANDING OF AN OLD PROBLEM

CHAPTER SEVENTEEN OVERVIEW

Pressure Ulcers: towards a New Understanding of an Old Problem

Caroline E. Fife

INTRODUCTION

A pressure sore is defined as an ulceration of the skin and/or deeper tissues due to unrelieved pressure. Wounds due to shear and frictional forces are also grouped with pressure sores even though they are not strictly due to pressure. Traditional teaching is that pressure ulcers are the result of external factors such as pressure, sheer, friction and moisture. Consequently, many lesions not caused by pressure are labeled "pressure ulcers," including maceration from incontinence, superficial erosions from friction, and erythema from shear-induced tearing of blood vessels. It is now understood that most superficial ulcers are not really pressure ulcers. All reliable data support the assertion that pressure ulcers result from deep tissue damage and form from the inside out. Older terms such as "decubitus ulcer" or "bed sore" are no longer considered appropriate since they imply an etiology limited to the supine position or bed confinement. Nevertheless, pressure sores are still classified as "decubitus ulcers" in the World Health Organization's ICD-9 (International Classification of Diseases) system. (The ICD-10, updated for morbidities in 2003 has yet to be implemented in the United States.)

Increased legislation and litigation have heightened awareness of the pressure ulcer problem, though they have done little to change its prevalence. Whether pressure ulcers develop in acute or chronic care settings, they have an impact on patients which can range from mild to severe. In addition to the quality of life issue, family lives are also disrupted, especially when members become intensively involved in the caregiving process. Further, pressure ulcers increase the cost of health care and lengthen any hospital or institutional stay, regardless of their severity, causing patients to run risks of developing complications, such as cellulitis, osteomyelitis, heterotopic bone formation, bacteremia, sepsis, and even death. Today, the term "pressure ulcer" has almost become synonymous with poor care, especially in nursing homes and long-term institutions, but are pressure ulcers always the result of poor care? In hope of providing an answer to this question, this chapter is devoted to a discussion of the most recent literature available on the pathogenesis and treatment of pressure ulcers.

THE SCOPE OF THE PROBLEM
Prevalence and Costs of Pressure Ulcers

In 1995, a national pressure ulcer (PU) survey conducted in 265 acute-care hospitals found a prevalence of 10.1%, of which 74% were Stage I and II (1). These results were similar to the previous four surveys. Four years later, an even larger survey of 42,817 patients conducted in acute-care facilities across the country determined an even higher prevalence of 14.8%, with a nosocomial PU prevalence of 7.1% (2). Another large retrospective study of hospitalized patients with PUs conducted in Washington State between 1987 and 2000 using ICD-9 diagnosis codes showed an incidence of 7.0 to 8.3 per 100,000 for primary diagnosis but a doubling from 34.5 to 71.6 per 100,000 during the period when a secondary diagnosis code was added (3). The problem of PU acquisition from hospitals has been also highlighted in a 1992-95 study of long-term-care Maryland patients, which showed that the proportion with one or more PUs admitted from a hospital was 11.9% versus 4.7% not admitted from a hospital (4).

In nursing homes, the long-standing issue of PUs was addressed as early as 1987 by the legislature in the Omnibus Budget Reconciliation Act (OBRA) (1987), but studies have shown that such legislative measures had little impact. In research carried out by Coleman et al. (5), two cross-sectional surveys conducted in 1992-94 and 1997-98 demonstrated that the unadjusted prevalence rates of all PUs were 8.5% in both cases, with Stage II PU prevalence rates of 5.3% and 5.65% respectively. Another review of 15,121 nursing home residents in Ohio, carried out in 1994 showed a similar result: the prevalence of PUs was 12%, with 8% having a Stage II or greater PU (6). A more recent, multisite, international study supported by Hill Rom found an average prevalence of 15.5% for PUs in facilities of all types, and is probably a good benchmark (*www.hill-rom.com/usa/offering/solutions/ wound_care.html*).

The situation is not any better in Europe. In Germany, for example, the PU prevalence determined from an extremely large national survey conducted during 2002–03 was found to be 24.6% in hospitals and 13.9% in nursing homes (7). In over half of the hospital patients the PUs were facility acquired compared to 60% for nursing home residents. In the Netherlands a similarly sized study found a mean PU prevalence of 23% in 16,344 patients present in 89 healthcare institutions (8).

In 1992, it was reported that 1.7 million patients developed pressure ulcers annually in the USA, with an associated cost of $8.5 billion (9). Sixty percent of these patients acquired their PUs while in acute-care hospitals. In 1999, Beckrich and Aronovich attempted another analysis and reported   a cost of $2.2–3.6 billion associated with 1.6 million pressure ulcers annually, with each Stage III or IV ulcer adding a cost of $14,000–23,000 to the cost of caring for a patient (10). Zhan and Miller calculated the cost of developing a pressure ulcer at $10,845, and noted that each ulcer added nearly four days to a hospital stay, and increased mortality by 7.2% (11). In fact, it is estimated that some 60,000 deaths a year nationally are attributable to complications arising from pressure ulcers (12), and pressure ulcers were among the three most common patient safety incidents reported during 37 million hospital admissions during 2002-2003 in a 2004 report by HealthGrades (*www.healthgrades.com/media/english/pdf/HG_Patient_Safety_Study_Final.pdf*).

A more recent assessment of the cost of pressure ulcers in the U.S. by Zulkowski et al. placed the figure at $9.1 to $11.6 billion annually in 2004 dollars (13).

For nursing homes, a 25% rate decline of PUs during 1991-95 was reported by Berlowitz et al. (14), but it has been hard to ascertain during the last ten years whether this trend has continued. Eckman (15) estimated a figure of 1.7 million hospitalized patients with PUs in 1989, and in 1999 Beckrich and Aronovitch (10) computed a figure of 2.5 million patients receiving treatment for PUs in acute-care settings. When the growth of the population is taken into account, especially the 70+ years subpopulation in which two thirds of PUs occur, this represents a stable incidence. Most wound care professionals agree that the overall prevalence of pressure ulcers has not significantly declined in the last 15 years despite new guidelines, legislation, and the increased threat of litigation. However, since patients with PUs tend to be older and sicker, this can also be viewed as a positive trend (13). Nevertheless it seems that the PU objective (1–16) of the Healthy People 2010 initiative (a 50% reduction in the prevalence of PUs in nursing home residents from 8/1000; *www.health.gov/healthypeople*) is unlikely to be met.

The Healthcare Cost and Utilization Project (HCUP) data reported by Russo and Elixhauser (Hospitalizations related to pressure sores, 2003; *www.hcup-us.ahrq.gov/reports/statbriefs/sb3.pdf*) found that in 2003 there was a 63% increase in PUs compared to 1992 but the total number of hospitalizations and number of stays of patients aged 65 years or older during this time period only increased by 11%, and 14% respectively. This suggests that hospitals are doing a worse job of preventing PU formation than a decade ago. Although one might think that a reduction in the nurse/patient staffing ratio is the crucial factor (leading to a poorer quality of care), a recent study casts doubt on this as the only factor (16). Most disturbing is the HCUP finding that stays were longest for the 18 to 44 age group, and shortest for the patients aged 85 years and older for hospitalizations primarily related to pressure ulcers (14.1 versus 10.2 days). Is this further evidence for the fact that older patients are being prematurely transferred to longer-term facilities, and that part of the perceived nursing home PU problem probably lies with newly admitted residents have more PUs derived from acute-care facilities? Julian and Fell agree that this is a likely scenario, and further point out that poor appreciation of incipient PUs in patients transferred from acute-care facilities is another factor that has contributed to higher litigation at nursing homes (17). Although lack of training and awareness of pressure ulcer development among acute-care staff is certainly one aspect (18), prevention during surgery (19) and transportation of patients are other causes that are not frequently addressed, and it is clear more research regarding their formation would be useful (20, 21).

Litigation, Nursing Homes, and the Role of the CMS

Since the population continues to slowly age, how then should we tackle this monumental problem? Given that the development of pressure ulcers is often perceived as lack of quality care by the public, the focus has tended to fall on nursing homes. The 1987 OBRA legislation was intended to promulgate a set of federal standards by which any Medicare-certified nursing home would be measured: a standard of care. Unfortunately, the standards were unrealistic, as Meehan and Hill (22) point out with this example: "[a] resident who enters the facility without a pressure sore does not develop pressure sores unless the individual's clinical condition demonstrates that they were unavoidable." The result was a vast increase in malpractice litigation. According to Bennett et al. (23), the median number of lawsuits increased almost tenfold by 1992 compared to five years prior to passage of the act. The foundation criteria for the litigation were often the clinical practice guidelines produced by the Agency of Healthcare Research and Quality (AHRQ), 85% of which were "C" rated in the treatment section and 81% in the prevention section (17). According to the AHRQ, a "C" rating requires one or more of the following: 1) the results of one controlled trial, 2) the results of at least two case series/descriptive studies on pressure ulcers in humans, or 3) expert opinion (24). Even today, pressure ulcer prevention is still based more on clinical practice than research, so it should hardly be surprising that these guidelines would prevent PU problems from occurring. For example, one of the AHRQ guidelines states that a Stage I ulcer need not progress to the deeper layers of tissue for at-risk patients (22). Implicit in this statement is a tenet that all patients at risk can be successfully identified, and that pressure ulcers naturally progress from lower stages to higher stages (i.e. "outside in") if untreated. Neither is true.

The enormous costs of litigation are being the most strongly felt in the long-term care industry, where it is becoming more common to settle out of court due to jury awards (the highest was $312 million in damages) and a high plaintiff recovery rate of 87% (25). For example, plaintiff compensation during 1996–98 for 28 out of 30 nursing home cases averaged nearly a million dollars (26). The Balanced Budget Act of 1997, which changed the way the Centers for Medicare and Medicaid Services (CMS) paid skilled nursing facilities, impacted care for both short-term and long-term residents at many nursing homes that depended on Medicare. Essentially the Act caused a payment decrease, which, in turn, resulted in staffing reductions and less quality care, according to a study carried out by Konetzka et al. (27). Grabowski and Angelelli also found a strong relationship between Medicaid payment and the quality of care in nursing homes in their research, especially those that were resource poor (28).

More recently, CMS has adopted a policy of issuing financial penalties to those facilities, which oversight surveys show are allowing the development of pressure sores in residents. The most important change has been the reinterpretation of F-314, which went into effect the same day it was issued on November 14, 2004. In terms of non-compliance, the number of deficiency levels was reduced by three, by eliminating the mildest (29). Although some changes have been helpful, there exists a potential problem with the regulation which states that the patient "…does not develop pressure sores unless the individual's clinical condition demonstrates that they were unavoidable." The definition for unavoidability is: "The resident developed a pressure ulcer even though the facility had evaluated the resident's clinical condition and pressure ulcer risk factors: defined and implemented interventions that are consistent with resident needs, resident goals, and recognized standards of practice; monitored and evaluated the impact of the interventions; and revised the approaches as appropriate (29)." For example, what happens when the risk evaluation "fails," i.e., the resident was evaluated as low risk but developed a PU anyway? Whose fault is that? According to CMS, it would be the provider's fault. Or take a situation in which the resident is approaching the end of life and forbids certain treatments. According to the reinterpretation of CMS Regulation F-314, this does not obviate the provider from having to prevent or treat PUs and document the process completely (29). Failure to do so will incur a financial penalty.

The issue of PU preventability is key. Litigation for pressure sores is a national epidemic based on the assumption that all pressure sores are preventable. Are all pressures sores preventable? If not, which ones can we prevent? Before we can begin to answer these questions, we must first understand the pathophysiology of tissue damage from pressure.

PRESSURE ULCER PATHOPHYSIOLOGY: INSIDE OUT VS. OUTSIDE IN

Confusion will continue to exist regarding the pathophysiological process and staging of wounds as long as wounds due to moisture and friction are grouped with those due to pressure. Frictional forces are due to the resistance of one body sliding, rolling, or flowing over another. These forces produce specific types of superficial tissue damage. Strain is the tissue deformation which happens in response to pressure. Shear forces are produced when contiguous tissues slide relative to each other in a direction parallel to their plane of contact, and can make a patient more vulnerable to subsequent pressure injury (30). Some investigators have suggested that shear contributes to all pressure sores.

With regard to pressure injury, for many years the standard explanation was that they occurred when tissues trapped between a bony prominence and a hard surface were exposed to tensions in excess of the mean capillary pressure (32 mm Hg), thus resulting in tissue ischemia and necrosis. However, histological studies by Witkowski and Parish demonstrated that the epidermis does not show any signs of necrosis until very late, and that the first evidence of tissue damage is in the subcutaneous tissue (31). It is known that epidermal cells are able to withstand prolonged absence of oxygen both *in vivo* and *in vitro*, whereas more metabolically active muscle cells can be more vulnerable to injury. Animal studies have shown that muscle is more sensitive to pressure than skin, suggesting that deeper tissues, such as muscle, will undergo necrosis under less severe conditions than the superficial tissues (32, 33). Moreover, recent studies using the rat model have shown that the mechanical properties of striated muscle can be used as an indicator of compression injury. Forces between 13 kPa (97 mm Hg) delivered for six hours and 40 kPa (299 mm Hg) delivered for two hours appear to represent an injury threshold; higher pressures result in increased muscle stiffness and necrosis, which can propagate to surrounding tissues if stresses are unrelieved (34).

The final common pathway to tissue injury is ischemia and hypoxia. Necrosis can occur more easily in tissues overlying a bony prominence (35), perhaps because in these areas, tissue oxygen tensions fall rapidly in response to pressure compared to soft tissues, such as the thigh (36). This finding might be due to the unique physics of pressure distribution. Shear stress also reduces the reduction in oxygen tension and accompanying ischemia in skin (37).

The tissues nearest to the bony prominence are thought to experience the most pressure, which then dissipates and spreads as the superficial layers are approached (38). Pressure is believed to be distributed in a triangular fashion with the point of the triangle located at the site nearest to the bony prominence. Animal studies have demonstrated that pressure increases both laterally and in depth as proximity to a bony prominence increased. In humans, Linder-Ganz and colleagues used MRI to assess the mechanical conditions in subdermal tissues and found that they do experience larger amounts of pressure during sitting, and demonstrated that the highest pressures were in the muscle next to the bone (39). It is therefore likely that despite maintaining low skin surface pressures, deeper tissues could experience higher pressures, leading to subsequent tissue damage and the formation of a cavity below the dermis. Stekelenburg and colleagues confirmed this, documenting that the first tissue damaged was the deep tissue (40). Furthermore, although the superficial layers experience the least amount of pressure, they are the layers with the largest area affected (an upside-down triangle). The critical point is that the damage from pressure occurs in the deeper tissue first, and progresses toward the surface. In other words, pressure sores form from the inside out, rather than from the outside in. This also means that the degree or depth of tissue damage might not be apparent by the condition of the overlying skin. Slow acceptance of this "inside out" model is probably due to deep roots in clinical practice in which education based on early staging methods and wound descriptions has predominated (41).

Even more surprising is the fact that urinary incontinence is not an independent predictor of pressure sores (42). Moisture can contribute to superficial wounds, but these are the least harmful and easiest to heal. It can also alter skin hardness and make tissues somewhat more susceptible to pressure, but there is no evidence that moisture, per se, significantly contributes to the formation of deep pressure sores. Friction and moisture appear to have little role in the development of Stage III and IV pressure sores.

Pressure loading of soft tissues for prolonged periods of time results in a variety of biochemical disturbances, which, if unrelieved, lead to cell damage (43). Using an indenter on the sacrum area of humans and transcutaneous electrochemical sensors, Knight et al. (43) established that a 60% drop in $TcpO_2$ is probably the threshold at which biochemical changes are initiated. Krouskop (44) has hypothesized that hypoxia results in the production of a water-soluble form of collagen that is subsequently washed out. Mechanical stress is then redistributed, increasing stress and decreasing nutrient transport to other elements. Interstitial fluid diminishes, resulting in cell-to-cell contact and possible rupture of the cells, thus dumping their contents into the intercellular space. Studies of spinal cord injury patients also suggest that increased collagen degradation occurs, reducing the tissue's ability to bear mechanical stresses (45, 46).

Krouskop (44) also postulates that glucocorticoids, released during stress, inhibit smooth muscle functioning in the lymphatic system. Impairment of lymphatic transport capacity, due to hypoxia or increased lymphatic load from glucocorticoids or other molecules, will subsequently result in the poisoning of tissue. The decrease in elastic fiber production, which occurs with increasing age (44), would result in a stiffening of tissue, thus increasing the risk of pressure damage. Seiler and Stahelin (45) also attribute the mechanism of tissue injury to a decrease in fibrinolytic activity leading to fibrin deposits in the capillaries and intercellular space, with subsequent vessel occlusion and tissue necrosis. Bader et al. (46) suggest that shear stress also causes a decrease in fibrinolytic activity. While these postulated mechanisms require further study, they explain the pattern of tissue necrosis in response to pressure better than the simplistic idea of decreased capillary perfusion caused by pressure.

Krouskop (44) also postulates that glucocorticoids, released during stress, inhibit smooth muscle functioning in the lymphatic system. Impairment of lymphatic transport capacity, due to hypoxia or increased lymphatic load from glucocorticoids or other molecules, will subsequently result in the poisoning of tissue. The decrease in elastic fiber production, which occurs with increasing age (47), would result in a stiffening of tissue, thus increasing the risk of pressure damage. Seiler and Stahelin (48) also attribute the mechanism of tissue injury to a decrease in fibrinolytic activity leading to fibrin deposits in the capillaries and intercellular space, with subsequent vessel occlusion and tissue necrosis. Bader et al. (49) suggest that shear stress also causes a decrease in fibrinolytic activity. A further factor which has not been recognized until recently is that of heat. Using porcine models, Kokate et al. demonstrated that even with the same pressure profiles, deep tissue damage occurred at temperatures of 35°C whereas no damage was observed at 25°C (50).

While all these postulated mechanisms require further study, they explain the pattern of tissue necrosis in response to pressure better than the simplistic idea of decreased capillary perfusion caused by pressure. Stress and strain, factors which are greatest near the bone, are integral to the process of tissue damage. This results in tissue ischemia, which, all experts now agree, is the final common pathway for pressure ulceration.

STAGING PRESSURE SORES

The National Pressure Ulcer Advisory Panel (NPUAP) pressure ulcer staging system has serious limitations and is currently under consideration for extensive revision. It consists of four stages.

Stage I

This is largely characterized by non-blanching erythema of the skin, which can be accompanied by changes in skin temperature, tissue consistency, and sensation. In patients with pigmented skin, a Stage I PU can take on persistent red, blue, or purple hues, but it can be difficult for even an experienced clinician to properly stage this kind of pressure ulcer (51). For example, a Dutch study showed a difference of 50% in the same-day assessment of Stage I PUs (52). There also exists an issue with the definition of Stage I, which can be misleading. Thus, in using the word "purple" one could document a PU as Stage I, when in fact there might be a deep tissue injury present (53). It is disheartening to know that, despite the recent CMS policy assessing monetary penalties for the development of Stage I "pressure ulcers," experts in the field are as yet unable to determine exactly what these skin changes represent or whether they result in any long-term tissue damage. They *do not* lead to higher-stage pressure ulcers.

Stage II

Stage II involves a partial-thickness skin loss involving the epidermis and possibly the dermis. This superficial ulcer presents clinically as an abrasion, blister, or shallow crater with the most common causes due to friction, trauma, or excoriation stemming from incontinence, and not necessarily pressure *per se* (53). Superficial erosions can make deeper injury more likely to become apparent at the surface, but are *not* the cause of higher-stage ulcers.

Stage III

A Stage III PU incorporates full-thickness skin loss involving damage or necrosis of subcutaneous tissue, which can extend down to *but not through the fascia*. It presents clinically as a deep crater with or without undermining present. Experts in the field argue that Stage III ulcers might not in fact, exist as a separate category but are part of the spectrum of deep tissue injury, which include Stage IV ulcers.

Stage IV

A PU at Stage IV presents as a full-thickness skin loss with extensive destruction, tissue necrosis, or damage to the muscle, bone, or supporting structures, such as the tendon, or joint capsule.

THE DEADLY SINS OF STAGING

There are serious limitations of the NPUAP staging system, even when it is used correctly, which often it is not. The most common limitations of the staging system, or common misconceptions regarding the pathophysiology of pressure sores, revolve around the following issues: a) "unstageable wound," b) deep tissue injury problem, c) reverse staging, d) shearing, and e) evolution of the stages.

The Unstageable Wound

A necrotic wound, that is a wound with an eschar, is "unstageable" since the base of the wound cannot be assessed. It is possible, particularly in heel pressure sores, for tissue necrosis to be superficial, but this is the exception.

The Deep Tissue Injury Problem

The NPUAP system does not provide a way to describe deep tissue injury (DTI), that is wounds caused by an infarction of the skin (common as the patient nears death, or in association with shock and multiorgan system failure). DTI presents classically as a purple non-blancheable area of intact skin. Demarcation of the dead tissue usually occurs within 24–48 hours and is due to deep underlying tissue destruction. Another way of looking at the problem is that the staging system refers *only* to the type of tissue observed at the base of the wound at its deepest depth. In other words, deeper tissue injury could be present, but since this is not visually observed, (more extensive investigation would be required) the PU could be staged as something less severe. Currently, NPUAP advises that clinicians document such cases as "pressure-related deep tissue injury under intact skin" or "deep tissue injury under intact skin" in order that proper treatment be undertaken, and for legal purposes (13).

It is common to find a large purple "bruise-like" area over the sacrum due to the death of subcutaneous tissue. The skin will eventually die and an eschar will form, but in the meantime, the "bruise-like" changes are often mistaken for a Stage I pressure sore. A not uncommon scenario is as follows (this is a summary of a true case): An abdominal aortic aneurysm began leaking in a 60-year-old diabetic woman. She was air-evacuated to a large medical center for emergency surgery, because no surgeon in her city had the skill to manage this problem. She first underwent angiography after which she was required to remain supine for five hours to prevent bleeding from the angiography site. She was then taken immediately to surgery, where she had a prolonged vascular procedure during which her abdominal aorta was clamped and she remained supine on the operating room table. She arrived at the intensive care unit in poor condition and required vasopressors to maintain her blood pressure. Attempts at turning caused her blood pressure to decrease. Approximately 72 hours after arriving at the hospital, she was stable enough to be turned and the nurses note a large purple discoloration over her sacrum. It was incorrectly documented as a "Stage I" pressure sore. Over the following week, as a result of the deep tissue infarction which likely occurred during surgery, but perhaps as early as the time the patient remained supine after angiography, the following events occurred: The overlying skin necrosed, the edges separated from the viable tissue at the margins, and foul-smelling, liquefied necrotic fat and subcutaneous tissue drained. The nurses described this as a Stage III "infected" wound due to the odor. The bone then became visible and the PU was documented as Stage IV.

The documentation (Stage I, Stage III "infected," and Stage IV, over a period of time) suggested that the wound had deteriorated and this progression was blamed on poor care by the staff. The patient had, in fact, suffered deep tissue death of all the skin and subcutaneous tissue over the sacrum, and the rest of the course was the natural *evolution* of an event, which occurred at a particular point in time, likely during the first few hours of hospitalization. Thus, the wound did not "progress" so much as "evolve" once damage had occurred. The patient later required a rotational flap for closure, which was successful, and died a year later of urosepsis. The family brought suit for pain and suffering, as well as wrongful death, intimating that the sepsis was due to the wound (The organisms grown from a small separation near the flap were different from the organisms grown from blood and urine cultures.), despite the fact that the patient survived a frequently fatal condition (a leaking aneurysm) thanks to the best of surgical intervention, and received a successful closure of the pressure sore. The defendant prevailed in court, *in spite* of the documentation by the hospital staff, rather than because of it. The documentation problems were due to the limitations of the NPUAP staging system, the nurses' inability to use it properly insofar as it was possible, and the common misconceptions that any wound, which eventually becomes a Stage IV, can be halted if earlier intervention is provided and that there can be adequate visible warning of the development of Stage IV ulcers. The data do not support the last two statements.

The accompanying photos illustrate these points (Figure 1). A 64-year-old woman with adult onset diabetes had undergone a below-the-knee amputation (BKA) on the right, and was undergoing intensive rehabilitation in hope of walking with a prosthesis. She developed an area of apparent "bruising" over the lateral BKA stump (Figure 1A). As a result, her ambulation program was immediately discontinued, the use of her prosthesis suspended, and she was placed back into her wheelchair. Despite this aggressive offloading, an eschar developed within approximately ten days (Figure 1B). When the eschar was debrided, a deep ulceration was apparent with exposed tendon (Figure 1C). Did this pressure ulcer "deteriorate?" No. This is an example of the *evolution* of tissue injury despite the immediate cessation of pressure once tissue damage was recognized.

Another example of the DTI syndrome is the Kennedy terminal ulcer. This is a pressure ulcer particularly identified with the dying. It is described

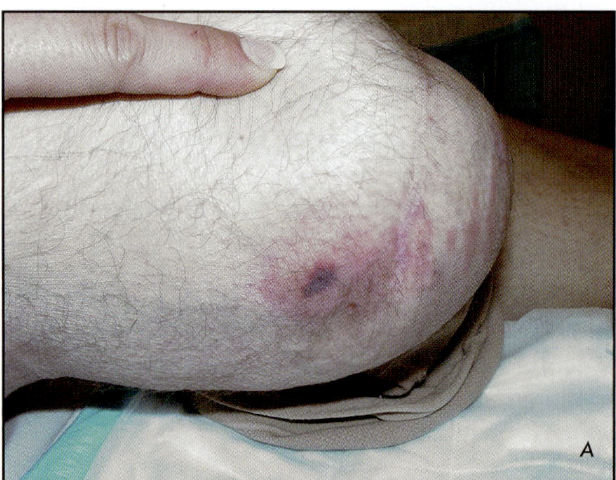

Figure 1A. A 64-year-old woman with adult onset diabetes had undergone a below-the-knee amputation (BKA) on the right, and was undergoing intensive rehabilitation in hope of walking with prosthesis. She developed an area of apparent "bruising" over the lateral BKA stump.

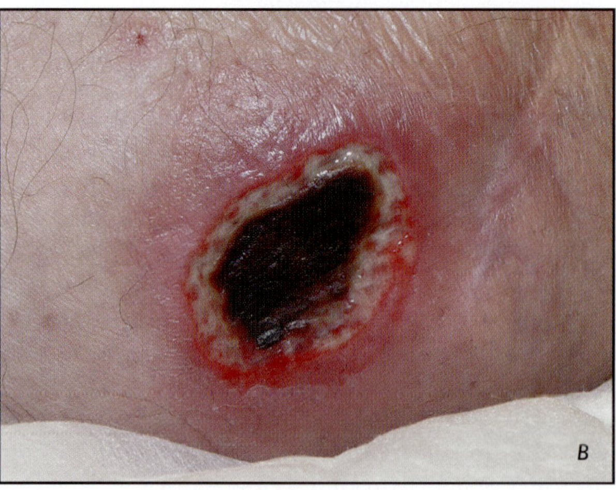

Figure 1B. As a result, her ambulation program was immediately discontinued, the use of her prosthesis suspended, and she was placed back into her wheelchair. Despite this aggressive off-loading, an eschar developed within approximately ten days.

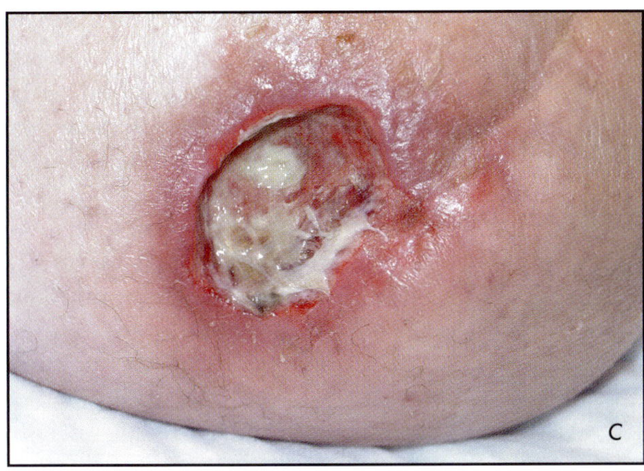

Figure 1C. When the eschar was debrided, a deep ulceration was apparent with exposed tendon. Did this pressure ulcer "deteriorate?" No. This is an example of the evolution of tissue injury despite the immediate cessation of pressure once tissue damage was recognized.

often as pear-shaped, with irregular borders, and is usually found on the sacrum. Its characteristic is sudden onset, with one nursing shift stating equivocally that the skin was intact and the next describing an extensive area of tissue injury. It is often a harbinger of death.

Reverse Staging

Another serious limitation of the NPUAP system is that it does not allow a mechanism for defining progress in healing. Reverse staging of full-thickness wounds is physiologically inaccurate, but is mandated by the Minimum Data Set (MDS) and OASIS (Outcomes and Assessment Information Set). The correct way to describe a pressure sore, which is healing, is a "healing Stage IV" even if the wound is now superficial and epithelializing.

Consider the following hypothetical case: if a patient has Stage III PU that has partially healed, i.e., it has not fully epithelialized, it might be restaged as a Stage II PU. However, if the original pressure ulcer was is not properly documented, a future healthcare worker might not realize the origin of the PU and properly take account of its history (13). The whole concept of reverse staging is invalid, because it suggests that severe ulcers heal back to normal in terms of anatomically functioning tissues, and this in incorrect; scar tissue has very different properties to uninjured normal tissue.

Since 1996, the NPUAP has developed and validated the Pressure Ulcer Scale for Healing tool (PUSH Tool) which it recommends be used to document pressure ulcer healing. At the February 2007 meeting, the NPUAP adopted a standard definition of suspected deep tissue injury as follows: "Purple or maroon localized area of discolored intact skin or blood-filled blister due to damage of underlying soft tissue from pressure and/or shear. The area may be proceded by tissue that is painful, firm, mushy, boggy, warmer or cooler as compared to adjacent tissue."

Shearing

The most common cause of "Stage II Pressure sores" is actually shearing or friction, and *not* pressure. This makes it even more impossible to argue that Stage III or IV ulcers have evolved "from" Stage II wounds, although they might occur over the same areas of the body. Friction and moisture have been shown to have little role in the development of Stage III and IV pressure ulcers.

The Evolution of the Stages

The most serious problem with the NPUAP system is that the numeric nature of staging implies that a Stage IV pressure ulcer is preceded by Stages I, II, and III. It cannot be overemphasized that the NPUAP stage refers *only* to the type of tissue visible at the base of the wound.

As has been discussed, deep pressure sores occur from the *inside out* (the way an apple rots). Payments of millions of dollars in settlements or jury awards have been based on the misconception that a Stage IV pressure sore must have been preceded by wounds of lesser stages, and that intervention at an earlier stage would have prevented the more severe wound from occurring. The concept that Stage III or IV pressure sores occur from the inside out, and might not be preceded by any visible evidence of tissue damage until it is too late, cannot be made clear from the current staging system.

MDS AND OASIS

The MDS was originally developed as a clinical tool for assessment of and care planning for patients entering long-term nursing facilities, and was an outcome of the 1987 OBRA Act. Its intent was to ensure patients do not develop avoidable pressure ulcers. In 1996, it was updated and became MDS-2. NPUAP took exception to it for several reasons: 1) It fails to acknowledge all the etiological factors of PUs and does not adequately define pressure ulcers, allowing misclassification; 2) It requires all PUs to be staged in a "one-size-fits-all scheme"; 3) It forces restaging during the progression of healing ulcers but does not permit documentation of ulcer healing or development; and 4) It has exceeded its original design by becoming a vehicle for quality assurance, reimbursement, long-term care recertification, and clinical database research (*www.npuap.org/positn3.html*). As a result, inappropriate citations are often issued, and it can lead to befuddled decision-making, particularly if this is the only tool used to assess patient risk of developing PUs. Moreover, a recent study showed that the MDS PU quality indicator is not a useful measure of quality care at nursing homes (54).

OASIS is a more recent data set designed to measure patient outcomes and improve the quality of patient care at home healthcare facilities (55). It is a 79-item form that must be completed at the start of care for any such facility utilizing Medicare payment. Although OASIS does not constitute a comprehensive assessment instrument (56), a study by Bergquist did show that it might be used as an adequate method for identifying elderly patients at risk of developing Stage I or II pressure ulcers (57). These tools fail to identify co-morbid conditions which can contribute to pressure sore development and will never be satisfactory as sole risk-assessment instruments.

SKIN FAILURE

In the context of CMS regulation F-314, if CMS perceives that the vast majority of pressure ulcers are avoidable and that the appearance of a PU is largely due to failure of care, serious legal and financial consequences can ensue. Thomas states that, "No intervention strategy has been reported that consistently and reproducibly reduces the incidence of pressure ulcers to zero. The published data on prevention of pressure ulcers do not support an assumption that all pressure ulcers are preventable (58)." A survey of 65 experts in the field of pressure ulcer care five years ago found that 62% of respondents agreed with the last statement (59). Although a great many studies have shown that the incidence of pressure ulcers can be considerably reduced when proper quality care is consistently implemented, there remains a core of patients in whom there is an apparent prevention failure. For this group, we introduce the term "skin failure," which is described in three types: acute, chronic, and end-stage. Not all clinicians subscribe to the end-stage skin failure concept (60).

The skin requires between one fourth and one third of the cardiac output, and comprising 10–15% of an individual's body weight, is the largest organ of the body (61, 62). It has huge nutritional, as well as perfusion requirements. Standard definitions exist for the failure of every other organ system (e.g., heart failure, liver failure, and renal failure) and when these occur, they are understood as the natural progression of underlying medical conditions, such as diabetes, and peripheral vascular disease. Healthcare providers are not assumed responsible for the failure of these organs. However, skin breakdown is often referred to as a "failure of care" regardless of the underlying health status of the patient who frequently is experiencing the failure of every other organ system. Due to the visible and often disturbing nature of skin breakdown, the emotional impact is understandable, although this impact is sometimes a greater issue for the family since the patient may be far along in the dying process. The challenge we currently face is how to separate those episodes of skin breakdown that are unavoidable from those which are, in fact, due to substandard care.

Skin failure can be defined as the loss of core temperature homeostasis with the concurrent cessation of the barrier properties of skin, i.e., prevention of water, electrolytes, and protein loss, and ingress of foreign materials. Acute skin failure can constitute a clinical emergency, requiring intensive care. It has a variety of primary dermatological causes, including erythroderma, dermatitis, psoriasis, cutaneous T-cell lymphoma, Stevens-Johnson syndrome, and infection (63), and can occur at any age. It can also result from the complications of severe illness, such as myocardial infarction, stroke, sepsis, or trauma, in which accompanying decreased perfusion, anemia, malnutrition, or immobilization significantly increases the risk of developing a pressure ulcer (62). However, provided the basal factors giving rise to the condition are understood and appropriately treated, the prognosis is generally excellent, and the patient will completely recover.

By contrast, chronic skin failure is a longitudinal condition arising from a chronic comorbidity in which skin and underlying tissue die from hypoperfusion, and usually afflicts older patients. Chronic skin failure should not be confused with the age-related general deterioration of the skin in which elasticity and skin vascularity diminish, thinner epithelial and fatty layers prevail, and the number of sweat glands decrease. When a patient approaches the end of life, it is possible that several organ systems can begin to fail simultaneously—including the skin—and this is termed end-stage skin failure. End-stage skin failure can be a sequitur of chronic skin failure, or the final and abrupt outcome of acute illness in which treatment is failing and multiple organs are shutting down.

When skin fails catastrophically, the development of pressure ulcers will not only be unavoidable, but their treatment will be problematic, i.e., they will be unlikely to heal regardless of the type of treatment. Thus, healing pressures ulcers at the end of life is not ordinarily a reasonable goal (62).

THE UNAVOIDABLE PRESSURE ULCER REVISITED

The CMS definition of an "unavoidable pressure ulcer" sets a standard that is almost impossible to meet. Even if impeccable care is provided, if the documentation of that care is inadequate at any point (e.g. failing to document a single episode of turning), the pressure ulcer cannot be considered "unavoidable" regardless of the extremity of the patient's medical condition. Conversely, it is possible to provide impeccable documentation ("paper compliance") without providing the actual care. Furthermore, turning every two hours has never been shown to prevent pressure sores, and in fact, might be inadequate in highly compromised patients, or in even simple cases in which strong shear forces are at work, such as a semi-reclining position in bed (64). As Salcido has recently pointed out, the so-called two-hour rule was largely instituted as a result of animal studies (65). What if studies were to show that pressure sores could be prevented by turning every 15 minutes? At what point does the patient become so debilitated that the care required cannot be realistically provided? In fact, recent studies in the rat have already shown that significant stiffening can occur within 30 minutes when 35 kPa (261 mm Hg) is applied, or 15 minutes if 70 kPa (523 mm Hg) is applied (62). Further modeling of these studies in the buttocks of wheelchair users showed that in 30 minutes the stiffening-stress-cell-death-injury spiral can already develop (66), indicating that some patients might need repositioning every half hour.

It has been proposed that the answer to the turning issue is to provide more and more technologically sophisticated beds. However, in general payers will not reimburse for beds until pressure sores have already occurred, so this is not a reasonable option for *prevention* given current healthcare policy. Yet, a common complaint when pressure sores occur is that the hospital or facility ought to have provided pressure-relieving mattresses as part of a preventive plan, even if payers would not have covered it. This shifts the cost of prevention to the facility, out of fear of litigation.

LOCATION, LOCATION, LOCATION

Areas most prone to development of pressure ulcers include the sacrum, greater trochanter, ischial tuberosity, calcaneus, parts of the head, the scapula, the elbow, and the iliac crest (67). However, the vast majority of PUs occur on the sacrum and heel (61, 68) In a large German post-mortem study (N = 3857) these PU locations constituted 76.7% in nursing home residents, and 72.6% in hospital patients (7).

Heel pressure sores are a significant cause of morbidity in the U.S. and a common cause of amputation (69). They usually occur in patients who have underlying peripheral vascular disease, but in acute-care facilities can result from elective hip surgery, or treatment of hip fractures (70, 71). Part of the problem, it is thought, is the use of epidural anesthesia or peripheral nerve blocks for operations involving the hips or knees (72, 73). The calcaneous has only a small amount of soft tissue overlying the fat pad, and it is possible to cause deep tissue trauma on the heels within an hour, especially, if any kind of skin failure is present (62), after which the damage is not reversible.

Figure 2 depicts a heel pressure sore that formed in the same patient with the BKA, as a result of neuropathy and pressure from her shoe while attempting to learn to ambulate with a prosthesis. The extent of the damage could not be appreciated with the blister intact (Figure 2A). Despite immediate off-loading with a wheelchair, an eschar developed and when debrided, the extent of the wound was apparent (Figure 2B). This is another example of the way in which these wounds "evolve" rather than progress after the injury has occurred. It would be easy to assume that appropriate interventions had not been put in place, but in fact, aggressive off-loading was introduced as soon as the blister was discovered. Patients with heel pressure sores must have a plan in place to prevent further trauma. In bedridden patients, L'NARD or multipodus boots are the gold standard as they keep the heels elevated off the bed or floor. It is also possible to use pillows placed under the calf to keep the heels elevated (67), but this might be impractical in patients who have limited capacity for movement.

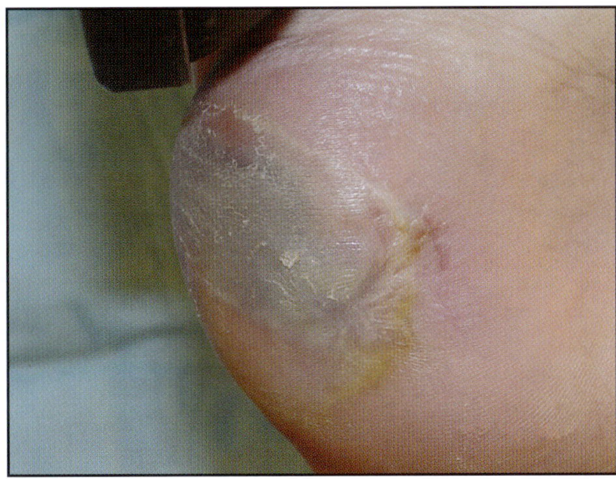

Figure 2A. Heel pressure sore blister as a result of pressure from her shoe. Extent of damage cannot be appreciated with blister intact.

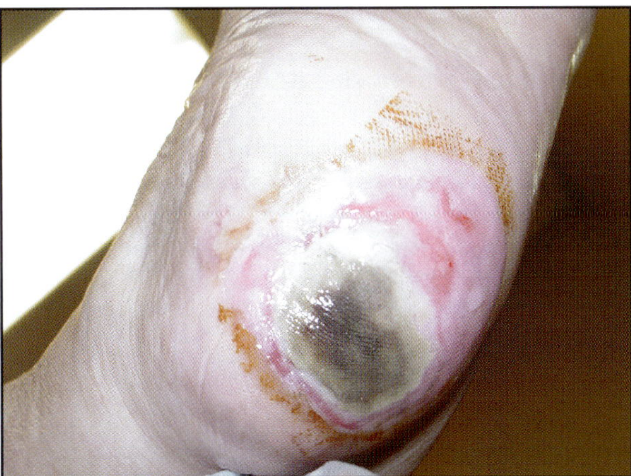

Figure 2B. Heel Pressure sore eschar. Despite immediate offloading an eschar developed and when debrided, the extent of the wound was apparent.

As part of developing a treatment plan for a pressure ulcer patient, the location of the pressure sore must be evaluated in relation to body position. For example, ischial pressure sores are usually due to unrelieved pressure during prolonged periods of sitting. Sacral pressure sores are usually, but not always, due to problems with supine positioning. The patient needs to be observed in his chair or bed if possible and a history taken regarding the length of time he or she remains in any particular position. There are many commercially available seat cushions designed to create an even pressure distribution during sitting. Generally, these cushions fall into four categories: foam, viscoelastic foam, gel, and fluid flotation. Each of these has advantages and disadvantages for a given patient. Interestingly, 8 cm (3.2") has been determined as the most optimal thickness for a foam cushion to reduce pressure over the ischial tuberosity (74).

Recently, pressure mapping has become available to assess the distribution of pressure in various positions and in response to such devices (75). Though the relationship between interfacial pressure and subcutaneous pressure varies—the latter is always larger than the former (69)—these devices can help in selecting the best method of reducing the interface pressure. It also helps to remember that deep muscle stresses (von Mises and internal principal compression) are an order of magnitude greater than interfacial contact stresses (34).

ASSESSING THE RISK FOR DEVELOPING PRESSURE ULCERS

A number of standard assessment tools exist for estimating the risk of developing PUs. The most common of these is the Braden Scale (76), which is a 6-parameter validated instrument (*http://www.bradenscale.com/braden.pdf*). A score of ≤ 18 for elderly and persons with darkly pigmented skin, and ≤ 16 for other adults is considered high risk. Its subgroups comprise: 1) Sensation, 2) Activity, 3) Mobility, 4) Moisture, 5) Friction and 6) Nutrition.

The Norton Scale (76), which is a 5-parameter, validated instrument, is also used commonly, sometimes in conjunction with the Braden, as the two instruments overlap, but cover different areas. Its five parameters include: 1) Physical condition, 2) Mental state, 3) Activity, 4) Mobility and 5) Continence. A score of ≤ 16 for an adult is regarded as the threshold for an increased risk of PU development.

The Braden Q Scale was adapted from the Braden Scale for use in pediatrics, and has seven parameters, although a modified Braden Q Scale with three parameters: 1) Mobility, 2) Sensory perception and 3) Tissue perfusion/oxygenation) is also used (77). The scores for the full and modified scales which identify patients at risk for developing PUs are 16, and seven respectively, with sensitivities and specificities of 0.88 and 0.58, and 0.92 and 0.59 respectively (77).

The purpose of these tools is to identify high-risk settings and patient groups to target interventions to minimize risk. For example, a Braden score of ≤ 13 has been found to be a good threshold for deciding which patients should receive a specialty bed in an ICU, since so many patients are at risk in that setting (78). However, despite that fact that these instruments attempt to assess such factors as moisture and turning, which do predict the development of wounds, they do not directly measure the physiological processes about which we are concerned, such as perfusion and tissue oxygen levels. Using technology, such as transcutaneous oxygen measurement, studies have attempted to define thresholds that are associated with the development of pressure sores (79). However, in practice, such thresholds are often surpassed by patients without apparent damage to tissue; there is yet no method proven to identify impending skin damage. A subset of patients scored as low risk by assessment tools continue to develop pressure sores, and some high-risk patients do not (80, 81).

The allocation of specialty beds and other interventions, even among high-risk patients, requires the development of better technology to evaluate the skin, which can also be used to follow patients longitudinally. Imaging studies on pressure sores have shown that such devices as radiography, computed tomography, and sonography can give information about deeper tissues and provide images showing any complications (82–86). Air cavities on imaging have suggested that in some cases, deep tissue injury might have occurred, which did not affect the skin. Surgeons performing flaps for subsequent wounds describe entering fluid-filled sacs, which are presumed to be areas of pressure injury that never caused visible changes to the skin.

Correlation studies have suggested that anticoagulation medication, low serum albumin level, low total lymphocyte count, fecal incontinence, fractures, increased age, increased length of paralysis, social state of the patient, and smoking have all been correlated with either the presence or worsening of pressure sores (42, 67, 87–89). Studies have also shown that some elderly subjects are not able to increase skin blood flow in response to a thermal stimulus (such as bathing) (90–92), suggesting that aging has an effect on the nervous regulatory mechanisms on blood flow, leading to a predisposition for PU development. Paralysis, in addition to its obvious effect on reducing mobility, might have other direct effects on tissue. Animal studies of denervated tissue showed a significant reduction in thickness of epidermal tissue below the level of paralysis beginning in as little as a week (93–95).

Clearly there is much research to be done to define the most significant physiological factors that increase the risk of developing pressure ulcers. However, with a better understanding of these factors will come better instruments to assess the overall risk.

CURRENT PROTOCOLS FOR TREATMENT OF PRESSURE ULCERS

Pressure sores are an international health problem and many excellent guidelines exist around the world. In the U.S.A., the most referenced document was published by the Agency for Healthcare Policy and Research, (now known as the Agency for Healthcare Research and Quality, AHRQ) AHCPR Clinical Practice Guideline Number 3: Pressure Ulcers in Adults: Prediction and Prevention (AHCPR #92-0047: May 1992). This was created in conjunction with AHCPR #95 Clinical Practice Guideline Number 15: Treatment of Pressure Ulcers (AHCPR #95-0652, Dec 1994). Both can still be ordered at the AHRQ web site (*www.ahrq.gov/news/pubcat/c_clin.htm#clin014*). More recently, the Wound Ostomy and Continence Nurses Association developed excellent guidelines on the prevention/ management of PUs (WOCN Guideline for prevention and management of pressure ulcers, 2003, 52 pp; order from *www.wocn.org*), a summary of which can be found at on the government web site (*www.guideline.gov/summary/pdf.aspx?doc_id=3860&stat=1&string=*).

Evidence-Based Guidelines

As part of the current emphasis on evidence-based medicine, the guidelines developed by the AHCPR and WOCN are rated according to the common Strength of Evidence Ratings Scale (Table 1). It is interesting to note that in the AHCPR guidelines, commonly referred to as the "Purple Book," over 80% of the guidelines are based on C-level evidence. In other words, the majority of treatment guidelines are based on expert opinion. Whether these guidelines reduce pressure ulcer formation is unclear, but following clinical practice guidelines may reduce malpractice lawsuits (96). Table 2 shows several guidelines based upon A and B-level evidence.

Nutrition

Little objective evidence of value exists regarding specific nutritional interventions on ulcer healing or prevention. Several trials (some RCTs) have been conducted with various nutritional regimes that showed essentially no or small positive changes (97–103). A meta-analysis conducted of 5 RCTs out of a total of 15 identified nutritional clinical trials concluded that nutritional interventions, especially those involving high-protein diets, can significantly reduce the risk of developing PUs by 25% (104). Despite this positive assessment, many larger and more well-controlled trials will need to be conducted with regard to the healing and prevention of PUs before the evidence for nutritional interventions can be firmly placed into the A category.

There is widespread acceptance that protein and calorie malnutrition or both, when present, should be addressed, with targets of 35–40 kcal/kg body weight/day for total calories and 1.0–1.5 g protein/kg body weight/day for total protein. However, data supporting specific vitamin administration or other specific supplements is scant. Arginine is often cited as a specific amino acid that should be included nutritional supplements on the basis that it was demonstrated in animals to increase collagen deposition in wound areas, and in the case of humans, simulated wound areas (105). However, accelerated actual wound healing with arginine alone has yet to be demonstrated. Concern that arginine administration might exacerbate inflammation via nitric oxide production appears to have been unwarranted (106). There might additionally be a role for essential fatty acids: a double-blind controlled study employing topical application of linoleic acid showed that it could substantially reduce the development of PUs, as well as maintain skin elasticity in elderly subjects fed a high-protein diet (107). Oxandrolone (anabolic steroid) can also facilitate weight gain but no data exists regarding the impact on wound healing outcome. In assessing dietary intake, albumin, pre-albumin, and transferrin levels should be measured at a minimum; a case might also be made for including C-reactive protein (88, 109).

TABLE 1. STRENGTH OF EVIDENCE RATINGS SCALE

Category	Description
A	The results of two or more randomized controlled clinical trials on pressure ulcers in humans that provide support.
B	The results of two or more controlled clinical trials on pressure ulcers in humans that provide support, or when appropriate, the results of two or more controlled trials in an animal model that provide indirect support.
C	The results of one controlled clinical trial or the results of at least two case studies/descriptive studies on pressure ulcers in humans, or expert opinion.

TABLE 2. SELECTION A-LEVEL AND B-LEVEL EVIDENCE RATINGS IN PURPLE BOOK

A-level Evidence	B-level Evidence
Two-week trial topical antibiotics for clean PUs healing or continuing to produce exudate after 2–4 weeks of optimal patient care	Ensure adequate dietary intake. (p.29)
Assess for recurrence of PUs as an ongoing component of care	Use static support surface if patient can assume a variety of positions without bearing weight on a PU and "bottoming out." (p.39)
	Use dynamic support surface if patient cannot assume a variety of positions without bearing weight on PU (p.39)
	Use enough irrigation pressure to enhance wound cleansing without causing trauma to wound bed. Safe/effective ulcer irrigation pressures range from 4–15psi. (p.51)
	Use dressings to keep ulcer bed continuously moist. Wet-to-dry dressings should be used only for debridement and are not considered continuously moist saline dressings. (p.53)
	Use clinical judgment to select type of moist wound dressing suitable for the ulcers. Studies of different types of moist wound dressings showed no differences in pressure ulcer healing. (p. 53)
	Do not use topical antiseptics (e.g., povidone iodine, iodophor, sodium hypochlorite (Dakin's solution, hydrogen peroxide, acetic acid) to reduce bacteria in wound tissue.

AHCPR guidelines.

Wound Care Principles

Sound wound-care principles are universally applicable to pressure sore management. First, debride the ulcer of devitalized tissue (either by sharp techniques at the bedside or in the operating room, or by enzymatic or autolytic methods. However, blood flow issues should be addressed before aggressively debriding heel PUs, or those of the lower extremities, particularly if end-stage arterial vascular disease or severe ischemia is present.

Second, bear in mind that no significant difference in overall PU healing rates or outcomes exists between types of wound care products. The core principle here is wound bed moisture balance maintenance without maceration of adjacent tissue. In utilizing products, consider caregiver time, ease of use, availability, and cost. In general, little information exists regarding the cost-effectiveness of wound-care products, although hopefully this situation will change as evidence-based medicine is applied to the field of wound care.

Management of the Bacterial Burden

Bacteria are believed to contribute to tissue breakdown and delay the healing of pressure sores. Since hypoxia is present in the final common pathway to tissue injury, a variety of aerobic or anaerobic microorganisms can accumulate, leading to infection, bacteremia, and further tissue damage. All chronic wounds are contaminated with bacteria and most are colonized, the latter referring to organized but noninvasive bacterial growth on the wound surface. However, the classic definition of infection is the presence of greater than 10^5 colony-forming units on a quantitative culture for each ml or gram of infected material. Note that the AHCPR guideline states that pressure sore infection can be diagnosed *only* by quantitative culture from tissue biopsy.

The value of topical antimicrobials in combating contamination and colonization is controversial, because such materials can cause allergic reactions or local hypersensitivity reactions, and some antimicrobials can be toxic to healthy granulation tissue. Systematic reviews on the subject also show that the methodology of clinical trials to date is generally poor (109, 110). As a guideline, a two-week topical course should be considered if the ulcer continues to produce exudate after two to four weeks of care. Silver and cadexomer iodine are commonly used dressings that can be used for this purpose (41). For cases of documented infection in which cellulitis, osteomyelitis, or bacteremia/septicemia are involved, systemic antibiotics should be employed, with attention to side effects, as well as antibiotic resistance. Thus, in one recent French study of methicillin-resistant *Staphylococcus aureus* (MRSA), it was noted that pressure ulcers were an independent risk factor (111). In addition, the practicing clinician should always be on the lookout for developing sepsis: for example, one large retrospective study found that of 114,380 persons whose cause of death was ascribed to pressure ulcers in the U.S. during 1990–2001, 39.7% had septicemia (112).

Pain Assessment

Rastinehead relates the stories of ten patients with painful pressure ulcers who were treated in an acute-care community hospital in a recent article (113). It is clear from their accounts that pain management of PUs is still an area to which we must pay careful attention. The first step is to engage in communication with the patient regarding pain, and observe for physical signs/symptoms in non-communicative patients. The second step is to manage the pain; failure to do so impairs the patient's ability to heal. Understanding the etiology of the ulcer and the nature of the pain—chronic, or associated with dressing changes or debridement—will help decide which approach should be used: topical or systemic administration of analgesics (114, 115) Topical application of morphine and diamorphine-infused gel can be particularly effective in patients receiving palliative care (116). Repositioning of patients and use of appropriate dressings can also assist in mitigating pain.

Closure of Pressure Ulcers

The best nonsurgical rates of healing reported to date are 40% healing for Stage III PUs in nursing homes and 45% in hospitals, and 34% healing for Stage IV PUs in nursing homes and 30.6% in hospitals (117–119) Stage III and IV PUs often will heal with deep tracts. Tracts lose the biochemical stimulatory effects needed for healing, so if they cannot be unroofed, or if there has been substantial loss of subcutaneous tissue, surgical closure, often with a muscle flap, will be necessary. A complete review of the surgical options for pressure ulcer closure is beyond the scope of this chapter but includes: a) direct closure, b) skin grafting, c) skin flaps, d) musculocutaneous flaps and e) free flaps.

The problem with surgical closure of pressure ulcers is that there is a 61% ulcer and 69% patient recurrence within 9.3 months (120), which translates only to a 31% successful long-term outcome for surgery (121). For a patient to be a candidate for plastic surgical closure, compliance with postoperative offloading, and adequate nutrition must occur. As a result, patients whose wound tracts contact to the bone or who otherwise cannot be expected to heal without surgery, but who are not surgical candidates, will fall into the palliative care category.

Adjunctive Therapies

Negative pressure wound therapy

Advanced adjunctive therapies are sometimes used in the treatment of pressure sores. Negative pressure wound therapy is commonly used if not to allow complete wound closure, at least to allow closure with a small flap rather than a large one (122). Two small-scale randomized controlled trials have been performed using the VAC (vacuum-assisted closure) in PU healing and have shown promising results (123, 124), but have been criticized on several grounds (125). Larger-scale, better controlled trials are in progress, but results are not expected soon. Hopefully, these trials will address some of the issues raised.

Other modalities

Other modalities which have undergone evaluation with randomized controlled trials in the case of pressure ulcers include growth factors, which showed an improvement in rate and total healing (126-130), and electrical stimulation (131). Bioengineered skin has shown great promise in RCTs with diabetic and venous leg ulcers (132, 133), yet despite the results of these trials, CMS does not cover the use of bioengineered skin in the management of pressure ulcers, and growth factor therapy would be considered off-label as well. Ultrasound showed no evidence of specific effectiveness as judged by a meta-analysis of trials conducted prior to 2000 (134), though a more recent RCT looks promising (135). Two RCT studies of noncontact normothermic

TABLE 3. AHCPR RECOMMENDATIONS CONCERNING PREVENTION OF PRESSURE ULCERS

Skin Care	Positioning
Assess skin daily	Turn/position bed-bound clients every two hours if consistent with overall care goals
Clean skin at time of soiling—avoid hot water and irritating cleaning agents	Use written schedule for turning/repositioning of clients
Use moisturizers on skin	Use pillows/other devices to keep bony prominences from direct contact with each other
Don't massage bony prominences	Raise heels of bed-bound clients off the bed; don't use donut-type devices
Protect skin of incontinent clients from exposure to moisture	Use a 30-degree lateral side lying position; don't place client directly on their trochanter
Use lubricants, protective dressings, and proper lifting techniques to avoid skin injury from friction/shear during transfer and turning of clients.	Keep head of bed at lowest height possible
	Use lifting devices (trapeze, bed linen) to move clients rather than dragging them in bed during transfers and position changes
	Use pressure-reducing devices (static air, alternating air, gel, water mattresses)
	Reposition chair—or wheelchair-bound clients — *every hour.* In addition, if clients are capable, have them perform small weight shifts every *15 minutes.*
	Use a pressure-reducing device (not a donut) for chair-bound

wound therapy also look promising, though further research might be required to substantiate this approach (136, 137).

Risk assessment

Standard nursing orders to prevent pressure ulcers recommend performing a risk assessment at regular intervals, as well as following AHCPR recommendations (see Table 3). The ulcer prevention program outlined by Hiser et al. (18) shows that when such a program is properly designed and implemented, significant improvements in outcomes can be obtained.

Nutrition and support surface assessment

When pressure ulcers are identified, nutritional assessment and an assessment of the support surface are both important aspects of patient evaluation regardless of whether the patient is an inpatient or an outpatient. The topic of support surfaces is a complex one and necessarily linked to third-party payment policy. Static support surfaces are not mechanically operated; dynamic support surfaces are for those patients who are unable to change positions without bearing weight on the pressure ulcer, completely compress a static support surface, or have no evidence of improvement with regard to the ulcer.

Low-air-loss mattresses contain air-permeable fabric pillows that are constantly inflated with air, whereas air-fluidized beds contain silicone-coated beads covered by an air-permeable fabric, and which liquefy when air is pumped through the bed, allowing the patient to float on them. These dynamic surfaces are for patients who have multiple Stage III or Stage IV ulcers on their turning surfaces and occasionally for patients who have excess moisture on intact skin.

Evaluating support surfaces has been difficult. The majority of studies have been too small, thereby harboring problems of effect size (type 2 error)—in other words they were not sufficiently large to discriminate on a statistical basis the relatively small effects between devices. In addition, many suffered from design flaws. An extensive meta-analysis carried out in 2001 by Cullum et al. (38) reported a significant reduction in pressure incidence (RR: 71%; 95% CI: 57–81) when standard hospital mattresses were replaced with foam alternatives (pooled results of 4 RCTs), however the conclusions were mixed regarding comparisons of different low-tech mattresses. Similar deductions were reached in a later meta-analysis review (139). When Cullum et al. (138) reviewed alternating pressure (AP) versus constant low pressure devices they found no significant differences between the two classes, though they cited one robust trial that provided evidence for the efficacy of air-fluidized bed over AP beds (140). A large well-controlled very recent RCT also concluded that there was no difference between AP mattresses and alternating pressure overlays in preventing PUs, but that AP types are more cost-effective and better tolerated by patients (141). Clearly, controversy exists over the use of high-tech pressure-reduction devices and until more data, especially cost-effectiveness data, is published, this class of beds will be only be utilized by high-risk patients. On the other hand, even for low-risk patients, foam alternative mattresses should be utilized in all healthcare settings.

Medicare Group Coverage Criteria for Support Surfaces

Medicare defines Group I support surfaces as static devices that are not electrically powered, Group 2 as those support surfaces powered by a pump or electricity and are dynamic in nature, and Group 3 as air-fluidized beds.

Group 1 support surfaces are covered under Medicare Part B if the patient is completely immobile or the patient has limited mobility or any stage ulcer on the trunk or pelvis, and has at least one of the following:
1. Impaired nutritional status.
2. Fecal or urinary incontinence.
3. Altered sensory perception.
4. Compromised circulatory status.

Group 2 support surfaces are covered if the patient meets: a) criteria 1, 2, and 3, b) criterion 4, or c) criteria 5 and 6:
1. Multiple Stage II pressure ulcers located on the trunk or pelvis.
2. Patient has been on a comprehensive ulcer treatment program for at least the past month, which has included the use of an appropriate Group 1 support surface.
3. The ulcers have worsened or remained the same over the past month.

4. Large or multiple Stage III or IV pressure ulcer(s) on the trunk or pelvis.
5. Recent myocutaneous flap or skin graft for a pressure ulcer on the trunk or pelvis (surgery within the past 60 days).
6. The patient has been on a Group 2 or 3 support surface prior to a recent discharge from a hospital or a skilled nursing facility.

Group 3 support surfaces are covered only if the patient meets 'the following criteria:
1. The patient has a Stage III or IV ulcer.
2. The patient is bedridden or chair bound as a result of severely limited mobility.
3. In the absence of an air-fluidized bed, the patient would require institutionalization.
4. The air-fluidized bed is ordered in writing by the patient's attending physician based upon a comprehensive assessment and evaluation.
5. A comprehensive ulcer treatment program, including the use of an appropriate Group II support surface, has been tried for at least one month with worsening or no improvement to the ulcer.
6. A trained adult caregiver is available to assist the patient with activities of daily living, repositioning, dietary and fluid needs, prescribed treatments, and management and support of the air-fluidized bed system and its problems.
7. A physician directs the home treatment regimen on a monthly basis.
8. All other alternative equipment has been considered and ruled out.

Coverage will be denied if: a) there is co-existing pulmonary disease, b) wet soaks or moist dressings are not protected with an impervious covering, c) the caregiver is unwilling or unable to provide the type of care required on an air-fluidized bed, d) the structure support is inadequate to support the weight of the air-fluidized bed, or e) the electrical system is insufficient for the anticipated increase in consumption.

MEASURING OUTCOMES

The National Quality Forum is a private, not-for-profit membership organization tasked with the endorsement of consensus-based national standards for measurement and public reporting of healthcare performance data. They have established a number of performance standards pertaining to pressure ulcers (order from *http://www.qualityforum.org*). Most of these pertain to institutionalized or hospitalized patients. As the Center for Medicare Services (CMS) evolves its policies relating to Pay for Performance standards for physicians and other reimbursement and quality issues, it can be assumed that facilities (e.g. hospitals, nursing homes) or outpatient wound centers will need to report on some or all of these measures. This will require the ability to track wound measurements and other forms of patient outcomes in an organized, prospective way. For those patients in whom palliative care is the goal, meaningful outcomes can still be measured in the form of wound drainage, rate of infection, pain control, and quality of life indices.

SUMMARY

Pressure ulcers form from the inside out so that the depth and extent of tissue trauma might not be apparent from the condition of the skin. The NPUAP staging system refers only to the depth of tissue in the base of the wound at the time it is assessed. Stage III and IV pressure sores are not preceded by Stage I and II pressure sores; indeed, the most common cause of a Stage II "pressure sore" is friction. While risk-assessment tools, such as the Braden scale, are an important method to identify high-risk patients, these tools evaluate surrogates for pressure ulcer formation. Among the critical factors that determine skin breakdown are perfusion, tissue oxygenation, vascular response to stress, cellular effects of aging, lymphostasis, cellular reparative processes, and other physiological factors for which there are no practical measurement tools at this time. The current definition of an "unpreventable pressure sore" is largely based on documentation of certain types of care, yet it is possible that the skin can "fail" in the same way that other organs can fail, although this concept has still to gain widespread traction. Until there is some mechanism for evaluating tissue response to stress, it is likely that pressure sores will continue to occur despite the best care, and that caregivers will be considered at fault for their formation. Pressure sores represent a multibillion-dollar healthcare problem in the U.S.A. There is little doubt that the problem will continue to grow as our population ages, and better methods of screening for, preventing, and treating pressure ulcers are needed.

OTHER RESOURCES

A number of other useful documents pertaining to pressure ulcers can be found at the National Quality Clearinghouse web site (available at: *http://www.qualitymeasures.ahrq.gov/Browse/DisplayOrganization.aspx?org_id=1750& doc=7405)*.

REFERENCES

1. Barczak CA, Barnett RI, Childs EJ, et al. Fourth national pressure ulcer survey. *Adv Wound Care* 1997; 10:18-26.

2. Amlung SR, Miller WL, Boslev LM. The 1999 national pressure ulcer survey: a benchmarking approach. *Adv Skin Wound Care* 2001; 14:297-301.

3. Scott JR, Gibran NS, Engrav LH, et al. Incidence and characteristics of hospitalized patients with pressure ulcers: State of Washington, 1987 to 2000. *Plast Reconstr Surg* 2006; 117:630-634.

4. Baumgarten M, Margolis D, Gruber-Baldini AL, et al. Pressure ulcers and the transition to long-term care. *Adv Skin Wound Care* 2003; 16:299-304.

5. Coleman EA, Martau JM, Lin MK, et al. Pressure ulcer prevalence in long-term nursing home residents since the implementation of OBRA '87. Omnibus Budget Reconciliation Act. *J Am Geriatr Soc* 2002; 50:728-732.

6. Spector WD, Fortinsky RH. Pressure ulcer prevalence in Ohio nursing homes: clinical and facility correlates. *J Aging Health* 1998; 10:62-80.

7. Lahmann NA, Halfens RJ, Dassen T. Pressure ulcers in German nursing homes and acute care hospitals: prevalence, frequency, and ulcer characteristics. *Ostomy Wound Manage* 2006;52:20-33.

8. Bours GJ, Halfens RJ, Abu-Saad HH, et al. Prevalence, prevention, and treatment of pressure ulcers: descriptive study in 89 institutions in the Netherlands. *Res Nurs Health* 2002; 25;99-100.

9. Kuhn BA, Coulter SJ. Balancing the pressure ulcer cost and quality equation. *Nurs Econ* 1992;10:353-359.

10. Beckrich K, Aronovitch SA. Hospital-acquired pressure ulcers: a comparison of costs in medical vs. surgical patients. *Nurs Econ* 1999; 17:263-271.

11. Zhan C, Miller MR. Excess length of stay, charges, and mortality attributable to medical injuries during hospitalization. *J Am Med Soc* 2003; 290:1868-1874.

12. Brem H, Lyder C. Protocol for the successful treatment of pressure ulcers. *Am J Surg* 2004; 188(Suppl):9S-17S.

13. Zulkowksi K, Langemo D, Posthauer ME, The National Pressure Ulcer Advisory Panel. Coming to consensus on deep tissue injury. *Adv Skin Wound Care* 2005; 18:28-29.

14. Berlowitz DR, Bezerra HQ, Brandeis GH, et al. Are we improving the quality of nursing home care: the case of pressure ulcers. *J Am Geriatr Soc* 2000; 48:59-62.

15. Eckman KL. The prevalence of dermal ulcers among persons in the U.S. who have died. *Decubitus* 1989; 2:36-40.

16. Mark BA, Harless DW, McCue M, et al. A longitudinal examination of hospital registered nurse staffing and quality of care. *Health Serv Res* 2004; 39:279-300.

17. Juliano EB, Fell JR. Medical information management in nursing home litigation. Pressure Ulcers (Part I of II). *Rev Med Info Manage Litig* 2000; 3:1-5.

18. Hiser B, Rochette J, Philbin S, et al. Implementing a pressure ulcer prevention program and enhancing the role of the CWOCN: Impact on outcomes. *Ostomy Wound Manage* 2006; 52:48-59.

19. Bliss M, Simini B. When are the seeds of postoperative pressure sores sown? Often during surgery. *Br Med J* 1999; 319:863-864.

20. Russell L, Reynolds T, Clark M. More research is needed into the origins of pressure sores. *Br Med J* 2000; 320:801.

21. Bliss M, Simini B. Authors' reply. *Br Med J* 2000;320:801.

22. Meehan M, Hill WM. Pressure ulcers in nursing homes: does negligence litigation exceed available evidence? *Ostomy Wound Manage* 2002;48:46-54.

23. Bennett RG, O'Sullivan J, DeVito EM, et al. The increasing medical malpractice risk related to pressure ulcers in the United States. *J Am Geriatr Soc* 2000; 48:73-81.

24. Bergstrom N, Bennet MA, Carlson CE, et al. Clinical Practice Guideline Number 15: Treatment of pressure ulcers. Rockville, MD: US Department of Health and Human Services. Agency of Health Care Policy and Research; 1994. AHQR publication No. 95-0652.

25. Voss AC, Bender SA, Ferguson ML, et al. Long-term care liability for pressure ulcers. *J Am Geriatr Soc* 2005; 53:1587–1592.

26. Rowe TA. Nursing home personal injury ot [sic] just nuisance-value cases. Indiana Lawyer 1999. November 10, 22.

27. Konetzka RT, Norton EC, Sloane PD, et al. Medicare prospective payment and the quality of care for long-stay nursing facility residents. *Med Care* 2006; 44:270-276.

28. Grabowski DC, Angelelli JJ. The relationship of Medicaid payment rates, bed constraint policies, and risk-adjusted pressure ulcers. *Health Serv Res* 2004; 39:793-812.

29. Lyder C, van Rijswijk L. Pressure ulcer prevention and care: preventing and managing pressure ulcers in long-term care: An overview of the revised federal regulation. *Ostomy Wound Manage* 2005; 51(4 Suppl):2-6.

30. Stewart S, Box-Panksepp JS. Preventing hospital-acquired pressure ulcers: a point prevalence study. *Ostomy Wound Manage* 2004;50:46-51.

31. Witkowski JE, Parish LC. Histopathology of the decubitus ulcer. *J Am Acad Dermatol* 1982; 6:1014-1021.

32. Daniel RK, Wheatley D, Priest D. Pressure sores and paraplegia. *Ann Plast Surg* 1985; 15:41-49.

33. Nola GT, Vistnes LM. Differential response of skin and muscle in the experimental production of pressure sores. *Plast Reconstr Surg* 1980; 66:728-733.

34. Linder-Ganz E, Gefen A. Mechanical compression-induced pressure sores in rat hindlimb: muscle stiffness, histology, and computational models. *J Appl Physiol* 2004; 96:2034-2049.

35. Newson TP, Pearcy MJ, Rolfe P. Skin surface PO2 measurement and the effect of externally applied pressure. *Arch Phys Med Rehabil* 1981; 62:390-392.

36. Seiler WO, Stahelin HB. Skin oxygen tension as a function of imposed skin pressure: implication for decubitus ulcer formation. *J Am Geriatr Soc* 1979;27:298-301.

37. Goossens RH, Zegers R, Hoek van Dijke GA, et al. Influence of shear on skin oxygen tension. *Clin Physiol* 1994; 14:111-118.

38. Crenshaw RP, Vistnes LM. A decade of pressure sore research:1977-1987. *J Rehabil Res Dev* 1989; 26:63-74.

39. Linder-Ganz E, Shabshin N, Itzchak Y, et al. Assessment of mechanical conditions in sub-dermal tissues during sitting: A combined experimental-MRI and finite element approach. *J Biomech* 2006; Aug 17; [Epub ahead of print].

40. Stekelenburg A, Oomens CW, Strijkers GJ, et al. Compression-induced deep tissue injury examined with magnetic resonance imaging and histology. *J Appl Physiol* 2006; 100:1946-1954.

41. Niezgoda JA, Mendez-Eastman S. The effective management of pressure ulcers. *Adv Skin Wound Care* 2006; 19(Suppl 1):3-15.

42. Horn S, Bender SA, Ferguson ML, et al. The National Pressure Ulcer Long-Term Care Study: Pressure ulcer development in long-term care residents. *J Am Geriatr Soc* 2004;52:359-367

43. Knight SL. Taylor RP, Polliack AA, et al. Establishing predictive indicators for the status of loaded soft tissues. *J Appl Physiol* 2001; 90:2231-2237.

44. Krouskop TA. A synthesis of the factors that contribute to pressure sore formation. *Med Hypotheses* 1983; 11:255-267.

45. Rodriguez GP, Claus-Walker J. Biochemical changes in skin composition in spinal cord injury: a possible contribution to decubitus ulcers. *Paraplegia* 1988; 26:302-309.

46. Rodriguez GP, Claus-Walker J, Kent MC, et al. Collagen metabolite excretion as predictor of bone-and-skin complications in spinal cord injury. *Arch Phys Med Rehabil* 1989; 70:442-444.

47. Perier C, Granouillet R, Chamson A, et al. Nutritional markers and tissue inhibitor of matrix metalloproteinase 1 in elderly patients with pressure sores. *Gerontology* 2002; 48;298-301.

48. Seiler WO, Stahelin HB. Recent findings on decubitus ulcer pathology: implications for care. *Geriatrics* 1986; 41:47-50,53-57,60.

49. Bader DL, Barnhill RL, Ryan TJ. Effect of externally applied skin surface forces on tissue vasculature. *Arch Phys Med Rehabil* 1986; 67:807-811.

50. Kokate JY, Leland KJ, Held AM, et al. Temperature-modulated pressure ulcers: a porcine model. *Arch Phys Med Rehabil* 1995;76:666-673.

51. Matas A, Sowa MG, Taylor V, et al. Eliminating the issue of skin color in assessment of the blanch response. *Adv Skin Wound Care* 2001; 14:180-188.

52. Halfens RJ, Bours GJ, Van Ast W. Relevance of the diagnosis of "stage 1 pressure ulcer": an empirical study of the clinical course of stage 1 ulcers in acute care and long-term care hospital populations. *J Clin Nurs* 2001; 10:748-757.

53. Posthauer ME, Zulkowski K. The NPUAP dual mission conference: reaching consensus on staging and deep tissue injury. *Ostomy Wound Manage* 2005; 51:34.

54. Bates-Jensen BM, Cadogan M, Osterweil D, et al. The minimum data set pressure ulcer indicator: does it reflect differences in care processes related to pressure ulcer prevention and treatment in nursing homes? *J Am Geriatr Soc* 2003; 51:1203-1212.

55. Adams CE, DeFrates DS, Wilson M. Data-driven quality improvement for HMO patients: one agency's experience with OASIS and OBQI. *J Nurs Adm* 1998; 28:20-25.

56. Shaughnessy PW, Crisler KS, Schlenker RE. Outcome-based quality improvement in home health care: the OASIS indicators. *Top Health Inf Manage* 1998; 18:59-69.

57. Bergquist S. Pressure ulcer prediction in older adults receiving home health care: implications for use with OASIS. *Adv Skin Wound Care* 2003; 16:132-139.

58. Thomas DR. Are all pressure ulcers avoidable? *J Am Med Dir Assoc* 2003; 4(2 Suppl):S43-S48.

59. Brandeis GH, Berlowitz DR, Katz P. Are pressure ulcers preventable? A survey of experts. *Adv Skin Wound Care* 2001; 14:244,245-248.

60. Byrne J. More on pressure ulcers and the standard of care. *Adv Skin Wound Care* 2005; 18:352-353. [Author (Olshansky K) reply]

61. Brown G. Long-term outcomes of full-thickness pressure ulcers: healing and mortality. *Ostomy Wound Manage* 2003; 49:42-50.

62. Langemo DK, Brown G. Skin fails too: acute, chronic, and end-stage skin failure. *Adv Skin Wound Care* 2006; 19:206-211.

63. Arun I, Aparna P. Acute skin failure: Concept, causes, consequences, and care. *Indian J Dermatol Venereol Leprol* 2006; 71:379-385.

64. Reichel S. Shearing force as a factor in decubitus ulcers in paraplegics. *J Am Med Assoc* 1958; 166:762-763.

65. Salcido R. Patient turning schedules: why and how often? *Adv Skin Wound Care* 2004; 17:156.

66. Gefen A, Gefen N, Linder-Ganz E, et al. In vivo muscle stiffening under bone compression promotes deep pressure sores. *J Biomech Eng* 2005; 127:512-24.

67. Dharmarajan TS, Ahmed S. The growing problem of pressure ulcers. *Postgrad Med* 2003; 113:77-90.

68. Tippett AW. Wounds at the end of life. *Wounds* 2005; 17:91-98.

69. Kerstein, M. D. Heel ulcerations in the diabetic patient. *Wounds* 2002; 14:212-216,

70. Versluysen M. Pressure sores in elderly patients: The epidemiology related to hip operations. *J Bone Joint Surg* 1985; 67-B:10-13.

71. Houwing RH, Rozendaal M, Wouters-Wesseling W, et al. Pressure ulcer risk in hip fracture patients. *Acta Orthop Scand* 2004; 75:390–393.

72. Edwards JL, Pandit H, Popat MT. Perioperative analgesia: a factor in the development of heel pressure ulcers? *Br J Nurs* 2006; 15:S20-S25.

73. Todkar M. Sciatic nerve block causing heel ulcer after total knee replacement in 36 patients. *Acta Orthop Belg* 2005; 71:724-725.

74. Ragan R, Kernozek TW, Bidar M, et al. Seat-interface pressures on various thicknesses of foam wheelchair cushions: a finite modeling approach. *Arch Phys Med Rehabil* 2002; 83:872-875.

75. Stinson MD, Porter-Armstrong AP, Eakin PA. Pressure mapping systems: reliability of pressure map interpretation. *Clin Rehabil* 2003; 17:504-511.

76. Lyder CH. Pressure ulcer prevention and management. *J Am Med Assoc* 2003; 289:223-226.

77. Curley MA, Razmus IS, Roberts KE, et al. Predicting pressure ulcer risk in pediatric patients: the Braden Q Scale. *Nurs Res* 2003; 52:22-33.

78. Fife C, Otto G, Capsuto EG, et al. Incidence of pressure ulcers in a neurologic intensive care unit. *Crit Care Med* 2001; 29:283-290.

79. Mawson AR, Siddiqui FH, Connolly BJ, et al. Sacral transcutaneous oxygen tension levels in the spinal cord injured: risk factors for pressure ulcers? *Arch Phys Med Rehabil* 1993; 74:745-751.

80. Defloor T, Grypdonck MF. Pressure ulcers: validation of two risk assessment scales. *J Clin Nurs* 2005; 14:373-382.

81. Gould D, Goldstone L, Gammon J, et al. Establishing the validity of pressure ulcer risk assessment scales: a novel approach using illustrated patient scenarios. *Int J Nurs Stud* 2002; 39:215-228.

82. Dyson M, Moodley S, Verjee L, et al. Wound healing assessment using 20 MHz ultrasound and photography. *Skin Res Technol* 2003; 9:116-121.

83. Schwartz SR, Murray RA. Assessment of epithelial thickness by ultrasonic imaging. *Decubitus* 1991; 4:29-30,32,34,passim.

84. Ruan CM, Escobedo E, Harrison S, et al. Magnetic resonance imaging of nonhealing pressure ulcers myocutaneous flaps. *Arch Phys Med Rehabil* 1998; 79:1080-1088.

85. Esposito G, Ziccardi P, Meoli S, et al. Multiple CT imaging in pressure sores. *Plast Reconstr Surg* 1994; 94:333-342.

86. Livesley NJ, Chow AW. Infected pressure ulcers in elderly patients. *Clin Infect Dis* 2002; 35:1390-1396.

87. Clever K, Smith G, Bowser C, et al. Evaluating the efficacy of a uniquely delivered skin protectant and its effect on the formation of sacral/buttock pressure ulcers. *Ostomy Wound Manage* 2002; 48:60-67.

88. Gengenbacher M, Stahelin HB, Scholer A, et al. Low biochemical nutritional parameters in acutely ill hospitalized elderly patients with and without Stage III to IV pressure ulcers. *Aging Clin Exp Res* 2002; 14:420-423.

89. Fisher AR, Wells G, Harrison MB. Factors associated with pressure ulcers in adults in acute care hospitals. *Adv Skin Wound Care* 2004; 17:80-90.

90. Ek AC, Lewis DH, Zetterqvist H, et al. Skin blood flow in an area at risk for pressure sore. *Scand J Rehabil Med* 1984; 16:85-89.

91. van Marcum RJ, Meijer JH, Ribbe MW. The relationship between pressure ulcers and skin blood flow response after a local cold provocation. *Arch Phys Med Rehabil* 2002; 83:40-43.

92. Smolander J. Effect of cold exposure on older humans. *Int J Sports Med* 2002; 23:86-92.

93. Hunang IT, Lin WM, Shun CT, et al. Influence of cutaneous nerves on keratinocyte proliferation and epidermal thickness in mice. *Neuroscience* 1999; 94:965-973.

94. Chiang HY, Huang IT, Chen WP, et al. Regional difference in epidermal thinning after skin denervation. *Exp Neurol* 1998; 154:137-145.

95. Li Y, Hsieh ST, Chien HF, et al. Sensory and motor denervation influence epidermal thickness in rat foot glabrous skin. *Exp Neurol* 1997; 147:452-462.

96. Goebel RH, Goebel MR. Clinical practice guidelines for pressure ulcer prevention can prevent malpractice lawsuits in older patients. *J Wound Ostomy Continence Nurs* 1999;26:175-184.

97. Frias SL, Lage Vazquez MA, Maristany CP, et al. The effectiveness of oral nutritional supplementation in the healing of pressure ulcers. *J Wound Care* 2004; 13:319-322.

98. Rypkema G, Adang E, Dicke H, et al. Cost-effectiveness of an interdisciplinary intervention in geriatric inpatients to prevent malnutrition. *J Nutr Health Aging* 2004; 8:122-127.

99. Houwing RH, Rozendaal M, Wouters-Wesseling W, et al. A randomised double-blind assessment of the effect of nutritional supplementation on the prevention of pressure ulcers in hip-fracture patients. *Clin Nutr* 2003; 22:401-405.

100. Bourdel-Marchasson I, Barateau M, Rondeau V, et al. A multi-center trial of the effects of oral nutritional supplementation in critically ill older inpatients. GAGE Group. Groupe Aquitain Geriatrique d'Evaluation. *Nutrition* 2000; 16:1-5.

101. Hartgrink HH, Wille J, Konig P, et al. Pressure sores and tube feeding in patients with a fracture of the hip: a randomized clinical trial. *Clin Nutr* 1998; 17:287-292.

102. Breslow RA, Hallfrisch J, Guy DG, et al. The importance of dietary protein in healing pressure ulcers. *J Am Geriatr Soc* 1993; 41:357-362.

103. Desneves KJ, Todorovic BE, Cassar A, et al. Treatment with supplementary arginine, vitamin C and zinc in patients with pressure ulcers: a randomised controlled trial. *Clin Nutr* 2005; 24:979-987.

104. Stratton RJ, Ek AC, Engfer M, et al. Enteral nutritional support in prevention and treatment of pressure ulcers: a systematic review and meta-analysis. *Ageing Re Rev* 2005; 4:422-450.

105. Williams JZ, Abumrad N, Barbul A. Effect of a specialized amino acid mixture on human collagen deposition. *Ann Surg* 2002; 236;369-374.

106. Stechmiller JK, Langkamp-Henken B, Childress B, et al. Arginine supplementation does not enhance serum nitric oxide levels in elderly nursing home residents with pressure ulcers. *Biol Res Nurs* 2005; 6:289-299.

107. Declair V. The usefulness of topical application of essential fatty acids (EFA) to prevent pressure ulcers. *Ostomy Wound Manage* 1997; 43:48-52,54.

108. Reynolds TM, Stokes A, Russell L. Assessment of a prognostic biochemical indicator of nutrition and inflammation for identification of pressure ulcer risk. *J Clin Pathol* 2006; 59:308-310.

109. O'Meara S, Cullum N, Majid M, et al. Systematic reviews of wound care management: (3) antimicrobial agents for chronic wounds; (4) diabetic foot ulceration. *Health Technol Assess* 2000;4:1-237.

110. O'Meara SM, Cullum NA, Majid M, et al. Systematic review of antimicrobial agents used for chronic wounds. *Br J Surg* 2001; 88:4-21.

111. Pittet D. Challenges, treatment strategies and clinical progression of MRSA bacteremia. *Presse Med* 2004; 10(12 Pt 2):2S10-17.

112. Redelings MD, Lee NE, Sorvillo F. Pressure ulcers: more lethal than we thought? *Adv Skin Wound Care* 2005; 18:367-372.

113. Rastinehead D. Pressure ulcer pain. *J Wound Ostomy Continence Nurs* 2006; 33:252-257.

114. Reddy M, Keast D, Fowler E, et al. Pain in pressure ulcers. *Ostomy Wound Manage* 2003; 49(4 Suppl):30-35.

115. Freedman G, Cean C, Duron V, et al. Pathogenesis and treatment of pain in patients with chronic wounds. *Surg Technol Int* 2003; 11:168-179.

116. Ashfield T. The use of topical opioids to relieve pressure ulcer pain. *Nurs Stand* 2005; 19:90-92.

117. Payne WG, Ochs DE, Meltzer DD, et al. Long-term outcome study of growth factor-treated pressure ulcers. *Am J Surg* 2001; 181:81-86.

118. Brandeis GH, Morris JN, Nash DJ, et al. The epidemiology and natural history of pressure ulcers in elderly nursing home residents. *J Am Med Assoc* 1990; 264:2905-2909.

119. Berlowitz DR, Brandeis GH, Anderson J, et al. Predictors of pressure ulcer healing among long-term care residents. *J Am Geriatr Soc* 1997; 45:30-34.

120. Disa JJ, Carlton JM, Goldberg NH. Efficacy of operative cure in pressure sore patients. *Plast Reconstr Surh* 1992; 89:272-278.

121. Payne WG, Wright TE, Ochs D, et al. Dermagraft Pressure Ulcer Study Group. An exploratory study of dermal replacement therapy in the treatment of Stage III pressure ulcers. *J Appl Res* 2004; 4:12-23.

122. Ferreira MC, Wada A, Tuma P Jr. The vacuum assisted closure of complex wounds; report of 3 cases. *Rev Hosp Clin Fac Med S Paulo* 2003; 58:227-230.

123. Ford CN, Reinhard ER, Yeh D, et al. Interim analysis of a prospective, randomized trial of vacuum-assisted closure versus the healthpoint system in the management of pressure ulcers. *Ann Plast Surg* 2002; 49:55-61.

124. Wanner MB, Schwarzl F, Strub B, et al. Vacuum-assisted wound closure for cheaper and more comfortable healing of pressure sores: a prospective study. *Scand J Plast Reconstr Surg Hand Surg* 2003; 37;28-33.

125. Samson D, Lefevre F, Aronson N. Wound-healing technologies; low-level laser and vacuum-assisted closure. Summary. Evidence Report/Technology Assessment No. 111, 2003. Rockville, MD: Agency for Healthcare Research and Quality, Publication No. 05-E005-1.

126. Landi F, Aloe L, Russo A, et al. Topical treatment of pressure ulcers with nerve growth factor: a randomized clinical trial. *Ann Intern Med* 2003; 139:635-641.

127. Hirschberg J, Coleman J, Marchant B, et al. TGF-beta3 in the treatment of pressure ulcers: a preliminary report. *Adv Skin Wound Care* 2001; 14:91-95.

128. Kallianinen LK, Hirschberg J, Marchant B, et al. Role of platelet derived growth factor as an adjunct to surgery in the management of pressure ulcers. *Plast Reconstr Surg* 2000; 106:1243-1248.

129. Rees RS, Robson MC, Smiell JM, et al. Becaplermin gel in the treatment of pressure ulcers: a phase II randomized, double-blind, placebo-controlled study. *Wound Repair Regen* 1999; 7:141-147.

130. Robson MC, Phillips LG, Robson LE, et al. Platelet-derived growth factor BB for the treatment of chronic pressure ulcers. *Lancet* 1992; 339:23-25.

131. Adunsky A, Ohry A, DDCT Group. Decubitus direct current treatment (DDCT) of pressure ulcers: results of a randomized double-blinded placebo controlled study. *Arch Gerontol Geriatr* 2005; 41:261-269.

132. Falanga V, Sabolinsky M. A bilayered living skin construct (APLIGRAF) accelerates complete closure of hard-to-heal venous ulcers. *Wound Repair Regen* 1999; 7;201-207.

133. Marston WA, Hanft J, Norwood P, et al. Dermagraft Foot Ulcer Study Group. The efficacy and safety of Dermagraft in improving the healing of chronic diabetic foot ulcers: results of a prospective randomized trial. *Diabetes Care* 2003; 26:1701-1705.

134. Flemming K, Cullum N. Therapeutic ultrasound for pressure sores. *Cochrane Database Syst Rev* 2000; 4:CD001275.

135. Ennis WJ, Foremann P, Mozen N, et al. Ultrasound therapy for recalcitrant diabetic foot ulcers: results of a randomized, double-blind, controlled, multicenter study. *Ostomy Wound Manage* 2005; 51:24-39.

136. Whitney JD, Salvadalena G, Higa L, et al. Treatment of pressure ulcers with noncontact normothermic wound therapy: healing and warming effects. *J Wound Ostomy Continence Nurs* 2001; 28:244-252.

137. Kloth LC, Berman JE, Nett M, et al. A randomized controlled clinical trial to evaluate the effects of noncontact normothermic wound therapy on chronic full-thickness pressure ulcers. *Adv Skin Wound Care* 2002; 15:270-276.

138. Cullum N, Nelson EA, Flemming K, et al. Systematic reviews of wound care management: (5) beds; (6) compression; (7) laser therapy, therapeutic ultrasound, electrotherapy, and electromagnetic therapy. *Health Technol Assess* 2001; 5:1-221.

139. Cullum N, McInnes E, Bell-Syer SE, et al. Support surfaces for pressure ulcer prevention. *Cochrane Database Syst Rev* 2004; 3:CD001735.

140. Allman RM, Keruly JC, Smith CR. Cost effectiveness of air-fluidized beds versus conventional therapy for pressure sores. *Clin Res* 1987; 35:A728.

141. Nixon J, Nelson EA, Cranny G, et al. Pressure relieving support surfaces: a randomised evaluation. *Health Technol Assess* 2006; 10:1-180.

REVIEW QUESTIONS

1.) Recent regulatory and treatment guidelines have led to a significant decrease in the incidence of pressure ulcers in U.S. patients.
    a. True
    b. False

2.) All of the following tools are used to identify high-risk settings and patient groups to target interventions to minimize risk for pressure ulcers EXCEPT:
    a. Braden Scale
    b. Norton Scale
    c. Braden Q Scale
    d. Wagner Scale

3.) In the opinion of the author, limitations of the current NPUAP pressure ulcer staging system include:
    a. The "unstageable wound"
    b. The deep tissue injury phenomenon for which the current staging system does not allow
    c. Reverse staging mandated by governmental policies for nursing homes
    d. The inclusion of superficial wounds due to friction with those actually due to pressure
    e. The misconception that pressure ulcers develop according to a numeric sequence, rather than the understanding that the "stage" represents only the depth of current wound
    f. All of the above.

4.) Which of the following statements about pressure injury is FALSE?
    a. Animal studies have shown that muscle is more sensitive to pressure than skin, suggesting that deeper tissues, such as muscle, will undergo necrosis under less severe conditions than the superficial tissues.
    b. The final common pathway to tissue injury is ischemia and hypoxia.
    c. Necrosis can occur more easily in tissues overlying a bony prominence
    d. Shear stress exacerbates the reduction in oxygen tension and accompanying ischemia in skin.
    e. Pressure sores form from the outside in, rather than from the inside out.

5.) According to the National Pressure Ulcer Advisory Panel (NPUAP) pressure ulcer staging system, which of the following is a Stage IV pressure ulcer?
    a. Non-blanching erythema of skin
    b. Partial-thickness skin loss (epidermis and possibly dermis)
    c. Full-thickness skin loss down to but not including fascia
    d. Full-thickness skin loss including muscle, bone, or supporting structures)

Answers: 1b, 2d, 3f, 4e, 5d.

NOTES

Chapter **18**

INTERVENTIONS IN MANAGING PRESSURE ULCERS

CHAPTER EIGHTEEN OVERVIEW

NOTES

INTERVENTIONS IN MANAGING PRESSURE ULCERS

Craig L. Broussard

PRESSURE ULCERS

Once referred to as "bed sores," pressure ulcers affect persons of all age groups, ethnicities, and economic backgrounds. Pressure ulcers are seen in severely debilitated individuals who are at the end of life as well as otherwise healthy, active individuals with spinal cord injury. The overwhelming commonality seen in persons that develop pressure ulcers is immobility, be it due to being permanently bed bound or as the result of a temporary period of immobility such as during an extended surgical procedure. This does not mean to suggest that all pressure ulcers are preventable or that pressure ulcers are a problem of nursing as has been frequently suggested.

A detailed discussion of the mechanisms of pressure sore formation is available in the chapter by CE Fife entitled "Pressure Ulcers: Towards a New Understanding of an Old Problem." This chapter will focus on the way in which good nursing care can mitigate the effects of numerous risk factors, specific issues related to documentation, and other aspects of care that are unique to nursing.

WHY NURSING CARE IS CRITICAL

In a report of the Medicare Coverage Advisory Panel in March 2005, it was reported that the number of patients with pressure ulcers is increasing by 5% annually. Between 3–10% of patients are hospitalized with pressure ulcers and in the general acute care setting, incidence rates of 7–38% are reported. The most commonly reported anatomic sites for pressure ulcer development are the sacrum and heels with a trend toward increasing heel ulcers. Critical care populations were reported to have an incidence of 8–40% with a prevalence of 22%. Incidence rates were clearly greater in patients on standard versus low-air-loss mattresses (40–79.9% vs.16–16.7%) in the critically ill patient.

Long-term care, nursing homes, and skilled nursing facilities were included in a 2001 National Pressure Advisory (NPUAP) report. Incidence rates of 2.2–23.9% are reported. These results are confounded by studies that report different ulcers stages. Studies whose reports included Stage I ulcers generally had higher incidence rates than those that reported only Stage II and higher. Good nursing care can have a positive impact on these staggering numbers. Three studies that support prevention programs in long-term care

are summarized in the NPUAP report and show decreases in incidence rates from 23.2–0.9% at 8-months post implementation of the prevention program, 15–1% at 6 months and 23.2–4.76% at 12 months.

There are other particularly vulnerable populations. For example, incidence rates for terminally ill persons receiving palliative care ranged from 13% to a high of 85% in terminally ill, institutionalized cancer patients. An incidence rate of 70% was found in one study that reviewed terminally ill non-cancer patients. Prevalence rates of 8.5–28% are reported. In addition, persons with hip fractures were reported in the past to have an incidence of 66%; however, this rate could not have been concluded from the original study as was reported by the 2001 NPUAP report. A more recent NPUAP report, updated November 2003, suggests an incidence rate of 19.1%. Of all pressure ulcer types, heel pressure ulcers may be most preventable with good nursing care.

Nurses must also be aware of the way in which skin color can affect the diagnosis of pressure ulcer formation. In studies where skin color is reported, dark skin persons have a lower prevalence of Stage I ulcers as compared to light skin persons, who have the highest prevalence of Stage I ulcers (19% vs. 46%). Dark skin persons identified as African-Americans are reported to have a prevalence of 16–41% of Stage II-IV ulcers. Nurses must be trained to evaluate subtle skin changes regardless of skin color.

NURSING CONSIDERATIONS IN THE ETIOLOGY OF PRESSURE SORES

Immobility remains the most important risk factor for the development of pressure sores. In addition, there are other components that contribute to the development of pressure ulcers including friction, sheer, and moisture. Pressure is the force placed on tissues in a specific area. Pressure that exceeds capillary filling pressures of 12–32 mm Hg for more than two hours will result in tissue death. The mechanism of tissue injury is now understood to be more complex than simple pressure alone. Nevertheless, turning remains the primary intervention for managing pressure. There have been no randomized controlled trials to provide evidence for the current standard of turning every two hours to prevent pressure sore formation. However, this remains the standard intervention in those patients who are not able to turn themselves. Argument continues over the best way to document that turning was provided. Given that pressure sores are a common reason for litigation, what may seem to be a trivial documentation matter (as compared, for example, to the administration of medications) the turning documentation may become the central focus of a court battle upon which millions of dollars depend. "Check charts" are often criticized because it is too easy to fill them in regardless of whether the turning is actually performed, or conversely, easy to omit a "check" despite providing the care. Written turning notes made every two hours are a burdensome demand on busy staff that may spend more time documenting care than providing it. Perhaps the best method continues to be a simple note at the end of the shift that turning was provided every two hours as ordered, unless there is evidence that the patient is turning himself.

Shearing is a factor that causes mechanical destruction of deep tissues. In essence, sheer occurs when underlying tissues are pulled in one direction due to gravity and skin tissues remain in place. When this occurs, blood vessels become either occluded or torn resulting in an ischemia to the skin and resultant tissue death. This can occur from a patient sliding in bed while in a high Fowler's position or when a patient is pulled across the surface of the bed. Damage due to shearing predisposes tissue to further damage from unrelieved pressure. Using draw sheets may substantially reduce wounds created due to shearing.

Another factor in pressure ulcer development is friction. Similar to shearing, friction occurs when skin is moved across a surface such as sheets. The result is an abrasion type wound with large amounts of exudate that contributes to adhesion of skin to a surface and thereby contributing to shear forces. It can be difficult to prevent these injuries, particularly in elderly patients with paper thin skin. Using lotions to prevent dryness and minimizing use of adhesive products such as tape are important.

Moisture also contributes to the risk of pressure ulcer development. Excess moisture from incontinence or diaphoresis leads to maceration of tissues. Macerated tissue is more prone to damage as the integrity of the tissue is compromised leading to tissue erosion. In addition, excess moisture removes protecting body oils and also contributes to friction and shear. The acidic nature of urinary and fecal incontinence leads to chemical damage of the skin and subsequent pressure ulcer development. Various skin barrier products are helpful here. It may also be necessary to utilize indwelling Foley catheters to control urinary incontinence, but this decision increases the possibility of urosepsis.

Finally, there are several risk factors that contribute to pressure ulcer development. While not necessarily independent risk factors, these factors increase the likelihood of pressure ulcer development and compromise ulcer prevention. These factors include malnutrition, age, spinal cord injury, neuropathy, and altered mental status. Malnutrition is frequently cited as a risk factor for not only pressure ulcer development, but also wound healing failure. Persons are at great risk of pressure ulcer development as they age. Persons in their eighties are at greatest risk for pressure ulcer development. Spinal cord injury contributes to immobility which in itself is a risk factor. Any condition that causes a decrease in sensation such as spinal cord injury or neuropathy increases risk as it is pain perception that typically motivates one to change position. Altered mentation contributes to risk by decreasing cognitive understanding of pain as well as appropriate decisions related to self-positioning.

Assessment and Staging

Pressure ulcers should be assessed as with any wound for size and viable and nonviable tissue. Recommendations for staging the wound are put forth by the National Pressure Ulcer Advisory Committee (NPUAC). Staging is discussed in detail by CE Fife in the chapter entitled "Pressure Ulcers: Towards a New Understanding of an Old Problem", along with some of the pitfalls inherent in the current National Pressure Ulcer Advisory Panel (NPUAP) staging system. Some wounds may not be stageable due to eschar. In addition, the NPUAP staging system does not provide a category for deep tissue injury which can manifest initially as "bruise like" skin changes. If there is any doubt as to how to designate the stage of the wound, the best option is to describe the wound in detail. The following factors need to be included in the nurse's note:

- **Measurements:** length, width and depth, by convention, in centimeters)
- Description of **Location**
    - o   Use proper terminology such as proximal and distal rather than "upper" or "lower")
    - o   Be consistent. Do not use "coccyx" one day and "sacrum" the next.
    - o   Be as specific as possible. If the wound is over the ischial spine, say so, rather than "buttocks"
- Describe the wound **Base**
- Describe the **Periwound Tissue:** (ie, macerated, erythematous, red)
- **Stage** the wound **If Possible**
- Describe the **Absence** of other wounds on high risk areas

CARE PLANS

It is imperative that the chart reflect that the risk factors for pressure sore formation were understood by the staff. Care plans should reflect efforts to mitigate these risk factors.

WOUND CARE

Wound care should focus on topical wound care and on removal of reasons for wound healing failure including correction of risk factors. Topical wound care should strive to maximize wound healing potential by optimizing the local wound environment to include maintaining the moist wound environment, removing necrotic tissue, and controlling bacterial infection. Topical wound care should be no different for the pressure ulcer than for any other wound. The goal of wound care is moist wound healing. Table 1 provides topical wound care options using common dressing types based on wound stage.

PRESSURE REDUCTION

In the pressure ulcer patient, perhaps more important than local wound care is the removal of the cause of wound healing failure. The primary cause of wound healing failure is failure to reduce or remove pressure from the ulcer. Pressure reduction can occur in a variety of manners. A simple regimen of turning a patient at least every two hours will reduce pressure to the affected site. Generally, turning is inadequate in itself to resolve pressure. Positioning the patient is of key importance in both preventing and treating pressure ulcers. The head of the bed should never be raised more than 30 degrees to prevent shearing. Pillow and or wedges should be used between the legs to prevent pressure when lying on the side. Heels should always be lifted and never allowed contact with the surface to prevent pressure ulcer development. Pillows may work in immobile patients, but in mobile patients, orthotics like Multipodus or L'Nard splints is the gold standard to prevent heel pressure. In addition to these interventions, one should also consider the support surface as another option for pressure reduction or pressure relief.

Support surfaces can be classified as either static or dynamic support surfaces. Static support surfaces comprise the most commonly used support surfaces for pressure ulcer prevention. These include foam, gel, and water mattress overlays. Foam mattresses have historically been the most popular choice of mattress overlay. Foam can be a good choice of pressure reduction;

however, most recommendations are that the foam must be at least four inches thick to prevent the patient from "bottoming out" or compressing the foam to the point where the body is in contact with the surface below the foam. Egg crate type foam overlays of less than four inches from the base of the foam to the valleys of the surface are comfort measures and do little to reduce pressure. They may, in fact, increase pressure when the peaks of the egg crate foam are compressed against a high pressure area. Gel or water filled overlays help to disperse pressure away from bony areas. Usually these overlays are compartmentalized to prevent the fluid from pooling due to gravity. Combination gel and foam overlays are also available. Another overlay product is the air overlay, which can take two forms, either a static overlay or a power controlled overlay. The principle behind these products is to redistribute weight as with the gel, foam, and water overlays.

Dynamic support surfaces are mattress replacements and consist of two types of mattresses. Low-air loss mattresses are designed to lose air at a low rate while maintaining enough volume to support the patient. Continuous airflow also helps to reduce skin moisture which helps to prevent shearing. Some low-air loss mattresses can adjust the airflow temperature in the mattress to provide for patient comfort. One concern related to these types of beds is the possibility of the patient becoming trapped between the mattress and the side rails. Care should be exercised to prevent this from occurring. Alternating pressure mattresses are composed of air-filled adjacent pillows. These pillows are designed to support the patient while inflating and deflating underneath the body, constantly changing the areas of high pressure. This permits perfusion and reoxygenation of the tissues by creating an environment similar to the high and low pressures that occur in people as a result of changes of position.

The final type of dynamic support surface is the air-fluidized bed. These beds consist of glass beads enclosed in a fabric. Air is blown through the beads causing them to resemble a "fluid" state, thus the name air-fluidized. Many consider this to be pressure relief in that capillary closing pressure approaches zero. It is considered to be the best selection to completely off-load a newly placed flap. Certain problems do exist with these beds. Due to the nature of the fluidization of the glass beads, the patient sinks into the bed making it difficult to maintain therapeutic positioning and to transfer the patient in and out of the bed.

Seated patients can be off-loaded with foam, gel, and alternating pressure seats. A difference in the seated versus the recombinant patient is that the surface area of the seated patient is much less and leads to greater forces being placed on the seated area. Pressure is concentrated in the ischial areas. Special attention should be given to postural control and stability so as not to further increase pressure to high pressure areas. A referral to a seating clinic or physical/rehabilitation therapy may be necessary to assist with appropriate seating selection (See Table 2 for a Pressure Reduction Care Plan).

OTHER TREATMENT

While pressure reduction is the key to pressure ulcer prevention and treatment, other causes of wound healing failure must also be addressed in this population. Frequently, nutrition is a factor as this population is often severely debilitated and/or critically ill. Screening for nutritional deficits through laboratory analysis of albumin and prealbumin levels will help to choose nutritional interventions. Due to the location of the most common ulcer site, the sacrum, pressure ulcers are often contaminated with fecal materials. Attention must be given to fecal and urinary continence. Due to contamination, infection is not uncommonly seen in these ulcers and appropriate topical and/or systemic antibiotic therapy should be given following wound cultures.

DOCUMENTATION ISSUES

Nurses should ensure that the following basic care issues are addressed for all pressure sore patients:

- Adequate nutrition (this may mean suggesting that the physician order a nutritional evaluation and at the very least, an albumin or pre-albumin)
- Appropriate support surface (many hospitals have "bed protocols" which define what surface is warranted on the basis of whether wounds are present, how many and at what stage, as well as how compromised the patient may be)
- Appropriate wound care (this may involve consulting the hospital "Enterostomal Therapy Nurse" for new wounds)
- An appropriate turning schedule (based on the mobility limitations of the patient, the support surface, etc)

The best way to ensure that these issues are addressed is via appropriate orders in the chart, signed by the attending physician. Many hospitals have created standard care plans which allow nurses to implement basic treatment and prevention measures even before the patient is seen by the physician. If your hospital does not have such an approach, consider helping to create them.

Many hospitals use "Skin Assessment Sheets" to document skin breakdown. One significant problem with the NPUAP staging system discussed by CE Fife in the chapter entitled "Pressure Ulcers: Towards a New Understanding of an Old Problem" is that the most common cause of Stage II "pressure sores" is actually friction and shear. Yet, these are documented on skin assessment sheets as "pressure sores" regardless of their etiology.

It is imperative that nurses document every time that a dressing is performed and the appearance of the wound at the time of the dressing, regardless of where in the chart that documentation is performed. It is also imperative that a note be made in the hospital chart of when the physician and the FAMILY were informed of any pressure related problems. It is wise to have the nurse actually show the family the pressure areas and explain that pressure sores form from the inside out so the appearance may worsen over time. That way, wounds that evolve into larger areas of tissue damage will not be a complete surprise to the family. Furthermore, in today's litigious society, notifying "risk management" or "patient relations" may be advisable whenever pressure sores are noted on a patient.

Many hospitals are uncomfortable with having photographs made of pressure sores, fearing that the photos will be used as a negative factor in litigation. For the most part, carefully taken photos may be the best defense a hospital has. It is possible to document the way in which certain wounds "evolve" rather than worsen, as well as documenting how severe the tissue damage was or was not at the time of discharge. Be assured that the family will have photos of their loved one taken at some later time.

One of the most important things that a nurse can do is to perform a complete skin assessment at the time a patient is admitted to his or her care. This is particularly critical if the nurse is performing the first skin assessment of the facility admission. On many occasions, a meticulous nurse has documented the presence of a pre-existing wound at the time of admission. Careful documentation is the best defense against frivolous litigation.

TABLE 1. TOPICAL WOUND CARE PLAN

Stage I Pressure Ulcer	
Characteristics:	Stage I is largely characterized by non-blanching erythema of the skin, which can be accompanied by changes in skin temperature, tissue consistency, and sensation.
Related Factors:	Mechanical factors such as pressure, friction, or shear. • Age • Poor nutrition • Prominent bony prominences • Immobility • Incontinence of bowel and/or bladder • Environmental moisture • Altered mentation • Paresthesia • Reactive erythema lasting longer than 1/2–3/4 the length of ischemic pressure time.
Symptoms: Stage I:	An observable pressure related alteration of intact skin whose indicators as compared to the adjacent or opposite area on the body may include changes in one or more of the following: skin temperature (warmth or coolness), tissue consistency (firm or boggy feel) and/or sensation (pain, itching). The ulcer appears as a defined area of persistent redness in lightly pigmented skin, whereas in darker skin tones, the ulcer may appear with persistent red, blue, or purple hues.
Expected Outcomes/Goals:	Skin will remain intact. Pressure relief is obtained within one week. Incontinence is managed within one week. Excess moisture is controlled within one week. Nutrition is optimized by evidence of adequate caloric intake within one week.

Intervention	Rationale
1. Perform a thorough assessment of the patient and document the changes. • Integumentary • Nutritional • Risk factors • Need for pressure relief	• Assessment is the initial step by which an appropriate plan of care can be developed.
2. Position patient off affected area and provide pressure distribution devices for the patient while in bed and while out of bed.	• Proper counter pressure can aid in preventing skin breakdown.
3. Keep skin clean, dry, and supple. Soaps should be avoided.	• Commercial soaps contain alkalis that excessively dry the skin and predispose the skin to further breakdown.
4. Moisturizers and skin emollients should be used judiciously on dry skin.	• Dry skin can lead to cracking that is a breach of the body's first line of defense. Excessive use of moisturizers may lead to maceration.
5. Apply a film dressing or hydrocolloid over the affected area while avoiding tension and skin wrinkling.	• These dressings reduce friction by acting as a protective layer over the skin. Tension or wrinkling of the skin may facilitate further breakdown.
6. DO NOT massage reddened areas.	• Massage of reddened areas is contraindicated as hyperemia heralds tissue damage and massage will cause further damage to compromised tissue.

TABLE 1. TOPICAL WOUND CARE PLAN (CONTINUED)

Stage II Pressure Ulcer

Characteristics:	Stage II is partial thickness skin loss involving the epidermis and possibly the dermis
Related Factors:	Mechanical factors such as pressure, friction, or shear. • Age • Poor nutrition • Prominent bony prominences • Immobility • Incontinence of bowel and/or bladder • Environmental moisture • Altered mentation • Paresthesia
Symptoms: Stage II:	Partial thickness skin loss involving the epidermis and/or dermis. The ulcer is superficial and presents clinically as an abrasion, blister of shallow crater.
Expected Outcomes/Goals:	Progressive healing as evidenced by epithelialization. Pressure relief is obtained within 1 week. Incontinence is managed within 1 week. Excess moisture is controlled within 1 week. Nutrition is optimized by evidence of adequate caloric intake within 1 week.

Intervention	Rationale
1. Perform a thorough assessment of the patient and document the changes. • Integumentary • Nutritional • Risk factors • Need for pressure relief	• Assessment is the initial step by which an appropriate plan of care can be developed.
2. Position patient off affected area and provide pressure distribution devices for the patient in bed and while out of bed.	• Proper counter pressure can aid in preventing skin breakdown.
3. Assess and document the dimension of the ulcer in centimeters: • Length • Width • Depth • Undermining • Sinus tracts • Tunneling • Fistulae • Odor • Drainage • Color • Necrosis • Slough • Eschar • Wound Margins • Granulation • Epithelialization	• Changes in a pressure ulcer can occur rapidly and will require prompt intervention with appropriate changes in the plan of care. Measurements should be done at least weekly and documented in the nursing progress note. Photographs, if appropriate, should be taken once a week or once every two weeks, depending on the progression or regression of the wound.
4. Assess peripheral skin: • Erythema • Induration • Maceration	• Peripheral skin erythema indicates inflammation. • Induration is an indication of venous congestion and is characterized by an abnormal firmness of tissue within a definite margin. • Maceration is a softening of tissue due to prolonged exposure to excess moisture.
5. Cleanse ulcer with normal saline or a dermal wound cleanser.	• Wound irrigation removes loose necrotic material and surface contaminants.
6. Cover ulcer with a dressing that maintains a moist wound environment.	• Wound healing occurs best in a moist environment by allowing epithelial cells to migrate across the wound surface unimpeded by scab formation.

Intervention	Rationale
a) Semipermiable polyurethane dressing (film dressing).	• Film dressings support autolytic debridement and help to prevent infections because of the hydrophobic outer surface of the dressing and bacteria cannot penetrate the dressing. However, wound contamination may occur from the surrounding skin. This dressing provides minimal insulation of the wound. Film dressings are gas permeable allowing some water vapor to pass from the wound out of the dressing which helps to prevent maceration. These dressings also allow ambient oxygen to diffuse into the wound. It is contraindicated in heavily exudating wounds and wounds with undermining or sinus tracts unless these areas are packed prior to the dressing application.
b) Hydrocolloid dressing	• Hydrocolloid dressings support autolytic debridement of wounds with dry eschar. They maintain a moist wound environment and provide insulation of the wound. These dressings are contraindicated in moderate to heavily exudating wounds as they do not provide enough absorption. Hydrocolloid dressings are generally occlusive and should be used with extreme caution on diabetic and arterial insufficiency wounds as they may increase the risk for anaerobic infection. However, the use of occlusive dressings has been associated with the elimination of certain bacteria, particularly Pseudomonas, and has been shown to be superior to gauze and transparent dressings in the prevention of secondary infections.
c) Moist normal saline dressing	• Moist saline gauze provides a continuously moist environment in order to promote granulation and epithelialization. A fine mesh gauze such as a 44/36 weave will allow new tissue growth without the tissue becoming entrapped in the mesh, thereby destroying the new growth. Care should be taken not to create an occlusive environment as this may promote anaerobic bacterial growth and/or Pseudomonas infection.
d) Foam dressing	• Foam dressings support autolytic debridement in wounds that are exudative. These dressing provide minimal to moderate absorption of exudate and help to maintain a moist wound environment. Foam dressings also insulate the wound. The nonadherant nature of this dressing is non-traumatic to the wound when removed. These dressings should be avoided in non-exudative wounds, wounds with a dry eschar, and wounds with sinus tracts unless appropriately packed.
7. Drying agents such as Maalox, heat lamps, or Milk of Magnesia should never be used.	• Wound healing is compromised and delayed in a dry environment. A dry environment promotes scab formation, which impedes epithelial movement. Heat increases the metabolic demand for oxygen at the wound site—an area already in need of increased oxygen. Antacids alter the normal pH of the skin therefore altering normal skin flora.

TABLE 1. TOPICAL WOUND CARE PLAN (CONTINUED)

Stage III and Stage IV Pressure Ulcer	
Characteristics:	Stage III incorporates full-thickness skin loss involving damage or necrosis of subcutaneous tissue, which can extend down to but not through the fascia. Stage IV presents as a full-thickness skin loss with extensive destruction, tissue necrosis, or damage to the muscle, bone, or supporting structures, such as the tendon, or joint capsules.
Related Factors:	Mechanical factors such as pressure, friction, or shear. • Age • Poor nutrition • Prominent bony prominences • Immobility • Incontinence of bowel and/or bladder • Environmental moisture • Altered mentation • Paresthesia
Symptoms:	Stage III: Full-thickness skin loss involving damage or necrosis of subcutaneous tissue that may extend down to, but not through, underlying fascia. The ulcer presents clinically as a deep crater with or without undermining of sinus tracts of adjacent tissue. Stage IV: Full-thickness skin loss with extensive destruction, tissue necrosis, or damage to muscle, one or supporting structures such as tendon, cartilage, or joint capsule.
Expected Outcomes/Goals:	Progressive healing as evidenced by granulation tissue and contraction of the wound. Pressure relief is obtained within one week. Incontinence is managed within one week. Excess moisture is controlled within one week. Nutrition is optimized by evidence of adequate caloric intake within one week.

Intervention	Rationale
1. Perform a thorough assessment of the patient and document the changes. • Integumentary • Nutritional • Risk factors • Need for pressure relief	• Assessment is the initial step by which an appropriate plan of care can be developed.
2. Position patient off affected area and provide pressure distribution devices for the patient in bed and while out of bed.	• Proper counter pressure can aid in preventing skin breakdown.
3. Assess and document the dimension of the ulcer in centimeters: • Length • Width • Depth • Undermining • Sinus tracts • Tunneling • Fistulae • Odor • Drainage • Color • Necrosis • Slough • Eschar • Wound Margins • Granulation • Epithelialization	• Changes in a pressure ulcer can occur rapidly and will require prompt intervention with appropriate changes in the plan of care. Measurements should be done at least weekly and documented in the nursing progress note. L x W x D helps to give a three dimensional representation of the wound. Photographs, if appropriate, should be taken once a week or once every two weeks, depending on the progression or regression of the wound. • Undermining, sinus tracts, fistulae, and tunneling indicate ulceration that cannot be visualized. • Drainage and odor may give indications of infection. • Color of the wound bed helps to determine the type of tissue present—granular tissue is beefy red, epithelial tissue is pearly pink, slough is yellow, brown, or gray, and eschar is leathery black or brown. • Granulation is indication of newly forming capillary beds. It is composed of collagen, hyaluronic acid, and fibronectin in a newly formed vascular network. • Epithelial tissue indicates new skin growth and skin cell migration across the wound bed.

Intervention	Rationale
4. Assess peripheral skin: • Erythema • Induration • Maceration	• Peripheral skin erythema indicates inflammation. • Induration is an indication of venous congestion and is characterized by an abnormal firmness of tissue within a definite margin. • Maceration is a softening of tissue due to prolonged exposure to excess moisture.
5. Cleanse ulcer with normal saline or a dermal wound cleanser.	• Wound irrigation removes loose necrotic material and surface contaminants.
6. Lightly pack undermined areas and sinus tracts with appropriate filler.	• Cotton dressing fillers is contraindicated for wound packing. The filling may act as a foreign body and cause the wound to enter into a chronic inflammatory phase, which would delay healing and possibly be detrimental to the wound healing process.
7. Fill dead space with the appropriate wound filler: • Gauze—wet, moist, dry • Alginates • Hydrogel • Hydrogel pastes • Hydrophilic powders	• It is essential that dead space in a wound be filled. The appropriate wound filler is determined by the amount of exudate.
8. In a non-draining ulcer use a dressing that maintains a moist wound environment and/or rehydrates the wound.	• Wound healing occurs best in a moist environment by allowing epithelial cells to migrate across the wound surface unimpeded by scab formation.
a) Semipermeable polyurethane dressing (film dressing).	• Film dressings support autolytic debridement and help to prevent infections because of the hydrophobic outer surface of the dressing and bacteria cannot penetrate the dressing. However, wound contamination may occur from the surrounding skin. This dressing provides minimal insulation of the wound. Film dressings are gas permeable allowing some water vapor to pass from the wound out of the dressing which helps to prevent maceration. These dressings also allow ambient oxygen to diffuse into the wound. It is contraindicated in heavily exudating wounds and wounds with undermining or sinus tracts unless these areas are packed prior to the dressing application.
b) Hydrocolloid dressing	• Hydrocolloid dressings support autolytic debridement of wounds with dry eschar. They maintain a moist wound environment and provide insulation of the wound. These dressings are contraindicated in moderate to heavily exudating wounds, as they do not provide enough absorption. Hydrocolloid dressings are generally occlusive and should be used with extreme caution on diabetic and arterial insufficiency wounds as they may increase the risk for anaerobic infection. However, the use of occlusive dressings has been associated with the elimination of certain bacteria, particularly *Pseudomonas,* and has been shown to be superior to gauze and transparent dressings in the prevention of secondary infections.

TABLE 1. TOPICAL WOUND CARE PLAN (CONTINUED)

Intervention	Rationale
c) Moist normal saline dressing	• Moist saline gauze provides a continuously moist environment in order to promote granulation and epithelialization. A fine mesh gauze such as a 44/36 weave will allow new tissue growth without the tissue becoming entrapped in the mesh, thereby destroying the new growth. Care should be taken not to create an occlusive environment as this may promote anaerobic bacterial growth and/or Pseudomonas infection.
d) Hydrogel dressing	• Hydrogel dressings support autolytic debridement due to the moisturizing effects of the dressing. These dressings are indicated for partial and full thickness wounds where wound hydration is a primary concern and autolytic debridement is an outcome. There are three types of hydrogel dressings: a gel form that is used to hydrate a wound, a granulate form that is used to pack full-thickness wounds with exudate, and a sheet form that is primarily used in partial-thickness wounds. Gel and sheet impregnated forms of this dressing often macerate surrounding skin. Therefore, the dressing should be changed frequently, especially if used for debridement. Contraindications are mainly influenced by maceration unless an alternate form of peripheral skin protection is appropriately provided.
9. In an exudating wound use an absorptive dressing that will maintain a moist wound environment while managing excess drainage without dehydrating the wound.	
a) Dry gauze	• Avoid dry cotton dressing fillers. These dressings may act as a foreign body and cause the wound to enter into a chronic inflammatory phase, which would delay healing and possibly be detrimental to the wound healing process.
b) Alginate dressings	• Alginate dressings support autolytic debridement as they provide for a moist wound environment. These dressing absorb up to 20 times their weight in exudate, making this an excellent choice for a heavily exudating wound. Alginate dressings may also be used as a wound packing eliminating dead space. They are indicated in moderately to heavily exudating wounds and may be used in wounds with undermining and sinus tracts as well as wounds with necrosis and infection. Alginate dressings are contraindicated in minimally exudating wounds, as they tend to dry the wound unless the alginate is premoistened with saline prior to application. Care should be taken not to mistake the gel of the alginate for wound infection. A secondary cover dressing is required.

Intervention	Rationale
c) Foam dressing	• Foam dressings support autolytic debridement in wounds that are exudative. These dressing provide minimal to moderate absorption of exudate and help to maintain a moist wound environment. Foam dressings also insulate the wound. The non-adherant nature of this dressing is non-traumatic to the wound when removed. These dressings should be avoided in non-exudative wounds, wounds with a dry eschar, and wounds with sinus tracts unless appropriately packed.
Negative Pressure Wound Therapy	• Negative pressure wound therapy provides a negative pressure gradient to improve tissue perfusion, reduce localized edema, remove excess drainage, increase localized blood flow, enhance epithelial migration and mechanically stabilize the wound by drawing the wound closed.

TABLE 2. PRESSURE REDUCTION CARE PLAN

Pressure Reduction	
Related Factors: Mechanical factors such as pressure, friction, or shear. • Age • Immobility • Environmental moisture • Paresthesia	• Prominent bony prominences • Incontinence of bowel and/or bladder • Altered mentation
Expected Outcomes/Goals: Progressive healing as evidenced by granulation tissue and contraction of the wound. Pressure reduction/relief is obtained within 1 week.	

Intervention	Rationale
1. Sheepskin pads, heel protectors, foam mattress overlays.	• Minimal to no risk for pressure ulcer development. Patient is able to turn self in bed. Patient may need protection from friction. Patient may be moved from bed to chair for periods of time. • No skin breakdown. • No issues with continence control.
2. Static support surfaces such as foam, gel, water or air overlay.	• Patient is at low risk for pressure ulcer development. Patient is confined to bed or may be confined to a chair for extended periods of time and may require some assistance to turn self or change positions.
3. Provide turning schedule in addition to static support surfaces such as foam, gel, water or air overlay.	• Patient is at moderate risk for pressure ulcer development. Patient is confined to bed and is unable to turn self or has altered sensorium/ mentation that prevents self turning. Heels may be at particular risk due to neuropathy as seen in diabetes. Patient requires assistance to turn. • Patient has Stage I or Stage II pressure ulcer(s).
4. Provide dynamic support surface such as low-air loss mattress, alternating pressure mattress.	• Patient is totally dependent for care and turning. • Patient has Stage III and/or Stage IV pressure ulcer(s).
5. Air-fluidized therapy	• Patient with surgical flap/graft intervention to repair pressure ulcer. • Patient has Stage III or Stage IV pressure ulcer(s).

CONCLUSION

Pressure ulcers are difficult wounds to treat. Patients with pressure ulcers are frequently severely debilitated. A rigorous prevention program should be established. The key to pressure ulcer treatment is removing repetitive trauma from pressure exerted on the wound site. Combining this with scrupulous topical dressing care, enhancing nutrition and treating infected wounds will provide the best possible outcomes.

REFERENCES

1. Allman, RM, Goode, PS, Burst, N, etal. Pressure ulcers, hospital complications, and disease severity: impact on hospital costs and length of stay. *Advances in Wound Care* 1999; 12(1), 22-30.

2. American Medical Directors Association. *Pressure ulcers* Columbia, MD: American Medical Directors Association, 1996.

3. Ayello EA. Preventing pressure ulcers and skin tears. In Mezey M, Fulmer, T, Abraham, I, and Zwicker, DA. (eds.). *Geriatric Nursing Protocols for Best Practice* 2nd ed. NY, NY: Springer Publishing Company, Inc, 2003.

4. Beckrich K. & Aronovitch SA. Hosptal-acquired pressure ulcers: a comparison of cost in medical vs. surgical patients. *Nursing Economics* 1999; 17, 263-271.

5. Bennett MA. Report of the task force on the implications for darkly pigmented intact skin in the prediction and prevention of pressure ulcers. *Advances in Wound Care* 1995; 8(6), 34-35.

6. Bergstrom N, Bennett MA, Carlson CE, et al. Treatment of pressure ulcers Clinical Practice Guidelines, No. 15. Rockville, MD: U. S. Department of Health and Human Services. Public Health Service, Agency for Health Care Policy and Research. AHCPR Publication No. 95-0652, 1994.

7. Bryant RA, Nix DP. *Acute and Chronic Wounds: Current Management Concepts* (3rd ed). St. Louis, MO: Mosby Elsevier, 2007.

8. Frantz R, Xakellis GC, Arteaga M. The effects of prolonged pressure on skin blood flow in elderly patients at risk for pressure ulcers. *Decubitus* 1993; 6(6), 16-20.

9. Kloth LC, McCulloch,JM. *Wound Healing: Alternatives in Management* (3rd ed) Philadelphia, PA: F. A. Davis Company, 2002.

10. Krasner DL, Rodeheaver GT, Sibbald RG. *Chronic Wound Care: A Clinical Source Book for Healthcare Professionals* (3rd ed) Wayne, PA: HMP Communications, 2001.

11. Maklebust J, Sieggreen MY. *Pressure Ulcers: Guidelines for Prevention and Management* (3rd ed.) Springhouse, PA: Springhouse Corporation, 2000.

12. National Pressure Advisory Panel (NPUAP). Cuddigan J, Ayello EA, Sussman C (eds) Pressure ulcers in America: prevalence, incidence, and implications for the future. Reston, VA: NPUAP, 2001.

13. Paralyzed Veterans of America. Pressure ulcer prevention and treatment following spinal cord injury: a clinical practice guideline for health-care professionals. *Journal Spinal Cord Medicine* 2001; 24(Suppl 1): S40-101.

14. Sussman C, Bates-Jensen BM. *Wound Care: A Collaborative Practice Manual for Health Professionals* (3rd ed) Philadelphia: Lippincott, Williams, & Wilkins, 2006.

15. van Rijswijk L, Braden BJ. Pressure ulcer patient and wound assessment: an AHCPR clinical practice guideline update. *Ostomy/Wound Management* 1999; 45(1A Suppl.), 56S-67S.

16. Wound, Ostomy, and Continence Nurses Society (WOCN). Guideline for prevention and management of pressure ulcers. Glenview, IL: Wound, Ostomy, and Continence Nurses Society (WOCN), 2003.

REVIEW QUESTIONS

1.) Static support surfaces such as foam, gel, water or air overlay may be appropriate for patients who are at what level of risk for pressure ulcer development?
    a. minimal or no risk
    b. low risk
    c. moderate risk
    d. high risk

2.) An inappropriate treatment for pressure ulcers includes the use of:
    a. a low air loss mattress
    b. nutritional support
    c. moisture barriers
    d. heat lamps

3.) An appropriate topical dressing for a pressure ulcer would include consideration of:
    a. the stage of the pressure ulcer
    b. patient mobility
    c. principles of moist wound healing
    d. pressure reduction

4.) Pressure reduction can occur by all of the following EXCEPT:
    a. Turning a patient at least every two hours
    b. Positioning the patient
    c. Raising the head of the bed to 45 degrees
    d. Placing pillows or wedges between the legs
    e. Lifting the heels to avoid contact with the surface

5.) The most common pressure ulcer site is the:
    a. sacrum
    b. elbow
    c. scalp
    d. shoulder
    e. ankle

Answers: 1b, 2d, 3c, 4c, 5a

Chapter **19**

Thermal Injury

CHAPTER NINETEEN OVERVIEW

NOTES

THERMAL INJURY

Clyde Ikeda, J. Benjamin Slade, Jr

INTRODUCTION

In the United States alone over 2 million burn injuries each year are brought to medical attention, 80,000 are hospitalized, 20,000 require admission to a specialized burn unit, and 14,000 die (1). According to the Executive Director of the American Burn Association (ABA), for patients who survive 60% total body surface area (TBSA) burns, charges for the hospital stay alone, not including operating room time, surgeons bill, artificial skin, rehabilitation, and other costs, averages $400,000 (in 2003 U.S. dollars). These costs can reach $500,000 for burns over 80% TBSA.

The evolution of burn care as a specialty of surgery has resulted in increased survival and quality of outcomes. The issues of burn shock, burn wound sepsis, and post burn deformity have been systematically addressed in recent years with substantial success. Burn shock is usually lethal in large burns during the first few post injury days. Burn wound sepsis kills survivors of shock during the first few post injury weeks. Post burn deformity occurs in survivors who heal their wounds by contraction and epithelialization.

As more patients survive even serious burn injuries, care of the burn wound has advanced to improve quality of function and cosmetic outcome. Burn care requires expertise, personnel, and equipment that are not cost effectively maintained in low-volume programs. These issues have led to the formation of the burn center verification program as a result of the combined efforts of the American Burn Association (ABA) and American College of Surgeons (ACS). This chapter represents the management philosophies and practices in one such burn center.

Burn Injury Physiology

Physiologic responses to a major burn include a fall in arterial pressure, an increased pulse rate, and a progressive decrease in cardiac output and stroke volume. Metabolic responses are complex and include metabolic acidosis and hyperventilation. Cellular adenosine triphosphate levels fall, resting cell membrane potential decreases, and cellular accumulation of sodium, calcium and water is paralleled by a loss of cellular potassium. Immunologic responses include alteration of macrophage function, and cellular and humoral immunity (1). The burn wound is a complex, dynamic injury characterized by a zone of coagulation (complete capillary occlusion), surrounded by an area of stasis, and bordered by an area of erythema. The zone of coagulation may progress by a factor of ten during the first 48 hours after injury.

Ischemic necrosis quickly follows. Edema is most prominent in directly involved burned tissues, but can also be found in distant, nonburned tissues, including muscle, intestine and lung. Some of the edema is due to intracellular swelling, but the major portion is caused by fluid collection in the interstitial space of burn tissue. Concurrent changes occur in the distant microvasculature, including red cell aggregation, white cell adhesion to venular walls, and platelet thromboemboli. Capillary or microvascular occlusion in deeper burns decreases perfusion of the burn tissue. There is decreased efficiency of the lymphatic network; dermal lymphatics are destroyed with a deeper burn wound, impairing absorption. Altered permeability is not caused by heat injury alone. Mediators released with the burn (including oxidants, prostaglandins, kinins and histamine) contribute to local and systemic hyperpermeability of the microcirculation, appear histologically as gaps in the venular and capillary endothelium, and render the permeability process amenable to the use of mediator inhibitors. A decrease in the edema process would have a marked positive proactive impact, especially on the early hemodynamic instability, as well as the later wound conversion, and is certainly worth pursuing (5). The continuing tissue damage in thermal injury is due to the failure of the surrounding tissue to supply borderline cells with oxygen and nutrients necessary to sustain viability.

The pathophysiologic changes within the burn wound show a striking similarity to those noted in the ischemia reperfusion model, i.e., depletion of ATP and production of xanthine oxidase, with subsequent generation of oxygen-free radicals (12–14).

INITIAL MANAGEMENT

The recommended initial management of burns is to ignore the burn and treat the victim like any trauma patient with evaluation of ABC's (airway, breathing, circulation). Airway security is the first priority. Complete examination of the injured is important to assess for concomitant injury, including life-threatening head injuries, cervical-spine, hemo/pneumothorax, and abdominal injury. There is significant morbidity to missed injuries. Liberal use of computerized tomographic scanning is justified if the mechanism of injury is consistent with head or abdominal injury.

A burn-specific secondary survey complements the trauma secondary survey. Immediate concerns are the management of the patient's airway and the need for escharotomies. If in doubt, and the patient has any signs of inhalation injury, the patient should be intubated (Figure 1) before the airway becomes occluded due to injury and fluid resuscitation that is required for these injuries. If the patient cannot be intubated, the next step is cricothyroidotomy, followed later by tracheotomy.

Constricting burns of the chest make it difficult to ventilate the patient adequately due to restricted chest excursions. Mid-lateral incisions are made to release the eschar, and the patient re-evaluated for adequacy of ventilation. If still not adequate, criss-cross incisions are then made to further release the tight eschar. This can be done along the costal margins.

Progressive soft tissue edema within non-elastic compartments or beneath overlying eschar can compromise extremity perfusion.

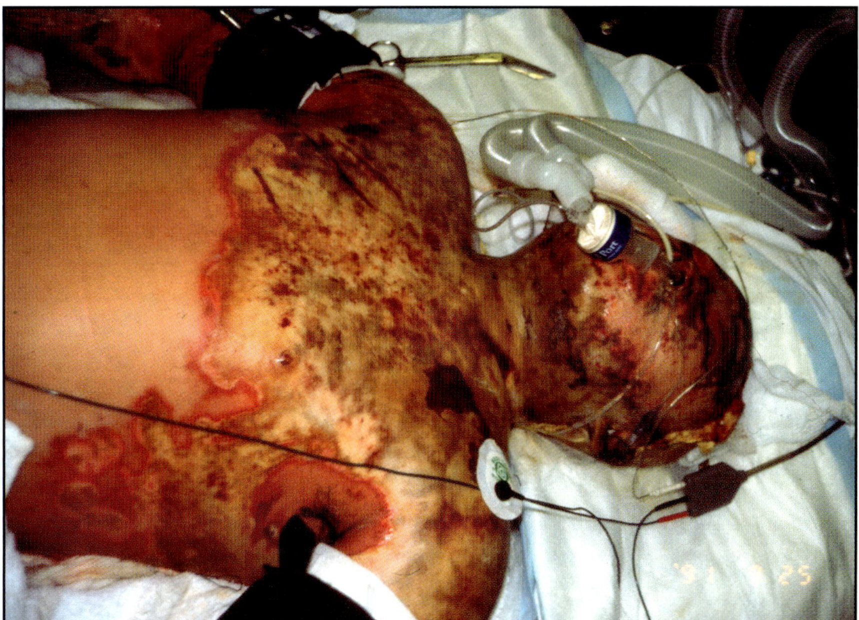

Figure 1. A male patient with massive burns to the upper torso and head.

Escharotomies can be done at the bedside or in the operating room. Anesthesia is seldom necessary when dealing with full thickness burns due to destruction of the pain fibers. A scalpel can be used, but electrocautery provides more effective hemostasis. Incisions are made proximal to distal along the entire length and depth of eschar, and perfusion is assessed before and after.

For the lower extremities, circumferential burn escharotomies are done through midlateral incisions, trying to avoid the peroneal nerves. Similarly in the upper extremities, midlateral incisions are made, trying to avoid the ulnar nerves along the elbow area.

Escharotomies of the hands are also done on an emergent basis. It is common for the extremity burns to involve the hands. The escharotomies of the digits are done on the mid-lateral, non-working side of the hands. In order to decompress the intrinsic muscles of the hand, incisions are made between the metacarpals, and bluntly dissected down to the interosseous muscles, resulting in fasciotomies. Recent recommendations promote the process of decompression in acute burns to replace the procedure of escharotomy. The process of decompression requires assessment, measurement and monitoring. The depth, extent and placement of surgical incisions should be based on anatomical considerations, with the aim of ensuring adequate tissue oxygenation via maintenance of the microcirculation. Decompression is considered for all body compartments where a rise in compartmental pressures can compromise vital function. Positioning of limbs and qualitative and quantitative fluid resuscitation are important considerations (2). American Burn Association guidelines for referral to a burn center are any partial thickness burn > 15% in an adult. In children and elderly persons, due to their delicate skin and comorbid illnesses, any partial thickness burn > 10% should

TABLE 1. ABA BURN CENTER TRANSFER CRITERIA

Partial thickness burns on > 10% of total body surface area (TBSA)
Burns that involve the face, hands, feet, genitalia, perineum, or major joints
Second and third degree burns that involve the face, hands, feet, genitalia, perineum, and major joints
Third degree burns > 5% of TBSA in any age group
Electrical burns, including lightening injury
Chemical burns
Inhalation injury
Burn injury in patients with pre-existing medical disorders that could complicate management, prolong recovery, or affect mortality
Any patients with burns and concomitant trauma (such as fractures) in which the burn injury poses the greatest risk of morbidity or mortality. In such cases, if the trauma poses the greater immediate risk, the patient may be initially stabilized in a trauma center before being transferred to a burn unit. Physician judgment will be necessary in such situations and should be in concert with the regional medical control plan and triage protocols.
Burned children in hospitals without qualified personnel or equipment for the care of children
Burn injury in patients who will require special social, emotional, or long-term rehabilitative intervention, including cases involving suspected child abuse and substance abuse

Excerpted from Guidelines for the Operations of Burn Units [pp. 55–62], Resources for Optimal Care of the Injured Patient: 1999, Committee on Trauma, American College of Surgeons.

be referred. Any patient with a full thickness burn > 5% TBSA at any age should be transferred to a burn center. Full thickness burns are more difficult to manage and will likely require grafting. Other indications for referral to a burn center include involvement of the face, hand, feet or perineum, electrical injuries, associated inhalation injury, any circumferential burns and patients that require pain control.

The two most important predictors of clinical outcome are the TBSA and depth of burn injury. Accurate assessment of TBSA determines both whether a specialist burn unit management will be required, and the magnitude of initial fluid resuscitation. The "Rule of Nines" and the Lund and Browder charts are the two most commonly used methods, but there is variability of burn size estimation with both methods. For the rule of 9's, the body is divided into dividends of 9's. The head is 9%, each upper extremity is 9%, the front and back of the torso and each lower extremity are 18% each, and the perineum 1%. The surface area of the palm is estimated to be approximately 1% of the TBSA, and is occasionally used to estimate burn surface area. First degree burns do not count in the calculation. Overestimation at the transferring ER is almost 100%. Computer-assisted assessments for determining burn surface area are far more consistent and accurate. Some include 3D graphics to increase accuracy, can compute fluid and nutritional requirements, and can include a permanent database for tracking statistics, mortality, morbidity and comparative treatment protocols. One such program, the Surface Area Graphic Evaluation (SAGE2) is accessible via the internet (*http://www.sagediagram.com/*).

Burn wound depth is difficult to determine. Even for experienced investigators, the differentiation between superficial and deep dermal burns is not always possible, and is highly inaccurate. Burns are dynamic, in a state of change for up to 72 hours after injury and local microcirculation compromised to the worst extent 12–24 hours post-burn. Other methods have been proposed to assess burn wound depth, some of which are promising, others with limitations and lacking validation, some experimental, and several not practical for routine clinical application. These methods include digital imaging, biopsy, tissue perfusion measurements, laser Doppler imaging (LDI) and laser Doppler perfusion imaging (LDPI), indocyanine green video angiography, fluorescein fluorescence, photo-optical measurements, fiber-optic confocal imaging, polarization-sensitive optical coherence tomography, Mueller-matrix optical coherence tomography, thermography, radioisotopes and nuclear magnetic resonance, and ultrasound.

Injury severity scoring systems for burn patients have considerable practical value to help recognize high-risk patients, indicate the setting in which the patient needs to be treated, and predict outcomes. While there is considerable agreement that risk factors include age, sex, TBSA burned, depth and presence of inhalation injury, the question of how to combine them into an accurate, simple scoring system has been problematic. Proposed scoring systems include the Abbreviated Burn Severity Index (ABSI), the Baux index (BI), and the DEMI score (Depth Extension Morbidity Inhalation) which is a tool for predicting mortality risk in burned children (1).

FLUID RESUSCITATION

Improved survival rates in modern burn care can largely be attributed to prompt, aggressive intravenous fluid infusions, although there are differing opinions about the type of fluids and rate of infusion. Most of the world's population does not have access to prompt advanced medical care and IV therapy. Volume resuscitation and the re-introduction of molecular oxygen into previously ischemic tissues cause reperfusion injury, and produces additional tissue damage (1).

There is a systemic capillary leak in the hours after a serious burn that typically "seals" after 18–24 hours if resuscitation has been successful. Who requires fluid resuscitation? Any adults with > 15%, and children with > 10% TBSA burns should be considered for fluid resuscitation. There may be increased fluid requirements proportionate with injury size, with associated inhalation injury, delay in resuscitation and unusually deep burns. Close monitoring of their fluid volume status is required. Patients with electrical injuries present special problems since the surface area is much smaller, but the amount of injury and the inflammatory response can be much greater. There are several formulas for fluid resuscitation of burn patients, but none accurately predict the volume requirements of individual patients. Physicians that manage burn wounds should know one formula well to adequately fluid resuscitate their patients. The Parkland formula is the method used by the author. It states that the fluid requirements for any patient with burns can be calculated by evaluating the extent of burns, total body surface area, and the weight of the patient. The formula for the first 24 hours is lactated ringers at 4cc/kg/%TBSA. For example, the 70 kg patient with a 50% TBSA burn would require (4cc X 70 kg X 50% = 14,000 cc) 14 liters of fluid in the first 24 hours. One-half is given in the first 8 post-injury hours, in this example almost a liter per hour, starting from the time of the burn injury. Should the resuscitation be delayed, this volume is administered so that infusion is completed by the end of the eighth post-injury hour. The other 1/2 of the calculated fluid requirements would be given over the next 16 hours. Ringer's lactate is the initial fluid of choice. Dextrose (D5LR) is not used because the dextrose in large volumes may cause hyperosmolar states.

The calculated fluid requirement is only a guideline and adjustments should be made according to clinical response which can be monitored by the urine output. Adequate output in the adult is 30–50 cc/hr (0.5 cc/kg/hr), and for a child 1–1.5 cc/kg/hr. The goal of fluid resuscitation is to restore and maintain perfusion and oxygenation while minimizing exogenous contribution to edema. Monitoring clinical response is more important than adhering to formulas.

Most resuscitation formulas recommend administration of colloid when capillary integrity returns, generally by day 2, since colloid is more likely to remain in the intravascular compartment at that time. Five percent albumin in isotonic crystalloid can be given at 0.3–0.5 cc/kg X TBSA. Using the prior example, the 70 kg patient with 50% TBSA burn would require about one-half of first day fluids on day 2, and one-half of that amount would be colloids. In order to calculate the remaining fluid volumes, the patient's normal maintenance and evaporative losses are used. Urine output should be closely monitored.

Fluid resuscitation does not always go well. It is important to avoid over-resuscitation. In any patient that requires > 150% of calculated fluid requirements, colloid should be started earlier (i.e., 8–12 hours post injury). In most other patients, colloid should be started at the 24 hours point or the second day post-burn. It is best to obtain more information regarding the status of the intravascular volume with a directed physical examination and by using central venous pressure or Swan-Ganz monitoring. The hematocrit is not a good way to follow adequacy of fluid resuscitation; there may be a delay of > 24 hours for the hematocrit to reflect changes in intravascular volume.

The importance of nutrition cannot be overemphasized. The significant benefits of early, enteral resuscitation in thermal injury have been established in animal and human research, though many present-day clinicians remain unaware of its utility. Enteral resuscitation is more effective when started within one hour after injury, increases intestinal blood flow, and results in better maintenance of gut barrier integrity to help inhibit bacterial translocation (5). The normal metabolic rate of 35–40 Kcal/M^2/hour and caloric demands can both double in burns > 50% TBSA. The indirect calorimeter remains the gold standard to determine resting energy expenditure and measure minute-by-minute protein and caloric needs of the patient to optimize wound healing.

INHALATION INJURY

In comparison with a comparable size burn alone, the combination of a body burn and smoke inhalation injury results in a marked increase in mortality and morbidity, an increase in hemodynamic instability, a 30–50% increase in initial fluid requirements, an accentuation of the degree of lung dysfunction, and a significant increase in burn wound edema (5).

Inhalation injury is primarily a clinical diagnosis and should always be suspected when there is a closed-space exposure, facial burns, oropharyngeal burns, singed nasal hairs, upper airway obstruction and carbonaceous debris in the mouth and pharynx or sputum.

The chest x-ray is routinely normal until complications occur. In the past, pulmonary function tests and ventilation-perfusion scans were ordered. Now, fiberoptic bronchoscopy is the gold standard for diagnosis, but is invasive, requires a skilled endoscopist, may worsen hypoxia, and a normal study does not exclude inhalation injury.

Virtual bronchoscopy, developed with use of high resolution, high-speed CT scanners may be useful in selected patients already going to CT, but will likely not replace flexible fiberoptic bronchoscopy. High frequency oscillatory ventilation was beneficial in improvement in partial pressure of oxygen/ fraction of inspired oxygen ratios in a group of severely burned adult patients with ARDS (3). Swelling is usually in the upper airway due to massive fluid hydration, and is maximal 2–6 hours post-burn. Intubation is recommended if there is any doubt about the diagnosis of inhalation injury since airway edema can be life threatening. Oxygen is always used for intubated patients. Arterial blood gas results include a carboxyhemoglobin level that can confirm a significant carbon monoxide (CO) exposure, but the clinical presentation is important to guide therapy. Cyanide and other toxic exposures are common in closed-space injuries.

CO poisoning can complicate burn injuries, especially in closed space fires, is associated with smoke inhalation, and can significantly increase morbidity and mortality. Smoke inhalation is associated with exposure to other toxins, causes asphyxia, generalized inflammation and airway and alveolar damage.

Indications for treatment of CO poisoning with hyperbaric oxygen (HBO2) include loss or alteration of consciousness, carboxyhemoglobin levels > 25%, evidence of myocardial injury, or metabolic acidosis. It may be difficult to determine whether symptoms and findings are due to carbon monoxide alone, or are part of the multiple pathologic consequences of smoke inhalation.

In a landmark randomized controlled clinical trial, Weaver and associates (41) demonstrated statistically significantly improved cognitive outcomes in CO poisoning victims treated with HBO2. Cognitive impairment was less frequent in the HBO2 group than in control patients at six weeks after treatment (25% vs. 46%, p < 0.007). It should be noted that while 8% of the patients in this study required intubation, no burn victims were included.

Mechanisms by which HBO2 might reduce cognitive sequelae after CO poisoning include increased oxygen content in the blood, accelerated elimination of CO from hemoglobin and other heme-proteins, preservation of adenosine triphosphate (ATP) activity, modulation of ischemia-reperfusion injury, and prevention of lipid peroxidation. Risks associated with HBO2 treatment include complications of patient transport, hyperoxic seizures and barotrauma.

WOUND MANAGEMENT AND TOPICAL ANTIBIOTICS

Immediate cooling of small wounds may help limit burn depth without causing systemic hypothermia, but this window of opportunity is quite small. Tar should be cooled with tap water and later removed with a lipophyllic solvent.

Initial wound management includes thorough cleaning, debridement of loose and necrotic tissue, appropriate splinting and positioning and the use of topical antibiotics.

The type of topical antimicrobials used in burn wounds depends on the depth, extent and location of the injury and are applied to control pain, decrease vapor loss and dessication, and slow bacterial growth. For superficial partial thickness burns (sunburn), minimal treatment is required and includes non-adherent gauze (Xeroform® & bacitracin ointment are recommended). In deep partial and full thickness burns, silver sulfadiazene (Silvadene®) is considered the gold standard. It's a white opaque cream, painless on application, fair to poor eschar penetration and no metabolic side effects. It is a good antimicrobial and antifungal agent, but can cause a transient neutropenia that peaks on burn day 3 and 4. Silvadene and other non-aqueous topicals can generate a free water requirement that can be added to enteral feedings. Extreme hypernatremia can be associated with adverse central nervous system events. Sulfamylon is recommended for cartilage (nose, ear) injuries due to its deeper eschar penetration. Patients with ear injuries can wear earmuffs to protect the vulnerable cartilage from pressure. In high-risk patients with greater than 40% TBSA burns, dressing changes should be done on a twice daily basis. Other patients can have daily dressing changes. Sulphur-containing topical antimicrobials can cause a reaction in allergic patients. Acticoat® (Smith and Nephew, Largo, FL), a silver-impregnated occlusive dressing, can be substituted in these patients. It has a broad spectrum of antibacterial activity that persists for 3 days. In a study of donor site healing, Acticoat donors healed 40% faster compared to donors dressed with antibiotic-soaked gauze dressings. Recent evidence in the literature shows that good hydration is the single most important external factor for optimal wound healing. Moisture-retentive ointments promote earlier functional recovery of regenerating keratinocytes and improve scar quality (1).

SURGICAL MANAGEMENT OF THE BURN WOUND

An early estimate of burn size and depth is useful for planning. Burns are classified as first, second, third or fourth degree (see Table 2). Examination by an experienced burn surgeon remains the most reliable and least expensive method of estimating burn depth and size, determining the probability of a burn wound healing and is central to operative planning. The clinical diagnosis of burn depth is easy for superficial injuries (sunburn) and full thickness (third degree) injuries. Sunburns are basically supported with pain medications. Full-thickness burns are characterized by complete destruction of the epidermis and dermis, are thick, leathery, charred, appear waxy white and are painless. These need to be excised and grafted.

Partial thickness burns are difficult to assess; both the healing potential and the thickness are indeterminate. A superficial partial-thickness burn involves destruction of the entire epidermis and no more than the upper third of the dermis. These are the most painful burns. A deep partial-thickness burn involves destruction of most of the dermal layer, with few viable epidermal cells remaining. Blood flow is compromised, increasing the risk of infection and conversion to full-thickness injury (6).

It is important to protect those areas that will heal, and surgically excise necrotic tissue as quickly as possible. By the end of the first post-burn week, it is usually quite clear which areas need to be excised and grafted. Operative management principles are that burns healing within 2–3 weeks will yield better cosmetic results with minimal scarring and will not need grafts. Unfortunately, if the burn is of indeterminate depth, the decision cannot be delayed 2–3 weeks, or the patient may become progressively more septic. There needs to be a plan to determine which areas to excise, and which areas to close as quickly as possible.

Tangential excision is for taking care of patients with indeterminate depth. Thin slices are removed until viable tissue is reached, marked by punctate dermal bleeding. If the tangential excision is deep, it is sometimes necessary to extend into viable fat or viable fascia. Endpoints for tangential excision include no more than 20% BSA at a time, transfusion requirement of less than ten units, core temperature less than 35°C, and operative time of less than two hours to avoid significant hypothermia. Blood loss during tangential excision should be minimized by the use of extremity tourniquets, dilute epinephrine injections or soaked sponges, and brisk operation pace.

Basic burn surgery principles are to expeditiously debride all dead tissue and provide coverage to protect the underlying wound. Advantages of early (first 2–3 days) excision include more rapid wound closure, less infection, less hospital time, earlier rehabilitation, fewer secondary reconstructions, and results are more satisfying to nurses, therapists and physicians. Excision on the first post-burn day minimizes blood loss. After that, disadvantages of early excision include increased blood loss, and increased anesthesia time. Whether early tangential excision decreases mortality remains controversial. Results can be disastrous if early excision is performed improperly.

TABLE 2. DEPTH OF BURN

First degree	red, dry, and painful
Second degree	red, wet, and very painful
Third degree	leathery in consistency, dry, insensate, and waxy
Fourth degree	involves underlying subcutaneous tissue, tendon or bone

PRIORITY OF EXCISION

The patient should be stabilized prior to excision. The first objective is to achieve bulk wound closure, generally with reharvested autograft. When this has been achieved, attention is turned to small, complex wounds, particularly the head and neck, hands, feet and genitalia. Though of small physiologic size, these areas are of immense functional and aesthetic importance. In large TBSA burns, the patient is placed in a prone position first - the large areas of the back are first excised to avoid having to turn the patient back and forth during subsequent operations. The hands are excised by about 14 days, allowing them to heal as much as possible. Facial excisions are done at the last possible point in time. An alternative to tangential excision is to go to the operating room and use electrocautery to excise through skin and subcutaneous tissue down to fascia. The fascia is usually very viable and provides a clean bed for autografting, expediting wound closure. There is less blood loss than tangential excision, and usually good graft take. Unfortunately, there may be undesirable cosmetic outcomes and significant functional compromise.

After tangential excision, prompt wound closure is desirable. Autografts from uninjured skin remains the mainstay of treatment, and can be meshed to expand the coverage area up to four times the donor site (1).

When autograft is exhausted, temporary biological closure is achieved with human cadaver allograft (HCAS), or other temporary closure material. HCAS provides a temporary biologic dressing, and can be used as a dressing to cover meshed autografts in large burns. Problems include limited supply, variable quality, and ultimate rejection.

Although no inexpensive, reliable and durable permanent skin substitute exists, recently developed devices can be classified as epidermal substitutes, dermal substitutes and composite substitutes. Options include tissue engineered bilayered substitutes (Apligraf), and cultured dermal substitutes (artificial skin), prepared by culturing fibroblasts on a two-layered spongy matrix of hyaluronic acid and atelo-collagen.

Bilaminar skin substitutes (Biobrane, Transcyte, Laserskin) may sometimes be used, especially when donor sites are limited. Dermal substitutes (Integra, Alloderm, Dermagraft, Terumo, Pelnac) have been available for clinical use in recent years.

In large burns, limited donor sites must be budgeted. The scalp is an excellent donor site, and can be harvested for split-thickness skin grafts every 3 days. Culture and transplantation of keratinocytes are a major advance in treatment of severe burns, are used in 50–60% TBSA burns with limited donor sites, and can be life-saving in massive full-thickness injuries. Disadvantages include clinically impractical delays in obtaining the product, fragility, unpredictable "take" and high costs. It is just epidermis without dermal ridges or pegs to allow for graft adherence to the skin, and is only 5–6 cells thick when delivered in the Petri dishes, and is difficult to handle, with a wet tissue paper consistency. A recent small, non-randomized study of 40% TBSA partial thickness burns showed a markedly shorter hospital length of stay in patients treated with operative debridement and covered with meshed cadaver skin. A similar 3-way randomized study of partial-thickness burns in children showed a shorter time to reepithelialization with TransCyte (Smith & Nephew) versus Biobrane (Mylan Bertex Pharmaceuticals) versus silver sulfadiazine (7.5 v. 9.5 v. 11.2 days, respectively). The TransCyte group also had fewer autografting procedures. Photochemical tissue bonding (PTB), an emerging laser technique, could have clinical applications in the future (9).

The mainstay for managing the dreaded complication of post-burn contractures is prevention. An integral part of the burn center team, occupational and physical therapists can provide daily range-of-motion and appropriate splints. Anti-deformity splinting helps by keeping injured areas in full extension if possible, in order to prevent burn scar contractures. Topical silicone gel has reduced hypertrophic scarring in many patients, though the mechanism of action is not known.

BURNS OF SPECIAL ANATOMIC AREAS

Suspected eye burns should be stained with fluorescein to rule out corneal injury, avoid dessication, and refer to an ophthalmologist. Full-thickness eyelid burns are rare. However, lower lid ectropion is common. Release and full-thickness skin grafting should be done as soon as possible. Multiple surgeries may be necessary to preserve the eye. Ear burns can result in perichondritis, which is easier to prevent than to treat. Superficial ear burns (Figure 2) are managed similarly to facial burns, but external pressure should not be applied to the helix, since the cartilage is already poorly vascularized (6). Sulfamylon should be used and pressure on the ear avoided until healed. Carefully monitor for infection; the usual pathogen in perichondritis is *pseudomonas*. Established perichondritis is a surgical emergency and needs to be aggressively managed with wide debridement of the cartilage and a drainage procedure and antibiotics.

Facial burns generally heal well due to the increased blood flow to the head and neck area. Facial burns need to be washed 2–3 times per day, and an ointment such as polysporin or bacitracin applied. Deep facial burns are problematic in terms of results obtained by tangential excision and grafting. The author prefers to leave the face last in order to perform excision of the non-viable tissues. Patients and their families are counseled extensively about what it means to have a burned face as well as what it means to have grafts of the face. Tangential excision to the face is very difficult and precludes the use of a tourniquet. Extensive bleeding occurs and must be carefully controlled. Excision of the face may need to be done in two stages; first, excise then temporize with biological dressing or allograft and then go back in 2–3 days for definitive grafting or sheet grafts. For best results, resurfacing should be done with thick split-thickness sheet grafts of optimal color match taken from closest to the burned area, namely the scalp, upper back or upper chest. The face should be

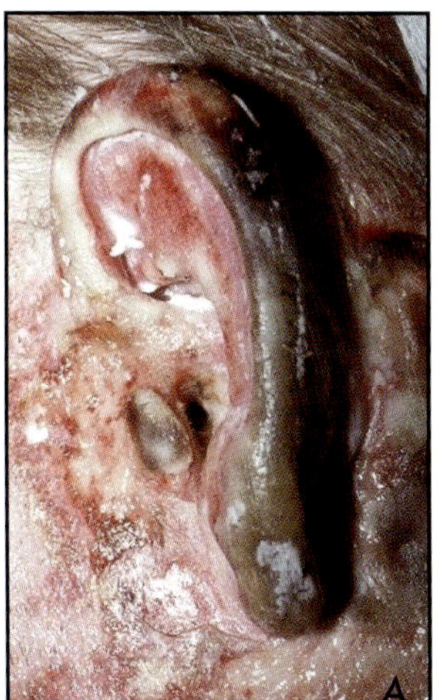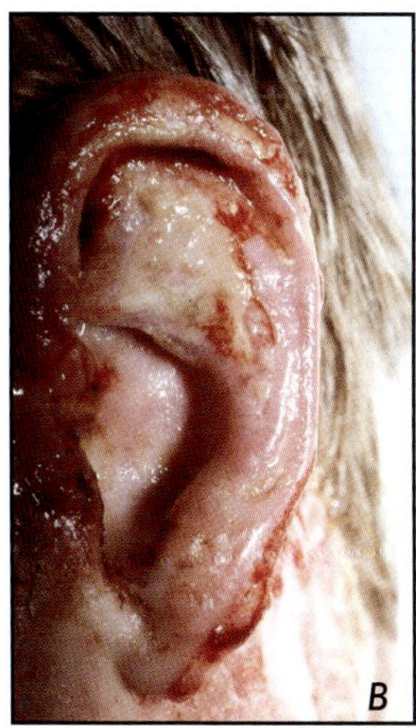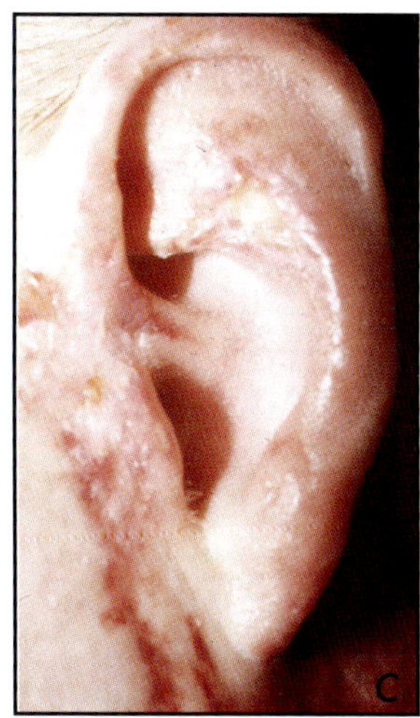

Figure 2 (A–C). Ear cartilage has a relatively poor blood supply. Burns to the ear are associated with a high risk of infection. Pressure on burned ears should be avoided. Adjunctive hyperbaric oxygen can be especially beneficial for burns in special anatomic areas for preservation of tissue and function.

rendered functional with good coverage of the globes and competence of the mouth. It is important to observe for globe exposure caused by retraction of burned peri-orbital tissues, and addressed promptly when it occurs due to the risk of loss of the globe through corneal ulceration and infection. Post-operative management of deep facial burns includes effective immobilization to prevent shearing or movement of the grafts. Most of the patients are already sedated, intubated, and on tube feedings. Patients should refrain from talking and grafts need to be rolled frequently to prevent seromas and hematomas. Once the graft takes, pressure garments like clear facemasks should be applied as soon as possible in order to reduce hypertrophic scarring.

Serious hand burns are especially difficult to manage and should be a focus of attention from the onset, or function can be severely compromised. Due to the joints involved, occupational and physical therapy are key adjuncts to avoid loss of small joint mobility and stiffness. If the burns appear to be deep partial thickness or full thickness, consider early tangential excision and sheet grafting. Sheet grafts should be used whenever possible to achieve better esthetic and functional results.

In a small group of human bilateral hand burns, early application of subatmospheric pressure with the VAC (Kinetics Concepts, Inc.) device helped prevent progression from partial to full thickness injury (8). Adjunctive hyperbaric oxygen should be considered for burns in special anatomical areas due to the potential for cosmetic and functional complications and compromise.

ELECTRICAL INJURY

Patients with electrical injuries should be treated like any other trauma victim, ruling out life-threatening injuries first. A general trauma evaluation should be done including assessment of the spinal cord and for long bone injury. Fasciotomy for compartment syndromes is emergent. Patients must be initially monitored for cardiac irritability. Neurovascular status should be assessed and neuro-sensory loss documented, if possible. However, neurological sequelae may not manifest for 1–2 years. Factors important in estimating the magnitude of injury include the voltage, resistance amperage, duration of contact, pathway, and whether the exposure was alternating current (AC) or direct current (DC). AC is more dangerous and associated with tetany. The victim cannot release the source of electricity, and often will go into ventricular fibrillation.

The electrical current causes the first component of injury. The resultant heat generated by bone is greatest due to increased resistance, followed in descending order by fat, tendon, skin, muscle, vessels, and nerves. Even though the superficial tissues may appear minimally injured, the most severe damage to muscle may be found near bone, and must be managed. Arcing can occur, generating enough heat to potentially vaporize metal. Arcing can also ignite the patient's clothing, causing flame burns.

After the diagnosis of electrical injury is made, management includes cardiac monitoring for 1–3 days in high (> 1000 volt) or intermediate (> 220 volt) exposures, determination of acid-base status, assessment of distal perfusion and neurovascular status and evaluation for compartment syndromes. Hospital admission is mandatory for high voltage injuries, urinary catheters should be placed to document myoglobinuria due to deep thermal injury and should be promptly treated with diuresis (1–2 cc/kg/hr) until the pigment load is decreased to avoid renal tubular injury. Volume replacement, mannitol, and sodium bicarbonate can be used in adults to keep urine output at 100 cc/hour until urine clears. Judicious use of bicarbonate may facilitate myoglobin clearance. Mannitol is rarely used, and can obscure urine output as an indicator of circulating volume. Fasciotomy and debridement should be performed as indicated. Compartment syndromes, loss of consciousness, or myoglobinuria are uncommon in patients exposed to < 500 volts. Fluid management basic principles are the same as in thermal injury but formulae are of no value. Crystalloids should be used initially, and increased as necessary to achieve adequate urine output. Colloid and blood may be needed for maintaining adequate perfusion. In electrical injuries, although the burn area is smaller, the inflammatory response is massive.

Wound Closure

All non-viable tissue must be debrided and the deep muscle compartments must be checked. Electrical injury is a staged project with many re-operations. It is difficult to get out of the zone of injury. Ancillary diagnostic tests can be used to assess the viability of the injured areas. Gallium is useful for identifying pockets of necrosis.

FROSTBITE INJURY

As burns were once thought merely to represent direct thermal injury to cells, the mechanism of frostbite injury has been thought to be a direct effect of freezing on the tissue cells.

Frostbite most commonly affects the extremities, and can be classified as superficial or deep. Superficial frostbite affects the skin and subcutaneous tissues; deep frostbite also affects bones, joints and tendons. The mechanism of frostbite injury on a cellular level is much more complex than previously believed. Cold damages tissue through cellular injury and vascular impairment.

Once body temperature drops more than a few degrees, the physiochemical processes of cells begin to fail, causing universal derangement. The metabolic rate declines by approximately 6% for each 1°C decrease in body temperature. A profound diuresis, vascular leakage, cardiac dysfunction and paradoxical vasodilatation combine to cause eventual circulatory collapse.

Cellular injury may be due to intracellular water crystallization, temperature-induced protein changes and membrane damage. Endothelial injury causes thrombosis that, combined with hemoconcentration and hyperviscosity, leads to thromboembolism.

When a frozen limb is initially thawed, it appears viable, and various studies have shown that blood flow is reinstituted after thawing.

As tissues thaw, marked edema occurs because of melting of water crystals, cellular damage, loss of endothelial integrity and thrombosis. Over time, necrosis and gangrene can result, depending on the severity of the injury. Rewarmed skin can have clear blisters in superficial frostbite, and hemorrhagic blisters in deep injury. Blister management is controversial; removal is advocated by some due to the high concentrations of prostaglandin

F2 alpha and thromboxane A2 in the exudates. If the blisters do not interfere with range-of-motion, it is reasonable to leave them intact. If ruptured or removed, the underlying area should be debrided and covered with a topical antimicrobial. Escharotomy may be necessary if there is vascular impairment. Mummification and auto-amputation may occur. Surgical amputation may be required many weeks after the injury.

Weeks may pass before demarcation appears between viable and nonviable tissues.

It is this progressive tissue injury that is interesting. Frostbite pathophysiology characteristics are very similar to ischemia-reperfusion injury, may be seen at different times in the injury process, and include neutrophil adhesion to damaged endothelial cells, breakdown of the endothelial cell membrane, erythrocyte and leukocyte extravasations, production of potent vasoconstrictors such as thromboxane A2 and prostaglandin F2 alpha, free radical generation, and the amelioration of some tissue damage with free radical scavengers such as deferoxamine and superoxide dismutase (SOD). Thrombus formation may play a significant role in the later stages of the ischemic injury process.

The primary therapy for hypothermia is rewarming. Adherent wet clothing should be removed. Rubbing affected areas worsens the tissue damage. Aggressive volume resuscitation is a requirement, best accomplished with large volumes of isotonic fluids that have been effectively warmed and are delivered rapidly.

In frostbite and other I-R injuries, the degree of tissue injury can vary from virtually uninjured to severely affected. In frostbite (but not other experimental I-R injury), the successful use of deferoxamine, superoxide dismutase, selective prostaglandin inhibitors, thromboxane A2 inhibitors and thrombolytics is encouraging. Emergent arteriography in recently thawed frostbite patients has shown significant vascular thrombus formation, even in larger arteries such as the dorsalis pedis. Thrombolytic therapy in small and microvascular structures is more difficult due to the limited surface area that the clot presents to the thrombolytic agent. Anticoagulation therapy, if given early in the process, may prevent the formation of microvascular thrombus. Presently, there is sufficient clinical and experimental evidence to support the use of selective prostaglandin inhibitors (ibuprofen), deferoxamine, thromboxane A2 inhibitors (topical aloe vera), and anticoagulation in certain frostbite patients. Selective thrombolytic therapy may be beneficial if there is arteriography-documented occlusion and the agent can be infused over many hours. The early and aggressive use of HBO2 therapy for frostbite may be beneficial when added to a regimen designed to minimize the production of vasoconstrictive agents and free radicals, limit endothelial damage, and prevent thrombosis. HBO2 has been shown to increase oxygen diffusion distance in ischemic tissue, helping to salvage marginal tissue until revascularization occurs. It has also been shown to preserve adenosine triphosphate levels, reduce free radical production, stabilize and reverse endothelial cell wall lipid peroxidation, and prevent or diminish neutrophil adhesion to the endothelium, a quantitatively major contributor to I-R injury. Hyperoxia-induced vasoconstriction only occurs in healthy tissue. HBO2 actually reverses vasoconstriction in ischemic tissue. In any case, the hyperoxia induced by HBO2 overwhelms any potential reduction in blood flow. The benefits of HBO2 greatly outweigh any potentially deleterious effects.

Though better understood than frostbite, it has been clinically difficult to treat I-R injury. A recent clinical study demonstrated HBO2-induced cardio-protection and attenuation of ischemia-reperfusion injury due to the generation of reactive oxygen species (ROS), resulting in the production of nitric oxide. HBO2-induced ROS are known to initiate gene expression, reduce neutrophil adhesion (via a decrease in CD11a/18 function, P-selectin, and down-regulation of intracellular adhesion molecule-1), decrease lipid peroxidation, stimulate neovascularization, and increase antioxidants, all resulting in cardioprotection (44). Understanding these mechanisms for cardio-protection helps clarify the mechanisms of benefit with HBO2 in other I-R injuries.

A cascade of causative factors are responsible for the injury in frostbite and different portions of the tissue are likely to be at different stages of injury. A combination of therapeutic agents may be necessary for optimal treatment. Amputation should be considered an outcome, not an intervention.

Case of Aviator with Frostbite of Face and Hand

A 35 YOM navigator was sucked out of the KC-135 aircraft up to his waist when the window failed at FL350 (flight altitude of 35,000 ft). Wind blast tore off his helmet, oxygen mask, and right glove, leaving his face and hand exposed to the frigid -67°F (-55°C) temperature outside the aircraft. (As one ascends in altitude, there is a steady decrease in atmospheric temperature of 3.5°F per 1,000 ft, or 6.5°C per km.) He was pulled back into the aircraft by other crewmembers in less than two minutes. The aircraft descended and landed at a nearby Air Force base where the navigator received treatment for severe frostbite. Figure 3 shows the frostbitten face (Photo A) and right hand (Photo B). Figure 4 shows the time to freezing of unprotected flesh. (Reference: Sheffield PJ, Aircrew Aerospace Physiology Course, Langley AFB VA, 1968).

HYPERBARIC OXYGEN THERAPY

Historical Considerations

Current use of adjunctive hyperbaric oxygen in the treatment of acute thermal injury is relatively rare, despite an abundance of experimental animal and human data, and clinical experience.

A significant body of experimental data supports the efficacy of hyperbaric oxygen in the treatment of thermal injury. The benefits of HBO2 for acute thermal injury in animals include a reduction of edema, healing time and infection, preservation of the microvasculature and earlier return of capillary patency. Other findings include improved collagen quality, prevention of conversion from partial to full-thickness injury, improved survival of dermal elements, more rapid epithelialization, preservation of adenosine triphosphate (ATP), reduction in burn shock, and overall increased survival.

Beginning in 1965, clinical studies have documented benefits of HBO2 that include statistically significant reductions in mortality, improved overall healing, faster healing of partial thickness burns, reduced number of

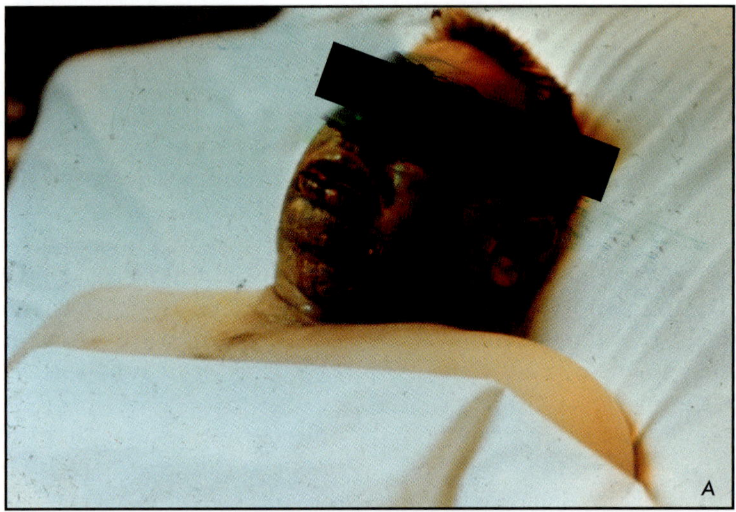

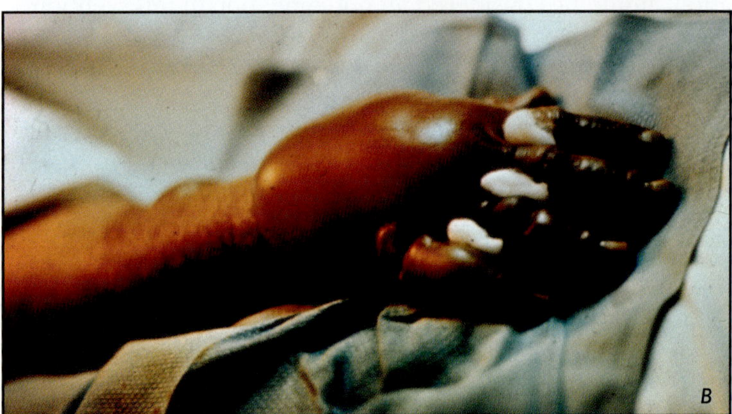

Figure 3 (A–B). Frostbite to unprotected face (3A) and right hand (3B) (photographs by Paul J. Sheffield).

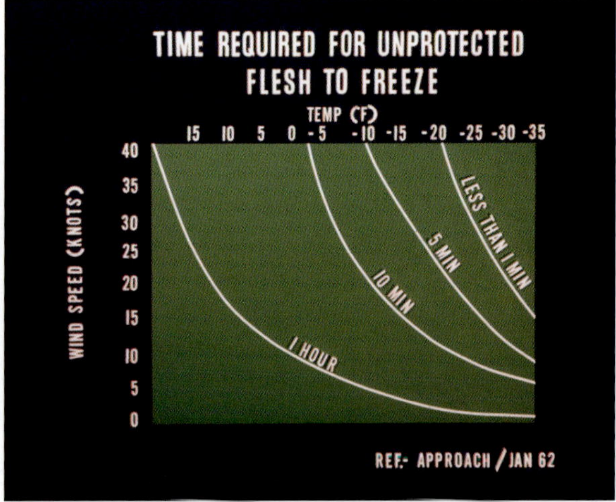

Figure 4. Time to freezing of unprotected flesh.

surgeries, reduced intensive care days and total hospital stay, reduced resuscitative weight gain, and lower incidence of wound sepsis.

In 1974, Hart (24) reported a controlled randomized series showing a reduction in fluid requirements, faster healing, and reduced mortality when HBO2-treated patients were compared to controls and to United States National Burn Information Exchange Standards.

Cianci (4) has reported multiple clinical studies on the benefits of HBO2, including a significant reduction in length of hospital stay in burns up to 39% TBSA, a reduction in the need for surgery, including grafting, and in one study, an average savings of $107,000 (36%) per case. Other findings include a reduction in resuscitative fluid requirements, a statistically significant reduction in maximum weight gain and percent weight gain in seriously burned (40–80% TBSA) patients treated with adjunctive HBO2 versus controls at a regional burn center.

Hammarlund (25) showed a reduction of edema and wound exudation in a carefully controlled series of human volunteers with ultraviolet (UV) irradiated blister wounds. In a similar study, Niezgoda (29) demonstrated in the HBO2-treated group a statistically significant reduction of wound size, hyperemia (measured by laser Doppler) and wound exudate. This was the first prospective, randomized, controlled, double-blinded trial comparing HBO2 with sham controls in a human burn model.

Cianci and Slade (19) conducted an evidenced-based review of the medical literature; data from the animal studies and clinical trials of the use of HBO2 in acute thermal injury was evaluated for benefit. The authors concluded that the American Heart Association therapeutic intervention classification for thermal injury merits a designation as a "Class IIa" indication (for HBO2). The British Medical Journal (BMJ) Clinical Evidence review of this indication would be "Beneficial" based on the multiple animal studies, randomized controlled trials and low incidence of "Harms." A Cochrane Database Systematic Review of the efficacy of HBO2 for thermal burns published in 2004 found that only two of four identified randomized controlled trials satisfied the inclusion criteria. One trial reported no differences in length of stay, mortality or number of surgeries between the control and HBO2-treated groups. The other trial reported shorter mean healing times in HBO2 patients (19.7 vs. 43.8 days). The reviewers stated that the trials were of poor methodological quality, making it difficult to have confidence in the individual results, and data pooling inappropriate. They concluded that there is insufficient evidence to support or refute the effectiveness of HBO2 for the management of thermal burns, and called for further research to better define a role for HBO2 (40).

Mechanisms of Action

Mechanisms of action of HBO2 include edema reduction, maintenance and preservation of the microcirculation, preservation of adenosine triphosphate (ATP), prevention of reperfusion injury, and reduction of bacterial translocation from the gastrointestinal tract and gut-related ischemia-reperfusion injury. Other demonstrated benefits include preservation of dermal elements, and improved collagen quality.

Data from Zamboni (45) demonstrate that HBO2 is a potent blocker of white cell adherence to endothelial cell walls, interrupting the ischemia-reperfusion cascade that causes vascular damage. The mechanism is an inhibitory effect on the CD18 locus on the surface of the neutrophil. Germonpre's (22) demonstration of a significantly reduced inflammatory response in HBO2-treated animals compared to controls supports this observation and may in part explain the beneficial effect of HBO2 therapy on the microcirculation observed by others.

Reduction of leukocyte (PMNL) killing ability in hypoxic tissue has been well documented. Mader and others (27) have demonstrated the ability of HBO2 to elevate tissue oxygen tension and to enhance PMNL killing in an O_2-enriched animal model. Bacterial translocation is felt to be a major source of burn wound infection. Tenenhaus and colleagues (35) showed reduction in mesenteric bacterial colonization in an HBO2-treated burned mouse model. More recently, Magnotti et al., (28) have proposed an evolution from bacterial translocation to gut ischemia-reperfusion injury after burn injury as the pathogenesis of multiple organ dysfunction syndrome.

Systemic inflammation, acute lung injury, and multiple organ failure after a major thermal injury are relatively common causes of morbidity and mortality. In the normal host, the intestinal mucosa functions as a major local defense barrier, a component of multiple defense mechanisms, that helps prevent bacteria that colonize the gut, as well as their products, from crossing the mucosal barrier. After a major thermal injury, and in other clinical and experimental circumstances, this intestinal barrier function becomes overwhelmed or impaired, resulting in the movement of bacteria and/or endotoxin to the mesenteric lymph nodes and systemic tissues, defined as bacterial translocation. The importance of this intestinal barrier function becomes clear when considering that the distal small bowel and colon contain 10^{10} concentrations of anaerobes and 10^5 to 10^8 each of Gram-positive and Gram-negative aerobic and facultative microorganisms per gram of tissue, and enough endotoxin to kill the host thousands of times over (28).

Loss of gut barrier function and a resultant gut inflammatory response, lead to the production of proinflammatory factors causing a septic state leading to distant organ failure. Splanchnic hypoperfusion leading to gut ischemia-reperfusion injury appears to be the dominant hemodynamic event triggering the release of biologically active factors into the mesenteric lymphatics. The benefits of the early use of hyperbaric oxygen in burn victims may in part be mediated through amelioration of gut reperfusion injury. The beneficial effects of HBO2 in ischemic-reperfused tissues have been demonstrated in intestine, (43) skeletal muscle, (30, 45) brain, (34, 36) and testicular tissue, (26) and myocardium (32, 33, 39, 43).

In a study of severely burned humans (> 30% TBSA), HBO2-treated patients compared to controls had increased levels of serum soluble interleukin 2 receptor (p < 0.05) and decreased plasma fibronectin (p < 0.01), resulting clinically in a lower incidence of sepsis (p < 0.05) (41).

On the basis of clinical and experimental experience, total enteral nutrition, starting as early as possible, is recommended for burn patients, (and results in decreased morbidity and mortality). Early enteral feeding after thermal injury supports intestinal structure and function, and has been shown to be superior to parenteral nutrition in burn patients.

Surgical Perspectives

In recent years, there is increased emphasis on aggressive surgical management of the burn wound with early tangential excision and grafting of the deep second-degree and probable third-degree burns, especially to functionally important parts of the body. Hyperbaric oxygen has allowed the surgeon yet another adjunctive modality of treatment for these burns, especially of the hands and fingers, face and ears, and other areas where the surgical excision is often challenging and coverage is sometimes difficult. If not obviously third degree, these often indeterminate wounds are best treated with topical antimicrobial agents, bedside and enzymatic debridements, wound care, and adjunctive HBO2, allowing the surgeon more time for healing to take place and for definition of the extent and depth of injury. In deep partial thickness burns, adjunctive HBO2 can prevent progression of injury, and minimize conversion of partial to full thickness injury. HBO2 has drastically reduced the healing time in the major burn injury.

Fourth-degree burns, most commonly seen in high voltage electrical injuries, are benefited by adjunctive HBO2 via reduction in fascial compartment pressure, as injured muscle edema is decreased by preservation of aerobic glycolysis and, later, by a reduction of anaerobic infection.

Finally, reconstruction utilizing flaps, full-thickness skin, and composite grafts, i.e., ear to nose grafts, has been greatly facilitated by using adjunctive HBO2.

Evidence of Benefit in Inhalation Injury

Considerable attention has been given to the use of hyperbaric oxygen in inhalation injury. In comparison with a comparable size burn without lung involvement, the combination of a body burn and smoke inhalation injury results in a marked increase in mortality and morbidity, an increase in hemodynamic instability, a 30–50% increase in initial fluid requirements, a significant increase in burn wound edema, and an accentuation of the degree of lung dysfunction, particularly in those patients maintained on high levels of inspired O_2.

Grim (23) studied products of lipid peroxidation in the exhaled gases in HBO2-treated burn patients and found no indication of oxidative stress. Thom (37) demonstrated in a rat model that HBO2 treatment after smoke exposure resulted in diminished neutrophil accumulation in the lung. His findings suggest mechanisms of HBO2 benefit in inhalation injury in ways other than by removal of carbon monoxide. Ray (31) analyzed serious burn patients being treated for concurrent inhalation injury, thermal injury, and adult respiratory distress syndrome. She noted no deleterious effect with HBO2, even in those patients on continuous high levels of inspired oxygen. More rapid weaning from mechanical ventilation was possible in the HBO2-treated group (5.3 days vs. 26 days, $p < 0.05$). There was a significant reduction in cost of care per case ($60,000) in the HBO2-treated patients ($p < 0.05$).

Conduct of HBO2 Treatments of Burn Patients

Patients can be treated in a multiplace or monoplace chamber configuration. Movement over long distances is not recommended, and patients should not be transported to a hyperbaric chamber that is not co-located in the same facility as the burn center. Units planning treatment of burn patients should be thoroughly versed in management of critical care patients in the hyperbaric setting and to specific problems of burn patients prior to initiation of a therapy program. Preferably personnel should be certified in burn care and hyperbaric oxygen therapy. The hyperbaric department should function as an extension of the burn unit and part of the "team approach" to burn management.

Optimally, treatment is begun within six hours, or as soon as possible after injury, often during initial resuscitation. Treatments are attempted three times within the first 24 hours and twice daily thereafter on a regimen of 90 minutes of 100% oxygen delivery at 2.0–2.4 atmospheres absolute (ATA). Children are treated for 45 minutes twice daily. Patients are monitored during initial treatment and as necessary thereafter. Blood pressure can be monitored via transducers or noninvasively using blood pressure cuffs. Patients can be maintained on ventilator support during either monoplace or multiplace treatment, which is frequently the case in larger burns with concurrent inhalation injury.

Careful attention to fluid management is mandatory. Initial requirements may be several liters per hour, and pumps capable of this delivery at pressure must be utilized in order to maintain appropriate fluid replacement in the hyperbaric chamber. In larger burn injuries, adequate fluid and electrolyte resuscitation during the first 24 hours can be problematic. Certain critically ill, volume depleted, and/or septic patients can develop hypotension on ascent or shortly after completing an HBO2 treatment presumably due to loss of vascular auto regulation in response to declining arterial oxygen levels.

Careful volume replacement and assessment of fluid status is mandatory prior to, during, and immediately after HBO2 treatment. Increasing fluids during ascent may help compensate for any hypovolemia unmasked by the hyperbaric oxygen exposure.

For burn patients treated with HBO2 whose wounds are infected or colonized with *vancomycin resistant Enterococcus* (VRE) or methicillin (oxacillin) resistant *Staph aureus* (MRSA), the wound dressings should be left intact during HBO2 therapy, and the chambers cleaned with an antimicrobial solution after each treatment. No additional or more specialized infection control measures are considered necessary.

Maintenance of a comfortable, ambient temperature must be accomplished. Thermal instability may be a problem within 1–2 hours of burn wound cleansing and dressing change (depending on the methods used), especially in large TBSA burns. These patients should be carefully assessed prior to an HBO2 exposure. Febrile patients must be closely monitored and fever controlled as oxygen toxicity is reported to be more common in this group.

In large burns (> 40%), treatment is rendered for 10–14 days in close consultation with the burn surgeon. Many partial thickness burns will heal without surgery during this time frame and obviate the need for grafting. Treatment beyond 20–30 sessions is usually utilized to optimize graft take. While there is no absolute limit to the total number of hyperbaric treatments, it is rare to exceed 40–50 sessions except in very unusual circumstances.

In larger TBSA burns, especially of the head and neck, otologic/sinus barotrauma may be a problem, and careful attention should be given to this potential complication. The HBO2 team should make use of early ENT consultation when indicated.

Patient Selection

Hyperbaric oxygen therapy is presently utilized to treat serious burns, i.e., greater than 20% total body surface area and/or with involvement of the hands, face, feet or perineum, that are deep partial or full thickness injury. Patients with superficial burns or those not expected to survive are not accepted for therapy.

SUMMARY

Ideal burn therapy should promote rapid healing, act as an anti-scarring therapy, enhance "positive" growth hormones and cytokines, and suppress "negative" factors. Inhibition of the immediate triggering of the inflammatory cascades that lead to prolonged metabolic imbalances would potentially enhance wound healing. HBO2 has recently been shown to mobilize stem/progenitor cells in humans and mice, via stimulation of nitric oxide synthesis causing the release of stem cell factor. The findings suggest that some of the cells mobilized from the bone marrow by HBO2 may function as endothelial progenitors, contributing to wound vasculogenesis. This study provides new insight into possible mechanisms for the known clinical benefits of hyperbaric oxygen in burn injury (38).

Another recent review discusses HBO2-induced cardio-protection and attenuation of ischemia-reperfusion injury due to the generation of reactive oxygen species (ROS). HBO2 pre-conditioning (inducing cellular tolerance and protection from ischemia) and adaptive responses are mediated by HBO2-induced ROS, a result of the production of nitric oxide.

HBO2-induced ROS are known to initiate gene expression, reduce neutrophil adhesion (via a decrease in CD11a/18 function, P-selectin, and down-regulation of intracellular adhesion molecule-1), decrease lipid peroxidation, stimulate neovascularization, and increase antioxidants, all resulting in cardioprotection (44). Better understanding of HBO2-induced cardio-protection may be helpful in clarifying some or all of the mechanisms of HBO2 benefit in acute thermal injury.

Current data show that hyperbaric oxygen therapy, when used as an adjunct in a comprehensive program of burn care, can significantly improve morbidity and mortality, reduce length of hospital stay, and lessen the need for surgery. It has been demonstrated to be safe in the hands of those thoroughly trained in rendering hyperbaric oxygen therapy in the critical care setting and with appropriate monitoring precautions. Careful patient selection and screening is mandatory.

REFERENCES

Thermal Burn

1. Atiyeh BS, Gunn SW, Hayek SN. State of the art in burn treatment. *World J Surg* 2005; 29(2):131-148.

2. Burd A, Noronha FV, Pang P. Decompression not escharotomy in acute burns. *Burns* 32(2006):284-292.

3. Cartotto R, Ellis S, Gomez M. High frequency oscillatory ventilation in burn patients with the acute respiratory distress syndrome. *Burns* 2004;30:453-463.

4. Cianci PE. Adjunctive hyperbaric oxygen therapy in the treatment of thermal burns and frostbite. In: Hyperbaric Surgery. Bakker DJ, Cramer FS (eds). Flagstaff, AZ: Best Publishing Company, 2002 ; 207-221.

5. Demling RH. The burn edema process: current concepts. *J Burn Care Rehabil* May/June 2005;26:207-227.

6. DeSanti L. Pathophysiology and current management of burn injury. *Advances in Skin and Wound Care* Jul/Aug 2005,18(6):323-332.

7. Heimbach D. What's new in general surgery: burns and metabolism. *J Amer College of Surgeons* Feb 2002; 194(2): 156-64.

8. Kamolz LP, Andel H, Haslik W. Use of subatmospheric pressure therapy to prevent burn wound progression in human: first experiences. *Burns* 2004;30:253-258.

9. Naoum JJ, Roehl DR, Herndon DN. The use of homograft compared to topical antimicrobial therapy in the treatment of second-degree burns of more than 40% total body surface area. *Burns* 2004;30:548-551

10. Saffle JR. What's new in general surgery: burns and metabolism. *Journal of the American College of Surgeons* Feb 2002;196(2): 267-89.

11. Sheridan RL. Burns *Critical Care Medicine* Nov 2002; 30(11 Suppl):S500-14.

12. Traystman RJ, Kirsch JR, Koehler RC. Oxygen radical mechanisms of brain injury following ischemia and reperfusion. *J Appl Physiol* 1991;71:1185-1195.

13. Ward PA, Mulligan MS. New insights into mechanisms of oxyradical and neutrophil medicated lung injury. Klin Wochenschr 1991;69:1009-1011.

14. Ward PA, Till GO. The autodestructive consequences of thermal injury. *J Burn Care Rehabil* 1985;6:251-255.

Frostbite

15. Biem J, Koehncke N, Dosman J. Out of the cold: management of hypothermia and frostbite. *Canadian Medical Association Journal* Feb 2003; 168(3):305-11.

16. Cianci PE. Adjunctive hyperbaric oxygen therapy in the treatment of thermal burns and frostbite. Hyperbaric Surgery. Bakker DJ, Cramer FS (eds). Flagstaff, AZ: Best Publishing Company, 2002; 222-230.

17. Corneli HM. Environmental emergencies. *Clinical Pediatric Emergency Medicine* Sep 2001; 2(3):179-91.

HBO2 and Burns

18. Brannen AL, Still J, Haynes M, et al. A randomized prospective trial of hyperbaric oxygen in a referral burn center population. *American Surgeon* 1997; 63:205-208.

19. Cianci P, Slade JB, Jr. Thermal burns. In: Feldmeier JJ. Hyperbaric Oxygen 2003: Indications and Results. Kensington, MD: Undersea and Hyperbaric Medical Society, 2003; 109-119.

20. Deitch EA, Xu DZ, Franko L, et al. Evidence favoring the role of the gut as a cytokine generating organ in rats subjected to hemorrhagic shock. *Shock* 1994:1:141-6.

21. Deitch EA. Role of the gut lymphatic system in multiple organ failure. *Current Opin Crit Care* 2001;7:92-8.

22. Germonpre' P, Reper P, Vanderkelen A. Hyperbaric oxygen therapy and piracetam decrease the early extension of deep partial thickness burns. *Burns* 1996;22(6):468-473.

23. Grim PS, Nahum A, Sznajder J, et al. Lack of measurable oxidative stress during HBO2 therapy in burn patients. *Undersea Biomed Res (Suppl)* 1989; 16: 22.

24. Hart GB, O'Reilly RR, Broussard ND, et al. Treatment of burns with hyperbaric oxygen. *Surg Gynecol Obstet* 1974; 139:693-696.

25. Hammarlund C, Svedman C, Svedman P. Hyperbaric oxygen treatment of healthy volunteers with UV-irradiated blister wounds. *Burns* 1991; 17:296-301.

26. Kolski JM, Mazolewski PJ, Stephenson LL, et al. Effect of hyperbaric oxygen therapy on testicular ischema-reperfusion injury. *J of Urology* Aug 1998;160:601-604.

27. Mader JT, Brown GL, Guckian JC, et al. A mechanism for the amelioration of hyperbaric oxygen of experimental staphylococcal osteomyelitis in rabbits. *J Inf Disease* 1980;142:915-922.

28. Magnotti LJ, Deitch EA. Burns, bacterial translocation, gut barrier function, and failure. *J of Burn Care Rehab* 2005;26(5):383-391.

29. Niezgoda JA, Cianci P, Folden BW, et al. The effect of hyperbaric oxygen therapy on a burn wound model in human volunteers. *Plast Reconstr Surg* 1997; 99(6):1620-1625.

30. Nylander G, Nordstrom H, Lewis D, et al. Metabolic effects of hyperbaric oxygen in postischemic muscle. *Plast Reconstr Surg* 1987;79:91-7.

31. Ray CS, Green G, Cianci P. Hyperbaric oxygen therapy in burn patients: Cost effective adjuvant therapy (abstract). *Undersea Biomed Res* 1991; 18(Suppl):77.

32. Shandling AH, Ellestad MH, Hart GB, et al. Hyperbaric oxygen and thrombolysis in myocardial infarction: The "HOT MI" pilot study. *Am Heart J* 1997:134:544-40.

33. Sharifi M, Fares W, Abdel-Karim I, et al. Usefulness of hyperbaric oxygen therapy to inhibit restenosis after percutaneous coronary intervention for acute myocardial infarction or unstable angina pectoris. *Am J Cardiol* 2004;93:1533-35.

34. Takahashi M, Iwatsuki N, Ono K, et al. Hyperbaric oxygen therapy accelerates neurologic recovery after 15-minute complete global cerebral ischemia in dogs. *Critical Care Medicine* November 1992;20(11):1588-1594.

35. Tenenhaus M, Hansbrough JF, Zapata-Sirvent R, et al. Treatment of burned mice with hyperbaric oxygen reduces mesenteric bacteria but not pulmonary neutrophil deposition. *Arch Surg* 1994; 129:1338-1342.

36. Thom SR. Functional inhibition of leukocyte B2 integrins by hyperbaric oxygen in carbon monoxide-mediated brain injury in rats. *Toxicology and Applied Pharmacology* 1993;123:248-256.

37. Thom SR, Mendiguren I, Fisher D. Smoke inhalation-induced alveolar lung injury is inhibited by hyperbaric oxygen. *Undersea Hyperb Med* 2001; 28:175-9.

38. Thom SR, Bhopale VM, Velazquez OC, et al. Stem cell mobilization by hyperbaric oxygen. *Am J Physiol Heart Circ Physiol* April 2006;290:H1378-H1386.

39. Thomas MP, Brown LA, Sponseller DR, et al. Myocardial infarct size reduction by the synergistic effect of hyperbaric oxygen and recombinant tissue plasminogen activator. *Am Heart J* 1990;120:791-800.

40. Villanueva E, Bennett MH, Wasiak J, et al. Hyperbaric oxygen therapy for thermal burns. *Cochrane Database Syst Rev* 2004; (3):CD004727.

41. Weaver LK, Hopkins RO, Chan KJ, et al. Hyperbaric oxygen for acute carbon monoxide poisoning. *N Engl J Med* 2002; 347:1057-67.

42. Xu N, Li Z, Luo X. Effects of hyperbaric oxygen therapy on the changes in serum sIL-2R and Fn in severe burn patients. Zhonghua Zheng Xing Shao Shang Wai Ke Za Zhi. 1999; 15(3):220-3.

43. Yamada T, Taguchi T, Hirata Y, et al. The protective effect of hyperbaric oxygenation on the small intestine in ischemia-reperfusion injury. *J Pediatr Surg* 1995;30:786-90.

44. Yogaratnam JZ, Laden G, Madden LA, et al. Hyperbaric oxygen: a new drug in myocardial revascularization and protection? *Cardiovascular Revascularization Medicine* 7 (2006):146-154.

45. Zamboni WA, Roth AC, Russell RC, et al. Morphological analysis of the microcirculation during reperfusion of ischemic skeletal muscle and the effect of hyperbaric oxygen. *Plast Reconstr Surg* 1993; 91:1110-1123.

REVIEW QUESTIONS

1.) Edema is not only present in directly burned tissues, but can be found in distant:
    a. muscle
    b. intestine
    c. lung
    d. all the above

2.) The two most important predictors of clinical outcome in burn injury are:
    a. Total body surface area (TBSA), depth of burn
    b. Patient age, TBSA
    c. Patient medical co-morbidities, depth of burn
    d. Time to arrival at burn unit, depth of burn

3.) The combination of a body burn and inhalation injury compared to only a body burn without inhalation injury results in:
    a. increased mortality and morbidity
    b. a 10% increase in fluid requirements
    c. a significant increase in burn wound edema
    d. A and C only

4.) Partial thickness burns
    a. appear waxy white
    b. are painful
    c. involve only the epidermis
    d. never convert to full thickness injury

5.) Mechanisms of benefit of HBO2 in burn injuries include:
    a. Decreased edema
    b. Preservation of the microcirculation
    c. Reduction in ischemia-reperfusion injury
    d. All the above

Answers: 1d, 2a, 3d, 4b, 5d

CHAPTER **20**

PROBLEM WOUNDS: THE IMPACT OF RADIATION THERAPY AND CHEMOTHERAPY

CHAPTER TWENTY OVERVIEW

NOTES

Problem Wounds: The Impact of Radiation Therapy and Chemotherapy

John J. Feldmeier, Michael J. Crotty, Shelley P. Godley

INTRODUCTION

Approximately, 1.2 million new cases of invasive cancers (not including basal and squamous skin cancers) are diagnosed annually in the United States (1). There are nearly 9 million cancer survivors alive today in America (2). About one half of all cancer patients will receive radiation therapy as treatment for their cancer. In some instances radiation is delivered as the sole modality of therapy. More and more frequently, with current treatment regimens, radiation is combined with surgery, chemotherapy or both as a component of a multi-modality approach to therapy. Chemotherapy is delivered to patients more and more frequently concurrently with radiation for both its own inherent anti-tumoral effect and its radiosensitization properties. The combined therapy is likely to enhance damaging effects in normal tissues as well as the tumor which is being targeted.

The radiation doses which are likely to eradicate gross or microscopic residual tumor for virtually all tumor histologies are well studied and established. Likewise, the tolerance of normal tissues that may be anatomically close to or even inseparable from the tumor is also well studied. Considerable individual idiosyncratic differences exist in tolerance to radiation doses and these sensitivities are distributed in a normal distribution. Certain genetic syndromes, most notably Ataxia Telangectasia, significantly enhance the likelihood of severe reactions and complications. Unfortunately, as yet there are no practical clinical tests available to predict which patients are especially at risk for radiation complications. Unlike chemotherapy or immunologic therapies, radiation therapy is a local-regional therapy. Both positive therapeutic effects and side effects will occur only within the treated radiation portals. The constant goal of the radiation oncologist is to irradiate adequately the entire target (which often includes the tumor plus any nearby sites of potential microscopic spread such as regional lymph nodes) and at the same time avoid overdosage of critical nearby normal tissues. This is frequently a difficult task. New imaging modalities that show tissue metabolic activity such as PET scanning can be combined with anatomically based imaging modalities such as CT or MRI to define the target. These imaging techniques are then combined with targeted radiation delivery techniques with tight anatomic margins of the radiation fields surrounding the defined target. New targeted therapy techniques are termed conformal radiation and intensity modulated radiation therapy. The most targeted radiation treatment is termed "stereotactic radiosurgery" which is most often used in the treatment of brain tumors. In order to achieve accuracies on the order of 1mm, a rigid head frame is fixed to the patient's calvarium establishing a 3D coordinate system. To guarantee the precise delivery of dose, this head frame is in turn itself fixed to a mounting bracket on the planning and treatment couches. All of these technologies will typically employ multiple intersecting shaped fields with tissue compensating filters and edge defining blocking. In this fashion, the target receives the full radiation dose, and adequate sparing of critical surrounding organs is achieved. The design of such radiation therapy plans requires the availability of image based systems that allow the 3D definition of both the target and sensitive anatomic structures coupled to powerful computers with calculation algorithms which generate treatment plans in an iterative fashion until the best combination of shaped and modulated fields is obtained. Frequently the accomplishment of these iterative calculations requires considerable dedicated computer time utilizing powerful modern computers.

A large variation of sensitivities for individual tumors has been observed. As previously mentioned, an idiosyncratic tolerance to radiation in terms of toxicities for individual patients is also seen. Tolerance varies widely from organ system to organ system and from patient to patient. Tolerance is dependent on several factors. The most obvious is total dose. It is very important also to consider the dose given per radiation treatment (dose per

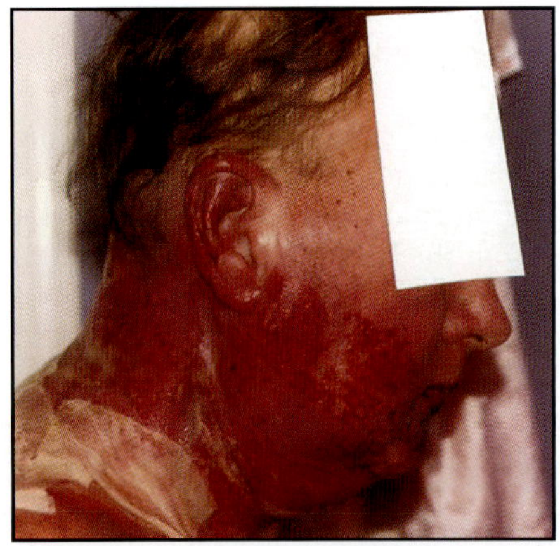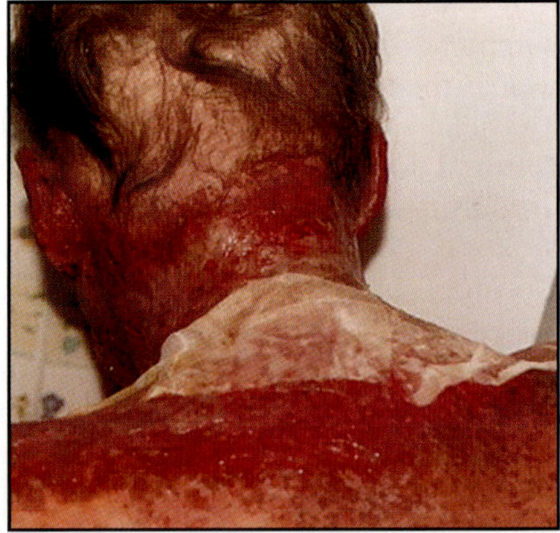

Figure 1A and 1B: Two views of this patient demonstrate an unusually severe skin reaction/ wound during radiation for a locally advanced head and neck cancer. This patient's reaction was so severe that his treatment was stopped at about 2/3's of the originally planned radiation dose. Fortunately, to date (about 2 years after treatment) the patient has no evidence of recurrence. No specific genetic or life style risks were identified as risk factors for this severe reaction.

fraction), the number of doses per day or week, and the volume or volume percentage of an individual organ that is included in the radiation treatment portals (3,4). Areas where skin contacts skin during treatment often show worse skin reactions.

Roentgen first discovered x-rays in 1895 and before the end of the 19th Century patients were receiving radiation therapy for cancers. Initially a wide variety of non-malignant pathologic entities were also treated though few non-malignant entities are treated now. Early observers found that cancer treatment was most successful and normal tissue reactions least severe when treatments were divided (or fractionated, as is said in the radiation oncology

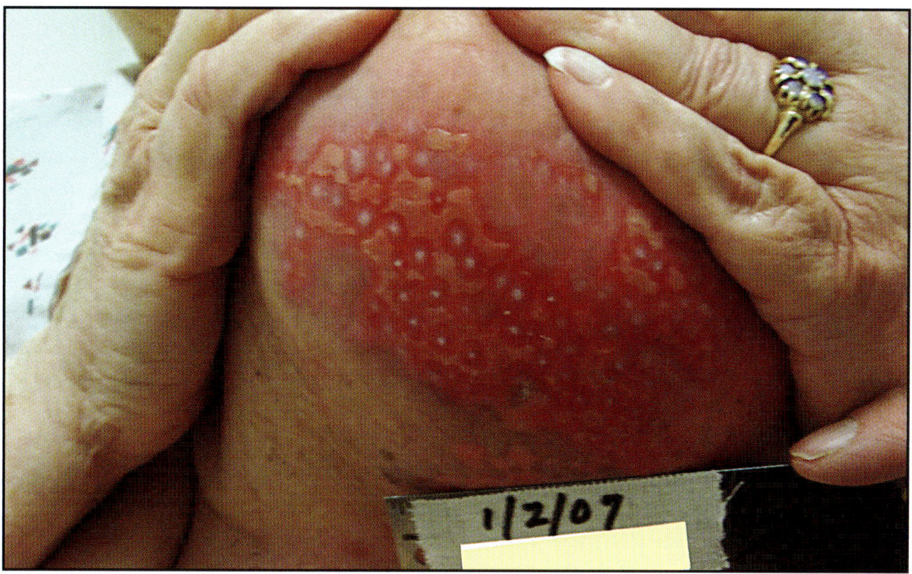

Figure 2. The photograph of this patient demonstrates a common location for marked skin reaction in patients treated for breast cancer. In the inframammary crease, this is skin against skin which increases the radiation dose and creates a moist area where perspiration collects. Careful examination of the photo demonstrates islands of epithelium seen as white "dots." Unlike other wounds where epithelial coverage must come across the wound from the wound edges, some epithelial cells survive radiation in the center of the wound and can proliferate in all directions leading to rapid wound coverage with epithelium.

community) over many daily treatments. Ever since it was introduced by the empiric methods of Coutard in France and others in the 1920's, the standard radiation therapy regimen for external radiation therapy is one treatment per day, five days per week at a daily dose of 180–200 cGy (centiGray) per day. Typical treatments for carcinomas require doses of 5,000–7,500 cGy over 5–8 weeks. The required dose depends to a large extent on whether the radiation is the sole local modality or whether radiation is to be combined with surgery. For other more radiosensitive malignant tumors such as lymphomas or germ cell tumors, radiation doses are reduced to the range of 2500–5000 cGy. For sarcomas doses required are on the order of 6000–7000 cGy. Because of normal tissue tolerance, total doses will rarely exceed 7000 cGy except in brachytherapy or implant radiation therapy treatments.

Brachytherapy or implant radiation consists of placing radioactive sources next to or within tumor masses. A common application for brachytherapy is gynecologic cancers where radioactive materials are placed through the vagina and sometimes into the uterus to treat cervical, endometrial or vaginal cancer. In these cases the sources are left only temporarily. An increasingly common treatment for prostate cancer is the implantation of Iodine-125 seeds. These seeds are left permanently. Usually 80–100 seeds will be implanted with transrectal ultrasound guidance. In brachytherapy applications doses often exceed the 7000 cGy referenced above for external beam treatments. However these doses are delivered to a very small volume and in the case of permanent iodine implants, they are delivered by the slow radioactive decay of a radioisotope which requires a full year to deliver the prescribed dose of 14,000–16,000 cGy.

Wounding within a radiated field can occur under several different circumstances. A patient may have radiation in a preoperative planned fashion as part of the initial approach to treatment of his or her cancer. A patient may have radiation following surgery, and the incompletely healed surgical wound may be included within the radiation field. A patient may undergo salvage or palliative surgery within an irradiated field if a recurrence occurs within those tissues previously irradiated. Many years following radiation the patient may require surgery within the irradiated field for either benign or oncologic indications which may or may not be related to his or her original cancer. Occasionally, spontaneous radiation necrosis (without precipitating surgery) occurs within the radiation field and a wound may result from this injury. To some extent, each of these circumstances presents a somewhat different challenge. In each case, however, wound healing is hampered and complications are higher as a result of the previous radiation exposure. The root cause of complications in any of these cases is usually an insult to both vascular and constitutive elements of the radiated tissues.

WOUND HEALING: A BRIEF REVIEW

The mechanisms of and biochemical reactions necessary to support wound healing are discussed in this text in other chapters and in many comprehensive discussions elsewhere (5,6). Briefly, the phases of wound healing will be discussed and delineated here since radiation before or after wounding can impact on the process during any stage of wound healing. What we know about the physiology of wound healing is based for the most part on the study of approximated surgical wounds. Three stages of wound healing have been recognized and described in the approximated surgical wound (7). In a chronic wound, including those which may develop within an irradiated field which heals by secondary intention or requires surgical debridement, grafts and or flaps, these stages are not as discrete as in the model of a surgically approximated wound and may overlap or even repeat themselves as surgical or other therapeutic intervention occurs. Though not always applicable to chronic wounds in terms of time and progression, this model of wound healing is useful in elucidating mechanisms and barriers to wound healing. The following three stages of healing have been described: 1) The Inflammatory Phase, 2) The Proliferative Phase, and 3) The Maturation or Remodeling Phase.

I. The Inflammatory Phase

In an approximated surgical wound, the first three or four days following wounding is dominated by an inflammatory response. During this time, hemostasis is established and formation of a matrix to which fibroblasts and monocytes are attracted is established. The fibrin clot gives the wound what integrity it has at this point and the wound typically has only five percent strength of a fully healed wound (7). For acute wounds including surgical wounds, this time period has been reported to be the most sensitive to inhibition by radiation or chemotherapy (8). Platelets, macrophages and granulocytes play major roles during this phase. Many cytokines are released from these cells and from other sources. Platelet derived growth factor (PDGF), transforming growth factor-beta and basic fibroblast growth factor are active in promoting mitogenesis and angiogenesis (5,7). Vascular dilation occurs which permits cellular and growth factor migration (7,9). Local fibroblasts increase in number and epithelialization begins with basal cell migration over the dermis (10). In the inflammatory phase macrophages play a vital role providing enzymes to remodel the extracellular matrix to prepare for continued remodeling (11).

II. The Proliferative Phase

The second identifiable stage in wound healing is the proliferative phase, which dominates for the next three weeks. During this phase there is an accelerated production of collagen enhanced by the presence of PDGF and TGF-beta (12). Fibroblasts migrate to the wound and proliferate under the influence of several cytokines. These actions are regulated by macrophage released bFGF (12,13) and further modulated by TGF-beta which also stimulates tissue inhibitors of metalloproteinases (TIMP) which are necessary to dissolve and allow remodeling of the wound matrix (14,15). Oxygen is a necessary substrate for healing during this phase since it is required for hydroxylation of proline and lysine and release of collagen from proliferating fibroblasts. Myofibroblasts appear during this phase, and their function is to provide wound contraction. In doing so, they reduce the size of the void into which proliferating cells must move and establish the collagen matrix of a healed wound. Basal keratinocytes migrate from the wound edge to accomplish epithelial coverage of the wound.

Collagen production peaks at about day seven after wounding but then continues at peak rate for about four weeks after wounding. Angiogenesis is stimulated by activated macrophages, which release many growth factors including vascular endothelial growth factor (VEGF) (5). Tissue hypoxia stimulates angiogenesis directly and through the production of lactic acid. By the end of the proliferative phase the wound has achieved about 30% of normal tissue strength (7).

III. Maturation Phase

The maturation or remodeling phase lasts for about the next two years. During this time collagen matures, and more crosslinkage occurs providing enhanced tensile strength to the wound. During the maturation phase there is a decrease in fibroblasts and macrophages in the wound. Collagen content progressively increases, as does the bursting strength of the wound (5). At the end of the maturation phase, the wound has achieved about 80% of the strength of surrounding normal tissues (7).

Some authors describe wound healing in four stages where the initiating stage is hemostasis, or the arrest of the loss of blood, see the chapter by Chin et al. entitled, "Biochemistry of Wound Healing in Wound Care Practice."

THE BROAD EFFECTS OF RADIATION ON WOUND HEALING

There is a general consensus that radiation inhibits wound healing by impairing vascularization and by directly depleting a number cell lines (fibroblasts, vascular endothelial cells and squamous cells) required for the healing process. Within the radiation oncology and surgical communities there is some controversy as to which of these two factors is dominant. Recently several investigators have demonstrated the prolonged effects of radiation on fibroblast numbers and function and the importance of these effects in impairing wound healing in radiated tissues (16). If we look at each of the above phases of wound healing, radiation can impact the progression of wound healing by specific mechanisms peculiar to that phase of wound healing. In addition to looking at each of these described phases of wound healing, it must be noted that the impact of radiation on wound healing is for the most part a permanent and probably progressive effect over time. Surgical wounding of irradiated tissues sometime after the completion of that irradiation for incidental reasons or for salvage of recurrent tumor presents a special problem. In this setting the vascular damage characterized by endarteritis, which progresses to a plateau within the first six to twelve months after irradiation, is well established, and the hypoxia that results from the resultant tissue ischemia presents significant difficulties in regard to wound closure. There continues to be some controversy within the radiation oncology community as to whether there is any recovery of the cellularity and vascularity of irradiated tissues with time. Most investigators who have studied these effects believe that there is no significant recovery of irradiated tissues with time and that indeed these effects are progressive with time. After the first 12–24 months, these changes probably progress at a much slower rate than they do initially. Further progression of these deleterious effects of radiation is consistent with the occasional occurrence of spontaneous tissue necrosis seen many years after radiation not associated with any identifiable precipitating insult. As the patient ages there are likely to be more intercurrent contributions to vascular injury including arteriosclerotic changes from hyperlipidemia.

Anscher and his co-investigators (17) in a review article have summarized and further clarified the cascade of events which follow therapeutic radiation and contribute to difficulties in wound healing. These authors explain that reactive oxygen species (ROS) initially affect the biologic damage to both benign and malignant cells. The immediate biochemical events trigger those injuries which we recognize both clinically and histologically through the release of proinflammatory cytokines, chemokines and profibrotic cytokines. Their "new paradigm" for delayed radiation tissue injury is that the initial

DNA damage carried out by ROS is followed by increased cellular permeability which results in edema and an accumulation of fibrin in the extracellular matrix. An inflammatory response follows with an accumulation and activation of macrophages. Macrophages release a broad range of cytokines. Hypoxia results from increased metabolic demand of the attracted macrophages and vascular damage caused by fibrosis. Hypoxia leads to additional ROS production with more tissue damage and fibrosis. TGF beta plays a major role in tissue fibrosis and in turn stimulates VEGF. Endothelial cells which have been damaged by the radiation are not able to respond normally to the VEGF produced, and they die as a result of prior damage and the stress of new stimuli for proliferation from VEGF. Hypoxia is therefore felt to perpetuate radiation induced tissue damage and interfere with healing. ROS continue to be generated along with tissue damaging cytokines. An evolving understanding of these mechanisms will potentially permit strategies for interrupting this continuum of events. Furthermore, the increasing elucidation of mechanisms may also explain the efficacy of hyperbaric oxygen including the production of free radical scavengers and the production of growth factors which can lead to the repair of radiation insulted tissues.

PRE-CLINICAL MODELS OF WOUND HEALING AND RADIATION

As already discussed, the first three days or so after wounding are dominated by an inflammatory response. If radiation occurs before or within this phase of wound healing, a depletion of those cells responsible for the inflammatory response, especially neutrophils and macrophages, is seen and wound healing is delayed. The decrease in these cells in large numbers within the wound environment in turn reduces the growth factors released by these cells which are so important in this first phase of wound healing.

In a clinical setting, external radiation is essentially never given during this time period. Clinicians are well aware of the risks of initiating radiation too close in time to surgery. There is experimental animal data that demonstrates the impact that radiation would have if given at this time. Also, there are instances in which brachytherapy or implant radiation sources are placed at the time of surgery. Initiation of the brachytherapy treatment immediately following surgery has been shown by some authors to be associated with a higher incidence of wound complications. This experience will be discussed in more detail later in this chapter.

Gu and associates have developed an animal model designed to investigate the effects of radiation during the inflammatory phase of wound healing (18). In a rat model they created consistent wounds of identical depth, width and length in the dorsal skin of study animals. One half of the animals served as controls. The other half of the animals were then immediately irradiated to a single dose of 15 Gy to a volume which included the wounded area with a 0.5 cm margin. The authors do not tell us whether this was the skin dose or the maximum dose within the radiation field (the so called given dose), Radiation with Cobalt 60 does provide some skin sparing with the surface dose typically about 80% of the given dose. These authors applied a number of analytic measures to the subsequent healing process. These included gross and microscopic morphometry, immunohistochemical assay of type III collagen, in situ hybridization assay of type I collagen and WBC and platelet measures.

These researchers found that both circulating white blood cell counts and platelets were decreased in irradiated animals but recovered by 12 days post irradiation. They reported reduced levels of both type I and III collagen in the wounds of irradiated animals on day 7 post wounding. By day 14, the levels of collagen increased in the irradiated animals to levels in excess of the non-irradiated controls.

In this model, gross examination of the wounds showed evidence of infection in 8 of 12 irradiated wounds at day seven and no sign of infection in the unirradiated controls. Microscopic examination of wounds showed decreased infiltration by neutrophils and macrophages and decreased granulation tissue in irradiated wounds versus control wounds at three days. At day 7, the radiated wounds showed much less and a thinner layer of granulation tissue. At day seven and again on day 14 after radiation, the irradiated wounds contained "radiation" fibroblasts and fibrocytes which lacked the activity and collagen production of normal fibroblasts.

Wang and colleagues have accomplished a study in rat skin employing both light and electron microscopy to determine the impact of radiation on the healing process (19). Electron irradiation was delivered to the animals' dorsal skin seven days prior to wounding. Radiation dose consisted of 9.6 Gy. Wounds were standardized, full thickness, incisional wounds. Animals were euthanized at various intervals after wounding (1, 3, 7 and 14 days). Examination showed depression of inflammatory cell and tissue exudate response in irradiated specimens compared to control. Investigators also observed a slowing of epithelial migration and decreased numbers of fibroblasts in the irradiated specimens. Granulation tissue was decreased up to the 7 day observation point in the radiated animals but had essentially recovered by day 14. The authors conclude that the healing process was delayed but not prevented in their model.

Bernstein and his co-workers have reported a study wherein guinea pigs were employed to study the effects of radiation on wound healing (20). Animals received 18 Gy orthovoltage irradiation to a skin flap which was isolated and extruded through a slit in a lead shielding box. In this model circular wounds of identical size were created in the dorsal skin of study animals utilizing a 6 mm skin biopsy punch two days after irradiation. A total of six such wounds were created in each animal. Half of these wounds were created in the irradiated tissues and one half in the contralateral unirradiated skin. These paired wounds were compared at 5, 7, 10 and 14 days after wounding. At 10 and 14 days the wounds within the irradiated area were larger in a statistically significant fashion as compared to the other side.

Another pre-clinical study by Yanase and colleagues demonstrates impairment in wound contraction as a result of radiation (21). This study examines the effects of radiation on fibroblast proliferation and function and therefore relates more specifically to the proliferative phase of wound healing. In this cell culture model, human oral mucosal fibroblasts were harvested, initially grown in cell culture and then subjected immediately to escalated single doses of radiation beginning at 2 Gy and increasing to 10 Gy. Some cells were then trypsinized and placed in a 3D collagen gel media. The diameters of this collagen gel media were measured at various times over 10 days for both irradiated and non-irradiated cells. No differences in contraction of the gels as determined by their average diameters were seen initially. However, at two weeks after irradiation the contraction of the gels wherein the irradiated cells had been cultured showed significantly less contraction in a dose dependent fashion. Gel diameters for unirradiated cells were only about 50% of those irradiated to doses of 6 Gy or greater. By eight weeks after irradiation there was some recovery with only about a 20% difference from irradiated to unirradiated controls.

This group also examined fibroblasts morphologically by staining for actin filaments. Again there was no significant difference between irradiated and control cells initially. However, at two weeks after radiation, the irradiated cells had an obvious decrease in actin filaments in a dose-related fashion. Cells irradiated to 6 Gy had very few identifiable actin filaments. By eight weeks after irradiation, the irradiated cells again showed a recovery with a considerable increase in actin filaments visible at that time.

The authors conclude that their model demonstrates a temporary but noteworthy inhibition of myofibroblasts in their ability to initiate wound contraction as a result of radiation and that the level of inhibition is radiation dose-dependent.

Aricini and associates have studied the effects of radiation on vascular microanastomoses in a rat model (22). One group of animals served as the control and had no radiation. One group had radiation two weeks before surgery; one group had radiation immediately followed by surgery. In a final study group, animals had surgery and then underwent radiation two weeks later. Study animals received a single dose of 20 Gy to groin fields including the femoral artery. All animals had identical surgery consisting of microvascular anastomoses of the femoral artery. One month after surgery, all animals were examined under anesthesia and the anastomotic site was removed for light and electron microscopy. No significant differences were detected in the patency of the anastomosis among groups. We do know of course that vascular changes typically require a latent period in patients of at least six months to become obvious. This model which shows no changes due to radiation may have failed to detect potential changes by not waiting an adequate time to elapse before animal euthanasia and microscopic examination of the femoral artery.

In another study, Doyle and co-workers (23) made use of a rat model employing polytetrafluroethylene (PTFE) sheet implants to investigate the effects of radiation on angiogenesis. Rats had either two or three fractions of irradiation at 24 hour intervals. Each radiation exposure consisted of 3 Gy. Animals receiving only two radiation exposures had no decrease in neovascularity in the PTFE sheets compared to unirradiated controls, while those animals that received three radiation exposures (9 Gy) did show a statistically significant decrease in neoangiogenesis compared to control.

In the above pre-clinical studies, researchers have concentrated on the effects of radiation on skin and subcutaneous tissues. The impact of radiation on other tissues and organs is of course very important and in most cases probably more important to the patient's survival and quality of life than is the skin. Several investigators have studied the impact of radiation on colonic anastomoses in irradiated animals.

Kuzu and associates (24) in 1998 reported a rat study wherein unirradiated controls were compared to animals who received 22 Gy of irradiation (4 fractions of 5.5 Gy) to their whole pelvis. All animals had left colon resection with primary anastomosis. The surgery followed the radiation by four days. Animals were assessed at three and seven days after surgery. No differences were seen between irradiated and control groups in adhesions or anastomotic failure. Strength of the anastomoses was determined by checking burst strength. Burst strength was reduced in irradiated animals at both three and seven days in a statistically significant way. In a similar study accomplished by the same group, the effects of 5-flurouracil chemotherapy combined with irradiation were investigated. This study likewise showed detrimental effects on healing in the left colonic anastomosis as demonstrated on histopathologic examination. However, even with combined chemotherapy and irradiation, there were no increased failures of the physical integrity of the anastomosis *in vivo*. Ceelen and co-workers (25) have studied the impact of radiation on colonic anastomosis as well. This also was a rat study. The difference in this study is that only one limb of the colonic anastomosis was irradiated. The other limb was shielded. Radiation consisted of standard daily doses of 2 Gy with total doses of 40, 60 or 80 Gy. An unirradiated control group was also studied. The anastomosis was accomplished the day after radiation and animals were euthanized ten days after radiation. These authors found no difference in peritonitis, anastomotic complications, burst strength of the anastomosis or hydroxyproline content. Irradiated animals did have lower weights than control animals. The authors conclude that irradiation does not affect anastomotic healing when one limb of the anastomosis is not irradiated.

Taken on the whole, these pre-clinical animal and cell culture studies help to elucidate the effects of radiation on wound healing. They consistently show diminishment of the typical initial inflammatory response by radiation and a delay in wound healing. These studies are somewhat limited in their value due to their design. Most involve radiation just before surgical wounding and do not mimic a clinical course where surgery is not accomplished for at least two and usually four weeks after radiation. Radiation dose fractionation is also often non-standard with many studies employing one large fraction. Nor are they appropriate models for surgery occurring before irradiation when there are still open wounds. Finally, they do not reflect the circumstance of surgery in an irradiated field many months or even years after radiation has been completed.

CLINICAL EXPERIENCE: RISKS AND PREDISPOSING FACTORS

The classic radiation pathology text book of Rubin and Casarett (3) published in 1968 continues to be a primary source for understanding of radiation injury to and tolerance of normal tissues. Emami and his colleagues (4) have updated certain information regarding the likelihood of radiation injury to normal tissues based on several factors. Identifiable factors include total radiation dose, dose per individual radiation treatments, number of treatments per week and volume of tissue or percentage of an individual organ included in the high dose region. A normal distribution of individual patient sensitivities to radiation injury is recognized. Certain organ systems are more susceptible to injury at lower doses than other organ systems. Some patients are unusually resistant to radiation injury while some are unusually sensitive. Intercurrent diseases such as diabetes or collagen vascular disease have been shown to increase the possibility of serious radiation complications (26). For example the presence of lupus erythematosis has been considered by some in the radiation oncology community to present an absolute contraindication for radiation following lumpectomy in early breast cancers (27). This author has himself attended a patient with a collagen vascular disorder who was treated with radiation for cervical cancer and cured of this disease who also rapidly succumbed to severe radiation complications including radiation enteritis, cystitis and proctitis. A similar case report of a radiation induced death due to extreme sensitivity to injury in a patient with lupus has been published (28).

The severity of acute skin injury in patients receiving radiation for breast cancer has been reviewed by Porock and her colleagues (29). This paper reports that injury is more likely to be severe in patients who smoke, patients with large breasts, patients who experience a lymphocele post operatively, patients taking Tamoxifen and patients with a past history of skin cancer.

When developing a treatment plan for a patient in whom combined surgical resection and radiation is planned, the optimal sequencing of the two modalities must be determined. There are theoretic advantages for the radiation preceding the surgery. These advantages include the possibility of preventing micrometastases which might be shed into the circulation at the time of surgical manipulation. If those cancer cells which are potentially released into the circulation have been sterilized by the radiation before surgery, metastases can be prevented. Well oxygenated cells which have not had their circulation disrupted by surgery are more radiosensitive, and radiation induced cancer cell kill is more pronounced, at least theoretically, by pre-operative radiation. Finally, tumors which are initially unresectable can often be made resectable by preoperative radiation.

In the clinic, it is not uncommon to consider pre-operative radiation in sarcomas, early stage but bulky cervical cancers, head and neck cancers, (especially those fixed to major vessels), and rectal cancers (especially those fixed in the pelvis). In these circumstances, the radiation dose is typically moderated with pre-operative doses typically not exceeding 5,000 cGy. If there is not a clear cut advantage for pre-operative radiation in terms of tumor control, the more usual practice in the United States is for the surgery to precede radiation if both are to be combined in a planned fashion in the initial management of malignancy. Because of the problems in wound healing caused by radiation, most surgeons prefer to accomplish the surgery first and follow with adjunctive radiation after the surgical wound has healed for at least two weeks (30).

The special circumstance of brachytherapy (implant radiation) in conjunction with resection of sarcomas has been briefly mentioned already. At many institutions, it is standard therapy to insert brachytherapy catheters into the resection bed after the tumor has been removed. These catheters are sewn into the tumor bed and one end of the catheter externalized for access to afterloading radioactive sources. At some time after the surgery, radiation treatment is initiated by manually loading radioactive isotopes in strands or ribbons into the catheters. Usually the isotope is Iridium 192. These sources are left for several days and the patient is isolated in a shielded room to prevent exposure to other patients or health care workers. We call this procedure low dose rate brachytherapy. An increasingly popular alternative treatment is to accomplish the catheter placement in the same fashion and then bring the patient to the radiation department and connect his or her catheters to a high dose rate brachytherapy unit. This unit contains a single very intense radiation source. The source is connected to a cable and can be programmed to move through each catheter sequentially to deliver the desired dose of radiation. In this way, the equivalent of one day's treatment with low dose rate brachytherapy is accomplished in less than one hour. For multiple interstitial catheters the patient must still be an in-patient, but he or she can receive visitors and not present a radiation exposure risk to nursing staff, other health care personnel and visitors. Again as discussed previously, this brachytherapy treatment is about the only time during which radiation might be delivered during the critical initiation of the inflammatory phase of wound healing. Several investigators have found that any problems associated with delayed wound healing due to the inflammation suppressing effects of radiation can be significantly reduced by not loading the appliance until five days or more after the surgical resection and wound closure.

Most delayed radiation complications occur after a latent period of six months or more. Animal studies have shown that the endarteritis associated with tissue hypoxia identified as a major risk factor for these complications is not fully expressed until several months after completion of clinically relevant exposures to fractionated radiation. When these complications result in open wounds, or when it is necessary to operate within the radiation field, wounds may become chronic and fail to heal or even progress to erode into important structures such as the carotid artery in head and neck cancer. Such complications impair quality of life and can progress to become life threatening.

On occasion, recurrent tumor may be discovered after radiation, and surgical intervention for potential salvage of the recurrence is often indicated. In protocols where pre-operative radiation and surgery are planned, it is generally recommended that surgery be done no later than six weeks after radiation is complete. If more than six weeks pass, the likelihood of significant complications and wound healing difficulties increase due to the progression of vascular compromise and tissue hypoxia and probably further cellular loss of fibroblasts. Of course, if and when a recurrence is discovered, often more than six weeks time has elapsed since the radiation, and the risk of surgical complications is a secondary consideration compared to the possibility of salvaging the patient by potentially curative surgery.

STRATEGIES TO DEAL WITH RADIATION-CAUSED OR COMPLICATED WOUNDS

As always, it is better to prevent complications than to deal with them when they occur. Several general guidelines will reduce the likelihood of wound healing complications as a result of radiation.

When radiation is given before surgery in a planned fashion, preferably at least 3–4 weeks should elapse between radiation and surgery. Under these conditions radiation should not depress the initial inflammatory response which is so necessary to initiate the healing process (30). If surgical closure requires flap creation, it is better whenever possible to avoid including the flap vasculature within the radiation portals. With this technique, the all important blood supply to the flap is not going to be subject to delayed radiation changes, including vascular compromise, as a result of radiation induced end-arteritis. In similar fashion, if surgery will require bowel resection, complications can be minimized when one limb of the anastomosis has not been irradiated.

When radiation follows surgery, at least two weeks and no more than six weeks time should pass before therapeutic radiation is begun (30, 31). This time interval is chosen based on balancing the dual concerns of having the greatest impact on any residual cancer remaining post-operatively and at the same time avoiding an unacceptable level of complications. Ideally in terms of tumor control, radiation should begin as soon after surgery as possible because theoretically any residual malignant cells will have the opportunity to divide until they are sterilized by radiation. In point of fact, it appears that there is no worsening of tumor control when radiation is given in the post-operative adjuvant setting as long as it is begun within six weeks of surgery (32). Occasionally, even at six weeks postoperatively the surgical wound is still open. A review of head and neck cancer patients treated at the University of Florida has shown that even when radiation is initiated before wound healing most of these wounds (67%) healed without surgical intervention while another 15% were successfully closed with additional surgery. The remaining patients died before healing was achieved or were lost to follow-up before the wounds had healed (31).

Sometime after completion of radiation and after enough time has elapsed for endarteritis and tissue fibrosis to occur, wounds may be encountered within the irradiated tissues either as the result of surgery through the radiated tissues or as a spontaneous delayed necrosis. In both cases, early intervention is indicated to prevent progression and enlargement of this difficult wound.

It may be necessary to operate through the region of heavily irradiated tissues for attempted surgical salvage of a recurrent tumor, for intervention designed to deal with radiation-induced injury or for a medical indication unrelated to the original malignancy. An example of the first of these circumstances includes a recurrent larynx cancer, previously radiated primarily, in which a potentially curative laryngectomy can be accomplished. For the second circumstance, we would include resection of radiation damaged small bowel some time after successful treatment of a rectal cancer.

The final situation would include a patient who developed bladder cancer after primary and successful radiation of a prostate cancer and who requires cystectomy.

Under all of these circumstances, several surgical principles have been recommended to avoid or minimize post-operative complications. Fascia and underlying muscle should be left attached to skin and subcutaneous tissues whenever possible. All potential dead space should be filled. Wounds should be closed without tension and drained. If a seroma or hematoma develops, it should be evacuated. Sutures should be left in place longer (some recommend up to 1 month). It has also been recommended that patients with lower extremity wounds maintain bedrest for an extra few days (7). In her review Tibbs recommends that when a complication occurs within two weeks of surgical wounding, the patients should be promptly returned to the operating room for intervention to include debridement or flap rotation or both (7). She also notes that if healing proceeds without complication during the first three to four weeks, the patient will most likely go on to heal without subsequent difficulties.

Hyperbaric oxygen has been employed in a pre-operative, post-operative or combined pre- and post operative fashion when surgical wounding has been planned within the radiated tissues. Hyperbaric oxygen is given with the intention of preventing wound complications. Marx was the first to propose this approach (33). He has shown success in reducing subsequent mandibular necrosis following dental extractions in a randomized controlled study which emphasized the importance of pre-operative hyperbaric oxygen consisting of 20 treatments at 2.4 atmospheres absolute pressure for 90 minutes of 100% oxygen. Following dental extractions, the patients completed an additional

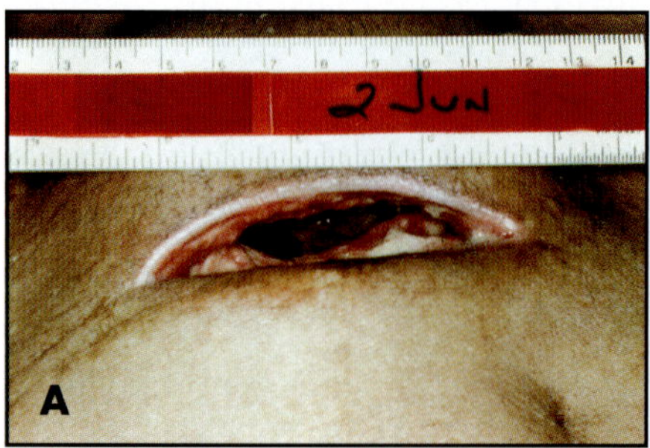

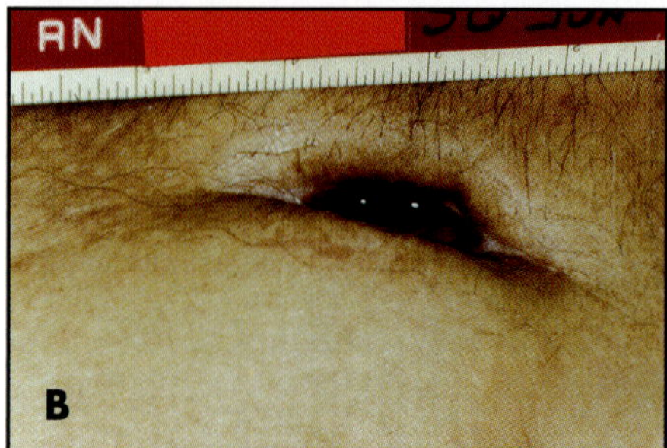

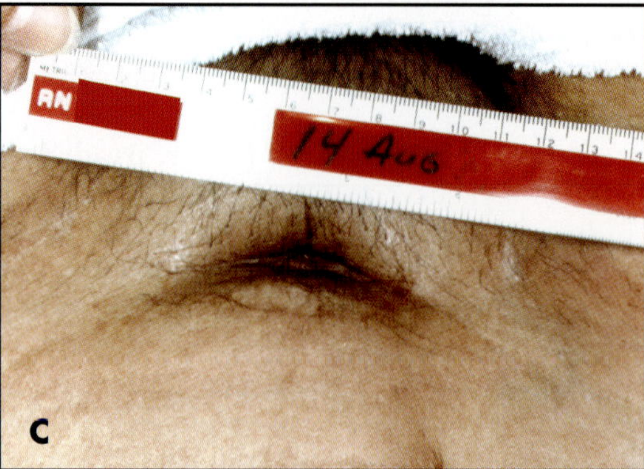

Figure 3 A-C. These figures demonstrate the response of a patient with radiation necrosis of the soft tissue overlying the bladder with a fistulous communication to the bladder itself. After ten weeks of daily hyperbaric oxygen treatments, the fistula has resolved and the wound is essentially closed. In this case of soft tissue radiation necrosis, surgery was not required to close the wound.

ten hyperbaric treatments. The treatment group which received hyperbaric oxygen had only a 5.4% incidence of mandibular necrosis while the control group experienced 29.9% likelihood of osteoradionecrosis. In an animal model, Marx has also shown that hyperbaric oxygen directly addresses one of the primary sources of delayed complications in irradiated wounds. In this model, Marx has shown that hyperbaric treatments enhance the vascularity of irradiated tissues (34). In an indirect fashion, he has also shown improvement in vascularity and subsequent oxygen supply by conducting serial transcutaneous oxygen measurements in irradiated patients receiving hyperbaric oxygen for their mandibular osteoradionecrosis (35).

Both Marx and Grandstrom have reported the benefit in supporting dental implants in radiated tissues with significant improvement in osseous integration of the dental implant and prevention of osteoradionecrosis in patients receiving hyperbaric oxygen (36, 37). In fact many clinicians will not attempt dental implants in heavily irradiated jaws due to the exceptionally high likelihood of failure and the possibility of precipitating osteoradionecrosis. These treatment protocols emphasize the importance of pre-surgical delivery of hyperbaric oxygen.

Feldmeier and associates have reported a similar successful experience in treating 32 patients with hyperbaric oxygen immediately postoperatively following resection of recurrent cancer within an irradiated field (38). In this group of patients a short course (10–15 treatments) of hyperbaric oxygen led to prompt healing in 87.5% of patients and no serious wound complications in any patient compared to published complication rates of 60% in patients not receiving hyperbaric oxygen. Historically, death due to carotid artery blowout is not an uncommon complication in patients receiving surgery for salvage of head and neck cancers after radiation.

When dealing with established open wounds complicated by radiation necrosis, surgical guidance is similar to the principles applied in the discussion above in preventing wound complications. The surgical literature emphasizes the importance of debriding all necrotic tissues. Marx and Feldmeier have reported the necessity of surgically eradicating necrotic bone in order to achieve healing (39, 40). In order to close these wounds, flaps (usually an axial flap based on a sizable artery) are utilized. Ideally, these should have their blood supply originate outside the radiation field. Rudolph (41) has reported a 100% failure rate when simple skin grafts have been applied to radionecrotic wounds. In the same paper he reported a 43% likelihood of complications in myocutaneous flaps employed to close radiation induced skin ulcers. Since this paper was published, many improvements have been made in flap design. Axial flaps based on at least a medium sized (and usually named) artery are preferred to random flaps in the reconstruction of radiated tissues. Arnold and his colleagues have reported their experience in employing myocutaneous flaps in the reconstruction of 100 radiation-related wounds (42). Roughly, one half of the flaps had had their blood supply irradiated and remainder were supported by unirradiated blood supply. The complication rate when the vasculature had been irradiated was 32% with complete loss of muscle in 14%. Complications in the group where flaps had their blood supply outside of the radiation field were 19% with none of these flaps completely lost. Free flaps have also been used to close defects in irradiated wounds with good success

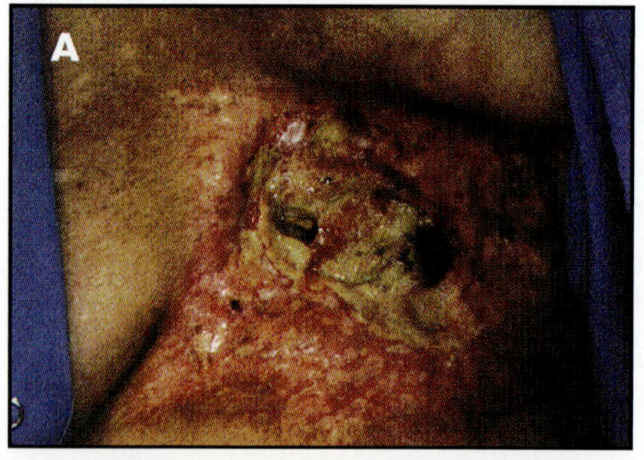
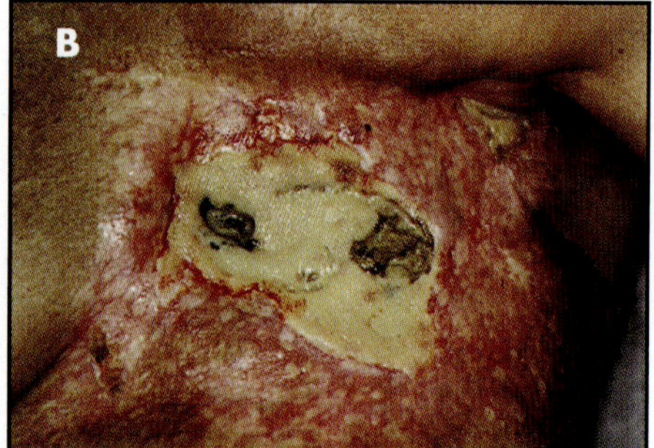
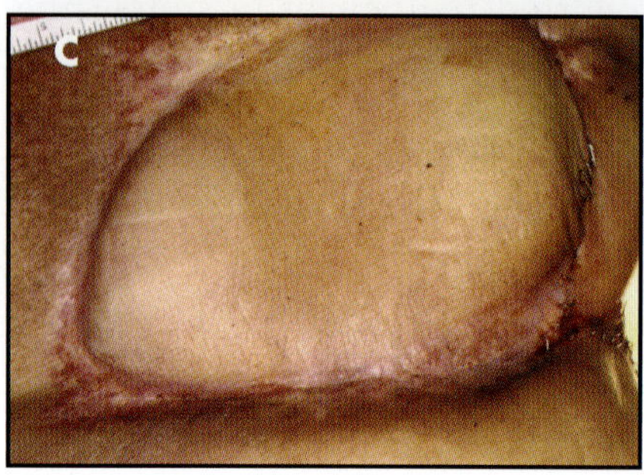

Figure 4 A-C. These figures demonstrate several principles involved in treating wounds due to radiation necrosis. This post-mastectomy, post-radiation patient received preoperative hyperbaric oxygen with the intent of providing improvement in tissues prior to surgical debridement and closure with an axial flap whose blood suppply originated outside of the radiation field. To insure resolution of the bony necrosis, the surgeon also debrided the necrotic bones.

reported. Teknos and his co-workers (43) have reported the results in using radial forearm free flaps in the reconstruction of the hypopharynx of patients undergoing surgical salvage after radiation. In this report 20% of patients (2/10) experienced post-operative wound complications.

An extensive body of literature now exists reporting the success in applying hyperbaric oxygen to tissues exhibiting radiation injury. In most cases these injuries also include a chronic open wound. Feldmeier and Hampson have recently conducted a review of 74 published reports dealing with this issue from an evidence based approach (44). This review includes discussions of wounds in the head and neck, chest wall, extremities and abdomen and pelvis. Results here are consistently positive with a successful resolution rate typically in the 65–85% range. One of the most impressive reports is that of Marx wherein he discusses the application of hyperbaric oxygen combining pre- and post-operative hyperbaric oxygen in a protocol identical to that already discussed above in regard to the prevention of mandibular necrosis (45). In this publication, Marx reports the results in 160 patients in whom surgery was planned for repair of radiation necrosis or resection of recurrent tumor. This study was controlled but not randomized. Marx reports the incidence of complications in the hyperbaric group vs the control group in the following fashion: 1) wound infection: 6 vs 24%, 2) wound dehiscence: 11 vs. 48%, 3) delayed wound healing: 11 vs 55%.

Another very successful study is that by Neovius and associates (46). In this report, the authors tell us of the results in applying hyperbaric oxygen to 15 patients with soft tissue wounds after pre-operative radiation doses of 64 Gy preceding surgical resection for laryngeal or pharyngeal cancers. Post operatively, these patients showed no evidence of healing and began hyperbaric oxygen. Typically, they were treated at pressures of 2.5 bar once daily. Treatments varied from 10–40 with most receiving 30 or more treatments.

Twelve of 15 healed completely and two improved. The authors contrasted these results with a historical control group who had not received hyperbaric oxygen. In this group only 7 of 15 healed without additional surgery. Two of these patients had severe postoperative hemorrhage, and in one of these, the patient died secondary to the hemorrhage.

In their review, Frank and colleagues extensively discuss wound dressing materials for the radiation associated wound (9). A full discussion of dressing materials is beyond the scope of this chapter and is discussed elsewhere in this text. This technology is rapidly developing. Frank does enumerate several characteristics that are desirable for dressings in an irradiated wound. It is recommended that wound dressing materials: 1) Optimize perfusion and oxygenation; 2) Optimize wound environment including pH and eradication of infection; 3) Retain serum to stimulate migration and adhesion of cellular constituents involved in healing; and 4) Protect the wound mechanically and reduce inflammation.

FUTURE POSSIBILITIES FOR INTERVENTION TO PREVENT OR TREAT RADIATION-ASSOCIATED WOUNDS

A number of pre-clinical studies have been conducted wherein the exogenous administration of growth factors or unirradiated fibroblasts have favorably impacted in healing in models of radiation associated wounds. Both Gorodetsky and colleagues (47) and Kruegler and co-workers (48) have shown in animal models that the injection of unirradiated syngenic fibroblasts directly into wounds enhances healing in these animals.

Platelet derived growth factor-BB (10) and transforming growth factor beta (13, 49) applied topically to irradiated wounds have been shown to promote healing in animal models. Anscher and colleagues (17) have discussed a number of potential therapeutic strategies including free radical scavengers, anticytokine antibodies, antichemokine antibodies and antiapoptotic agents.

Certainly, these promising results must be validated in clinical trials. Clinical trials are underway to investigate the effects of ACE inhibitors which block the renin-angiotensin system and where radiation protection has been demonstrated in pre-clinical models.

CHEMOTHERAPEUTIC EFFECTS ON WOUND HEALING

There are few papers discussing the effects of chemotherapy. Chemotherapeutic agents are systemic both in their therapeutic and toxic effects on wound healing. Traditional cytotoxic chemotherapy agents are generally divided into groups according to their mechanism of action. Group I agents are termed alkylators. Common or prototype alkylators are Cyclophosphamide and Nitrogen Mustard. Group II agents are called antimetabolites. Common examples are 5-Flurouracil and Capecitibine. Group III are termed antibiotics. This group includes Adriamycin and Bleomycin. There are a number of miscellaneous agents including Cis-platinum and the Taxanes (Taxol and Taxotere) which do not fit well in one of the three classes. Regardless of their mechanism of action, these agents work to impair DNA synthesis or function and in doing so inhibit the growth of neoplasms. These agents commonly cause myelosuppression and alopecia. Nausea and vomiting, much feared complications of chemotherapy, are now commonly controlled with new strategies including the use of a new class of serotonin antagonists, trade names Zofran and Kytril.

Recent developments in systemic cancer therapy have included the development of new agents. Many of these are agents designed to interfere with angiogenesis in the neoplasm. Judah Folkman (50) of Harvard has promoted the concept of anti-angiogenic therapy since the 1970's and has shown that ten cancer cells will be prevented for each vascular endothelial cell which is prevented.

Cytotoxic chemotherapeutic drugs preferentially impact the rapidly dividing cells of the body, and do not discriminate between malignant cells and the normal cells. The effects of chemotherapeutics are often determined by which cells internalize them. Initially, this ability is spread fairly evenly between malignant and normal cells. However, cancerous cells are more prone to mutations, and this genetic instability all too often leads to drug resistance. This resistance can be a result of down-regulating the mechanism of uptake or up-regulating the ability to pump out toxic material. As normal cells do not typically develop these avoidance strategies, normal cells may be disproportionately damaged by chemotherapy. Consequently, it is expected that these agents will interfere with the mechanics of wound healing by damaging the cells necessary for initiating and promoting healing. Many cell types are involved in wound healing, including mediators of the immune system. Although chemotherapy targets all rapidly dividing cells, mediators of the immune system are particularly sensitive.

White blood cells levels must be monitored during chemotherapeutic regimens to ensure levels do not fall to critical values (leucopenia), leaving the patient vulnerable to infection and other complications. Leucopenia may necessitate suspension or termination of therapy. Acute infection becomes more likely when absolute neutrophil counts fall below 1,000 per deciliter. Among the diverse cell types necessary for wound healing, macrophages and fibroblasts are prominent in their roles. Depletion of these cells leads to impaired wound healing.

PRE-CLINICAL STUDIES OF CHEMOTHERAPY AND WOUND HEALING

There are various pre-clinical studies demonstrating the negative impact of chemotherapy on wound healing. Salm et al. (51) examined the effects of the FAM regimen (5-fluorouracil, adriamycin and mitomycin C) on gastrointestinal anastomoses in a rat model. They found these drugs affected the initial stages of wound healing and that their use immediately before surgery promoted the evolution of problem wounds. However, once fibroblast proliferation and collagen synthesis had increased the mechanical strength of the wound, no negative effects on wound healing were induced by the FAM regimen. The authors conclude that the early inflammatory phase of wound healing is most vulnerable to inhibition by the administration of chemotherapy.

A more recent murine study by Asmis and colleagues (52) also supports the premise that macrophage dysfunction induced by chemotherapy contributes to wound healing delays. Adriamycin-treated mice demonstrated increased production of ROS and decreased production of cytokines (IL-1beta and TNF-alpha, among others), as well as a decreased overall number of macrophages. Adriamycin was given as eight injections over 38 days with the last dose ten days prior to production of an experimental wound. Compared to animals receiving saline injections as a control group, those animals receiving adriamycin experienced wound healing delays.

A third pre-clinical study examined the effects of chemotherapeutic agents post-operatively. Shirafuji and colleagues (53) studied two groups of rats which received chemotherapy three days or seven days after a bronchial anastomosis was performed. The authors detected a delay in wound healing which coincided with leukopenia and reduced macrophage infiltration. However, the suppression of wound healing appeared to be transient.

Occasionally, chemotherapeutic agents are administered after surgery for cancers of the GI tract or ovarian cancers. In a rat study performed by Uzunkoy and associates (54), if was found that intraperitoneal mitomycin-c significantly impairs healing of intestinal sites of anastomoses if given before the fifth post-operative day.

Gulcelik and associates (55) demonstrated that local injections of granulocyte-macrophage colony-stimulating factor (GM-CSF) improved the impaired wound healing caused by adriamycin in rats. These studies support the importance of macrophages during the inflammatory phase of wound healing and demonstrate the disruption of wound healing by chemotherapy if drugs are administered in close proximity to wounding in such a way as to cause immune suppression.

CLINICAL GUIDANCE FOR CHEMOTHERAPY AND WOUND HEALING

The studies discussed so far are pre-clinical animal studies. There are a few clinical trials which help to elucidate the effects of chemotherapy on wound healing.

Colleoni et al. (56) presented a study of 49 patients with Stage II through Stage III breast cancer who received perioperative chemotherapy defined as preoperative chemotherapy consisting of a three drug regimen (vinorelbine, cisplatin and 5-flurouracil) for up to six cycles. Thirty nine of the 49 patients demonstrated a complete or partial response. In this group of patients, additional chemotherapy was delivered until 30 minutes before and immediately after surgery (actually beginning in the operating room) for 15 days following surgery. No wound infections or delays in wound healing were detected.

Kolb and colleagues (57) reported a retrospective review of 100 patients treated with cytoreductive surgery followed by chemotherapy for their ovarian cancers. These authors found that wound complications were no more common in patients who began their chemotherapy from day 1 to day 10 postoperatively compared to those who began chemotherapy between days 11 to 20 or after day 20. Chemotherapy was multi-agent and platinum based.

The incidence of wound complications in the entire group was 11%. This rate of complications was not significantly different from other women undergoing surgery for other malignancies (13%) at their institution who did not receive chemotherapy. The authors conclude that significant delays in initiating chemotherapy following debulking surgery for ovarian cancer are not justifiable on the basis of fears of wound complications and should be initiated sooner rather than later to have the optimal anti-cancer effect.

Some new systemic agents employed in cancer treatment do not function by killing rapidly dividing cells (traditional cytotoxic chemotherapy) but rather produce their effects by blocking a step (or steps) in a signaling cascade(s). A recently introduced agent, Bevacizumab (Avastin), is a monoclonal antibody against vascular endothelial growth factor (VEGF) that functions in this manner. VEGF plays a critical role in the growth of new blood vessels (angiogenesis). Increased expression of VEGF in human cancers is associated with increased microvascular density, tumor growth, metastasis, and a poor prognosis. Bevacizumab blocks VEGF from binding its receptors, and consequently prevents the initiation of a signal cascade which would culminate in angiogenesis. By preventing the growth of new vasculature in a tumor, expansion and growth can be greatly inhibited. Bevacizumab, in combination with 5-fluorouracil, has been found to significantly prolong survival of patients with certain types of cancer. However, like many chemotherapeutic agents, bevacizumab is not specific for tumor vasculature and inhibits the growth of all new blood vessels, including those involved in wound healing.

Scappaticci and associates (58) reported on wound healing in patients treated with a combination of 5-fluorouracil and bevacizumab for metastatic colorectal cancer. In this report, they studied patients receiving major surgery in the midst of their chemotherapeutic regimen as well as those who received major surgery 28–60 days prior to initiating chemotherapy. These patients were then followed for up to 60 days to assess wound healing. Significant wound healing complications were found in the group receiving chemotherapy while undergoing surgery (13% versus only 3.4% in non-chemotherapy control patients), but not in those who had surgery more than four weeks before the initiation of chemotherapy. These results indicate that surgery should not be accomplished during an ongoing chemotherapy regimen that includes bevacizumab.

In the authors' search for published guidelines giving direction in terms of the optimal interval between chemotherapy and surgery, no clear cut concise published guidelines were discovered. In the absence of such guidelines, we conducted an informal survey of practice policies at our institution among our medical and gynecologic oncologists. Gynecologic oncologists as both surgeons and chemotherapists are especially aware of these issues since any wound complications experienced as the result of chemotherapy are serious problems for them as well as for the patient. Leaks in intestinal anastomoses or bleeds or wound dehiscence will likely require re-operation. Senior specialists as well as more recently trained faculty were queried. Their responses to our questions were fairly consistent though the gynecologic oncologists tended to be a bit more aggressive. After surgery, the medical oncology group would characteristically wait at least two weeks to initiate chemotherapy. This group felt that ideally at least four weeks should intervene between surgery and the initiation of chemotherapy if a bowel resection and re-anastomosis had occurred. With agents such as Avastin, this group felt that ideally an eight week healing period should take place before initiating treatment agents are designed to impair angiogenesis in the tumor since they also interfere with angiogenesis in a healing wound.

The senior gynecologic oncologist indicated that in aggressive tumors such as advanced and rapidly proliferating ovarian cancer she is comfortable initiating chemotherapy on the third day following surgical staging and debulking as long as a bowel resection has not occurred. If a bowel resection/anastomosis has occurred, it is his policy to wait at least two weeks before initiating chemotherapy. His feeling was that agents such as Avastin were potentially more likely to cause complications but he felt comfortable initiating therapy to include Avastin at two weeks post surgery even if a bowel resection has occurred.

Genentech, the manufacturer of Avastin, includes in their promotional literature warnings in regard to the use of Avastin in conjunction with surgery. They state that the "appropriate interval between the termination of Avastin and subsequent elective surgery has not been determined." In addition they indicate that in the clinical studies of Avastin leading to FDA approval, at least 28 days elapsed after surgery before initiating Avastin treatment. The manufacturer notes that the calculated half life of the drug is 20 days and suggests that this prolonged half life be considered in preoperative regimens of Avastin prior to planned surgical resection. The manufacturer also notes that wound healing complications occurred in 15% of patients receiving both Avastin and 5-Flurouracil as opposed to 4% in patients receiving 5-Flurouracil only.

Cetuximab (trade name Erbitux) is another new drug now being commonly employed in head and neck cancer and colorectal cancer. Like Avastin, it is not a traditional cytotoxic agent. Erbitux is a monoclonal antibody against epidermal growth factor receptor (EGFR). EGFR has been shown to be over-expressed in some squamous cancers of the head and neck and in some colorectal cancers. Since EGFR also plays a role in wound healing, there are obvious concerns in regard to employing this agent in conjunction with surgery. A report by Harari and associates (59) published in abstract form did show an increase in hospital stay following neck dissection for patients receiving Erbitux compared to those who had not (2.8 versus 2.1 days). Time to drain removal was longer in the Erbitux group (3.3 versus 3.1 days). No major wound complications were seen in either group though the authors point out that generally 6–8 weeks transpired between the last dose of Erbitux and neck dissection.

SUMMARY

Radiation and chemotherapy present significant difficulties and require special considerations when dealing with associated wounds. An understanding of the complex biochemical processes associated with wound healing and an appreciation for the stepwise progression of the healing process allow us to combine radiation and chemotherapy and surgery in an optimum fashion when these treatments are employed in the multidisciplinary management of cancer. Both pre-clinical studies and clinical experience have confirmed the importance of these concerns and have provided practical guidelines for the clinical management of radiation associated wounds. Pre-clinical studies and mechanistic considerations suggest that similar concerns should apply to chemotherapy and surgical wounding. A careful search of the medical literature suggests that the problem of chemotherapy and wound healing is a less serious and less common concern than the difficulties in integrating radiation therapy and surgery. Pre-clinical work suggests that the addition of growth factors or untreated fibroblasts can reverse some difficulties identified during the early phases of wound healing, namely delayed angiogenesis and wound contraction. Well established surgical principles emphasize the use of flaps especially those whose vascular supply originates outside the radiation portals. Hyperbaric oxygen has proven to be very effective as an adjunct when approaching wounds in heavily irradiated tissues. Marx has emphasized the importance of giving most of the hyperbaric treatments prior to surgical wounding to improve the vascularity and inherent quality of the tissues prior to surgical wounding. Both animal studies and clinical reports show an improvement in vascularity and a reduction of fibrosis as a result of hyperbaric oxygen. A fertile area for future studies is the combination of growth factors and hyperbaric oxygen for the treatment and prevention of radiation associated wounds. Based on the scientific information available, delaying chemotherapy for at least a few days after surgery not involving bowel resections and two weeks for surgeries where the bowel is resected will likely prevent an increase in wound complications. New agents including Avastin and Erbitux which employ antibodies or other strategies to block growth factors including angiogenetic growth factors will have to be used for a longer period of time before any definite conclusions can be made as to the optimal timing between these agents and surgery. As always in oncology, concerns related to the toxicities of treatment need to be balanced against the efficacy of such treatments in regard to their ability to control the cancer.

REFERENCES

1. Jemal A, Murray T, Samuels A, et al. *Cancer Statistics* 2003. CA 2003;53(1):5-26.

2. Cancer Facts and Figures 2003. *American Cancer Society Website* 2003;1

3. Rubin P, Cassarett GW, eds. Clinical Radiation Pathology. Philadelphia, WB Saunders;1968

4. Emami B, Lyman J, Brown A, et al. Tolerance of normal tissue to therapeutic radiation. I*nt J Radiat Oncol Biol Phys* 1998;21 (1):109-22.

5. Hunt TK, Hopf H, Hussain Z. Physiology of wound healing. *Adv Skin Wound Care* 2000;13(2 Suppl):6-11.

6. Witte MB, Barbul A. General principles of wound healing. *Surg Clin North Am* 1997;77:509-28.

7. Tibbs MK. Wound healing following radiation therapy: a review. *Radiotherapy and Oncology* 1997;42:99-106.

8. Drake DB, Oishi SN. Wound healing considerations in chemotherapy and radiation therapy. C*linics in Plastic Surgery* 1995;22(1):31-37.

9. Frank J, Barker JH, Marzi I, et al. *Strahlentherapie und Onkologie* 1998;174 (sup3):69-73.

10. Mustoe TA, Purdy J, Gramates P, et al. Reversal of impaired wound healing by platelet-derived growth factor-BB. *Am J Surg* 1989;158:345-50.

11. Tokarek R, Bernstein EF, Sullivan F, et al. Effect of therapeutic radiation on wound healing. *Clin Dermatol* 1994;12:57-70.

12. Pierce GF, Tarpley JE, Yangihara D, et al. Platelet derived growth factor (BB homodimer), transforming growth factor-beta 1 and basic fibroblast growth factor in dermal wound healing: neovessel and matrix formation and cessation of repair. *Am J Pathol* 1992;140:1375-88.

13. Bernstein EF, Harisiadis L, Salomon G, et al. Transforming growth factor beta improves healing of radiation-impaired wounds. *J Invest Dermatol* 1991;97:430-434.

14. Wahl SM, Wong H, McCartney-Francis N. Role of growth factors in inflammation and repair. *J Cell Biochem* 1989;40:193-199.

15. Armstrong FG, Jude EB. The role of matrix metalloproteinases in wound healing. *J Am Podiatr Med Assoc* 2002;92:12-8.

16. Miller SH, Rudolph R. Healing in the irradiated wound. *Clin Plast Surg* 1990;17(3):503-8.

17. Anscher MS, Chen L, Rabbani Z, et al. Recent progress in defining mechanisms and potential targets for prevention of normal tissue injury after radiation therapy. *Int J Radiat Oncol Biol Phys* 2005;62(1):255-9.

18. Gu Q, Wang D, Cui C, et al. Effects of radiation on wound healing. *Journal of Environmental Pathology, Toxicology and Oncology* 1998;17(2):117-23.

19. Wang Q, Dickson GR, Abram WP, et al. Electron irradiation slows down wound repair in rat skin: a morphologic investigation. *Br J Dermatol* 1994;130:551-60.

20. Bernstein EF Harisiadis L, Salomon G, et al. Healing impairment of open wounds by skin irradiation. *Dermatol Surg Oncol* 1994;20:757-60.

21. Yanase A, Ueda M, Kaneda T, et al. Irradiation effects on wound contraction using a connective tissue model. *Ann Plast Surg* 1993;30:435-440.

22. Arcini A, Topalan M, Aydin I, et al. Effects of early pre- and postoperative radiation on the healing of microvascular anastomoses. *J Reconstr Microsurg* 2000;16(7):573-6.

23. Doyle JW, Ya-Qi L, Salloum A, et al. The effects of radiation on neovascularization in a rat model. *Plast Reconstr Surg* 1998;98:129-35.

24. Kuzu MA, Koksoy C, Akyol FH, et al. Effects of preoperative irradiation on left colonic anastomoses in the rat. *Dis Colon Rectum* 1998;41:370-6 .

25. Ceelen W, El Malt M, Cardon A, et al. Influence of preoperative radiotherapy on postoperative outcome of colonic anastomotic healing: experimental study in the rat. *Dis Colon Rectum* 2001;44(5):717-21.

26. Linengood CH, Soper JT, Clarke-Pearsson DL, et al. Necrotizing fasciitis in irradiated tissue from diabetic women: a report of two cases. *J Reprod Med* 1991;36:455-458.

27. Fleck R, McNeese MD, Ellerbroek NA, et al. Consequences of breast irradiation in patients with pre-existing collagen vascular diseases. *Int J Radiation Oncology Biol Phys* 1989;17:829-33.

28. Olivotto IA, Fairey RN, Gillies JH, et al. Fatal outcome of pelvic radiotherapy for carcinoma of the cervix in a patient with systemic lupus erythematosis. *Clinical Radiology* 1989;40:83-4.

29. Porock D, Kristjanson l, Nikoletti S, et al. Predicting the severity of radiation skin reactions in women with breast cancer. *ONF* 1998;25(6):1019-2929.

30. Sause WT. Principles of combining radiation therapy and surgery,IN: *Moss' Radiation Oncology: Rationale, Technique, Results*. James Cox ed., Mosby, St. Louis, Missouri, 1994.

31. Isaacs JH, Siles WA, Cassisi NJ, et al. Postoperative radiation of open head and neck wounds-updated. *Head and Neck* 1997;19:194-9.

32. Vikram B, Shaw EW, Shah J et al. Failure in the neck following multimodality treatment for advanced head and neck cancer. *Head Neck Surg* 1984;6:724-9.

33. Marx RE, Johnson RP, Kline SN. Prevention of osteoradionecrosis: A randomized prospective clinical trial of hyperbaric oxygen versus penicillin. *J Am Dent Assoc* 1985;11:49-54.

34. Marx RE, Ehler WJ, Tayapongsak P, et al. Relationship of oxygen dose to angiogenesis induction in irradiated tissue. *Am J Surg* 1990;160:519-524.

35. Marx RE. Radiation injury to tissue. In: Kindwall EP, ed. *Hyperbaric Medicine Practice, Second Edition*. Flagstaff, Best Publishing, 1999, pp 668-673.

36. Marx RE. Radiation injury to tissue. In: Kindwall EP, ed. *Hyperbaric Medicine Practice, Second Edition*. Flagstaff, Best Publishing, 1999, pp 693-697.

37. Granstrom G, Jacobsson M, Tjellstrom A. Titanium implants in irradiated tissue: benefits from hyperbaric oxygen. *Int J Oral Maxillofac Implant* 1992;7(1):15-25.

38. Feldmeier JJ, Newman R, Davolt DA, et al. Prophylactic hyperbaric oxygen for patients undergoing salvage for recurrent head and neck cancers following full course irradiation (abstract). *Undersea Hyper Med* 1998;25(Suppl):10.

39. Marx RE. Radiation injury to tissue. In: Kindwall EP, ed. *Hyperbaric Medicine Practice, Second Edition*. Flagstaff, Best Publishing, 1999, pp 703-715.

40. Feldmeier JJ, Heimbach RD, Davolt DA, et al. Hyperbaric oxygen as an adjunctive treatment for delayed radiation injury of the chest wall: a retrospective review of 23 cases. *Undersea Hyperb Med* 1995;22:383-393.

41. Rudolph R. Complications of surgery for radiotherapy skin damage. *Plast Reconstr Surg* 1982;70(2):179-85.

42. Arnold PG, Lovich SF, Pairolero PC. Muscle flaps in irradiated wounds: an account of 100 consecutive cases. *Plast Reconstr Surg* 1994;93:324-326.

43. Teknos TN, Myers LL, Bradford CR, et al. Free tissue reconstruction of the hypopharynx after organ preservation therapy: analysis of wound complications. *Laryngoscope* 2001;111:1192-6.

44. Feldmeier JJ, Hampson NB. A systematic review of the literature reporting the application of hyperbaric oxygen prevention and treatment of delayed radiation injuries: an evidence based approach. *UHM* 2002;29:10-30.

45. Marx RE. Radiation injury to tissue. In: Kindwall EP, ed. *Hyperbaric Medicine Practice, Second Edition*. Flagstaff, Best Publishing, 1999, pp 682-689.

46. Neovius EB, Lind MG, Lind FG. Hyperbaric oxygen therapy for wound complications after surgery in the irradiated head and neck: a review of the literature and a report of 15 consecutive patients. *Head and Neck* 1997;19:315-322.

47. Gorodetsky R, Mc Bride WH, Withers HR, et al. Effect of fibroblast implants on wound healing of irradiated skin: assay of wound strength and quantitative immunohistology of collagen. *Radiat Res* 1991;125:181-6.

48. Kruegler WWO, Goepfert H, Romsdahl M, et al. Fibroblast implantation enhances wound healing as indicated by breaking strength determinations. *Otolaryngology* 1978;86:804-11.

49. Cromack DT, Porras-Reyes B, Purdy J, et al. Acceleration of tissue repair by transforming growth factor beta1: identification of an in vivo mechanism of action with radiotherapy-induced specific healing deficits. *Surgery* 1993;113:36-42.

50. Folkman J. Tumor angiogenesis: therapeutic implications. *N Engl J Med* 1971; 285:1182-6.

51. Salm R, Wullich B, Kiefer G, et al. Effects of a three-drug antineoplastic protocol of wound healing in rats: a biomechanical and histologic study on gastrointestinal anastomoses and laparotomy wounds. *J Surg Oncol* 1991;47(1):5-11.

52. Asmiks R, Qiao M, Rossi RR, et al. Adriamycin promotes macrophage dysfunction in mice. *Free Radical Biology & Medicine* 2006;41:165-74.

53. Shirafuji T, Oka T, Sawada T, et al. The importance of peripheral blood leukocytes and macrophage infiltration on bronchial wound healing in rats treated preoperatively with anticancer agents. *Surgery Today* 2001;31:308-16.

54. Uzunkoy A, Bolukbas C, Horoz M et al. The optimal starting time of postoperative intraperioneal mitomycin-C therapy with preserved intestinal wound healing. *BMC Cancer* 2005;5:31-6.

55. Gucelik MA, Dinc S, Dinc M et al. Local granulocyte-macrophage colony-stimulating factor improves incisional wound healing in adriamycin-treated rats. *Surgery Today* 2006;36:47-51.

56. Colleoni M, Curgliano G, Minchella I et al. Preoperative and perioperative chemotherapy with 5-flurouracil as continuous infusion in operable breast cancer expressing a high proliferation fraction: cytotoxic treatment during the surgical phase. *Annals of Oncology* 2003;14:1477-83.

57. Kolb BA, Miller RE, Connor JP, et al. Effects of early postoperative chemotherapy on wound healing. *Obstet Gynecol* 1992;1979:988-92.

58. Scappaticci FA, Fehrenbacher L, Cartwright T, et al. Surgical wound healing in metastatic colorectal cancer patients treated with bevacizumab. *J Surg Oncol* 2005;91:173-80.

59. Harari PM, Chinnaiyan W, Durland W, et al. Surgical wound healing in advanced head and neck cancer patients undergoing neck dissection following high dose radiation +/- cetuximab. *Int J Radiat Oncol Biol Phys* 2003;57(sup):S245-6.

REVIEW QUESTIONS

1.) Which of the following is true about the effects of chemotherapy and radiation therapy in regard to their impact on wound healing?
   a. Neither cancer treatment impacts significantly on wound healing and no special considerations are necessary when combining surgery and other anti-cancer treatments.
   b. It is common to initiate chemotherapy and/or radiation immediately after surgery.
   c. Chemotherapy and radiation therapy should always follow surgery by at least six weeks to prevent serious wound healing problems.
   d. Whether given before or after surgery, chemotherapy and radiation therapy can significantly impact wound healing and careful consideration should be given to the timing of the various therapies.

2.) In regard to the timing of radiation alone relative to surgery which statement is most correct?
   a. Radiation should be given right up to the day of surgery to have the best impact on cancer control.
   b. Radiation should be given immediately after surgery (preferably the same day) to have the optimal impact on tumor control.
   c. Typically radiation should follow only after surgical healing is well established and usually this means at least 2 weeks after surgery.
   d. It is mandatory that at least 8 weeks separate surgery and radiation otherwise postoperative radiation will cause wound breakdown in a majority of patients.

3.) Which of the following is most correct in regard to the impact of radiation on wound healing?
   a. Radiation has its biggest impact on wound healing during the "Maturation" Phase of Wound Healing.
   b. Radiation has little impact on wound healing during the "Inflammatory" phase of wound healing because neutrophils and macrophages are known to be exceptionally radioresistant.
   c. Timing makes no difference for pre-operative radiation but for postoperative radiation it is essential that the wound be completely healed for at least one month.
   d. Postoperative radiation can impact on wound healing during any phase of wound healing but practically speaking can follow surgery by 2 to 4 weeks without causing an increase in wound breakdown if the wound is healing appropriately before the radiation is started.

4.) Which of the following is most correct in regard to wound healing and chemotherapy?
   a. There is a much larger body of literature describing wound complications and chemotherapy.
   b. Overall, chemotherapy probably has less impact on wound healing compared to the radiation effects.

    c. Chemotherapy is always given in the postoperative setting to prevent wound healing difficulties.

    d. The newer antiangiogenic agents such as Avastin are likely to have less negative effects on wound healing

5.) Which of the following is not correct in regard to wound healing problems as the result of radiation therapy?

    a. Careful surgical technique including the design of flaps with their blood supply outside the radiation field can prevent wound problems.

    b. Experimental studies have shown that that the topical application of certain growth factors are likely to enhance wound healing in radiated wounds.

    c. Hyperbaric oxygen has been shown to have role in preventing wound healing difficulties and should be considered when surgery needs to be accomplished within the radiation field.

    d. When radiated wounds begin to breakdown in the immediate post operative time period, the surgeon should not intervene because these complications always occur and most are self limited.

Answers: 1d, 2c, 3d, 4b, 5d.

NOTES

CHAPTER 21

MANAGEMENT OF WOUNDS OF THE SCALP, SKULL AND BRAIN

CHAPTER TWENTY-ONE OVERVIEW

Management of Wounds of the Scalp, Skull and Brain

Herbert B. Newton

ABSTRACT

Wound healing problems are generally uncommon in neuro-oncology patients. When they do occur, an underlying infection is the most likely cause. Standard wound care is appropriate for non-healing wounds of the scalp and craniofacial region, including meticulous debridement, appropriate dressings, cultures of bacteria, and other microorganisms, judicious use of antibiotics, and the use of skin grafts or skin substitutes. Wound infections are dangerous because of the potential for lethal complications such as meningitis, osteomyelitis, brain abscess, epidural abscess, and subdural empyema. Surgical drainage and the use of antibiotics, based on culture results, are the mainstays of treatment for these forms of suppurative infection. Hyperbaric oxygen therapy may be of benefit in carefully selected patients with non-healing wounds and suppurative infection that remain refractory to standard treatment modalities.

INTRODUCTION

Because the scalp usually has an excellent blood supply, delayed wound healing is relatively uncommon in Neuro-Oncology patients and most often occurs because of an infection of the facial region, scalp, skull, meninges, or brain (1–3). Wounds of this type usually arise in the context of specific surgical procedures, such as craniotomy, craniofacial reconstruction, or repair of damage from head trauma, but can be idiopathic in some cases (1, 4–6). In addition, various treatment modalities for brain tumors or malignancies of the head and neck, such as external beam irradiation and chemotherapy, can impair the wound healing capacity of underlying tissues and render them more susceptible to chronic infection (7–9). The initial treatment of a slowly healing wound of the scalp or craniofacial region is similar to the care of chronic wounds elsewhere on the body, including aggressive debridement, treatment of regional infection, use of proper wound dressings, primary closure with or without skin flaps and, when necessary, grafting of skin or application of skin substitutes (9–13). The rest of this chapter will review some general principles of wound care that are applicable to the cranial cavity, skull, and head and neck region, as well as cover related topics including infections after craniotomy and craniofacial surgery, meningitis, osteomyelitis of the skull, intracranial abscess, epidural abscess, and subdural empyema. In addition, the application of hyperbaric oxygen treatment to these disease entities will be discussed.

OVERVIEW OF WOUND CARE

Meticulous "sharp" debridement of all necrotic and nonviable tissue is crucial to provide an environment for proper wound healing of the scalp and craniofacial region (10, 12). Proper debridement will convert the non-healing wound into a healthier, acute wound that can proceed through all of the phases of normal healing (i.e., hemostasis, inflammation, proliferation, remodeling). The area should be debrided until the wound edges and base consist only of normal, soft, well-vascularized, healthy tissue. Only a "sharp" atraumatic technique should be used to avoid damaging the underlying healthy tissues (i.e., by crushing or burning), which is critical to minimize scarring and cosmetic damage to the face and scalp. For a more detailed discussion of debridement and related techniques, see the chapters entitled "Principles of Surgical Wound Management" by Greer and colleagues and "Wound Debridement" by Emhoff and Ferro.

During debridement sessions, tissue should be removed under aseptic conditions and sent for appropriate bacterial cultures. The specimen should be large enough (i.e., 200–250 mg) to allow for proper preparation, dilution, and inoculation onto culture plates (13). Cultures of non-healing wounds are usually polymicrobial, with a mean number of species per wound ranging from 1.6 up to 4.4 (13, 14). The most common microbial isolates from non-healing wounds are *Staphylococcus aureus*, coagulase-negative staphylococci, and *Pseudomonas aeruginosa*. *S. aureus* has been reported in 43% of infected leg ulcers and 88% of non-infected leg ulcers, while *Staphylococcus epidermidis* has been noted in 14% of venous ulcers and 21% of diabetic foot ulcers. *P. aeruginosa* has been reported to be present in 7% to 33% of isolates from various types of ulcers. Other aerobic species that have been reported include *Escherichia coli*, *Enterobacter cloacae*, and several varieties of *Klebsiella* and *Proteus* species. Anaerobic bacterial species are also commonly identified in wounds, although the frequency varies widely from study to study (approximately 10% to 25% of chronic leg ulcer samples) (13, 14). The most commonly isolated anaerobes include *Peptostreptococcus* species, *Prevotella/Porphyromonas* species (pigmented and non-pigmented varieties), and *Finegoldia magna*.

The presence of bacteria in a non-healing wound of the scalp or head and neck is not an absolute indication of infection (10–14). Wounds can be contaminated and colonized by bacteria, without causing an active infection within the tissues, as outlined in detail by JL LeFrock in the chapter entitled "Post-Operative Sugical Site Infections and Non-Necrotizing Skin and Soft Tissue Infections." At the stage of "critical colonization," the bacterial load becomes large enough to adversely affect wound healing and may progress to active infection if the bacterial counts exceeds 10^5 CFU per gram of tissue (15). An exception to this rule is infection with Group A β–hemolytic streptococcus infection, in which active infection and poor wound healing can be associated with bacterial loads of less than 10^5 CFU per gram of tissue (16). At the stage of "critical colonization" and during active infection, the wound remains in the inflammatory phase, with the release of numerous proteins, cytokines, and oxidants, and cannot progress to the proliferative and remodeling phases (16, 17).

The use of antibiotics during the treatment of non-healing wounds of the scalp and craniofacial region remains controversial (13, 14). Further debate exists over the use of systemic antibiotics in addition to, or instead of, localized topical antibiotics. Despite the controversy, antibiotics remain in widespread use (18). A recent meta-analysis supports the use of topical preparations such as silver sulfadiazine, silver zinc allantoinate, and DMSO powder, which are able to attain high local concentrations without regard to regional vascular supply (19). However, the analysis did not support the routine use of systemic antibiotics. If there is evidence for an acute wound infection, with or without an associated cellulitis, experts are in agreement that the use of systemic antibiotics is appropriate, as guided by wound cultures and antibiotic sensitivities (13, 14, 19).

After the wound has been thoroughly debrided of all necrotic tissues and appropriate treatment has been instigated for any associated infection, a suitable dressing must be applied to the area (10). Wounds tend to heal best in a moist environment; dry, desiccated wounds are prone to poor healing. However, persistent edema is also detrimental to wound healing and should be minimized. The use of wet-to-dry dressings are recommended by many clinicians, and have the advantage of repeated intrinsic debridements after each dressing change. In selected patients, the use of skin grafts or skin substitutes may be necessary to allow for complete healing and wound closure (9, 10). More in-depth discussion of wound dressings and skin grafting techniques can be found in the chapter entitled "Principles of Surgical Wound Management" by Greer and co-workers.

DELAYED WOUND HEALING AFTER CRANIOTOMY AND CRANIOFACIAL SURGERY

In most patients, incisions following craniotomy and craniofacial surgery heal in a timely fashion and are not associated with any complications (1, 4, 5). Delayed healing is more likely in patients undergoing a repeat procedure (e.g., resection of recurrent brain tumor) or in those cases that have been previously exposed to irradiation and/or chemotherapy, are immunosuppressed for other medical reasons (e.g., chronic corticosteroid usage), have very poor nutritional status, or have developed a wound infection (2, 7, 8). In general, the presence of an underlying wound infection is the most likely cause of delayed healing in this cohort of patients. However, postoperative infections are not common in neurosurgical and craniofacial patients, with an incidence that ranges between 2.5% to 6% in most series. The incidence of true incisional infections and related complications is even lower than this rate because these figures often include other types of infections, such as involvement of the urinary tract and pneumonia (1, 4, 5). Contributing factors to the development of postoperative infection include re-operation, prolonged duration of surgery, advanced patient age, and the presence of a cerebrospinal (CSF) leak. Although it remains controversial, some authors contend that prophylactic, perioperative use of antibiotics can reduce the risk of infection, based on randomized clinical trial data (20). The most significant factor across all studies appears to be the presence of a CSF leak, which can evolve into a CSF fistula and provide a route for bacterial spread deep into the wound and underlying tissues. In many cases of CSF leak, extra stitches in the involved region of skin will solve the problem. More persistent leaks will require the placement of a spinal lumbar drain or repeated spinal taps to reduce intrathecal pressure and stop CSF flow through the leak, thereby allowing the fistula to scar over. If the CSF leak persists despite lumbar drainage, then primary repair of the dural tear will be necessary, using a pericranial patch graft approach. Although there is no definitive data, many authors recommend culturing the CSF and then instituting prophylactic antibiotics with activity against skin flora.

Even a seemingly benign, superficial wound infection should be treated very aggressively as outlined above because of the potential for spread to the surrounding scalp (i.e., scalp cellulitis) and, more importantly, spread into the deeper tissues. Deep tissue spread of infection can lead to severe complications with adverse neurological sequelae, including meningitis, epidural abscess, subdural empyema, bone flap infection and osteomyelitis, and brain abscess. In general, topical and systemic antibiotics should be avoided in the early stages of scalp and craniofacial wound healing. However, due to the severity of neurological complications that develop in patients with deep wound infections after these procedures, antibiotics should be instituted once there is unequivocal evidence of early infection and all appropriate cultures have been drawn. In addition to bacterial and fungal cultures, some authors recommend obtaining an erythrocyte sedimentation rate (ESR) and a C-reactive protein (CRP) in patients with a possible scalp wound infection (4). Both tests are useful indicators of infection, although they are nonspecific. The CRP is an acute phase protein reactant in the albumen fraction that is very labile and can rise and fall depending on the status of an acute infection. Daily CRP levels in patients with an elevated temperature are suggested because a secondary rise in level is highly correlated with acute infection. The levels begin to decline within 24 to 48 hours after successful treatment of the infection. The ESR rises and subsides more slowly than the CRP; however, a highly elevated ESR (above 75 mm/hr) indicates a deep, persistent infection such as osteomyelitis.

POSTOPERATIVE MENINGITIS

Postoperative meningitis after craniotomy or craniofacial surgery is uncommon, occurring in 0.5% to 1.5% of cases (1, 4, 5, 21). It can arise acutely after the surgical procedure, or in the setting of a slowly healing, chronic wound that develops an infection and spreads into the deeper tissues, transgressing the dura (Figure 1). Although meningitis is uncommon, it is a potentially lethal complication if the diagnosis is delayed or if the infection is left untreated. The most common symptoms include persistent or rising fever, progressive decline in level of consciousness, headache, neck stiffness, and the

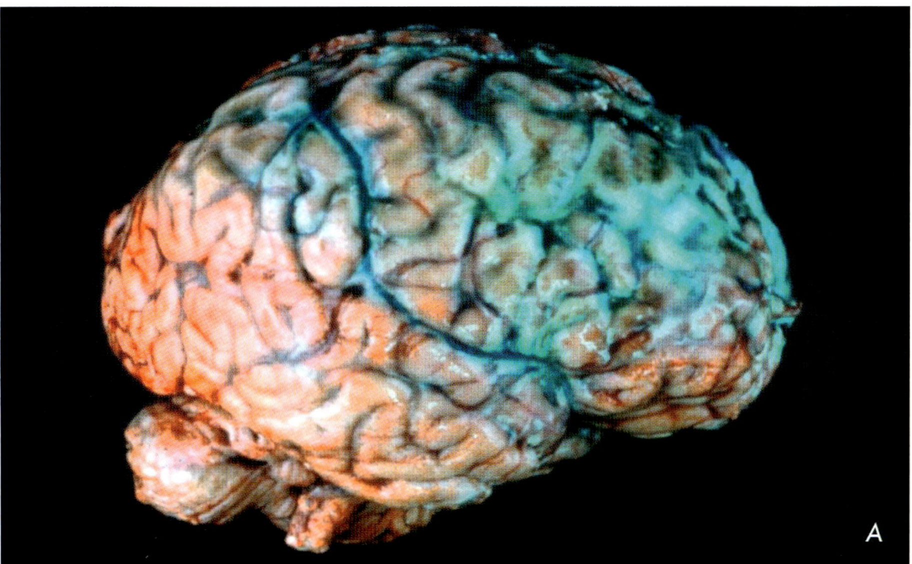

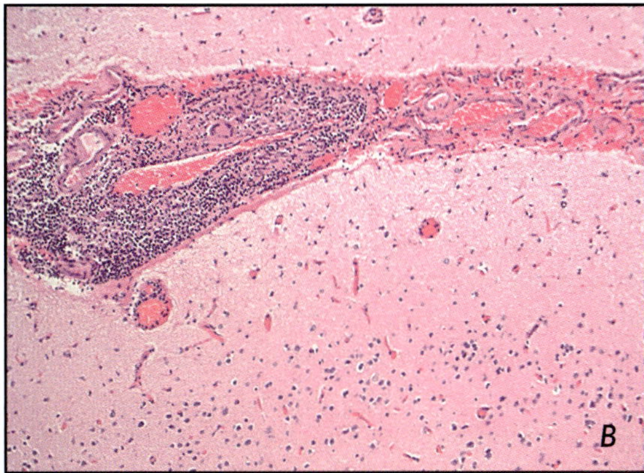

Figure 1. Acute meningitis.
(A) Gross specimen, demonstrating dense patchy areas of suppurative exudate overlying exudate overlying the frontal, parietal, and anterior temporal lobes.
(B) Low power view of inflammatory infiltrates expanding the meninges in between two gyri (hematoxylin and eosin @ 100x). Also note the inflammation surrounding some of the blood vessels in the superficial regions of cortex.

onset of new neurological deficits (e.g., cranial nerve palsies) (21). Any postoperative patient suspected of having meningitis should undergo a lumbar puncture for analysis of CSF parameters (i.e., cell count, differential, protein, glucose, lactate level, gram stain) and to obtain CSF for screening cultures (bacterial, fungal). The CSF typically demonstrates a pleocytosis (> 1,000 WBC cells/mm^3), with a predominance of neutrophils, an elevated protein level, and a reduced glucose level. In bacterial meningitis, the gram stain will be positive for the causative organism in 80% or more of cases. The most common pathogens include *S. aureus*, coagulase negative staphylococci, *P. aeruginosa*, *E. coli*, and *Acinetobacter baumannii* (4, 21). If the infection develops after craniofacial surgery involving the ear or nose, the pathogenic profile may be different (e.g., *Streptococcus pneumoniae*, *Haemophilus influenzae*, *Streptococcus*).

In some early postoperative patients it may be difficult to differentiate between bacterial meningitis and chemical meningitis because both can present with headache, photophobia, and nuchal rigidity (22). Chemical meningitis can develop secondary to meningeal irritation from the surgical procedure and hemolyzed blood products. In a large series of 70 neurosurgical patients described by Forgacs and colleagues, the cohort of 30 patients diagnosed with chemical meningitis rarely had a temperature above 39.4° C, a CSF leak, or an inflamed or purulent surgical site (22). In addition, chemical meningitis was not associated with delerium, seizures, coma, or spinal fluid CSF with a WBC above 7,500/microliter or a glucose level below 10 mg/dl.

Because CSF cultures require 48 to 72 hours to complete, the patient should be placed on empiric antibiotics. Delay in empiric treatment of postoperative meningitis has been associated with increased neurologic morbidity and mortality. A combination regimen should be implemented that is directed at the most likely pathogens. Once culture results have been finalized, a more exact regimen can be formulated. Several empiric regimens are appropriate in the setting of postoperative meningitis. For most neurosurgical or craniofacial patients the recommended regimen consists of intravenous (IV) vancomycin 1 gm every 12 hours, plus ceftazidime 2 gm IV every 8 hours for a two to three week course. Another regimen that would be appropriate for adults 18 to 50 years of age includes vancomycin 1 gm IV every 12 hours, plus cefotaxime 2 gm IV every 6 hours or ceftriaxone 2 gm IV every 12 hours. Vancomycin is active against skin pathogens, including drug-resistant *S. aureus*, while third-generation cephalosporins have good CSF penetration and are usually active against hospital-acquired gram-negative bacilli. Some authors have suggested using prophylactic perioperative antibiotics to reduce the risk of postoperative meningitis. However, recent data would suggest that although this approach may reduce the incidence of localized incisional infections, it does not prevent meningitis and will select for resistant organisms (23). In patients with clinical evidence for elevated intracranial pressure, high-dose IV dexamethasone and/or hyperosmolar agents (i.e., mannitol) may be necessary.

BONE FLAP INFECTION & OSTEOMYELITIS OF THE SKULL

Neurosurgical and craniofacial patients that develop incisional infections are at risk for underlying bone flap infections and regional osteomyelitis of the skull (4, 5, 24). Following craniotomy, the bone flap is essentially devascularized and devitalized, reducing its natural resistance to infection. A pure bone flap infection may cause persistent fevers, with marked inflammation and suppuration of the overlying scalp. In other patients it may be more subtle, presenting instead as a fistula, with continuous drainage through a non-healing wound. If the infection spreads to the surrounding skull, regional osteomyelitis can develop (Figure 2). Osteomyelitis usually presents acutely, with fever, headache, seizures and, if the infection involves the skull base, focal neurological deficits such as cranial nerve palsies (24). In some cases, the symptoms may also be due to an underlying brain abscess (see below), which is often noted in many patients with skull osteomyelitis. In rare cases, the patient can remain asymptomatic except for local signs of swelling and tenderness. In most patients, the white blood cell (WBC) count does not

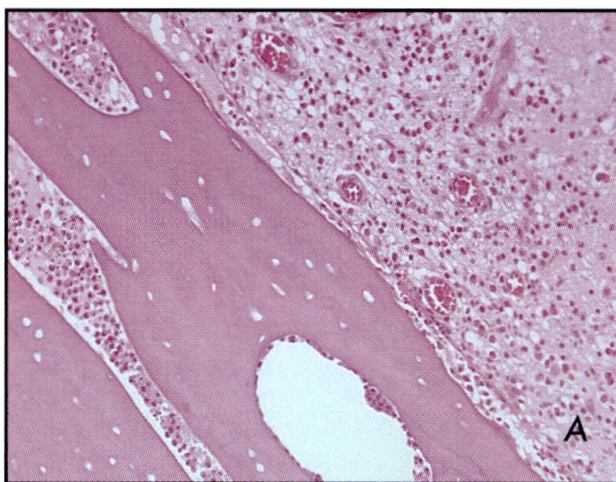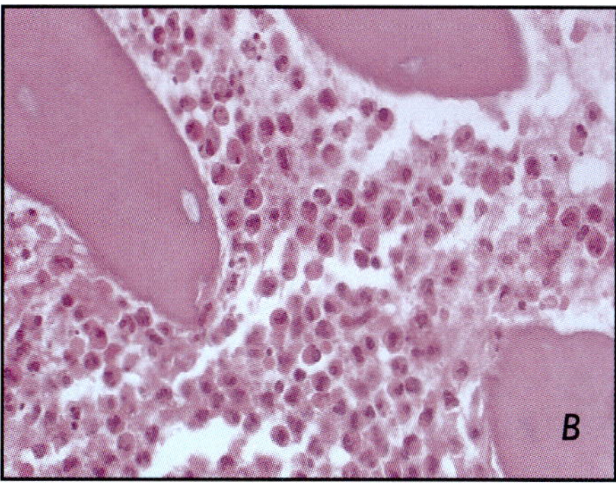

Figure 2. Acute osteomyelitis of the frontal bone. (A) Medium power demonstrating bone spicule surrounded by inflammatory cells (hematoxylin and eosin @ 200x). (B) High power view of bone spicules, revealing a dense concentration of polymorphonuclear leukocytes and inflammtory exudate (hematoxylin and eosin @ 600x).

develop a significant leukocytosis. However, the ESR is usually elevated and may be accompanied by a rise in the CRP. Gadolinium-enhanced MRI is a very sensitive method for detecting early osteomyelitis of the skull (24). The typical features include enhancement of the dura overlying the involved region, as well as loss of the normal T1-weighted signal from the fatty marrow of the infected bone. The MRI scan will also screen for the presence of a brain abscess.

The initial treatment for a simple bone flap infection is to remove the infected flap, draw cultures from the specimen, and then proceed with a course of antibiotics (approximately 4 weeks for most patients) as dictated by culture results (4). The most commonly involved bacteria include *S. aureus, S. epidermidis*, and *P. acnes*. Further local debridement in the area may also be of benefit. Cranioplasty of the region can be performed several months later, after complete resolution of the bone flap infection. In the case of skull osteomyelitis, a biopsy of the involved region of bone is often necessary to obtain cultures of the causative organism and to rule out a neoplasm (24). Surgical debridement of the region should also be performed, if possible. The profile of involved bacteria is similar to that of bone flap infections, with *S. aureus* being most common. However, various *Salmonella* species have also been known to cause osteomyelitis of the skull (25). A course of intravenous antibiotics, based on the culture results, should be implemented and continued until one week after both MRI and gallium scans demonstrate complete resolution of the infection (approximately four to six weeks in most patients).

BRAIN ABSCESS

Brain abscess is a relatively uncommon infection that affects 0.3–1.3 per 100,000 people per year, with a male predominance (1, 4, 26). It is most likely to develop in the context of pulmonary arteriovenous malformation, penetrating craniocerebral trauma, bone marrow transplantation, acute sinusitis, congenital heart disease, and adjacent infections (e.g., meningitis). Following craniotomy, brain abscess is somewhat rare, occurring in less than 1% of neurosurgical and craniofacial patients (27). Abscess development can occur in the setting of a chronic, non-healing wound of the scalp or craniofacial region, or can arise spontaneously underneath a properly healing incision. Pathologically, there are several stages to abscess formation, including the cerebritis, early capsule, and late capsule stages. In the early phase of the cerebritis stage (days 1–3) there is evidence for bacterial invasion, with acute inflammation and cerebral edema. As the degree of cerebritis becomes more advanced (days 4–9), the zone of inflammation expands, with the development of necrosis and pus in the center of the lesion. The early capsular stage (days 10–13) demonstrates the initial formation of a surrounding collagenous capsule, along with a diminution in the degree of cerebritis and edema. In the late capsule stage (days 14 and beyond), the capsule has become thick and mature, with extensive extracapsular gliosis and residual edema (Figure 3). The bacteriology of a brain abscess is quite variable depending on the clinical setting and source of infection. Following craniotomy, the most common species are *S. aureus*, methicillin-resistant *S. aureus, S. epidermidis, streptococci*, and anaerobes (26).

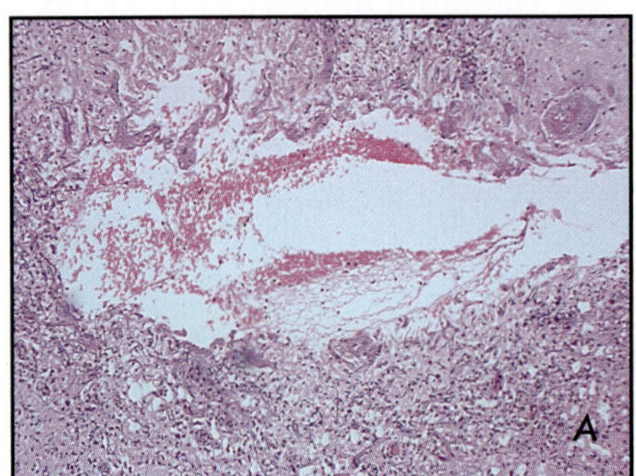
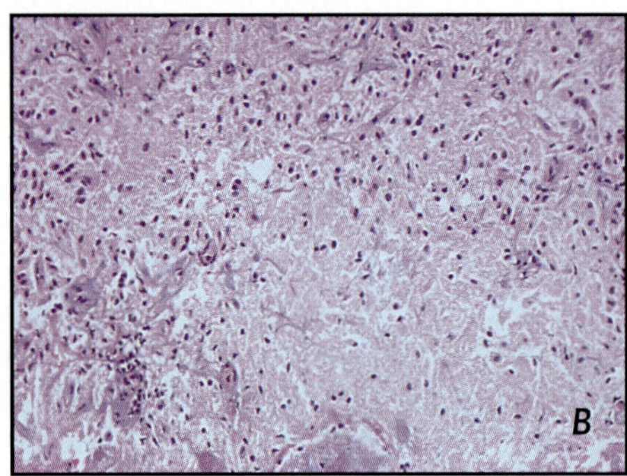

Figure 3. Brain abcess of the parietal lobe. Low power view demonstrating the whole abscess, including the fibrous wall, with granulation tissue and inflammatory cells, as well as the central region of necrotic inflammatory cells, including lymphocytes and foamy macrophages, along with capillaries and some necrotic debris toward the center of the field (hematoxylin and eosin @ 200x).

Neuro-imaging with both computed tomography (CT) and MRI can reveal the presence of an intracranial abscess (4, 26,28). However, MRI has superior sensitivity for the presence and extent of an abscess, especially in the early phases of growth. During the initial stage of infection (i.e., cerebritis phase), imaging reveals a diffuse high signal abnormality that may or may not enhance (28). Once the abscess has matured beyond the cerebritis stage, it will develop a well-defined capsule and present on MRI as a ring-enhancing lesion with significant surrounding edema (Figure 4). On T2-weighted and FLAIR images, the capsule usually appears hypointense in comparison to surrounding brain. The only MRI modality with the ability to differentiate abscess from tumor is diffusion-weighted imaging (DWI). DWI relies on the molecular motion of water within the tissues of interest to provide contrast; lesions with restricted water diffusion are hyperintense (i.e. very bright). Several studies have shown that on DWI, abscesses tend to demonstrate hyperintense signal, similar to an acute infarct. This may be due to the high viscosity of the pus, which results in a restriction of water movement within the abscess cavity. In contrast, the majority of brain tumors are hypointense (i.e., dark) on DWI.

Most patients with a brain abscess are symptomatic for one to two weeks, with a variable clinical presentation that depends on the size and location of the mass, the virulence of the causative agent, and the amount of cerebral edema (4, 26). Headache is the most common symptom. It is noted in 70% to 80% of patients. Alterations of consciousness, emesis, and fever are each noted in 45% to 55% of cases. Focal neurologic signs will depend on the location of the abscess; hemiparesis is the most common and can be demonstrated in 30% to 35% of patients. Seizures and neck stiffness are also noted in 20% to 25% of cases. Most patients will have an elevation of the peripheral WBC, ESR, and CRP. However, these labs may be normal in some cases and blood cultures are not always positive in this cohort. Because of an increased risk for brain herniation, it is not advisable to perform a lumbar puncture on a patient suspected of harboring a brain abscess.

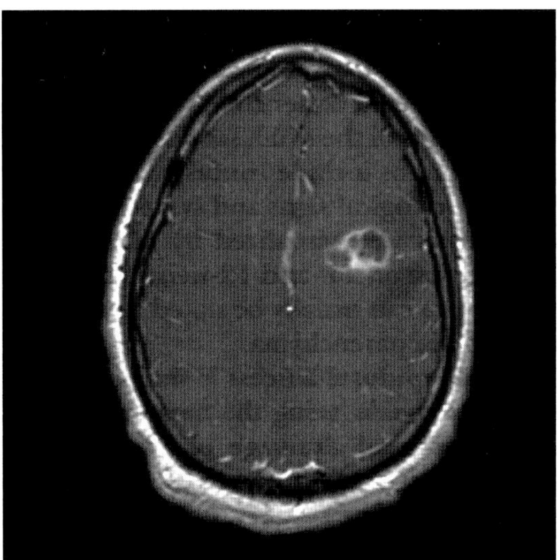

Figure 4. T1-weighted, gadolinium enhanced MRI scan of a patient with a right frontal brain abscess. Note the ring enhancement surrounding edema as well as the lack of enhancement in the necrotic central regions of the mass. There is also some mild midline shift.

The treatment of a brain abscess requires a collaboration between the neurosurgeon, neurologist, infectious disease specialist, and neuroradiologist (1, 4, 26, 28). Empiric antibiotics are usually started as the patient is being prepared for surgical drainage of the lesion in order to impede spread of the infection within the CNS and eradicate residual foci of infection following aspiration. For patients with an abscess following craniotomy, active regimens include vancomycin (1 gm IV q 12 hours), plus ceftazidime (2 gm IV q 8 hours) or vancomycin plus meropenem (1 gm IV q 8 hours). Surgical drainage of the abscess is necessary for any lesion larger than 2.0 cm in diameter. Image-guided, stereotactic needle aspiration is the method of choice for most patients, with a diagnostic yield of 95% and low morbidity. Open craniotomy with aspiration and resection is only necessary in selected patients; in particular, those patients with large lesions and significant mass affect. At the time of aspiration and drainage, definitive cultures should be obtained, including aerobic and anaerobic bacterial cultures, gram stain, and fungal cultures. Corticosteriods (i.e., dexamethasone) should not be used unless there are unequivocal signs of increased intracranial pressure because laboratory studies suggest reduced efficacy for antimicrobial therapy when used in combination with this class of drugs (26). The duration of antimicrobial therapy is variable, but most patients will require six to eight weeks of continuous treatment and serial monitoring with MRI scans.

EPIDURAL ABSCESS

Epidural abscess is a suppurative infection that develops between the dura and the inner table of the skull (1, 4, 26). It is less common than brain abscess and subdural empyema and accounts for less than 1.8% of all intracranial infections. In the postoperative setting after craniotomy, epidural abscess is strongly associated with wound infection, occurring concomitantly in 95.7% of cases in one series (29). Other conditions that predispose to epidural abscess include osteomyelitis of the skull, subdural empyema, and meningitis. The most common symptoms include confusion and encephalopathy, fever, and headache. Focal neurological signs and symptoms are infrequent in most series. Epidural abscess is well visualized by MRI, which demonstrates a hyperintense fluid collection on T1- and T2-weighted images in comparison to ventricular CSF. The dura can usually be noted as a thin line separating the abscess fluid from the brain parenchyma.

The bacteriology of epidural abscess is similar to that of brain abscess, with *S. aureus* and *S. epidermidis* being the most common pathogens (4, 26). Treatment consists of surgical drainage of the abscess via burr hole or craniotomy, as well as appropriate antimicrobial therapy. Empiric antibiotic coverage should be started before surgery, using the same drug combinations as suggested for brain abscess (as noted above), followed by a more definitive antibiotic regimen based on the results of cultures drawn at the time of surgical drainage. The duration of antibiotic treatment will be four to six weeks in most patients.

SUBDURAL EMPYEMA

Subdural empyema is a suppurative infection that occurs within the subdural space, between the dura mater and the arachnoid (Figure 5) (1, 4, 26, 29). It is termed an empyema because the subdural compartment is a normal, pre-existing intracranial space. Within the subdural space, the infection can spread rapidly and often extends through the arachnoid into the subarachnoid space, which is in direct contact with the brain. Subdural empyema accounts for approximately 15% of all intracranial infections, including a sub-group that can arise after craniotomy. In this setting, it is more likely to occur in a patient with an overlying wound infection and can, occasionally, develop after meningitis. If left untreated, subdural empyema can lead to severe complications, including brain abscess, epidural abscess,

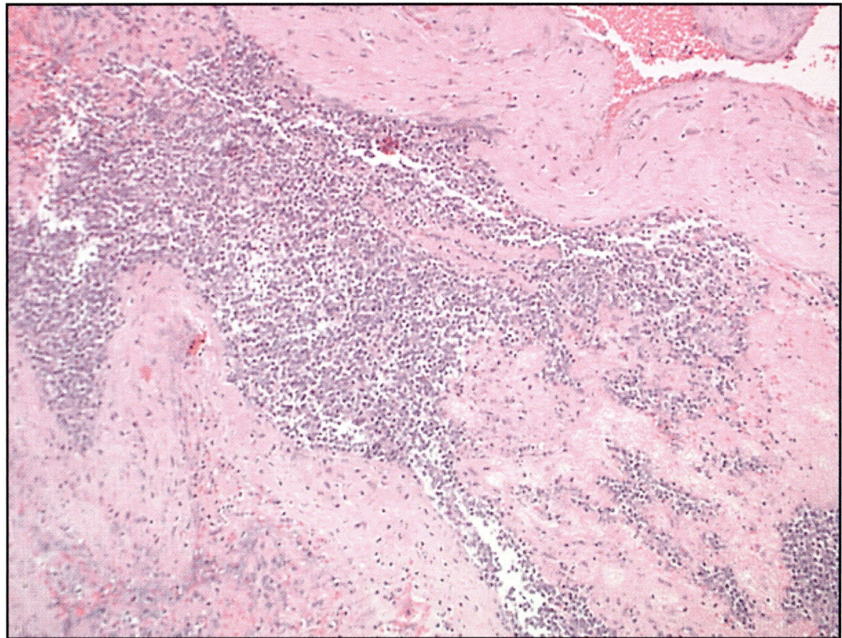

Figure 5. Specimen from a patient requiring surgical drainage and resection of a subdural empyema. Note the dense inflammatory cell infiltrate underlying the thick fibrous tissue of the dura mater (hematoxylin and eosin @ 100x). Regions of inflammatory cell debris are also present.

osteomyelitis of the skull, cerebral infarction, and cerebral venous thrombosis. The most common symptoms are fever and headache. Focal neurological deficits (e.g., hemiparesis), focal seizures, and signs of elevated intracranial pressure often develop as the infection enlarges within the subdural space. MRI is very sensitive to the presence of a subdural empyema, clearly demonstrating the presence of a subdural fluid collection that is hyperintense on T1- and T2-weighted images in comparison to ventricular CSF. Laboratory studies such as the WBC, ESR, and CRP are typically elevated.

The bacteriology of postoperative subdural empyema is similar to that of brain abscess and epidural abscess, with *S. aureus* and *S. epidermidis* as the most common organisms (4, 26, 29). Patients must be treated immediately with empiric antibiotics and surgical drainage of the subdural fluid collection through a burr hole or craniotomy. The method of drainage does not seem to be critical; retrospective analyses suggest that patient outcomes are similar when more invasive and less invasive approaches are compared (26). During the drainage procedure, fluid should be sent for Gram's stain and cultures (aerobic and anaerobic, fungal). Antimicrobial therapy should continue for three to six weeks, using a regimen based on the culture results.

APPLICATIONS OF HYPERBARIC OXYGEN THERAPY

Hyperbaric oxygen therapy (HBO2) is defined by the Undersea and Hyperbaric Medical Society (UHMS) as a treatment in which a patient intermittently breathes 100% oxygen within a chamber that is pressurized to greater than 1 atmosphere absolute (ATA) (30, 31). For a more detailed review of the basic principles of HBO2 see the chapter entitled "Hyperbaric Oxygen Therapy Applications in Wound Care" by Fife. Several of the disease entities mentioned above are currently recommended by the UHMS as appropriate for HBO2 (e.g., wound healing, brain abscess, osteomyelitis) based on available evidence in the literature and clinical experience (30). In addition, there are numerous other neurological and neurosurgical diseases that are under study for possible responsiveness to HBO2, including cerebral ischemia and stroke, multiple sclerosis, head injury, spinal cord trauma, migraine and cluster headaches, cerebral palsy, radiation-induced brain necrosis, and brain tumors (32–35).

Wound healing has become one of the most favorable indications for HBO2 as an adjunct to traditional wound care techniques, with HBO2 able to enhance local oxygenation, fibroblast production, collagen synthesis, epithelialization and neovascularization, bactericidal activity, and toxicity to anaerobes (30, 31, 36). Currently, the UHMS recommendations for HBO2 of non-healing wounds is 2.0–2.5 ATA for 90–120 minutes once or twice daily, for 30 sessions (30). The molecular basis for the ability of HBO2 to enhance wound healing is now becoming elucidated (37). HBO2 is able to induce neoangiogenesis via increased production of vascular endothelial growth factor (VEGF) and nitric oxide (NO). Fibroblast growth factor (FGF) is upregulated, which stimulates fibroblast activity and collagen synthesis. There are also immunosuppressive and anti-inflammatory effects mediated by reduced secretion of interleukin-1 (IL-1), prostaglandins, TNF-α, interferon-g (IFN-g), and IL-6. HBO2 has demonstrated efficacy in improving the healing capacity of chronic ulcers from diabetic patients, including significant phase III randomized clinical trial data (31, 36). It has also been applied to irradiated head and neck cancer patients and neurosurgical patients with poorly healing wounds (38, 39). Neovius and colleagues reviewed the results of a series of 15 consecutive head and neck cancer patients who had previously undergone irradiation, and then subsequently had surgery with poorly healing soft tissue wounds who were treated with HBO2 (38). Healing appeared to be initiated and accelerated by HBO2; 12 of 15 patients healed completely, two healed partially, and one did not heal at all. Previously non-healing wounds were noted to demonstrate significant amounts of well-vascularized granulation tissue after one to five weeks of HBO2 (monoplace chamber; 2.5–2.8 ATA x 30 sessions). In a similar group of 15 control irradiated head and neck cancer patients with non-healing wounds that did not receive HBO2, complete healing was noted in only 7 of 15 patients. In a consecutive series of 39 neurosurgical patients that developed infections after craniotomy or laminectomy, Larsson and co-workers reviewed their experience with HBO2 (39). In the cohort of 31 patients with osteomyelitis and an overlying wound infection, 28 patients had complete healing of the wound following HBO2 (monoplace chamber; 2.5–2.8 ATA x 40 sessions).

Refractory osteomyelitis (including the skull) that is unresponsive to surgical drainage and antibiotics is a UHMS approved diagnosis for the application of HBO2 (30, 31). The current UHMS recommendations for HBO2 in these patients are 2.0–2.5 ATA for 90–120 minutes daily for 40 sessions. The benefit of HBO2 in refractory osteomyelitis is mediated by increasing oxygen tension in ischemic and hypoxic tissues, enhancing osteoclastic activity to remove necrotic bone, enhancing osteogenesis and neovascularization in regions of necrotic tissue, enhancing leukocyte-mediated bacterial killing and toxicity to anaerobes, and by reducing edema and inflammation. Although there is no Class I evidence (i.e., phase III randomized, controlled trials) to prove benefit of HBO2 in refractory osteomyelitis, several uncontrolled studies have demonstrated very positive results (31, 33). More recently, the report by Larsson and co-workers included 31 patients with refractory osteomyelitis of the skull who had undergone HBO2 (39). Fifteen of the patients had an infection confined to the bone flap, while the other 16 had an infection involving the bone flap or surrounding skull, or an acrylic flap, as well as involvement of regional soft tissues in several cases. In the cohort with infection confined to a bone flap, HBO2 resulted in resolution of the infection without removal of the bone flap in 12 of 15 patients. In the cohort with more complicated infections, HBO2 resulted in the retention of three of six acrylic cranioplasties and three of four free bone flaps. In this paper there were also seven patients with refractory osteomyelitis of the spine, some of whom also had regional soft tissue infections. After treatment with HBO2, all of the patients had resolution of osteomyelitis and concomitant soft tissue infection, with retention of all spinal fixation materials in five of seven cases.

Brain abscesses that remain refractory to surgical drainage and antibiotics, are multifocal or located in eloquent regions of the brain, or that occur in immunocompromised patients, are another UHMS approved indication for HBO2 (30, 31). The current UHMS recommendations are 2.0 to 2.5 ATA, once or twice daily for 60 to 90 minutes, for 10 to 20 sessions. The rationale for the use of HBO2 in these patients include enhanced immune activity and bacterial killing, especially of anaerobic species, the synergistic effect of HBO2 with the antibiotics used for the treatment of abscess, reduction of cerebral edema around the abscess cavity, and improved entry of antibiotics into the abscess cavity due to intermittent opening of the blood-brain barrier. Although the benefit of HBO2 for treatment of brain abscess has not been proven in randomized phase III trials, there is substantial evidence of activity in animal models and uncontrolled clinical studies (33).

CONCLUSION

In Neuro-Oncology patients, non-healing wounds and wound infections are relatively uncommon after craniotomy and other forms of surgery. When they do occur, wound infections must be diagnosed and treated very aggressively because of the high morbidity and mortality of potential complications that can arise if the infection spreads into the deeper tissues and gains access to the brain and CNS. Meticulous debridement and other standard wound care techniques, along with the use of antibiotics in carefully selected cases, should be adequate for the treatment of most non-healing wounds and wound infections in this patient population. HBO2 should be considered for patients with persistent wounds that have not responded to standard techniques, as well as for refractory infections of the scalp, skull, and CNS.

ACKNOWLEDGMENTS

The author would like to thank Dr. Abhik Ray-Chaudhury for the preparation of the neuropathological materials, Drs. Hank Weed (Infectious Diseases) and Atom Sarkar (Neurosurgery) for critically reviewing the manuscript, and Julia Shekunov for research assistance. Dr. Newton was supported in part by National Cancer Institute grant, CA 16058 and the Dardinger Neuro-Oncology Center Endowment Fund.

REFERENCES

1. Warnick RE. Complications of surgery. In: Bernstein M, Berger MS (Eds.). *Neuro-Oncology: The Essentials*. Thieme Medical Publishers, New York 2000; 14:148-157.

2. Kingsley A. The wound infection continuum and its application to clinical practice. *Ostomy Wound Manage* 2003; 49:1-7.

3. Ovington L. Bacterial toxins and wound healing. *Ostomy Wound Manage* 2003; 49:8-12.

4. Blomstedt GC. Craniotomy infections. *Neurosurg Clin N Am* 1992; 3:375-385.

5. Stieg PE, Mulliken JB. Neurosurgical complications of craniofacial surgery. *Neurosurg Clin N Am* 1991; 2:703-708.

6. Cohen-Gadol AA, Pichelmann MA, Manno EM. Management of head trauma and spinal cord injury in adults. In: Noseworthy J (Ed.). *Neurological Therapeutics: Principles and Practice*. Volume 1. Martin Dunitz, London 2003;108:1221-1237.

7. Dormand EL, Banwell PE, Goodacre TE. Radiotherapy and wound healing. *Int Wound J* 2005; 2:112-127.

8. Lefor AT. Perioperative management of the patient with cancer. *Chest* 1999; 115:165s-171s.

9. Oishi SN, Luce EA. The difficult scalp and skull wound. *Clin Plastic Surg* 1995; 22:51-59.

10. Izadi K, Ganchi P. Chronic wounds. *Clin Plastic Surg* 2005; 32:209-222.

11. Mustoe TA, O'Shaughnessy K, Kloeters O. Chronic wound pathogenesis and current treatment strategies: A unifying hypothesis. *Plast Reconstr Surg* 2006; 117:35s-41s.

12. Attinger CE, Janis JE, Steinberg J, et al. Clinical approach to wounds: Debridement and wound bed preparation including the use of dressings and wound-healing adjuvants. *Plast Reconstr Surg* 2006; 117:72s-108s.

13. Heggers JP. Assessing and controlling wound infection. *Clin Plastic Surg* 2003; 30:25-35.

14. Howell-Jones RS, Wilson MJ, Hill KE, et al. A review of the microbiology, antibiotic usage and resistance in chronic skin wounds. *J Antimicrob Chemo* 2005; 55:143-149.

15. Robson MC. Wound infection: a failure of wound healing caused by an imbalance of bacteria. *Surg Clin N Am* 1997; 77:637-650.

16. Steed DL. Wound-healing trajectories. *Surg Clin N Am* 2003; 83:547-555.

17. Diegelmann RF, Evans MC. Wound healing: An overview of acute, fibrotic, and delayed healing. *Front Biosci* 2004; 9:283-289.

18. Tammelin A, Lindholm C, Hambraeus A. Chronic ulcers and antibiotic treatment. *J Wound Care* 1998; 7:435-437.

19. O'Meara SM, Cullum NA, Majid M, et al. Systematic review of antimicrobial agents used for chronic wounds. *Br J Surg* 2001; 88:4-21.

20. Haines SJ. Antibiotic prophylaxis in neurosurgery: The controlled trials. In: Haines SJ, Hall WA (Eds.). *Infections in Neurological Surgery*. W. B. Saunders, Philadelphia; 1992: 355-358.

21. Wang KW, Chang WN, Huang CR, et al. Post-neurosurgical nosocomial bacterial meningitis in adults: microbiology, clinical features, and outcomes. *J Clin Neurosci* 2005; 12:647-650.

22. Forgacs P, Geyer CA, Freidberg SR. Characterization of chemical meningitis after neurological surgery. *Clin Infect Dis* 2002; 34:556-558.

23. Korinek AM, Baugnon T, Golmard JL, et al. Risk factors for adult nosocomial meningitis after craniotomy: role of antibiotic prophylaxis. *Neurosurg* 2006; 59:126-133.

24. Malone DG, O'Boynick PL, Ziegler DK, et al. Osteomyelitis of the skull. *Neurosurg* 1992; 30:426-431.

25. Kamarulzaman A, Briggs RJS, Fabinyi G, et al. Skull osteomyelitis due to Salmonella species: Two case reports and review. *Clin Infectious Dis* 1996; 22:638-641.

26. Kastenbauer S. Infectious intracranial mass lesions. In: Noseworthy J (Ed.). *Neurological Therapeutics: Principles and Practice*. Volume 1. Martin Dunitz, London 2003; 78:874-888.

27. Korinek AM and The French Study Group of Neurosurgical Infections tSatC-CP-NSEHeP. Risk factors for neurosurgical site infections after craniotomy: a prospective multicenter study of 2944 patients. *Neurosurg* 1997; 41:1073-1079.

28. Nguyen JB, Black BR, Leimkuehler MM, et al. Intracranial pyogenic abscess: imaging diagnosis utilizing recent advances in computed tomography and magnetic resonance imaging. *Crit Rev Comput Tomogr* 2004; 45:181-224.

29. Hlavin ML, Kaminski JH, Fenstermaker RA, et al. Intracranial suppuration: a modern decade of postoperative subdural empyema and epidural abscess. *Neurosurg* 1994; 34:974-980.

30. Feldmeier JJ (Ed.). Hyperbaric Oxygen 2003: Indications and Results. The Hyperbaric Oxygen Therapy Committee Report. Kensington, MD, *Undersea and Hyperbaric Medical Society*, 2003.

31. Gill AL, Bell CN. Hyperbaric oxygen: its uses, mechanisms of action and outcomes. *Q J Med* 2004; 97:385-395.

32. Jain KK. The use of HBO2 in treating neurological disorders. In: Jain KK (Ed.). *Textbook of Hyperbaric Medicine*. 4th Edition. Hogrefe & Huber, Cambridge 2004; 16:179-194.

33. Sukoff M, Jain KK. HBO2 therapy in neurosurgery. In: Jain KK (Ed.). *Textbook of Hyperbaric Medicine*. 4th Edition. Hogrefe & Huber, Cambridge 2004; 19:263-278.

34. Al-Waili NS, Butler GJ, Beale J, et al. Hyperbaric oxygen in the treatment of patients with cerebral stroke, brain trauma, and neurologic disease. *Adv Ther* 2005; 22:659-678.

35. Al-Waili NS, Butler GJ, Beale J, et al. Hyperbaric oxygen and malignancies: a potential role in radiotherapy, chemotherapy, tumor surgery and phototherapy. *Med Sci Monit* 2005; 11:RA279-289.

36. Roeckl-Wiedmann I, Bennett M, Kranke P. Systematic review of hyperbaric oxygen in the management of chronic wounds. *Br J Surg* 2005; 92:24-32.

37. Al-Waili NS, Butler GJ. Effects of hyperbaric oxygen on inflammatory response to wound and trauma: Possible mechanisms of action. *TheScientificWorldJOURNAL* 2006: 6:425-441.

38. Neovius EB, Lind MG, Lind FG. Hyperbaric oxygen therapy for wound complications after surgery in the irradiated head and neck: A review of the literature and a report of 15 consecutive patients. *Head Neck* 1997; 19:315-322.

39. Larsson A, Engström M, Uusijärvi J, et al. Hyperbaric oxygen treatment of postoperative neurosurgical infections. *Neurosurg* 2002; 50:287-296.

REVIEW QUESTIONS

1.) Delayed healing after craniotomy for a brain tumor would be related to all of the following factors EXCEPT:
    a. chemotherapy
    b. prior irradiation
    c. wound infection
    d. dexamethasone
    e. initial resection

2.) Spread of infection from a craniotomy scalp wound into the deeper tissues can lead to all of the following complications EXCEPT:
    a. brain abscess
    b. osteomyelitis of the skull
    c. cerebal vasculitis
    d. subdural empyema
    e. epidural abscess

3.) The most common species of bacteria cultured from postoperative suppurative infections of the CNS is:
    a. streptococci
    b. S. epidermidis
    c. P. acnes
    d. S. aureus
    e. Salmonella

4.) UHMS approved indications for the use of HBO2 in Neuro-Oncology patients include all of the following EXCEPT:
    a. brain abscess
    b. wound ulcer of the scalp
    c. osteomyelitis of the skull
    d. acute meningitis
    e. compromised skin graft of scalp

5.) All of the following statements regarding neuro-imaging of brain abscess are accurate EXCEPT:
    a. MRI has superior sensitivity to CT
    b. a mature abscess capsule will demonstrate ring enhancement
    c. MRI of cerebritis reveals a region of high signal abnormality with variable enhancement
    d. diffusion-weighted imaging can differentiate cerebral abscess from a brain tumor
    e. diffusion-weighted imaging of an abscess typically reveals a hypointense lesion in the brain

Answers: 1e, 2c, 3d, 4d, 5e

NOTES

CHAPTER 22

NECROTIC WOUNDS PRODUCED BY SPIDER BITES

CHAPTER TWENTY-TWO OVERVIEW

NOTES

NECROTIC WOUNDS PRODUCED BY SPIDER BITES

Clyde O. Hagood, Jr., Judy R. Wilson

INTRODUCTION

Necrotic wounds produced by certain spiders continue to present significant challenges to physicians. The primary problem has been finding the cause of the lesions that were first described in Chile as the "Chilean black spots." In 1872, a Chilean biologist found that these lesions were caused by the bite of the Chilean Brown Spider *(Loxosceles laeta)* (1). The *Loxosceles laeta* is now known to inhabit a large part of South America and its bite has caused problems in many of these areas.

There are many species of *Loxosceles* world-wide, thirteen of which reside in the United States. Four of these are capable of producing necrotic wounds, but usually not as severe as the bite of the *Loxosceles reclusa*. They are the *L. unicolor, L. arizonica, L. deserta* and *L. rufescens. Loxosceles* species have also been documented in China, Australia, Russia, Japan, the Mediterranean region, especially Israel, Brazil, Paraguay, and Africa. The Brazilian Wolf Spiders *(Lycosa raptoria and erythrognatha)*, also found in Uruguay, are poisonous and produce a necrotic wound and share a habitat with *Loxosceles laeta* (2).

In 1957, a series of necrotic skin lesions occurred in the United States that were caused by the bite of the Brown Recluse Spider *(Loxosceles reclusa)*. These bites occurred in the Midwestern state of Missouri (3). Since that time numerous cases have been reported. Those substantiated as Brown Recluse Spider bites through identification by an arachnologist have been located in the Midwestern and southern United States, including Texas.

In 1970, in the Northeastern United States, several necrotic wounds were seen that were attributed to spider bites, namely the Brown Recluse Spider. It was soon realized that Boston, Massachusetts was not in the habitat range of the Brown Recluse Spider. Further investigation revealed the lesions were caused by the bite of the Yellow Sac Spider *(Cheiracanthium inclusum)*, a rather widely distributed spider in the Northeastern United States (4).

In 1987, in the Northwestern United States several necrotic spider bites were thought to be due to the Brown Recluse Spider. Its habitat does not extend to that part of the country, and it was found that the wounds were caused by the bite of the "Hobo Spider" *(Tegenanaria agrestis)* (5).

The diagnosis of a necrotic wound as being caused by a spider bite can only absolutely be made if the spider is seen to bite the victim, and then if the spider is identified by an arachnologist as a spider capable of causing a necrotic wound.

There are a number of spiders in the world that are poisonous to humans such as the Black Widow Spider *(Latrodectus mactans)* or the South American Banana Spider *(Phoneutria nigriventer)*. These spiders inject poison that cause illness and in some cases death, but rarely, if ever, produce a necrotic wound. Since the chapter in this book is "Necrotic Wounds Produced by Spider Bites," these other spiders will not be discussed.

THE VENOMOUS SPIDERS

Loxosceles. The *Loxosceles* are unique in that they have a violin-like marking on the cephalothorax and only have six eyes where most spiders have eight.

Loxosceles laeta (Araneae: Sicariidae) (Figure 1) was the first spider described in 1872 whose bite produced a necrotic wound. It is about the size of a silver dollar, a bit larger than the *L. reclusa*. It is said the venom of the *laeta* is more powerful than that of the *L. reclusa* and produces a more serious wound. It is found primarily in the southern two thirds of South America. In Chile it is known as "the spider in the corner." It has now been identified in the United States (6).

Loxosceles reclusa (Aranaea: Sicariidae) (Figure 2) is about the size of a half-dollar. The abdomen is cream-tan and the body is about 6–10 mm long. The violin pattern is fairly consistent, but it should be pointed out that because of its size it may be unrecognizable without magnification. The habitat includes the entire Midwest, deep South, and Texas. It is seldom found north of Ohio. It is very non-aggressive and will only bite if trapped or pressed between, for example, clothing and skin. The peak incidence of bites occurs in April and continues on until October. It prefers a warm, dark and dry environment such as in closets, under beds, in wood piles, and in vacant buildings (6).

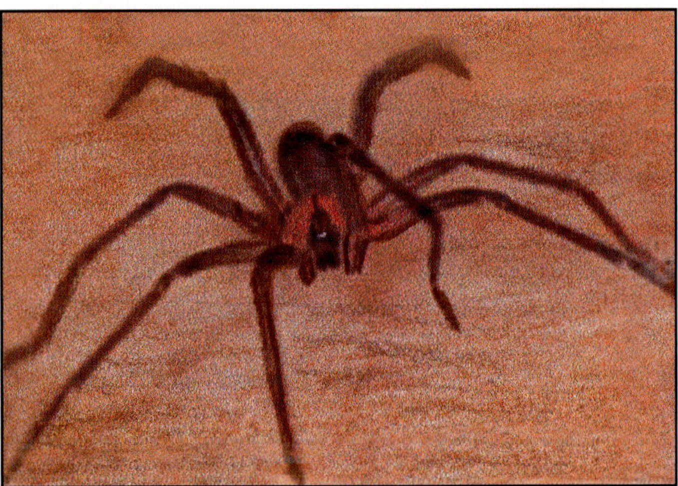

Figure 1. Chilean Brown Spider (Loxosceles laeta). Drawing courtesy of Pamela Hall-Hagood.

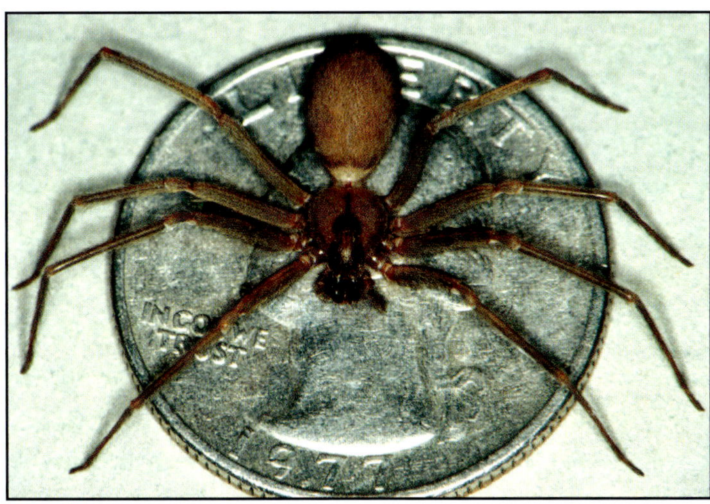

Figure 2. Brown Recluse Spider (Loxosceles reclusa). The spider is somewhat flattened making it appear larger than normal. Photo courtesy of University of Nebraska Department of Entomology.

Loxosceles unicolor is the only indigenous *Loxosceles* in California. Its violin markings are different in that they are not always as distinct. Its bite is immediately painful. There have only been three confirmed cases of bites by the *L. unicolor* (6).

Loxosceles arizonica is found in the desserts of Arizona, New Mexico, and West Texas. They are strictly desert dwellers and are not found around irrigated areas. They may be found around houses where cactus skeleton wood is brought in for firewood. *L. arizonica* prefers dry, dark places such as under rocks and wood.

Loxosceles deserta is similar in most ways to *L. arizonica* in regard to habitats, behavior, and wound type (6).

Loxosceles rufescens has been documented in a number of areas in the United States. It is similar to the other *Loxosceles* as far as markings, size, and habits. Its bite is less potent than that of the *L. reclusa*, still it is important in a number of other areas of the world, especially in the entire Mediterranean region, Australia, and southern South America because of the necrotic wounds it produces (6).

Cheiracanthium inclusum and ***mildei*** *(Araneae: Clubionidae)* (Figure 3) are both called Yellow Sac Spiders. They are small, yellow spiders with their bodies measuring about 8 mm in length. An interesting feature is that their first legs are much longer than the others, and these first legs end with tiny claws for grasping their prey. They are different in two ways from the *Loxosceles*. They are extremely aggressive and their bite is instantly painful like a wasp sting (4).

Tegenaria agrestis *(Araneae: Agelinidae)* (Figures 4 and 5) is found in the northwestern section of the United States. It is a rather large spider, having a body measuring approximately 18 mm in length; it would sit comfortably on a silver dollar. It is brown in color and has chevron markings on its abdomen. It, like the *Loxosceles,* is very non-aggressive and will only bite when cornered, pressed, injured or immobilized. The males apparently do the biting. It

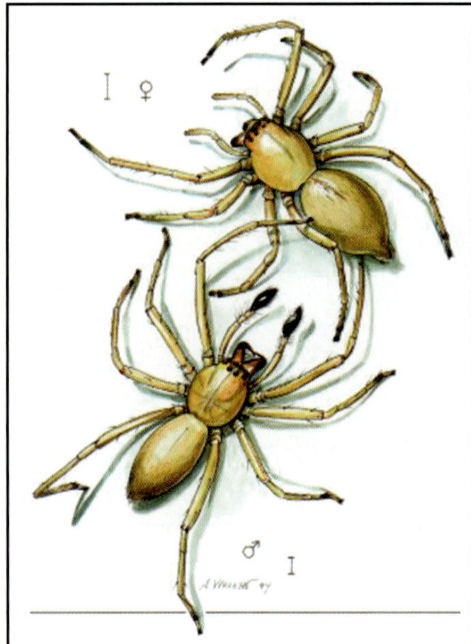

Figure 3. Yellow Sac Spider (Cheiracanthium inclusum). Photo courtesy of the National Pest Control Association.

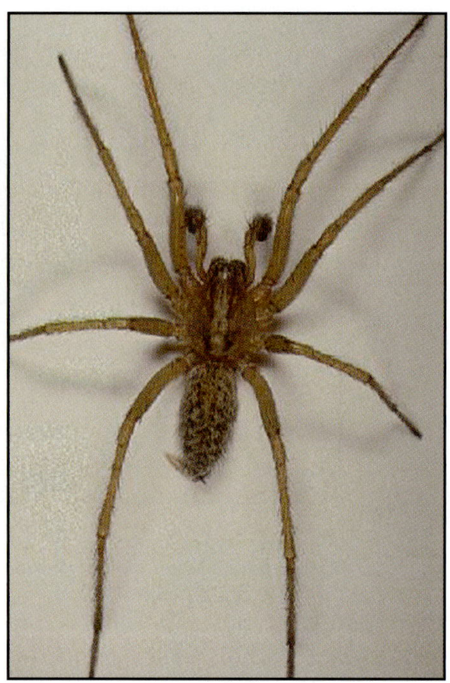

Figure 4. Male Hobo Spider (Tegenaria agrestis). Notice the "boxing gloves" on the pedipalps and the chevron marking on the abdomen. Photo courtesy of the Eagle Research Center and the Vest Family.

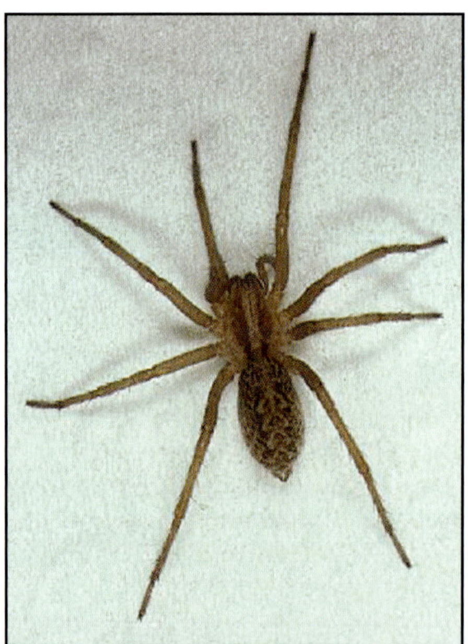

Figure 5. Female Hobo Spider (Tegenaria agrestis). The chevron markings on the abdomen are more pronounced than on the male. Photo courtesy of the Eagle Research Center and the Vest Family.

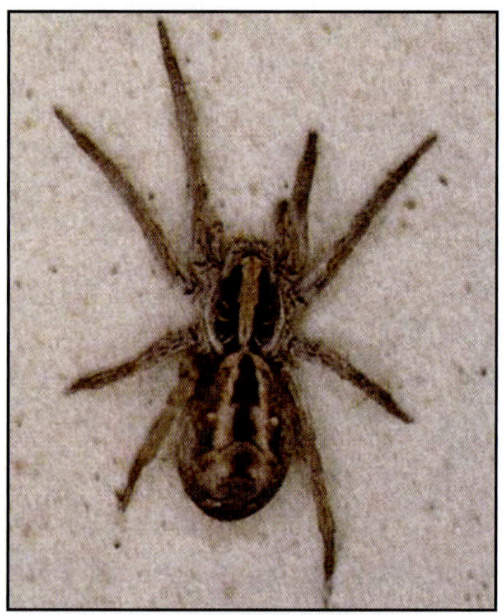

Figure 6. Brazilian Wolf Spider (Lycosa raporia and erythrognatha). These spiders are almost identical and can only be told apart by an Arachnologist. Photo courtesy of the institute of Biological Investigations, Merciful Stable, Uruguay.

prefers dark places like crawl spaces, under rocks, wood piles and yard ornaments, and is seldom seen in houses (5).

Lycosa raptoria and ***erythrognatha*** *(Araneae: Lycosidae)* (Figure 6) or Brazilian Wolf Spiders. *Lycosa raptoria* is more common in Uruguay and *Lycosa erythrognatha* is more common in Brazil. Both spiders are about 30–40 mm across including legs. They have two longitudinal light stripes down their dark brown bodies. They are found in houses, yards, and gardens and they are both equally venomous (7).

THE VENOM

The venom from the genus *Loxosceles* is the best studied of the four genera discussed in this chapter. It is a biochemically complex venom that is capable of inducing dermal necrotic ulcerations that are difficult to heal and can be disfiguring. It was realized early on that to study the complex mechanism of the action of the venom, the various components of the venom would have to be isolated. It is most likely that these first efforts were carried out in South America, but the authors have been unable to find any references to these efforts in the literature or on the internet. In 1968, using electrophoretic techniques, O'Dell determined there were five to seven components to the venom consisting of proteins and nucleotides (8). It was already known that the venom contained enzymes so this additional discovery provided valuable information.

More advanced techniques have identified at least eight subcomponents including a protease, alkaline phosphatase activity, lipase activity, Sphyngomyelinase D and hyaluronadase activity. Forrester, in 1978, was the first to demonstrate that Sphyngomyelinase D was the major component of the venom that caused cell lysis and death, including those in the endothelial system, red cells, and platelets (9).

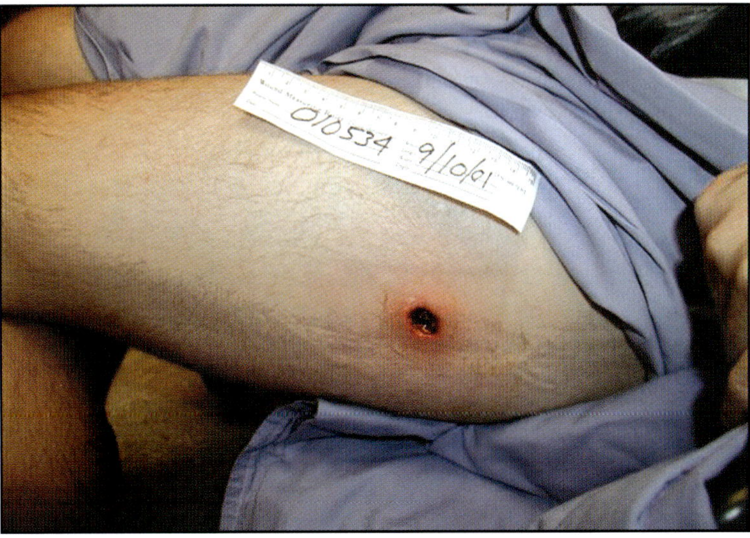

Figure 7. Brown recluse spider bite on thigh several days old seen for the first time in Wound Management Clinic. Only home treatment before. Photo courtesy of Paula Alexander, RNC, Wound Management Treatment Center, Memorial Hospital, Gulfport, MS.

The pathology of the wound reveals an intense infiltration of leucocytes. There is marked endothelial destruction and plugging of the capillaries and arterioles with leucocytes obstructing blood flow causing distal ischemia and gangrene. It has been shown *in vitro* that the venom from *L. reclusa* does not stimulate or attract leucocytes by itself. On envenomation, Gomez postulates from his animal work, that dermal, epithelial, and endothelial cells are stimulated to secrete the chemokines interleukin-8, growth-related oncogene-alpha, and monocyte chemoatractant protein-1. Endothelial cells secrete the cytokine granulocyte/macrophage-colony-stimulating factor and express the adhesion molecule E-selectin on the cell surface. Neutrophils migrate to the bite site and adhere to the intercellular junctions via the resulting inflammatory process and necrosis. Gomez's studies also show that the process is confined fairly closely to the area of the venom spread, so the chemokine activation is a much localized phenomenon. This work is also interesting in that the antivenom developed so far has been for intradermal injection. After four to eight hours the venom will have diffused away from the initial envenomation site, and the antivenom would no longer be effective. It seems that further development should be toward a parenteral antivenom (10–14).

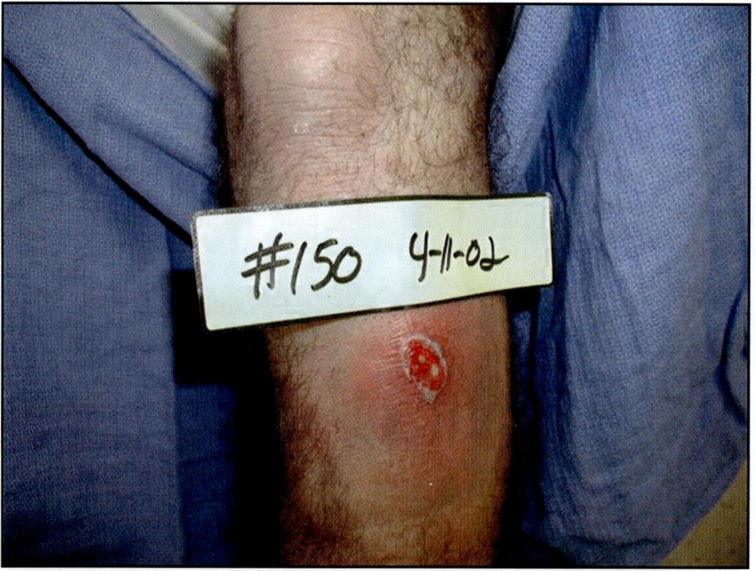

Figure 8. Brown recluse spider bite on medial leg at one week after three hyperbaric oxygen treatments and wound care. Photo courtesy of Paula Alexander, RNC, Wound Management Treatment Center, Memorial Hospital, Gulfport, MS.

THE WOUNDS

Brown Recluse Spider Bites

The wounds of the Brown Recluse Spider will be discussed first because more is known about them than the other spiders.

Those patients seen in the Emergency Room with classic findings of gangrenous ulcerations are most likely only the minority of the bites that occur.

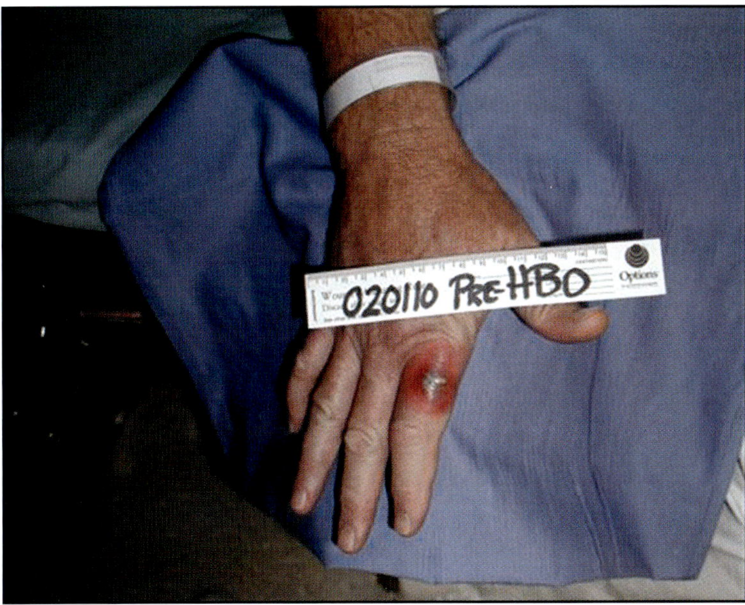

Figure 9. Brown recluse spider bite on right index finger being seen for the first time approximately 48 hours after bite. Very painful. Uses hands in his work. Will receive hyperbaric oxygen therapy because of proximity to tendons, nerves, vessel, and joints. Photo courtesy of Paula Alexander, RNC, Wound Management Treatment Center, Memorial Hospital, Gulfport, MS.

The majority of bites are probably never seen in the Emergency Room or by a physician (15).

A common scenario is the victims see a spider bite and kill the spider. The bite only becomes a small red "spot" that goes away in a few days with minimal treatment and with never having seen a doctor.

Another scenario is the victims are bitten by a spider and kill it, thinking it may be a Brown Recluse Spider. The area where they were bitten doesn't bother them a great deal, but it's red, about 1.5 cm, indurated, and itches. They apply some medicine from their medicine cabinet; it doesn't get any worse and goes away after nine or ten days.

Next are the victims who are bitten by a spider, kill the spider, and think it is a Brown Recluse Spider. That evening they notice that the area itches quite a bit and is uncomfortable. The next day it is red, sore and about 3 cm, so they go to their local doctor who gives them some cortisone, antibiotics and a tetanus shot, some Neosporin cream and a band aid, and tells them if it gets worse to come back. The area of the bite resolves over the next couple of weeks (Figure 7).

In the more serious bite, the victims, many times, do not know they have been bitten. On occasion, they may feel a slight stick or pain at the site or something crawling and hit it. At night the victims usually roll over on the spider. Then six to twelve hours later they begin to feel pain in the area of the bite. The pain increases in intensity and the area around the bite becomes red and swollen. Early on, with magnification, it is possible to see the fang marks. Within the next few hours, depending on the severity of the

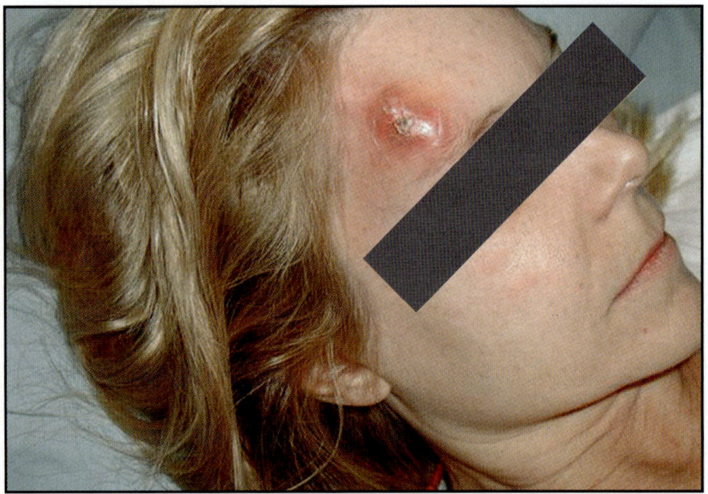

Figure 10. Brown recluse spider bite on forehead approximately 48 hours after bite. Note secondary infections with edema in orbit and in upper face with erythema. Photo courtesy of Paula Alexander, RNC, Wound Management Treatment Center, Memorial Hospital, Gulfport, MS.

bite, it will either stabilize or continue to worsen. The redness, edema, and pain will increase, and an area of paleness in the center will develop, followed by blistering, which sometimes becomes hemorrhagic. The center area will gradually begin to sink and the border will be irregular.

If it is not hemorrhagic, the center will be bluish in color surrounded by a ring of pale, then the red color, giving the wound a "bull's-eye target" appearance (16). Over the next few days, the bluish or hemorrhagic, center area will break down and become gangrenous. The wound may be anywhere from three to twenty centimeters in diameter; however, it is unusual for the wounds to exceed six to seven centimeters (Figures 7–10). The gangrenous area gradually dries, becoming an eschar. This slough may extend all the way down to the fascia. The eschar will eventually slough allowing the wound to granulate and heal. The healing may take many months.

If a spider was not identified as the cause of the wound, some of the more common other lesions that resemble Brown Recluse Spider bites must be considered as the diagnosis such as basal cell carcinoma, cellulitis, drug eruptions, ecthyma, herpes simplex, pyoderma gangrenosum, squamous cell carcinoma, and facticious ulceration (16).

The most serious complication of the bite wound is systemic involvement. One author (COH) speculates that at the time of the bite, the venom is injected either directly into a capillary or immediately adjacent to one so that it is easily absorbed into the circulation. Patients with the systemic reaction usually become ill rather quickly or within a day or so after the bite. An interesting phenomenon is noted with the systemic reaction. That is, the more severe the systemic reaction, the less severe the cutaneous wound seems to be. The reverse is also true, lending more credence to the first author's theory. The patient becomes extremely ill with fever, nausea, vomiting, and malaise, and develops a generalized punctate rash. The venom is a powerful hemolytic agent. When the red cells begin breaking down, the patients begin passing dark urine (hemaglobinurea or "Black Water Fever"). With the loss of red cells, they become anemic (17).

The wounds from the other *Loxosceles* are not as severe; however, there is a case report of a bite from a *L. arizonica* that was associated with shock. The spider was identified by an entomologist. The bite occurred on a 15-year-old girl, and shock was documented in the ICU approximately nine hours after the bite. It required massive fluid replacement and Dopamine to maintain her blood pressure for 56 hours. During that time she had the characteristic rash and a superficial ulcer at the bite site that healed in three weeks without a skin graft (18).

Cheiracanthium inclusum and *mildei* Bites

The bite of Yellow Sac Spiders is extremely painful, whereas the *Loxosceles reclusa* as a group is usually painless. There maybe some pain with the *L. unicolor*, but none with the others. There were no systemic reactions found in the literature. The cutaneous wounds are usually superficial and heal with simple wound care (4).

Lycosa raptoria and *erythrognatha* Bites

Little could be found regarding the wounds produced by *Lycosa raptoria* and *erythrognatha* spiders except that they were similar to the *Loxosceles reclusa* wounds and sometimes larger.

MECHANISM OF INJURY

The spiders discussed in this chapter create their injury by a bite and not a sting. Other arthropods envenomate by stinging, i.e., wasps, bees or scorpions. These spiders have modified mouth parts called chelicerae that are curved hollow fang-like apparatuses that act like hypodermic needles. The bases are connected to their venom glands in the cephalothorax. When the spider bites, the chelicerae come together in a pincer-like motion penetrating the skin and injecting the venom (6).

TREATMENT

Over the years, various treatments have been tried, but no single form of therapy seems to be ideal. Various antihistamines have been tried with little or no effect. Immediate and total excision of the bite wound was in vogue for a short while, but was found to be too destructive, frequently removing far more tissue than was necessary and has been abandoned. Steroids were tried with little success.

Wounds With Minor Symptoms

The patients state that they have been bitten by a Brown Recluse Spider, but may or may not bring in the spider. These patients will have a wound that will be 2–3 cm with erythema and induration. There might be an area of paleness with some cyanosis in the center or a blister. The blister on occasion may be hemorrhagic, and the area may be painful. They usually have no other symptoms, except on occasion a minor punctuate rash around the wound. These patients need to be given a tetanus booster injection or if they have never been immunized against tetanus begin the tetanus immunization series. Wound care consists of cleansing and applying an antibiotic cream and a sterile dressing. An antibiotic in the form of a Cephalosporin or Azithromycin should be given to stop any infection that may have begun. Analgesia in the form of a non-steroidal anti-inflammatory or acetaminophen should suffice (2, 16). *The most important thing about this wound is to follow up in 24 hours.*

Upon return, if there is no change or improvement in the wound, continued good wound care and debridement as necessary is usually all that will be required to heal the wound. Only rarely will the wound be large enough to require grafting. If the wound has become larger or the patient has developed further systemic symptoms, then they will fall into the category discussed in the next paragraph and should be admitted to the hospital.

Wounds With Major Symptoms

The patients state that they have been bitten by a Brown Recluse Spider and they may or may not have brought in the spider with them. These patients will have a wound that will be any size from 2–20 cm. It may be anything from the "bulls-eye target" lesion with the red outer ring, white middle ring and blue center to the classic gangrenous, necrotic wound that one would see on the patient who did not come in until a number of days after the bite. They may have fever, a punctuate, rash all over their body, and just not feel well. When questioned, they are eating, their urine is normal color, they have no shortness of breath, and they just feel "sick." These patients should be admitted to the hospital.

First, wound evaluation should be done to determine the extent of the wounding. This would include determining the length, width, and borders (regular or irregular), is the center gangrenous (yes or no)? If yes, has an eschar formed? Is there any cellulitis around the wound? Get a complete blood count, platelet count, and chemistry panel to include electrolytes and kidney functions. If temperature is elevated above 100.0 °F, get a blood culture. Do a urinalysis and urine for possible hemaglobinuria and draw a blood sample for a glucose 6 phosphate dehydrogenase test stat before any consideration for starting Dapsone (16).

Treatment of the wound at this time is simple wound care consisting of cleaning with normal saline under normal pressure, and applying moist healing dressings.

Intravenous antibiotics, with second or third generation Cephalosporins or Azithromycin in Ringers Lactate to maintain at least 1000 cc urine output per 12 hours are also important to prevent renal shut down.

Dapsone

Dapsone (Avlosulfon), an antibacterial Sulfone drug, was developed to treat Hanson's Disease. It has been tried with some success in the treatment of Loxoscelism. Dapsone is an antileucocyte drug that helps prevent the massive concentration of leucocytes at the bite site. The drug is relatively safe. It does have some major drawbacks. If a patient has a glucose-6-phosphate dehydrogenase (G-6-PD) deficiency, and is given Dapsone, it could prove fatal. All patients taking Dapsone develop methemaglobinemia. It may become elevated enough that the patient becomes so short of breath that the drug must be stopped. It requires frequent monitoring. Occasionally, a patient will develop a hypersensitivity reaction to the drug that may cause a severe hepatitis that can be fatal. One other complication is agranulocytosis, which needs to be monitored closely. Dapsone is also contraindicated if the patient is taking Trimethoprim or Probenicid. There has been one reported fatality in a patient treated with Dapsone for a Brown Recluse Spider bite (16).

Patients who believe they have been bitten by a spider should be strongly encouraged to bring the spider with them to the doctor or Emergency Room. Even a crushed spider can possibly be identified by an entomologist. When the patient is first seen, it is very important to obtain as good a history as possible of what happened. The doctor should ask specific questions:

- Where did it happen exactly, closet, bedroom, garage, wood-pile, etc?
- What were you doing? Getting dressed, reaching in the closet or tool chest, picking up dirty clothes or gathering wood.
- Did you feel a bite or sting or just something crawling around? Be specific.
- Did you bring in the spider?
- Is this the first time you have been bitten by a spider? There is some suggestion that a prior bite may confer some degree of immunity.

The patient's condition at the time of admission to treatment is important. Those having systemic reactions will require urgent care which will be discussed later.

Hyperbaric oxygen therapy

If hyperbaric oxygen therapy is available in the facility or immediate vicinity, the authors recommend treatment with hyperbaric oxygen therapy. A minimum number of 14 treatments are recommended at a pressure of two atmospheres absolute for two hours each (21). There are some risks with hyperbaric oxygen therapy such as sinus pain or ear pain or, at worse, sinus or ear bleeding. There is also the possibility of an oxygen seizure, which is rare, and an even rarer event, a pneumothorax (20). One of the theories put forth is that hyperbaric oxygen therapy breaks down the sulfhydryl chain to disulfide on the cysteine side chain on the Sphyngomyelinase D molecule. That molecule is thought to be the culprit that causes the breakdown of tissue and gangrene. Hyperbaric oxygen also quickly demarcates the area of gangrene around the bite area and prepares the area for accepting any future skin grafts as well.

Even though there are no controlled studies showing hyperbaric oxygen therapy is better than Dapsone, there are numerous anecdotal reports showing excellent results (20).

If there are no hyperbaric chambers in the facility or local area, then Dapsone should be considered if the G-6-PD is negative and there are no other contraindications. Dapsone 200 mg/ day for 10 days should be started. Daily monitoring should be done of the patient's blood gases for pO_2, methemaglobin, along with a CBC to monitor for Agranulocytosis. Midway through, liver functions should be checked. Rarely should a wound less than 2.5 cm be treated with Dapsone unless the patient is exhibiting systemic reaction. Debridement and grafting should be done as it becomes necessary.

Hyperbaric oxygen therapy has been tried with some success, but has been met with resistance because of lack of prospective, controlled blinded studies documenting outcome of this form of treatment. Medicare does not reimburse for hyperbaric oxygen therapy for brown recluse spider bites, therefore, private insurers also usually do not reimburse for hyperbaric oxygen therapy (19–21). For more information see the chapter by CE Fife entitled "Hyperbaric Oxygen Therapy Applications in Wound Care."

High Voltage, Low Amperage (HVLA) Therapy

Another form of therapy described first by Osborne from Oklahoma is called high voltage, low amperage or "Stun Gun" therapy (22). This idea came about when Guderian et al. (1986) (23) described successfully treating venomous snake bite victims in South America with HVLA electricity. Osborne applied this technique to Brown Recluse Spider bite victims with some success.

Work with HVLA therapy has been carried on by Abrams of Texas, who has treated a number of people with the HVLA technique and reported great success. It is interesting that he has reported successful treatment of wounds in all stages including some several years old. He does not include any patients with systemic symptoms. Abrams uses a mini stun gun (Figure 11) and attaches a cable to one pole and uses it as ground wire on the opposite side of the extremity. If the bite is on the abdomen or back, he places the ground wire 10" away from the wound. The other pole of the mini stun gun is then applied at five clock positions, with the sixth position being in the center of the wound. One-second stimulation with the "stun gun" is applied at each position. Apparently it is tolerated well by the patients. It is said to be "about like bumping against an electric fence." In Abrams' experience the pain subsides in one to two hours, and in two days beginning of healing should be noted (24).

Moss, in Granbury, Texas, has been treating Brown Recluse Spider bites with the "Stun Gun" since 1994, and she states that of the nearly 60 patients she has treated, none has required skin grafting and have healed with minimal scarring. She also shocks five sites equally spaced around the wound and once in the center, for one second each site (Figure 12). If the bite is recent, one treatment usually suffices. If the bite is several days old, two or more treatments may be required. Pain relief occurs shortly after the treatment. Moss points out that it is contraindicated in patients with pacemakers or other implantable pumps (Hagood, CO. Personal Communication, Dr. Judith Moss: Use of "Stun Gun" to Treat Brown Recluse Spider Bites; 2006).

The theoretical basis of the shock treatment is that the current will influence the hydrogen bonds of the enzymes and destroy their secondary and tertiary structures. The application of HVLA current will reduce metal ions (zinc, copper, magnesium, iron and calcium), which are firmly bound to some venom enzymes, and are mandatory cofactors for these enzymes. The electric particles interfere with the membrane as well as the positively charged polypeptides, decreasing their cytotoxic properties (24). There has been one controlled study (Barrett et al. 1993) comparing the "stun gun" and Dapsone

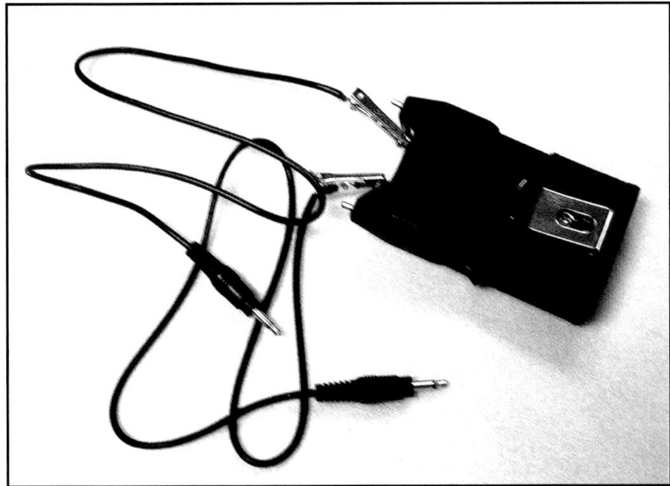

Figure 11. High Voltage, Low Amperage (HVLA) Therapy, or use of "Stun Gun" therapy to treat Brown Recluse spider bite. First described by Osborne in 1990. Photo courtesy of Dr. C.O. Hagood.

with a finding that Dapsone was superior (25). Only four quadrants of the wound were treated in the Barrett et al. study compared to the six quadrants done in the Abrams protocol. As of this writing, HVLA therapy is not being reimbursed by Medicare or the insurance companies. The "Gold Standard" for the treatment of the cutaneous spider bite wound remains centered around aggressive wound care (26).

Patients with Systemic Symptoms

Patients seen in the Emergency Room with systemic symptoms and no history of a spider bite can present quite a challenge. There will usually be a cutaneous bite site of some consequence on either the torso or an extremity. The patients will be quite ill with fever, headache, rash, nausea ,and vomiting. They will be pale and complaining of dark or "Coca-Cola" urine. Their pulse rate will usually be elevated and their blood pressure low. If all of these findings are present along with a cutaneous lesion, compatible with a Brown Recluse Spider bite, then a tentative diagnosis of *Loxoscelism* is warranted (17).

The patient should have a complete blood count and platelet count done and a complete blood chemistry panel to include electrolytes, kidney functions, 6-Glucose Phosphate Dehydrogenase, and a urinalysis. If at the time the urine specimen is obtained, there is gross hemaglobinurea, then a Foley catheter should be put in place. An I.V. should be started with a large bore needle with Ringers Lactate to run at a rate to keep the urine flow at 100cc per hour to prevent renal failure from blockage of the kidneys by hemoglobinemia. Blood should also be drawn for type and cross-matched for transfusion of whole blood in case the serum hemoglobin falls below 8 gms. The fever and headache can usually be controlled with Acetaminophen, and the nausea and vomiting with prochlorperazine. A second or third generation Cephalosporin or Azithromycin antibiotic should be given I.V. for 24 hrs, then by mouth for another six days. From the time the patient is stabilized, the

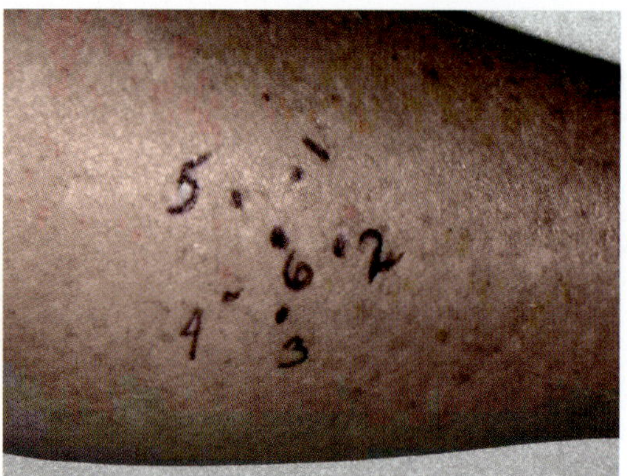

Figure 12. Treatment protocol outline of Dr. Judith Moss on a human forearm. Five sites around the bite and the sixth over the bite, one second each. Photo courtesy of Dr. C.O. Hagood.

treatment is supportive on a frequent basis until it is obvious that the symptoms are receding and the hemoglobin is beginning to rise.

The cutaneous wound can be managed with simple moist wound care. When the patient is stable, a tetanus booster should be given.

Even though rare, the combination of a large cutaneous gangrenous wound combined with systemic symptoms does occur. It is important to carefully watch the cutaneous wound and be prepared to use Dapsone or hyperbaric oxygen therapy if necessary.

CONCLUSION

Wounds produced by spider bites continue to be a problem mainly because of the problem of diagnosis of the borderline wounds and the various recommended forms of therapy. Perhaps the most important thing to remember is to closely follow the progress of the wound during the first 48–72 hours after the patient presents to see how the wound progresses. This will provide the information needed to best treat the wound. So far as the wound itself, the Golden Rule is "Good Moist Wound Care." If a progressive, gangrenous wound occurs and hyperbaric oxygen therapy is available, it is the opinion of the authors that HBO2 is the treatment of choice. Withhold Dapsone unless there is a progressive, gangrenous wound present. If there is only intense inflammation and induration with no progression, then simple wound care usually resolves the problem. When a Brown Recluse Spider bite victim develops a full blown systemic reaction with "Black Water" urine, fever, rash, nausea, vomiting, and anemia, aggressive in-hospital, intensive-care treatment is necessary. Remember, only a very few Brown Recluse spider bites ever develop into what is described as the classic necrotic wound.

REFERENCES

1. *http://www.sabramsmd.com/brs/brs_prof.html.*

2. Gendron BP. Loxosceles recluse envenomation. *Am J Emerg Med* 1990; 8(1):51-54.

3. Atkins JA, Wingo C W, Sodeman W A. Probable cause of necrotic spider bites in the Midwest. *Science* 1957;126: 73.

4. *http://www.srv.net/-dkv/hobospider/yellowsac.html.*

5. Vest DK. Necrotic Arachnadism in the northwest United States and its probable relationship to Tegenaria agrestis (Walkenauer) spiders. *Toxicon* 1987; 25(2):175-184.

6. *http://www.entomology.ucr.edu/ebeling/ebely-1.html.*

7. Capocasale PM. The dangerous spiders of Uruguay. *Institute of Biological Investigations, Merciful Stable* 1978;1-26.

8. O'Dell G, Nazhat N, Grothaus R, et al. Protein components of Loxosceles reclusa venom. *Proc Okla Acad Sci* 1968;47: 263.

9. Forrester LJ, Barrett JT, Campbell BJ. Red blood cell lysis induced by the venom of the Brown Recluse Spider: the role of Sphyngomyelinase D. *Arch Biochem Biophys* 1978;187:355-365.

10. Gomez HF, Miller MJ, Desai A, et al. Loxosceles spider venom induces the production of alpha and beta chemokines: implications for the pathogenesis of dermonecrotic arachnadism. *Inflammation* 1999; 23(3):207-215.

11. Gomez HF, Greenfield DM, Miller MJ, et al. Direct correlation between diffusion of Loxosceles recluse venom and extent of dermal inflammation. *Acad Emerg Med* 2001; 8(4):309-314.

12. Jong YS, Norment BR, Heitz JR. Separation and characterization of venom components in the Brown Recluse Spider (Loxosceles reclusa) -I- Preparative disc electrophoresis. *Toxicon*; 17:307-312.

13. Patel KD, Modur V, Zimmerman GA, et al. The necrotic venom of the recluse spider induces dysregulated endothelial cell dependant neutrophil activation. Differential Induction of GM-CSF, IL-8 and E-Selectin Expression. *J Clin Invest* 1994;(2):631-642.

14. Jong YS, Norment BR, Heitz JR. Separation and characterization of venom components in Loxosceles reclusa –II. Protease enzyme activity. *Toxicon*; 17:529-537.

15. Berger RS. The unremarkable Brown Recluse Spider bite. *JAMA* 1973; 225(9):1109-1111.

16. Stibitch AS, Schwartz RA. Brown recluse spider bite. *eMedicine J* 2001;2(6):sections 1-11:1-12. *http://www.emedicine.com/derm/topic598.htm.*

17. Bernstein B, Ehrlich F. Brown recluse spider bites. *Jour Emerg Med* 4;457-462.

18. Bey TA, Walter FG, Leber W, Schmidt J, et al. Loxosceles arizonica bite associated with shock. *An Emerg Med* 1997; 30(5):701-703.

19. Reilman GJ, Winslow CL, Teslow TW. For those who treat spider or suspected spider bites. *Toxicon* 1983; 21 (3):337-339.

20. Svendsen FJ. Treatment of clinically diagnosed Brown Recluse Spider bites with hyperbaric oxygen: a clinical observation. *J Ark Med Soc* 1986; 83(5):199-204.

21. Hobbs GD, Anderson AP, Yealy DM. Comparison of hyperbaric oxygen and Dapsone therapy for Loxosceles envenomation. *Acad Emerg Med* 1996; 3:758-761.

22. Osborne CD. Treatment of Venomous bite by high voltage direct current. *Jour Okla State Med Assoc* 1990; 83(1):9-14.

23. Guderian R, et al. High voltage shock treatment for snake bite. *Lancet* 1986; 2: 229.

24. *http://www.spiderbitetreatment.com/minisguse.htm.* Abrams S. Brown recluse spider bites (Loxosceles reclusa). 1998.

25. Barrett SM, Romine-Jenkins M. Dapsone or electric shock therapy of Brown Recluse Spider envenomation? *Ann Emerg Med* 1994; 24(1):21-25.

26. Merigian KS, Blaho K. Envenomation from the Brown Recluse Spider: review of mechanism and treatment options. *Amer J Therapy* 1996;3(3):724-734.

REVIEW QUESTIONS

1.) In the Brown Recluse Spider bite wound, tissue gangrene is caused by:
    a. Infection
    b. E-selectin
    c. Sphyngomyelinase D
    d. Interleukin-8

2.) The Brown Recluse Spider is found in:
    a. Central US through deep South and Texas
    b. Oregon
    c. Wisconsin
    d. New York

3.) The wound of the Brown Recluse Spider can be:
    a. Rather insignificant
    b. Large with a rash, nausea and fever
    c. Accompanied by the patient having "Coca-Cola" urine
    d. All of the above

4.) Treatment with hyperbaric oxygen therapy can:
    a. Rapidly demarcate the gangrenous area of the wound
    b. Increase the pO_2 of the circulating blood at wound site
    c. Prepare a good granulation bed in preparation for grafting in future
    d. All of the above

5.) Dapsone therapy for Brown Recluse Spider bites:
    a. 200 mg per day for ten days
    b. Contraindicated in 6-G-PD deficiency
    c. Contraindicated if patient is taking Trimethoprim
    d. All of the above

Answers: 1c, 2a, 3d, 4d, 5d

CHAPTER **23**

APPROACH TO COMMONLY MISDIAGNOSED WOUNDS AND UNUSUAL LEG ULCERS

CHAPTER TWENTY-THREE OVERVIEW

Approach to Commonly Misdiagnosed Wounds and Unusual Leg Ulcers

Jayesh B. Shah

INTRODUCTION

Some wounds demonstrate difficulty with healing despite seemingly appropriate management. In such situations, physicians should step back and look at the wound afresh. One should refocus at the complete history and physical and consider performing a wound biopsy, because often, failure to heal is a result of misdiagnosis. Sometimes, misdiagnosis occurs as a result of unusual presentation of a common condition, and in some instances, an unusual systemic condition presents as a wound.

Most often, misdiagnosis results from overlooking simple clues. As the first step to healing a wound is to make an accurate diagnosis, the wound care physician, like a detective, should gather all the clues and try to put them together to make a correct diagnosis.

CLINICAL CLUES TOWARDS DIAGNOSIS

Inability to heal may be due to local or systemic factors.

Local factors may include the following:

a. Repeated external trauma because of inappropriate offloading
b. Foot deformity causing abnormal pressure areas
c. Uncontrolled edema
d. Injury from use of toxic substances
e. Inappropriate measures for exudate control
f. Inappropriate infection control
g. Tissue tension
h. Hematoma formation
i. Undebrided wound
j. Poor blood supply
h. Hypoxia

Systemic factors may include the following:
  a. Arterial insufficiency
  b. Venous insufficiency
  c. Systemic conditions (collagen vascular disease, sickle cell disease, hemoglobinopathies, uremia, diabetes, jaundice)
  d. Immunosuppresive drugs (systemic corticosteroids, anticancer drugs, NSAIDS)
  e. Immunosuppressive diseases (HIV)
  f. Local or systemic malignancy
  g. Exposure to radiation
  h. Malnutrition
  i. Old age
  j. Systemic Infection

All these local and systemic factors need to be looked at when taking history of a patient with wound.

CLUES FROM A GOOD HISTORY

Even with the technological innovations of the twenty-first century, history taking still remains the best and cheapest tool to make a good diagnosis. Recognizing clues from patient's history can give important information about the patient's wound.

CLUES FROM EXAMINATION

"Simple attention to the clinical clues is really a good start, before you even touch the wound." Vincent Falanga, MD

General Appearance
- Cushingoid appearance—Corticosteroid use, disease with excessive release of corticosteroids
- Rheumatoid joints—Pyoderma gangrenosum, rheumatoid ulcer, vasculitis
- Cachexia—Malnutrition, AIDS, cancer, other infectious etiologies (tuberculosis)
- Scleroderma face (purse string mouth)—Calcinosis, Raynaud's phenomena
- Abnormal affect, posture, facial expression—Factitious disorder
- Facial palsy, weakness in one or more extremities—Cerebrovascular accident. If bed bound or wheelchair bound, more prone to pressure ulceration

Appearance of the Extremity/Extremities
- Edema—Venous disease, deep vein thrombosis, lymphedema, congestive heart failure with dependent edema
- Foot deformities—Neuropathic wounds, diabetes with autonomic neuropathy, osteomyelitis, rheumatoid arthritis
- Cyanosis—Arterial disease, Raynaud's syndrome

- Dependent rubor—Arterial disease
- Erythema—Infection, contact dermatitis
- Livedo Reticularis—Cholesterol emboli, collagen vascular disease, cryoglobulinemia
- Sclerodactyly—Scleroderma, Raynaud's disease
- Lipodermatosclerosis/ hemosiderin pigmentation—Venous disease
- Eczema—Irritation arising from previous treatments

Appearance of the Wound

Configuration/Wound edge
- Undermining edge—Pressure, pyoderma gangrenosum
- Irregular edge/intact fascia—Venous
- Undulating/Scalloped—Rheumatoid ulcer
- Linear/Geometric—Factitious
- Fenestrated—Pyoderma gangrenosum
- Eschar—Ischemia, pressure
- Irregular, raised, discolored—Malignancy

Wound base
- Green—Pseudomonas infection
- Pale—Pressure, ischemia
- Black—Arterial insufficiency
- Red—Good granulation/ vascularity
- Exposed tendon—Pressure, shear, tension, fistula
- Exposed bone—Osteomyelitis, pressure

Location of Wound
- Weightbearing surface—Neuropathic wound, pressure
- Digital Ulcers—Ischemia
- Gaiter area—Venous disease
- Tibial area—Arterial disease, Necrobiosis lipoidica diabeticorum
- Vaginal ulcers—Behcet's Disease
- Underlying internal viscera—Fistula, abscess, Crohn's disease, radiation injury

Surrounding Skin
- Edge necrosis—Pyoderma gangrenosum, vasculitis, ischemia
- Redness around the wound—Vasculitis, arterial disease, contact dermatitis
- Purpura—Vasculitis
- Purple discoloration—Pyoderma gangrenosum, vasculitis, cryoglobulinemia, cryofibrinogenemia,
- Micro livedo—Cryoglobulinemia, cryofibrinogenemia, antiphospholipid syndrome
- Red/yellow—Necrobiosis lipoidica diabeticorum

WOUND BIOPSY

"When in doubt, consider wound biopsy." Jayesh Shah, MD

Wound biopsy is a simple bedside procedure performed to establish a definitive diagnosis in a chronic nonhealing wound.

Correct time to obtain a biopsy of a wound base and its margins remains controversial. Some clinicians advocate performing biopsies of wounds that have been present for longer than three months and wounds that have not responded to standard therapy. Some clinicians routinely biopsy all wounds. Considering the uncommon nature of malignant wounds, some authors suggest that only suspicious wounds undergo biopsy. Following indications can serve as general guidelines for performing a biopsy.

Indications

1. Quantitative culture of infected wound
2. Chronic wound refractory to healing by standard wound care
3. Wounds that have increased in size despite appropriate treatment
4. Malodorous wounds
5. Painful wounds
6. Wounds with excess granulation tissue that extends beyond the margins
7. Wounds with irregular base or margin.
8. Wounds that experience a change in drainage, excess bleeding, or exophytic growth

Procedure

Wound biopsy can be done surgically in an operating room or can be done in a clinic depending on the type of wound with punch biopsy (biopsy in which the tissue is obtained by a punch) (Figure 1); or wedge biopsy (biopsy in which the tissue is removed by surgical cutting) (Figure 2). Optimally, wound biopsy should include wound bed and the surrounding skin. Wedge biopsy is indicated if cancer is suspected. Biopsy should be extended well beyond the wound perimeter. Also, multiple wound biopsies from different areas of the wound should be performed. A biopsy should also be taken from the center of the wound bed (Figure 1). If biopsy results do not match the clinical findings then repeat biopsy should be performed.

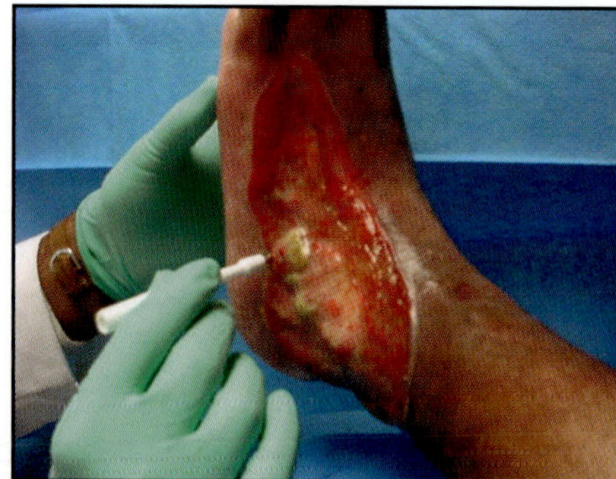

Figure 1. Physician performing quantitative wound culture by punch biopsy.

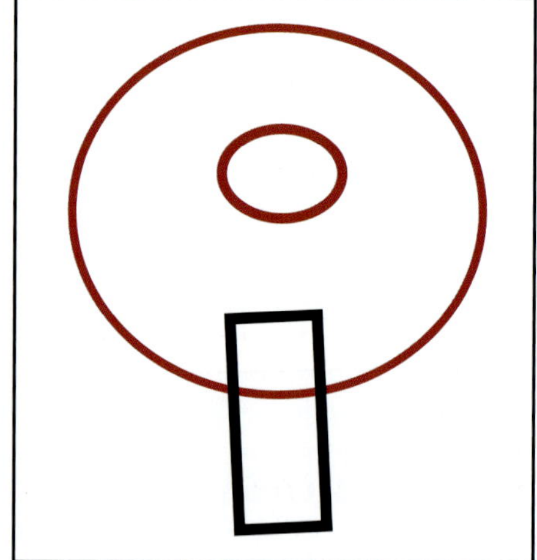

Figure 2. Sketch of wound sites for wedge biopsy.

Complications

Biopsy sites in wounds usually heal and do not generally worsen the condition. Most common complication from biopsy can be bleeding from the biopsy site, which in most cases, can be stopped with chemical cauterization.

Relative Contraindications

1. Blood dyscrasia
2. Extremely vascular wounds or venous congestion
3. Anticoagulation medications

COMMONLY MISDIAGNOSED WOUNDS AND UNUSUAL LEG ULCERS

Malignancy

Chronic nonhealing wounds of two to three months duration, especially those which are refractory to healing, should be looked at with high index of suspicion for malignancy. Malignancies and wounds can be related in two ways: there can be malignant degeneration of chronic wound into cancer or, malignancy can present as chronic wound. Malignancy found within chronic wound, though rare, is well documented.

The following clues should make a wound care physician suspicious of malignancy.

1. History of repeated trauma
2. Wound with no obvious etiology
3. Wound at unusual location
4. Asymmetric wound
5. Exuberant granulation tissue
6. Rolled out edges
7. Fungating growth
8. Purple red color around the ulcer
9. Ulcer in center of pigmented lesion (suspect melanoma)
10. Wounds secondary to burns, trauma, radiotherapy and diabetes, are at a risk for malignant degeneration

Malignant wounds are more common in older patients with advanced cancer, although they can develop in patients with localized cancer and can be present for several years. In general, malignant wounds will not heal unless the malignancy is amenable to treatment with anticancer therapy. For basal or squamous cell cancer, complete excision or Mohs micrographic surgery is the treatment of choice.

Basal cell carcinoma

Basal cell carcinoma is a malignancy arising from epidermal basal cells. In a study by Hansson et al, basal cell cancer was found to be the most common malignancy (13). Usually, basal cell cancer presents as a wound, outgrows its blood supply and erodes, and subsequently, ulcerates (Figures 3 and 4). Often, this ulcer remains misdiagnosed for a long time, unless a wound biopsy is done early on.

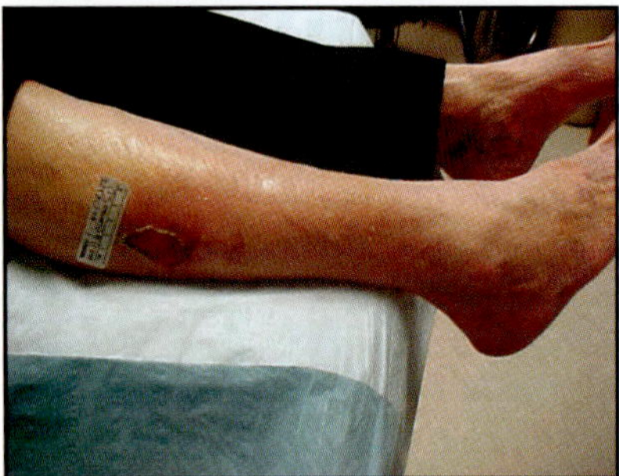

Figure 3. Basal cell carcinoma initially presented as an ulcer of leg.

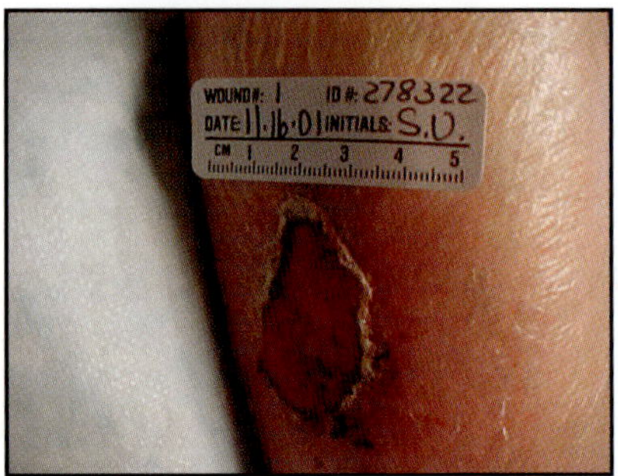

Figure 4. Basal cell carcinoma.

Squamous cell carcinoma

Primary cutaneous squamous cell carcinoma is a malignant neoplasm of keratinizing epidermal cells (Figure 5). Unlike basal cell carcinoma, which have a very low metastatic potential, squamous cell carcinoma can metastasize and grow very rapidly. Marjolin (9) was the first to report that borders of a chronic wound underwent malignant changes. The development of squamous cell carcinoma has been reported in chronic wounds secondary to burns, trauma, hidradenitis suppurativa, radiotherapy, diabetes, draining sinus tract of chronic osteomyelitis. It appears that squamous cell carcinomas occur more frequently than basal cell carcinoma within a venous ulcer. Until recently, amputation had been the treatment of choice for squamous cell carcinomas that arose within chronic wounds associated with chronic osteomyelitis; however, other reports have shown that other methods of ensuring complete local excision are also useful.

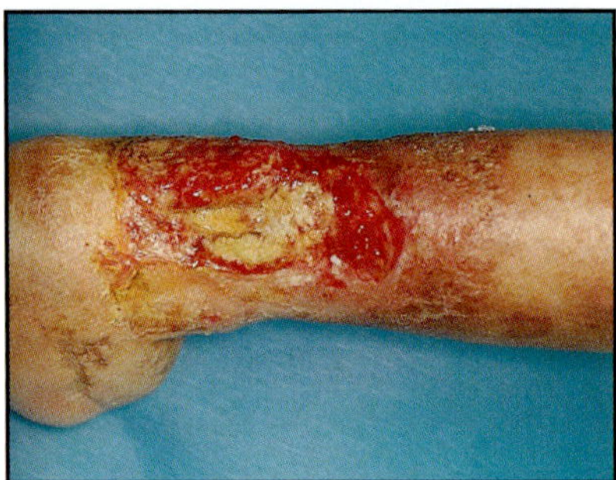

Figure 5. Non-healing wound diagnosed as squamous cell carcinoma.

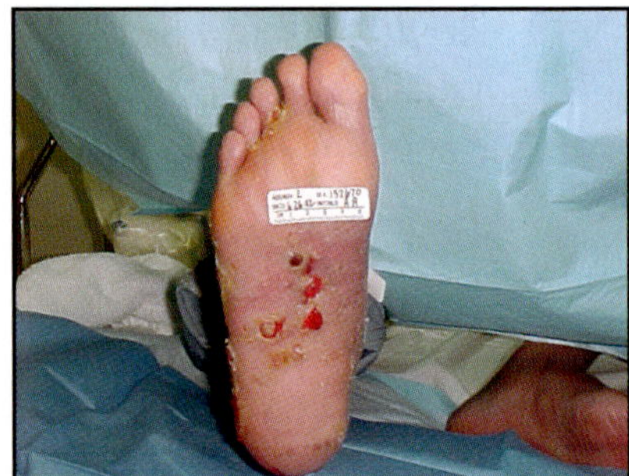

Figure 6. Kaposi's sarcoma that initially presented as a diabetic foot ulcer in a non HIV patient.

Kaposi's sarcoma

Kaposi's sarcoma is highly associated with HIV and herpes simplex infection. It is mainly associated with AIDS. Kaposi's sarcoma, though rare, is reported to present as an ulcer (Figure 6) associated with diabetes. Treatment mainly includes observation, surgical excision, radiation therapy, intralesion chemotherapy, systemic chemotherapy, using a combination of chemotherapy. Recently topical treatment with 9-cis-Retinoic acid (alitretinoin gel) has been proven superior to vehicle gel.

Cutaneous lymphomas

Cutaneous lymphoma may present as various types of skin lesions, and rarely as an ulcer (Figure 7). Ulcerative cutaneous lymphomas are associated with poor prognosis. They are increasingly seen in severely immunocompromised patients. Many of these lymphomas appear to be B-cell lymphomas, but occasionally, T-cell lymphoma can also be seen (Figure 8).

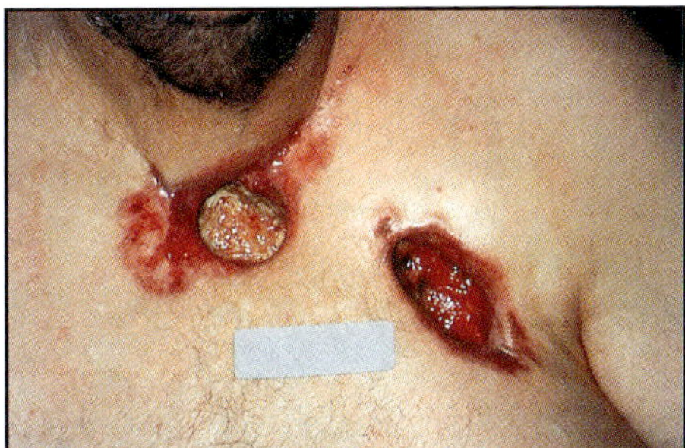
Figure 7. Patient with non-healing wound diagnosed with non-Hodgkin's lymphoma.

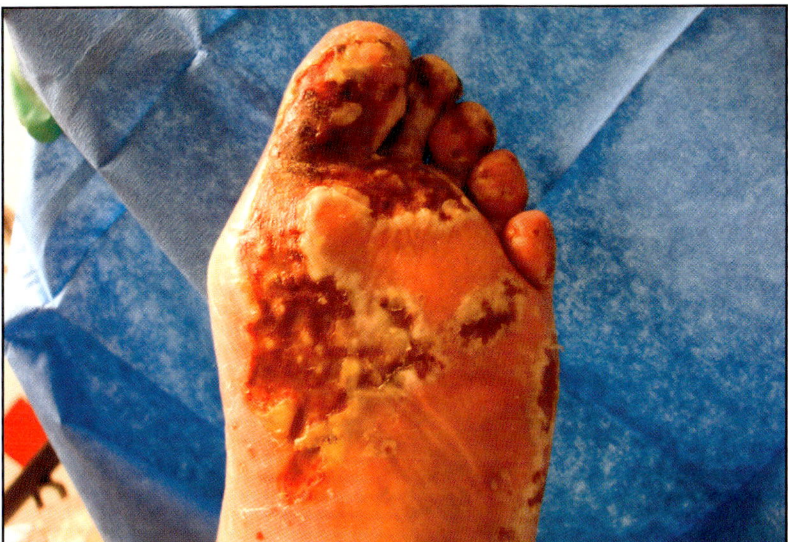
Figure 8. Wound on foot diagnosed as cutanous T-cell lymphoma.

INFECTION

Any wound can be infected with usual organisms such as staphylococci, streptococci, pseudomonas, etc. Some of the unusual infections associated with wounds are discussed below.

Actinomycosis

Clinical types of actinomycosis are predominantly cervico—facial, abdominal or thoracic. Actinomycosis of foot is very rare with only a couple of case reports in the literature. Actinomycosis israelli is the most common cause of actinomycosis in humans. Actinomyces organisms are gram positive, non spore forming anaerobic bacilli. Typical course of development is a painless swelling of the soft tissue that becomes indurated, followed by a period of apparent inactivity; then draining sinuses appear, followed by sinus tracts and osteomyelitis (Figure 9).

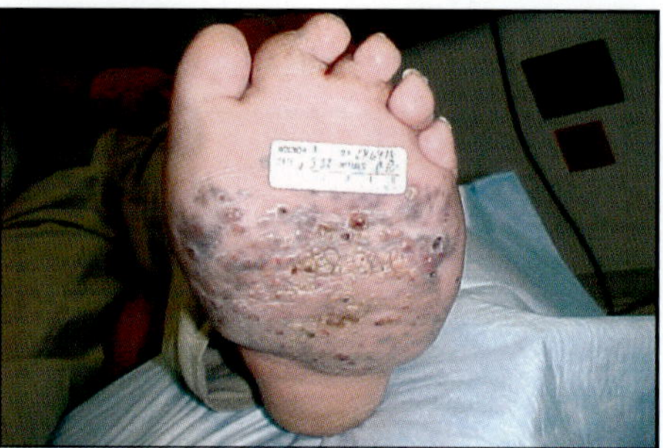

Figure 9. Chronic actinomycosis that initially presented as multiple ulcers of leg.

Recommended treatment is surgical excision of all necrotic tissue, sinus tracts, and infected bone, followed by a post operative course of antibiotics for minimum of six months; Ampicillin is the first drug of choice, followed by clindamycin and chloramphenicol.

Tuberculosis (Mycobacterium tuberculli)

Tuberculosis is caused by bacteria belonging to the mycobacterium tuberculosis complex. The disease usually affects the lungs, but, in some instances, it can cause cutaneous manifestations like abscesses, chronic ulcers, scrofuloderma, lupus vulguris, milliary lesions and erythema nodusum.

Nontuberculous Mycobacteria

Nontuberculous mycobacteria are bacteria except Mycobacterium leprae and Mycobacterium tuberculli.

Swimming pool and fish tank granuloma

After contact with contaminated tropical fish tanks, swimming pool, or saltwater fish for a period from one week up to two months, a small violet nodule or pustule may appear at the site of minor trauma. The lesion may evolve to form a crusted ulcer or small abscess. It is usually caused by M. marinum. Lesions often heal spontaneously, however, in case of persistence, lesions should be treated with rifampin in combination with ethambutol, Trimethoprim-sulfamethoxazole, or minocycline for a period of at least three months.

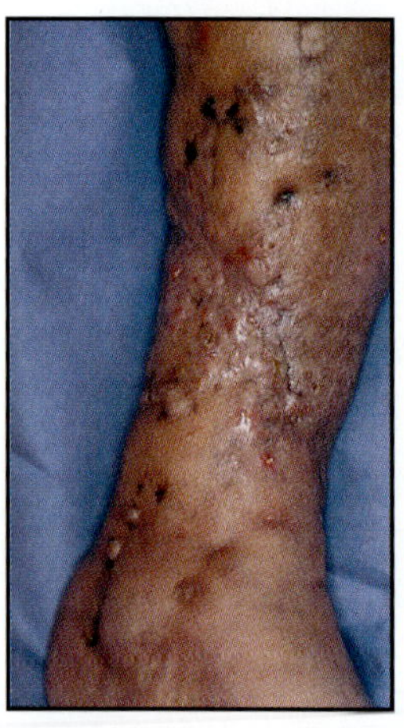

Figure 10. Buruli ulcer.

Buruli ulcer

In many tropical areas throughout the world, M. ulcerans may cause an itching nodule on arms or legs, which then breaks down to form a shallow ulcer of variable size (Figure 10). Treatment usually consists of excision, or treatment with rifampin, clofazimine or trimethoprim sulfamethaxole.

Nodular Skin Lesions Associated with **M. Fortuitum**

Occasionally, these kind of mycobacteria are isolated from nodular skin lesions (Figure 11) of hospitalized patients, particularly those who are immunosuppressed and diabetics. In some instances, there is associated lymphatic spread. They are rapidly growing mycobacteria and are known to be resistant to most antituberculous drugs.

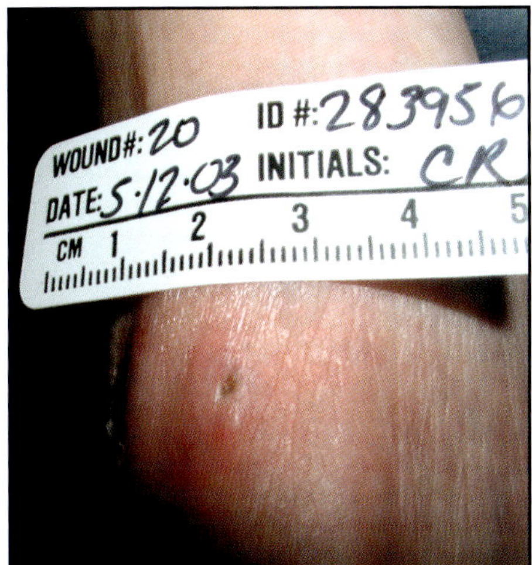

Figure 11. Nodular skin lesion diagnosed with *M. fortuitum* infection.

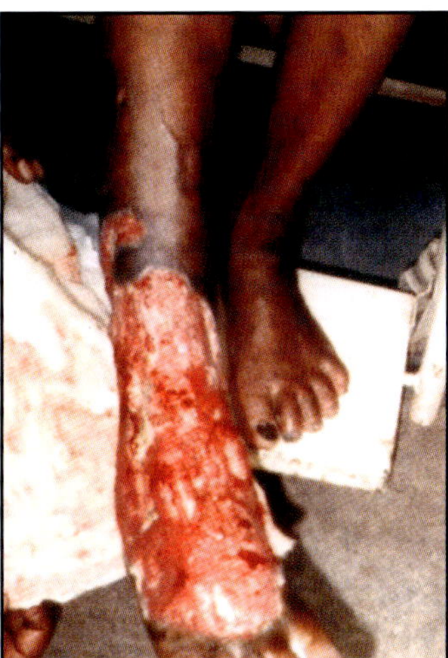

Figure 12. Patient with leprosy presenting with ulcer.

Leprosy

Leprosy (Hansen's disease) is a chronic granulomatous disease caused by Mycobacterium leprae, that attacks superficial tissues, especially the skin and peripheral nerves (Figure 12). Leprosy still remains as a common cause of non-healing wounds in developing countries like India, Brazil, Bangladesh, Indonesia, and Myanmar.

Sporotrichosis

Infection results from inoculation of S. *schenckii* (fungus) into subcutaneous tissue via minor trauma. Nursery workers, florists and gardeners acquire this illness from roses, sphagnum moss, and other plants. It usually presents as non tender red maculopapular granuloma confined to the site of inoculation which sometimes ulcerates. Usually treatment consists of either saturated solution of potassium iodide, or oral itraconozole.

Other rare infections to consider in patients with non-healing wounds are coccidiomycosis, histoplasmosis, syphillis, viral infections such as herpes simplex or cytomegalovirus, and protozoal infections like leishmaniasis, to name a few.

For more information about infection management see the chapters by JL Le Frock entitled, "Skin, Skin Structure, and Muscle Infections" and "Post-Operative Surgical Site Infections (SSIs) and Non-Necrotizing Skin and Soft Tissue Infections."

WOUNDS ASSOCIATED WITH VASCULITIS AND CONNECTIVE TISSUE DISORDERS

This section will focus on inflammatory causes of leg ulcers with emphasis on connective tissue disorders, pyoderma gangrenosum, vasculitis and microthrombotic disease.

Pyoderma Gangrenosum

Pyoderma gangrenosum is a noninfectious neutrophilic dermatosis that usually starts with sterile pustules, which rapidly progresses to painful ulcers of variable depth and size with undermined violaceous borders. Pyoderma gangrenosum is most commonly associated with an underlying disease such as inflammatory bowel disease, rheumatologic disease, hematological disease, or, malignancy. Diagnosis of pyoderma gangrenosum is based upon any underlying disease, typical presentation, histopathology, and exclusion of other diseases that can lead to a similar appearance.

The four different types of pyoderma gangrenosum include: ulcerative, pustular, bullous, and vegetative. In general, ulcerative variant is most common, has an association with inflammatory bowel disease and arthritis, and tends to evolve rapidly (Figure 13). Clinically, it is described as ulceration with a purulent base, undermined borders, and surrounding erythema. Pustular pyoderma gangrenosum is most commonly associated with active inflammatory bowel disease. Clinically, the lesions consist of discrete pustules with an inflammatory border occurring on the normal skin. Bullous pyoderma gangrenosum is often noted in patients with leukemia and other myeloproliferative disorders. It is characterized by superficial and painful bullae with progression to erosion and ulceration. Vegetative pyoderma gangrenosum is the most indolent of the four clinical variants. Clinically, it is more superficial ulceration without any undermining border and purulent base as opposed to the more common ulcerative type.

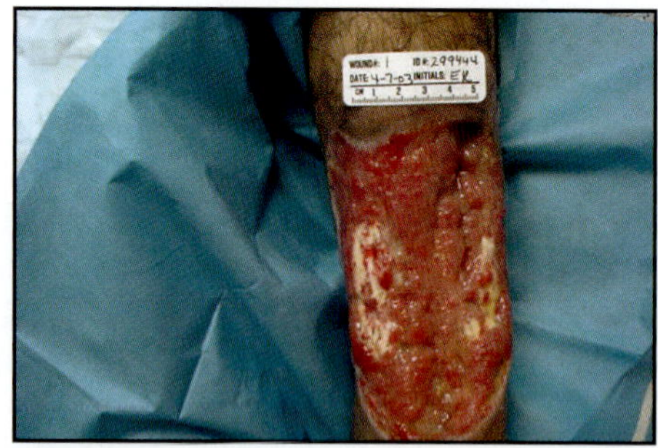

Figure 13. Ulcerative variant of pyoderma gangrenosum.

Treatment of pyoderma gangrenosum includes systemic corticosteroids 100–200 mg/day; combination of corticosteroids with cytotoxic drugs; combination of corticosteroids with sulfa drugs, such as Dapsone, clofazimine, minocycline and thalidomide.

Alternative treatments may include local application of granulocyte–macrophage colony stimulating factor; intravenous immunoglobulins; plamapheresis; skin transplants; application of bioengineered skin; hyperbaric oxygen therapy.

Rheumatoid Arthritis and Ulceration

Rheumatoid arthritis is a systemic autoimmune disorder of unknown etiology. The cutaneous manifestations include rheumatoid nodules over pressure points in 25–30% of patients with vasculitic lesions and leg ulceration in approximately 8–9 % of patients.

Typically, the ulcer in rheumatoid arthritis is smooth, undulating, with irregular "geographic" shape and is extremely painful (Figure 14). Accompanying cutaneous findings include palpable purpura and livedo reticularis. Occasionally there is histological evidence of leukocytoclastic vasculitis.

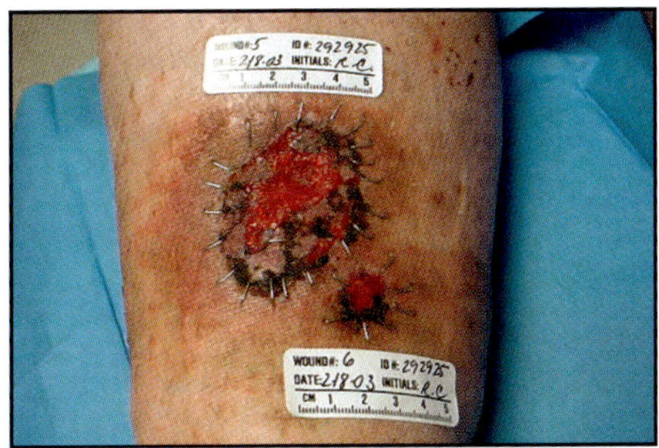

Figure 14. Ulceration in rheumotoid arthritis patient.

Some rheumatoid arthritis patients with several nodules have a constellation of symptoms collectively known as Felty's syndrome. This syndrome is described as the combination of rheumatoid arthritis, splenomegaly, granulocytopenia, and leg ulcers.

Treatment of rheumatoid ulcers often requires high dose corticosteroids, cyclophosphamide, Dapsone, alone or with colchicines and certain disease modifying drugs.

Wound treatment includes, standard wound care plus growth factors or bio-engineered skin.

Systemic Lupus Erythematosus (SLE)

The incidence of leg ulceration in SLE patients is between 2–8%. These ulcers can be extremely painful and are typically found over the pretibial surface and malleolar area. The ulcers may precede the diagnosis of SLE by many years. They are characterized by well defined margins with a purulent bed and varying amount of granulation tissue (Figure 15). Surrounding skin may be normal in appearance or erythematous with

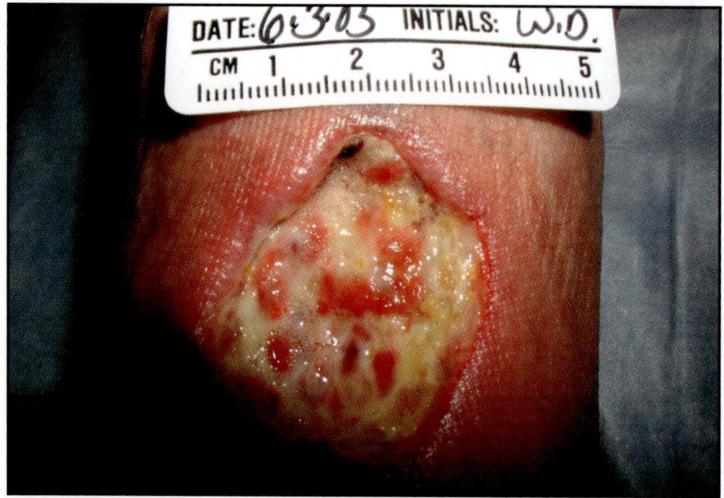

Figure 15. Ulceration in a systemic lupus erythematosus (SLE) patient.

evidence of atrophie blanche. Livedo reticularis is often observed in SLE and is associated with the antiphospholipid syndrome.

Treatment is often challenging, topical retinoic acid has been shown to improve granulation tissue in patients on systemic corticosteroids. Patients with antiphospholipid syndrome have shown promising results with stanozolol. Intralesional triamcinolone acetonide (5 mg/ml) has also been used with success.

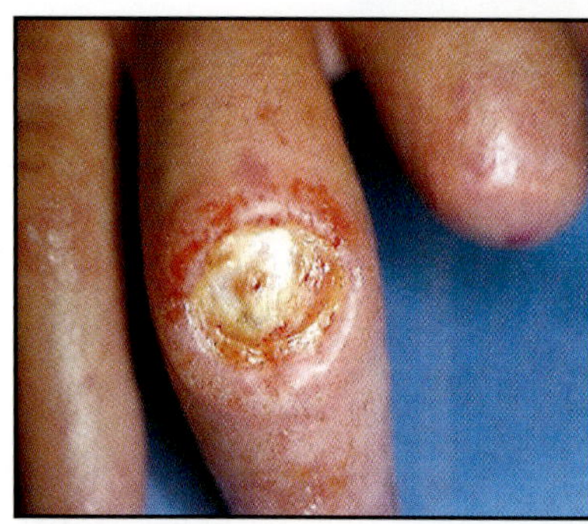

Figure 16. Scleroderma

Scleroderma

Scleroderma is an autoimmune disorder of unknown etiology. Often, patients will have a "purse–string mouth," and unusually smooth facial skin. Sclerodactyly is a hallmark and ulcers usually develop over the digits and overlying bony prominences (Figure 16). Digital ulcers are difficult to reepithelialize and are usually refractory to healing. Occlusive dressings may provide pain relief.

Vasculitis

Vasculitis, or inflammation of blood vessels, plays a crucial role in a number of collagen vascular disorders. Treatment depends on accurate diagnosis of the underlying cause and is directed at eliminating the underlying cause, in addition to local and/or systemic anti-inflammatory and immunosuppressive agents. Vasculitis usually affects males and females equally and is most common in the elderly.

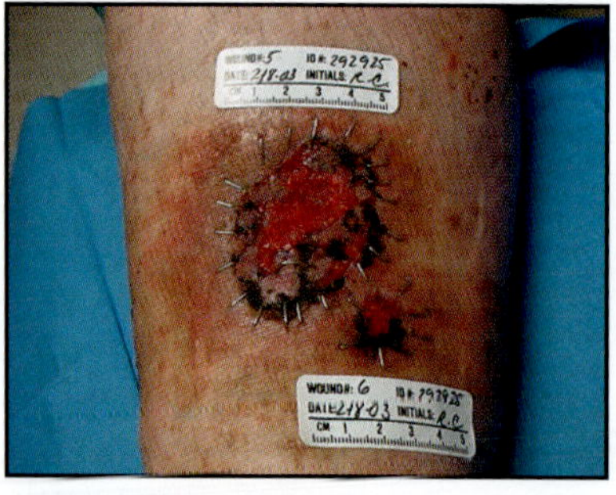

Figure 17. Vasculitis

Vasculitic wounds usually presents as flat red macules, nodules or purpura anywhere on the body, but most frequently appears on the back, hands, buttocks, inside of forearms and lower extremities, extensor surfaces of the joints. These lesions can ulcerate and present as non-healing wounds (Figure 17).

Classification of vasculitis (Adapted from Cupps TR, Fauci AS) (3)
1. Polyarteritis nodosa group
   • Classic polyarteritis nodosa (classic PAN)
   • Allergic angitis and granulomatosis
   • Systemic necrotizing vasculitis 'overlap syndrome'
2. Hypersensitivity vasculitis
   • Vasculitis associated with
        a. Infections
        b. Chemical/drug exposure
        c. Connective tissue disease
   • Serum sickness
   • Henoch– Schonlein purpura
   • Erythema elevatum diutinum
   • Mixed essential cryoglobulinemia with vasculitis
   • Vasculitis associated with other primary disorders
3. Wegener's granulomatosis
4. Lymphomatoid granulomatosis
5. Giant cell arteritis (Temporal, Takayasu's)
6. Other
   • Mucocutaneous lymph node syndrome
   • Thromboangiitis obliterans (Buerger's disease)
   • Central nervous system vasculitis

ULCERS DUE TO DERMAL THROMBI OR MICROTHROMBOTIC DISEASE

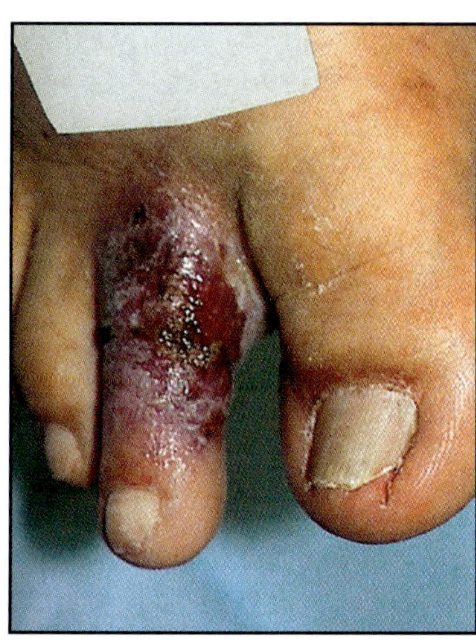

Figure 18. Antiphospholipid syndrome.

Disorders such as antiphospholipid syndrome, cryofibrinogenemia, cryoglobulinemia, cholesterol embolization, thrombocytosis and warfarin necrosis can cause thrombi within the microvasculature, resulting in ulceration.

Usually patients with microthrombotic disease presents with livedo reticularis pattern, purple discoloration of surrounding skin with cyanosis. Patients experience intense pain out of proportion to the size of the wound.

Antiphospholipid syndrome

Antiphospholipid syndrome (Figure 18) is associated with a multitude of disease states, and involves both lupus anticoagulant and/or anticardiolipin antibodies, occurring in an idiopathic form, or with collagen vascular disease.

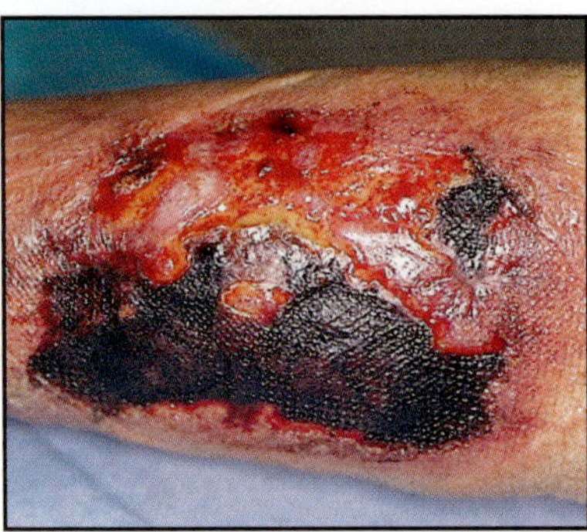

Figure 19. Cryofibrinogemia.

Cryofibrinogemia

Cryofibrinogemia (Figure 19) is a disease associated with the presence of cryofibrinogen in plasma. It can be a primary process or secondary to a neoplastic, infectious, thrombotic or connective tissue disorder.

Cryoglobulinemia

Cryoglobulinemia is a condition in which serum proteins precipitate at cold temperatures. It is often associated with hepatitis C, collagen vascular diseases, vasculitis, lymphomas and myeloproliferative disorders.

Cholesterol emboli

Cholesterol emboli results from the dissolution of cholesterol plaques. Cutaneous manifestations resemble vasculitis. There is often a history of recent surgical manipulation, angiography, or the commencement of anticoagulant therapy.

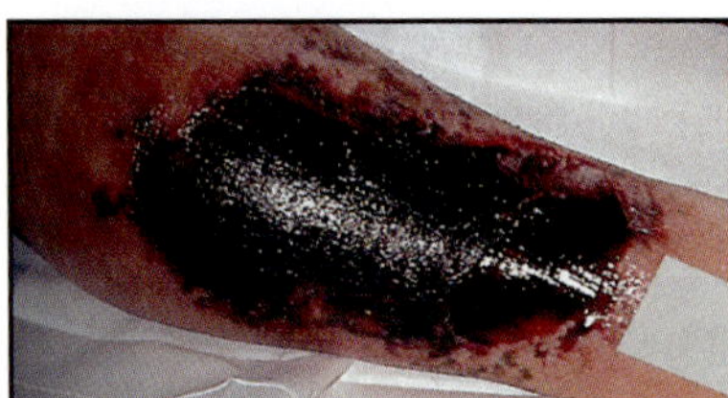

Figure 20. Warfarin necrosis.

Warfarin necrosis

Warfarin necrosis (Figure 20) may occur with initiation of warfarin (Coumadin®) therapy (within the first week) or secondary to protein C deficiency. The ulcerations usually appear on the trunk.

OTHER UNUSUAL WOUND CONDITIONS

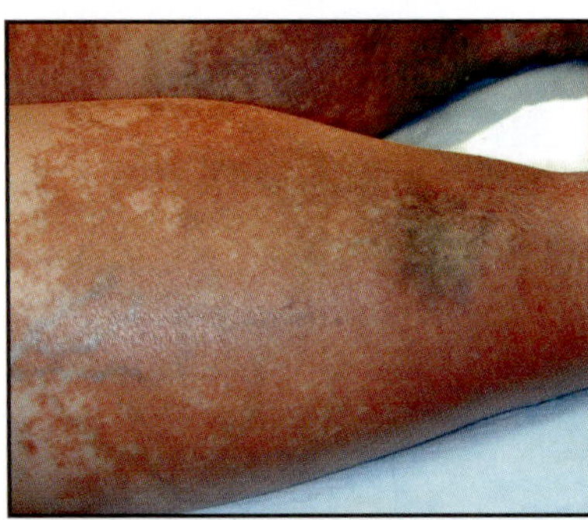

Figure 21. Lipodermatosclerosis.

Lipodermatosclerosis

Lipodermatosclerosis (Figure 21) is manifested by indurated skin that usually occurs on the medial aspect of the lower leg in patients with venous disease. In the acute phase, the skin is intensely red with scaling and exquisitely painful. In the chronic phase, there is pronounced hyperpigmentation and painless induration.

Necrobiosis Lipoidica Diabeticorum

Necrobiosis lipoidica diabeticorum (Figure 22) is a skin lesion or ulceration typically located on the shins and is usually associated with diabetes. The typical lesion is an irregular ovoid reddish- brown plaque with a shiny yellow center and a violaceous indurated border. Typically, the lesions occur over

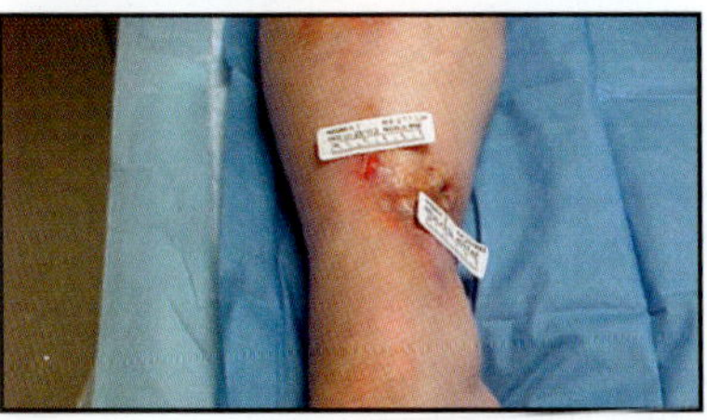

Figure 22. Necrobiosis lipoidica diabeticorum.

the anterior aspect of the lower extremities bilaterally but not symmetrically. The size and depth may vary. Treatment includes intralesional corticosteroid injections, topical cortico-steroids, perilesional heparin, aspirin and nicotinamide.

Radiation Injury

Injury can occur from therapeutic doses of radiation that, over time, can impair one or more phases involved in wound healing. Usually, radiation wounds show atrophy of tissues and show no evidence of independent healing capability (Figure 23). Fibrosis and poor wound bed is commonly seen. Biopsy of the wound bed should be performed to rule out cancer, particularly squamous cell cancer. Treatment of radiation induced wound includes a complete excisional debridement and closure with an appropriate skin or muscle flap. Hyperbaric oxygen therapy and growth factors has been shown to augment healing of radiation wounds. For more information see the Feldmeier et al. chapter entitled, "Problem Wounds: The Impact of Radiation Therapy and Chemotherapy."

Chemical Wounds

Chemical wounds can arise from drugs like cancer drugs, hydroxyurea (Figure 24), radium, etc. Also, chemical wounds can arise from spider bites, ant bites, or snake bites. Spider bites are very common in certain endemic areas of United States. Brown recluse bite is prevalent in the Southern, Western, and Midwestern United States. The toxins of a spider can cause a chemical wound following envenomation. Usually the wound starts with a blister and then progresses to areas of necrosis. Patient usually does not experience pain at the site of the bite.

Usual treatment of a spider bite includes initial ice application to the wound area, appropriate excision of the wound. Dapsone, 50–100mg/day may be used to limit the immediate zone of ischemia, if given within 48 hours of the spider bite.

For more details on spider bites, see the chapter entitled "Necrotic Wounds Produced by Spider Bites" by CO Hagood and JR Wilson.

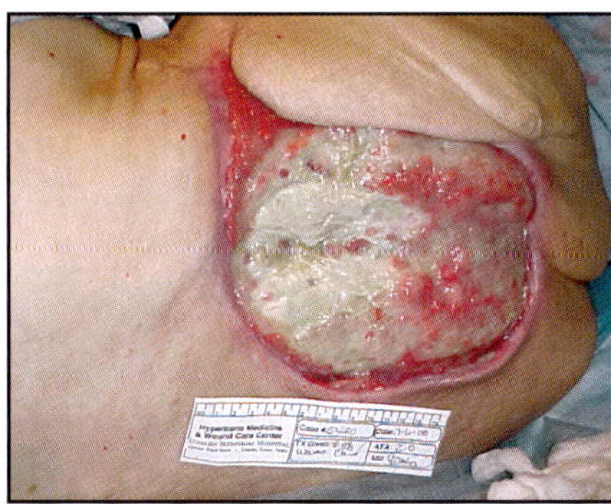

Figure 23. Radiation injury.

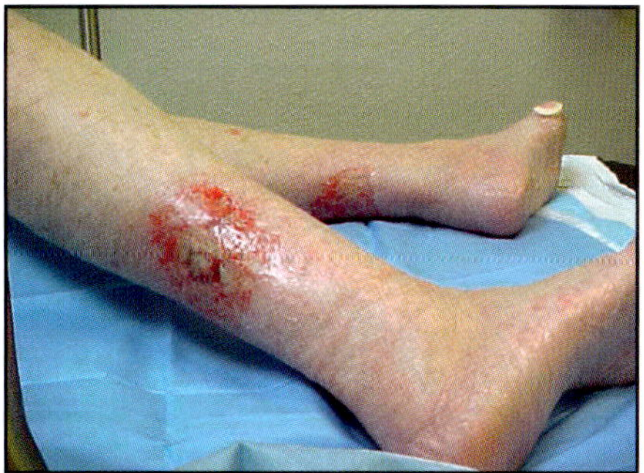

Figure 24. Chemical wound secondary to drug hydroxyurea

Sickle Cell Ulcers

Sickle cell disease (Figure 25) is an inherited hemoglobinapathy wherein sickle shaped red blood cells are formed that clogs the capillaries and prevents normal flow to the tissues, which can lead to local hypoxia, thrombosis and ischemia. Sickle cell patients are prone to ulceration and the ulceration can become chronic in nature. These ulcers are painful, debilitating, difficult to treat and prone to recurrence. Sickle cell ulcers frequently become infected or heavily colonized with bacteria.

This disease affects about 0.6% of the African American population in the United States, approximately 50,000 cases are reported every year. The trait is present in approximately 40% of the general population in some areas of Africa, descendents of Asiatic Indians, Italians, Greeks, or Mediterraneans.

Calciphylaxis

Calcific uraemic arteriopathy (calciphylaxis) (Figure 26) is a rare necrotizing cutaneous abnormality which is now increasingly recognized in the dialysis patient. It is usually associated with secondary hyperparathyroidism in the presence of advanced renal failure and high calcium/phosphate product. Treatment is difficult and often unsuccessful with high mortality rate of 50–100%. Ulcerations associated with calciphylaxis can be located on the heels, fingers, and toes and may manifest ischemic and gangrenous changes (Figure 26). Usually they are sudden in presentation. Patient usually has a black eshar. Ischemia can extend from skin to skeletal muscles. Skin biopsy will show calcium deposition.

Treatment includes standard wound care, parathyroidectomy, and hyperbaric oxygen. Low doses of warfarin or calcium channel blockers may be helpful. Also, low calcium hemodialysis is also found to be promising.

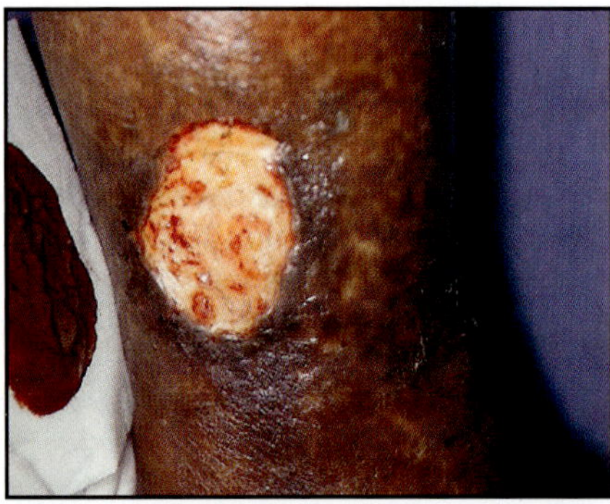

Figure 25. Ulceration secondary to sickle cell disease.

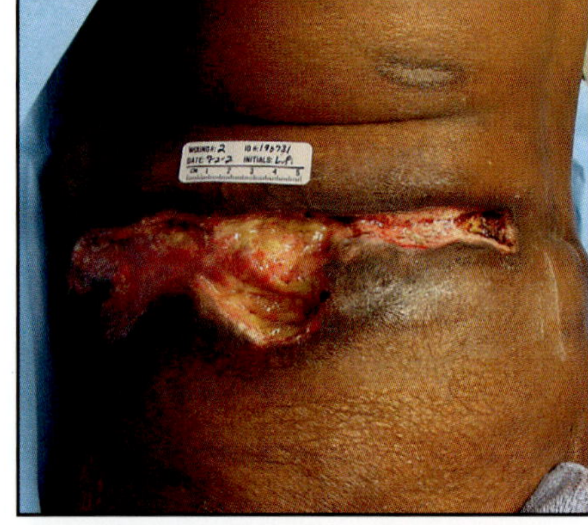

Figure 26. Calciphylaxis.

Factitious Disorder

This group of patients usually have unexplained urge to scratch and harm themselves. These patients have an associated psychiatric disorder. Ulcers have geometric edges and good granulation tissue on the wound base (Figure 27). Diagnosis sometimes is made after excluding all other diagnosis.

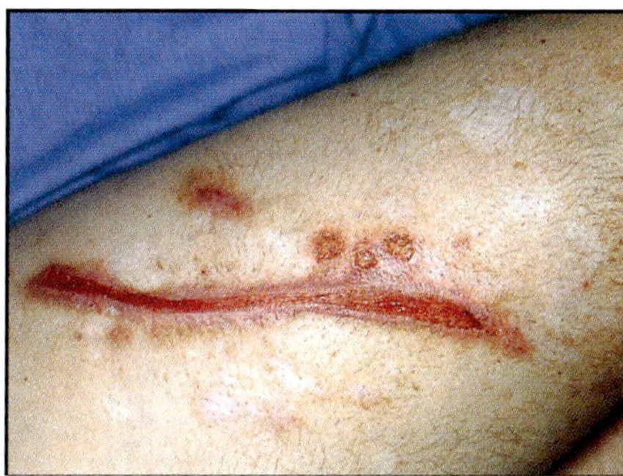

Figure 27. Factitious disorder.

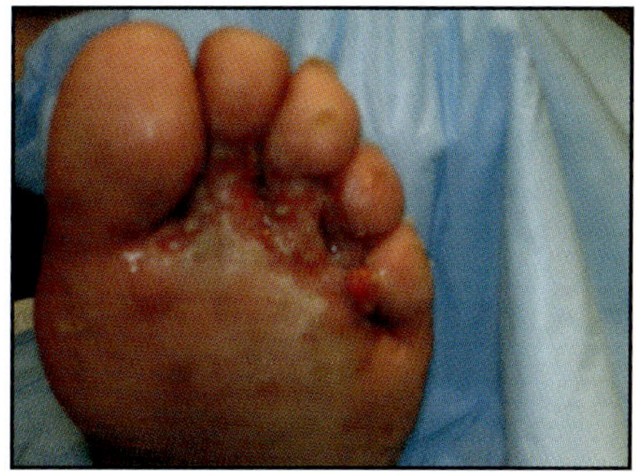

Figure 28. Pyogenic granuloma on 5th toe.

Pyogenic Granuloma

Pyogenic granuloma (Figure 28) is a relatively common skin growth and should not be confused with pyoderma gangrenosum. It is usually a small red, oozing and bleeding bump that looks like raw hamburger meat. It is an acquired vascular lesion which may follow a laceration or skin puncture and grows rapidly over a period of a few weeks. The head, neck, upper trunk and hands and feet are the most common sites. Treatment usually is by cauterization with silver nitrate, cautery, curettage, or laser removal (28, 29)

SUMMARY

This chapter focuses on the importance of a complete history and physical for initiation of the wound healing process. It implies that if the wound does not heal in a reasonable amount of time, it should be reassessed for any misdiagnosis and for a possible need of wound biopsy. An attempt has been made to identify a variety of disorders that can be ongoing with a non healing wound. Underlying systemic condition needs to be treated before the wound can be healed.

A non-healing wound that does not heal after four to six weeks of standard wound care, should be referred to a specialty wound center for a comprehensive evaluation.

TABLE 1. SIGNIFICANCE OF PATIENT HISTORY

Important Clues Found in the Patient History	Significance to the Patient's Wound
General History	
Age and sex	Leg ulcers more common in older woman; Some rheumatic disease more common in women
Initial injury	Spontaneous or gradual appearance; Trauma from accident, shoes, insect bite
Duration of wound	Acute—less than one week Subacute—one week to four weeks Chronic—more than four weeks
History of recurrence	Venous ulcers likely to be current
History of previous DVT	Predisposing factor to venous disease
Previous vein surgery or pelvic trauma	Indicative of venous disease
Intermittent claudication	Indicative of arterial disease
Rest pain	Indicative of arterial disease
Systemic symptoms	Indicative of systemic disease leading to ulcers
Arthralgia	Associated with some ulcers associated with systemic disease
Social History	
Smoking	Predisposes to or worsens arterial disease
Alcohol	Vitamin deficiency
IV drug use	HIV or ulcers related to IV drug use
Past Medical History	
Diabetes	Wound could be related to neuropathy or arterial disease associated with diabetes
Connective tissue disease	Wound could be related to vasculitis, pyoderma gangrenosum, cryoglobinemia
Sickle cell disease	Increased risk of small vessel occlusion
Dietary History	Some vitamin deficiencies common in a vegetarian diet; poor nutrition and obesity influences healing
Drug History	Steroids delay healing, hydroxyurea interferes with healing
Travel History or geographic location of patient	For example, leprosy still remains a common cause for non healing wounds in India; spider bites are only endemic in South, Western and Midwestern areas of USA.
Allergies	Contact dressings, bandages, and ointment can add to existing skin damage

REFERENCES

1. Alarcon–Segovia D, Deleze M, Oria C. Antiphospholipid antibodies and the antiphospholipid syndrome in systemic lupus erythematosus: a prospective analysis of 500 consecutive cases. *Medicine* 1989; 68: 353-365.

2. Coates T, Kirkland G, Dymock R, et al. Cutaneous necrosis from calcific uremic arteriolopathy. *American Journal of Kidney Diseases* 1998; 32 (3): 384–391.

3. Cupps TR, Fauci AS. The vasculitides. *Major Probl Intern Med* 1981;21:1-211.

4. Creighton R. Actinomycosis: a rare pedal infection. *JAPMA* 1993; 83: 637.

5. Falabella A, Falanga V. Uncommon causes of ulcers. *Clinical Plastic Surgery* 1998; 25: 467–479.

6. Falanga V. *Cutaneous Wound Healing*. London, UK: Martin Dunitz Ltd, 2001; 247–263.

7. Falanga V, Phillips T, Harding K, et al. *Text Atlas of Wound Management*. London, UK: Martin Dunitz Ltd, 2000; 61-97, 189–227.

8. Fauci A, Braunwald E, Isselbacher, et al. *Harrison's Principles of Internal Medicine* New York: McGraw Hill, 1998; 989-991, 1004–1019.

9. Fleming M, Hunt J, Purdue G, Sandstad J. Marjolin's Ulcer: A review and reevaluation of a difficult problem. *J Burn Care Rehabilitation* 1990; 11: 460–469.

10. Franco R. Basal and squamous cell carcinoma associated with chronic venous leg ulcer. *Intern J Dermatol* 2001; 40: 539–544.

11. Goldman M. Nonhealing leg ulcers: a manifestation of basal cell carcinoma. *J Am Acad Dermatol* 1992; 26:791-792.

12. Hafner J, Schneider E, Gunter B, et al. Management of leg ulcers in patients with rheumatoid arthritis or systemic sclerosis: The importance of concomitant arterial and venous disease. *Journal of Vascular Surgery* 2000; 32(2): 322–329.

13. Hansson C, Anderson E. Malignant skin lesions on the legs and feet at a dermatological leg ulcer clinic during five years. *Acta Derm Venereol* 1998; 78: 147-148.

14. Helfman T, Falanga V. Stanazolal as a novel therapeutic agent in dermatology. *J Am Acad Dermatol* 1995; 33: 254-258.

15. Kirsner R, Spencer J, Falanga V, et al. Squamous cell carcinoma arising in osteomyelitis and chronic wounds. Treatment with Mohs microsurgery versus amputation. *Dermatology Surgery* 1996; 22: 1015-1028.

16. Lawley T, Kubota Y. Vasculitis. *Dermatology Clin* 1990; 8: 681-687.

17. Lowitt M, Dover J. Necrobiosis Lipoidica. *J Am Acad Dermatol* 1991; 25: 735– 748.

18. Mahgoub E, Yacoub A. Primary actinomycosis of the foot and leg: report of a case. *J Trop Med Hyg* 1968; 71: 256.

19. Naylor W. Malignant wounds: Aetiology and principles of management. *Nursing Standard* 2002; 16 (52): 45–54.

20. Podymow T, Wherrett C, Burns K. Hyperbaric oxygen in the treatment of calciphlaxis: a case series. *Nephrology Dialysis Transplantation* 2001; 16: 2176-2180.

21. Powell F, Su W, Perry H. Pyoderma gangrenosum: Classification and Management. *J Am Acad Dermatol* 1996; 34: 395–409.

22. Taniguchi S, Kono T, Tanii T, et al. Secondary T-cell lymphoma presenting as a giant ulcer. *Clin Exp Dermatol* 1992;17: 379–381.

23. Thurtle O, Cawley M. The frequency of leg ulceration in rheumatoid arthritis: a survey. *J Rheumatology* 1983; 10: 507-509.

24. Trent J, Kirsner R. Wounds and malignancy. *Advances in skin and wound care* 2003; 16: 31-33.

25. Vassa N, Twardowski Z, Campbell J. Hyperbaric oxygen therapy in calciphylaxis- induced skin necrosis in a peritoneal dialysis patient. *American Journal of Kidney Diseases* 1994; 23 (6): 878–881.

26. Vogen K. A case report on actinomycosis of foot. *Journal of the American Podiatric Association* 1996; 86: 238-240.

27. Wollina, Uwe. Clinical management of pyoderma gangrenosum. *American Journal of Clinical Dermatology* 2002; 3 (3): 149–158.

28. Gill K., Shah J. Kaposi sarcoma in patients with diabetes and wounds. *Advances in skin and wound care* 2006:19(4):196-201

29. Silverstein LH,Hanes PJ, Garnick JJ. Pyogenic granuloma, *J Fam Pract*1995 Aug:41(2):196.

30. Wheeless' Text book of Orthopaedics. *http://www.wheelessonline.com*

REVIEW QUESTIONS

1.) All of the following are local factors contributing to nonhealing wound **Except:**
    a. Hypoxia
    b. Edema
    c. Microvascular disease
    d. Malnutrition
    e. Necrosis

2.) Malignancy should be suspected with
    a. History of repeated trauma
    b. Exuberant granulation tissue
    c. Rolled out edges
    d. Purple red color around the ulcer
    e. Wounds secondary to burns
    f. All of the above.

3.) Match the following

a. Basal Cell Cancer	1. Arises from keratinizing epidermal cells
b. Marjolin's Ulcer	2. Arises from epidermal basal cells
c. Kaposi's Sarcoma	3. Associated with hyperparathyroidism.
d. Pyoderma Gangrenosum	4. Malignant changes in edges of chronic wound
e. Calciphylaxis	5. Associated with inflammatory bowel disease.
	6. Associated with AIDS

4.) Match the following

a. Fish tank granuloma	1. S. schenckii
b. Buruli ulcer	2. Gram +, non spore forming anaerobic bacteria
c. Actinomycosis	3. Mycobacteria laprae
d. Hansen's disease	4. Mycobacteria marinum
e. Sporotrichosis	5. Mycobacteria ulcerans

Answers: 1d, 2f, 3a-2, 3b-1 and 4, 3c-6, 3d-5, 3e-3, 4a-4, 4b-5, 4c-2, 4d-3, 4e-1

NOTES

NOTES

NOTES

NOTES

NOTES

NOTES

NOTES

Volume One: pages 1–601 • Volume Two: pages 603–1210

C

Volume One: pages 1–601 • Volume Two: pages 603–1210

Volume One: pages 1–601 • Volume Two: pages 603–1210

Volume One: pages 1–601 • Volume Two: pages 603–1210

J

Volume One: pages 1–601 • Volume Two: pages 603–1210

Volume One: pages 1–601 • Volume Two: pages 603–1210

Volume One: pages 1–601 • Volume Two: pages 603–1210

Volume One: pages 1–601 • Volume Two: pages 603–1210

Volume One: pages 1–601 • Volume Two: pages 603–1210

NOTES